Thieme

Diagnostic Imaging of the Chest

Dag Wormanns, MD
Medical Director
Head of Department of Radiology
ELK Berlin Chest Hospital
Berlin, Germany;
Medical Faculty
Institute for Clinical Radiology
University of Münster
Münster, Germany

644 illustrations

Thieme
Stuttgart • New York • Delhi • Rio de Janeiro

Library of Congress Cataloging-in-Publication Data is available from the publisher

Translator: Sarah Venkata, London, UK

Important note: Medicine is an ever-changing science undergoing continual development. Research and clinical experience are continually expanding our knowledge, in particular our knowledge of proper treatment and drug therapy. Insofar as this book mentions any dosage or application, readers may rest assured that the authors, editors, and publishers have made every effort to ensure that such references are in accordance with **the state of knowledge at the time of production of the book.**

Nevertheless, this does not involve, imply, or express any guarantee or responsibilityon the part of the publishers in respect to any dosage instructions and forms of applications stated in the book. **Every user is requested to examine carefully** the manufacturers' leaflets accompanying each drug and to check, if necessary in consultation with a physician or specialist, whether the dosage schedules mentioned therein or the contraindications stated by the manufacturers differ from the statements made in the present book. Such examination is particularly important with drugs that are either rarely used or have been newly released on the market. Every dosage schedule or every form of application used is entirely at the user's ownrisk and responsibility. The authors and publishers request every user to report to the publishers any discrepancies or inaccuracies noticed. If errors in this work are found after publication, errata will be posted at www.thieme.com on the product description page.

Some of the product names, patents, and registered designs referred to in this book are in fact registered trademarks or proprietary names even though specific reference to this fact is not always made in the text. Therefore, the appearance of a name without designation as proprietary is not to be construed as a representation by the publisher that it is in the public domain.

Georg Thieme Verlag KG
Rüdigerstrasse 14, 70469 Stuttgart, Germany
+49 [0]711 8931 421, customerservice@thieme.de

Thieme Publishers New York
333 Seventh Avenue, New York, NY 10001, USA
+1-800-782-3488, customerservice@thieme.com

Thieme Publishers Delhi
A-12, Second Floor, Sector-2, Noida-201301
Uttar Pradesh, India
+91 120 45 566 00, customerservice@thieme.in

Thieme Publishers Rio de Janeiro,
Thieme Publicações Ltda.
Edifício Rodolpho de Paoli, 25º andar
Av. Nilo Peçanha, 50 – Sala 2508
Rio de Janeiro 20020-906 Brasil
+55 21 3172 2297 / +55 21 3172 1896

Cover design: Thieme Publishing Group
Typesetting by DiTech Process Solutions, India

Printed in Germany by CPI Books 5 4 3 2 1

ISBN 978-3-13-241565-2

Also available as an e-book:
eISBN 978-3-13-241566-9

Contents

Preface

No radiologist can get away from diagnostic imaging of the thorax. After all, chest radiography is the most common imaging examination. As such, all radiologists do in fact have practical experience in this area. Nonetheless, lectures on topics such as HRCT or parenchymal lung diseases regularly attract record audiences. Presumably, while radiologists do time and again come across these issues, they are too rare to become established routine practice.

This book provides information on virtually all the key questions related to diagnostic imaging of the thorax arising in the everyday clinical setting. The systematic organization of the sections of the book contains descriptions of all common diseases affecting the chest organs. It is based on the European Society of Radiology Training Curriculum for Subspecialisation in Radiology. The summary at the end of chapters comprises the subject matter featured in the curriculum, thus assuring efficient preparation of examination for trainee radiologists.

Furthermore, this book is intended as a useful reference for radiologists, with its *synoptic section* serving as a rapid guide through the diagnostic maze. Differential diagnoses and clinical management of frequently encountered findings are presented. For diffuse parenchymal lung diseases, there is a diagnostic guide structured like an identification book. The main findings quickly signpost the most probable differential diagnosis, which are shown in tables and figures.

The Fleischner Society's *Glossary of Terms for Thoracic Imaging* is featured at the end of the book.

In general, diagnostic imaging plays a pivotal role in diagnosis of thoracic diseases. Diagnosis of several diseases is exclusively confirmed on the basis of the imaging findings. This includes well-known diseases such as community-acquired pneumonia or usual interstitial pneumonia as well as rare disorders like lymphangioleiomyomatosis. Hence, the corresponding diagnostic criteria are an important component of this book. Thanks to our imaging data, we as radiologists are able to make the diagnosis, and it is up to us not to leave that task to the clinicians.

Encouraged by the success of the first German edition of this book which was published in late 2016, the idea of an English translation was born. It soon became obvious that this project comprises more than a simple translation. References to German guidelines had to be replaced by their international (and at times inconsistent) counterparts, and some classifications had to be updated. Hence, the translation turned into an updated second edition to the first German edition.

I would like to thank Thieme Publishers, especially Ms. Angelika Findgott and Mr. Marcus Laithangbam, for their kind and competent assistance in making this book happen. Ms. Sarah Venkata deserves my special thanks for translating the book, very rapidly and successfully acquainting herself with the specific vocabulary of chest radiology and shaping a straightforward English from the more complicated German language.

Finally, I thank my wife Ms. Anita Wormanns for her continued support and patience while this book was being written.

Dag Wormanns, MD, PD

Contributors

Jürgen Biederer, MD
Professor
Department of Diagnostic and Interventional Radiology
University Hospital Heidelberg
Heidelberg, Germany

Beate Rehbock, MD
Consultant
Diagnostic Radiology with Specialty Thoracic Radiology
Berlin, Germany

Dag Wormanns, MD
Medical Director
Head of Department of Radiology
ELK Berlin Chest Hospital
Berlin, Germany;
Medical Faculty
Institute for Clinical Radiology
University of Münster
Münster, Germany

Abbreviations

AAH	atypical adenomatous hyperplasia
AEP	acute eosinophilic pneumonia
AIDS	acquired immunodeficiency syndrome
AIP	acute interstitial pneumonia
AIS	adenocarcinoma in situ
ANA	antinuclear antibody
ANCA	antineutrophil cytoplasmic antibodies
c-ANCA	cytoplasmic antineutrophil cytoplasmic antibodies
p-ANCA	perinuclear antineutrophil cytoplasmic antibodies
AP	anteroposterior
ARDS	adult respiratory distress syndrome
BALT	bronchus-associated lymphatic tissue
BG	bronchocentric granulomatosis
BiVAD	biventricular assist devices
BOOP	bronchiolitis obliterans with organizing pneumonia
CAD	computer-assisted diagnostic
CEP	chronic eosinophilic pneumonia
COP	cryptogenic organizing pneumonia
CPAM	congenital pulmonary airway malformation
CT	computed tomography
CTA	computed tomography angiography
CTED	chronic thromboembolic disease
CTEPH	chronic thromboembolic pulmonary hypertension
CTPA	computed tomography pulmonary angiography
CUP	cancer of unknown primary
CWP	coal workers' pneumoconiosis
DAD	diffuse alveolar damage
DECT	dual-energy computed tomography
DIP	desquamative interstitial pneumonia
DVT	deep vein thrombosis
DWI	diffusion-weighted imaging
ECMO	extracorporeal lung assist device
FDG	^{18}F-fludeoxyglucose/fluorodeoxyglucose
FEV1	forced expiratory volume in 1 second
FSE	fast spin-echo
FVC	forced vital capacity
GE	gradient echo
GGO	ground-glass opacities
GvHD	graft-versus-host disease
HIV	human immunodeficiency virus
HRCT	high-resolution computed tomography
HU	Hounsfield units
IABP	intra-aortic balloon pump
IASLC	International Association for the Study of Lung Cancer
ICD	implantable cardioverter defibrillator
ICOERD	International Classification of HRCT for Occupational and Environmental Respiratory Diseases
ICU	intensive care unit
IGRA	interferon-γ release assay
IHS	idiopathic hypereosinophilic syndrome
IIPs	idiopathic interstitial pneumonias
ILO	International Labour Organization
IPAF	interstitial pneumonia with autoimmune features
IPF	idiopathic pulmonary fibrosis
IPS	idiopathic pneumonia syndrome
IV	intravenous
LAM	lymphangioleiomyomatosis/lymphangiomyomatosis
LDH	lactate dehydrogenase level
LIP	lymphoid interstitial pneumonia
LPAs	lepidic predominant adenocarcinomas
LV	left ventricle
LVAD	left ventricular assist devices
MAC	*Mycobacterium avium* complex
MCTD	mixed connective tissue disease
MDR-TB	multidrug-resistant tuberculosis
MIA	minimally invasive adenocarcinoma
MinIP	minimum intensity projection
MIP	maximum intensity projection
MOTT	mycobacteria other than tuberculosis
MPO	myeloperoxidase
MPR	multiplanar reformation
MRA	magnetic imaging angiography
MRI	magnetic resonance imaging
NK	natural killer
NLST	National Lung Screening Trial
NSIP	nonspecific interstitial pneumonia
OP	organizing pneumonia
PA	posteroanterior
PAP	pulmonary alveolar proteinosis
PAVM	pulmonary arteriovenous malformation
PCH	pulmonary capillary hemangiomatosis
PCT	pulmonary cytolytic thrombi
PEEP	positive end-expiratory pressure
PET-CT	positron emission tomography–computed tomography
PFT	pulmonary function testing
PLCH	pulmonary Langerhans cell histiocytosis
PMF	progressive massive fibrosis
PPFE	pleuroparenchymal fibroelastosis
PVOD	pulmonary veno-occlusive disease
RA	rheumatoid arthritis
RB	respiratory bronchiolitis
RB-ILD	respiratory bronchiolitis-interstitial lung disease
RECIST	Response Evaluation Criteria in Solid Tumors
RV	right ventricle
RVAD	right ventricular assist devices
SAPHO	synovitis, acne, palmoplantar pustolosis, hyperostosis, and osteitis
SARS	severe acute respiratory syndrome
SFT	solitary fibrous tumor
SSc	systemic sclerosis
SLE	systemic lupus erythematosus
SPE	simple pulmonary eosinophilia
STIR	short-tau inversion recovery
SUV	standard uptake value
T1w	T1-weighted
T2w	T2-weighted
UIP	usual interstitial pneumonia
VQ	ventilation/perfusion
VRT	volume rendering technique
XDR-TB	extensively drug-resistant tuberculosis

Part I

Fundamentals of Diagnostic Thoracic Imaging

Chapter 1

Examination Technique

1 Examination Technique

This chapter describes specific aspects of examining the chest organs with the different imaging modalities. It is outside the scope of this textbook to give a comprehensive overview of the technical aspects of the equipment or the positioning techniques. These details can be consulted in the pertinent literature.[1,2]

1.1 Projection Radiography

The following descriptions relate to digital radiography (flat panel detector or image plate). By now this is available in most radiology institutions. This chapter does not take account of older, conventional screen-film radiography systems but many aspects are very similar to that of digital radiography.

For almost all chest diseases, chest radiography constitutes the first step in diagnostic imaging. The few exceptions to that rule (e.g., suspected pulmonary embolism) will be pointed out in the relevant sections.

1.1.1 Standing Position

Patients are X-rayed in a standing position, whenever their condition permits. The standing patient is X-rayed in the PA (posteroanterior) beam path with the chest placed against the detector (*PA image*), while the focus detector distance is 1.4 to 2 m. ▶Table 1.1 summarizes the technical radiographic parameters. To avoid overlapping of the pulmonary fields, the scapulae must be rotated laterally. To that effect, the patient places his/her hands on the hips while rotating the elbows anteriorly as far as possible. Alternatively, the patient clasps the detector with their arms; this, too, assures anterior rotation of the scapulae.

If because of the patient's general condition an X-ray cannot be taken in a standing position, this can be done with the patient sitting down. The patient leans his/her back against the detector; the beam path is therefore oriented in an AP direction (anteroposterior; *AP image*). As a result, the diaphragm will be positioned at a higher level than seen in a standing radiograph, the inspiration depth is reduced, and, accordingly, the basal lung segments are less well ventilated.

Likewise, a *lateral radiograph* is obtained with the patient standing and the arms raised. Normally, the patient's left side rests against the detector. In general, a clearer image will be obtained of the lung closer to the detector compared with that farther away from the detector. If the clinical diagnostic indication calls for maximum image quality and the critical details are difficult to identify, in certain cases to visualize a right-sided pathology it may be advisable to take an image with the right side placed against the detector.

All radiographs of the chest organs should be obtained in deep inspiration. The *expiratory image* usually used in the past to exclude pneumothorax is now obsolete for several reasons[3,4]:

- The expiratory radiograph does not permit assessment of the cardiopulmonary status since the lung is inadequately ventilated and the pulmonary vessels appear dilated. This can obscure other relevant findings, e.g., small pulmonary infiltrates or incipient congestive heart failure.
- Comparability with previous or subsequent radiographs is not possible.
- With modern digital equipment technology, a pneumothorax of clinically relevant size can also be recognized on an inspiratory radiograph.

The European Guidelines on Quality Criteria for Diagnostic Radiographic Images issued by the European Commission define criteria to be met by radiographs.[5] ▶Table 1.2 lists the criteria specified for the image quality of overview chest radiographs.

> **Note**
>
> For radiographic diagnosis of chest organs, a *high-energy X-ray* taken with a high tube voltage is used. Calcified structures will appear radiolucent on such radiographs. This reduces the otherwise disruptive overlying of the pulmonary fields by the ribs (▶Fig. 1.1). Besides, osseous structures allow only limited assessment. Therefore, for diagnostic issues related to the thoracic skeleton, e.g., exclusion of rib fractures, a *low-energy X-ray* is needed with 60 to 75 kV tube voltage.

1.1.2 Supine Radiographs

For diagnostic imaging of bedridden patients, in particular in intensive care settings, supine radiographs are normally

Table 1.1 Radiographic parameters for PA and lateral radiographs[5]

Imaging parameters	PA projection	Lateral projection
Scanner type	Vertical stand with stationary or moving grid	Vertical stand with stationary or moving grid
Tube voltage	125 kV	125 kV
Focal spot value	≤1.3	≤1.3
Total filtration	≥3.0 mm Al equivalent	≥3.0 mm Al equivalent
Focus detector distance	180 cm (140–200 cm)	180 cm (140–200 cm)
Automatic exposure control	Right lateral chamber selected	Central chamber selected
Exposure time	<20 ms	<20 ms
Antiscatter grid	r = 10; 40/cm	r = 10; 40/cm
Nominal speed class	SC 400	SC 400
Entrance surface dose for standard- sized patient	0.3 mGy	1.5 mGy

I

Table 1.2 Quality requirements for chest radiographs[5]

Requirements	PA/AP thorax	Lateral thorax
Image criteria	• Performed at full inspiration (as assessed by the position of the ribs above the diaphragm—either 6 anteriorly or 10 posteriorly) and with suspended respiration • Symmetrical reproduction of the thorax as shown by central position of the spinous process between the medial ends of the clavicles • Medial border of the scapulae should be projected outside the lung fields • Reproduction of the whole rib cage above the diaphragm • Visually sharp reproduction of the vascular pattern in the whole lung, particularly the peripheral vessels • Visually sharp reproduction of: – The trachea and proximal bronchi – The borders of the heart and aorta – The diaphragm and lateral costophrenic angles • Visualization of the retrocardiac lung and the mediastinum	• Performed at full inspiration and with suspended respiration • Arms should be raised clear of the thorax • Superimposition of the posterior lung borders • Reproduction of the trachea • Reproduction of the costophrenic angles • Visually sharp reproduction of the posterior border of the heart, the aorta, mediastinum, diaphragm, sternum, and thoracic spine
Important image details	• Small round details in the whole lung, including the retrocardiac areas: – High contrast: 0.7 mm diameter – Low contrast: 2 mm diameter • Linear and reticular details out to the lung periphery: – High contrast: 0.3 mm in width – Low contrast: 2 mm in width	• Small round details in the whole lung: – High contrast: 0.7 mm diameter – Low contrast: 2 mm diameter • Linear and reticular details out to the lung periphery: – High contrast: 0.3 mm in width – Low contrast: 2 mm in width

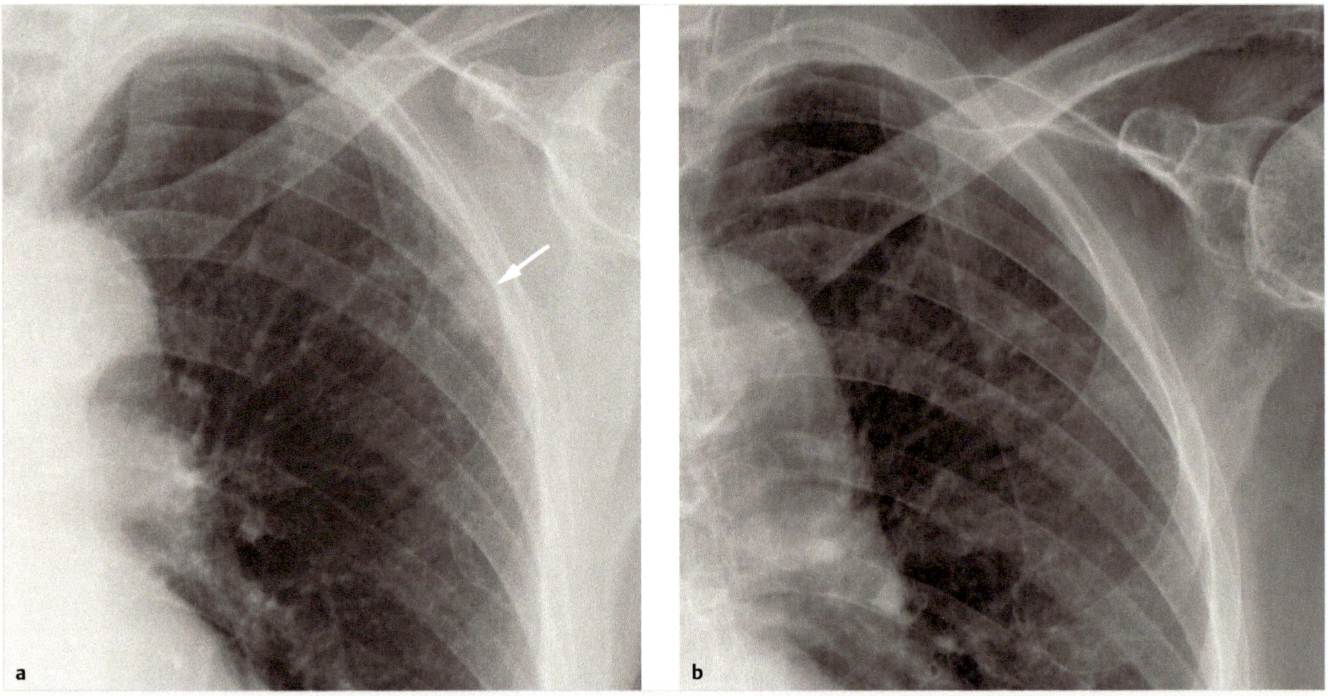

Fig. 1.1 **High-energy and low-energy chest radiographs.** Different detectability of bone structures. Bronchopneumonia in the left upper lobe is much easier to detect on the high-energy radiograph (**a,** *arrow*). **(a)** High-energy radiograph with 125 kV tube voltage. **(b)** Low-energy radiograph with 70 kV tube voltage.

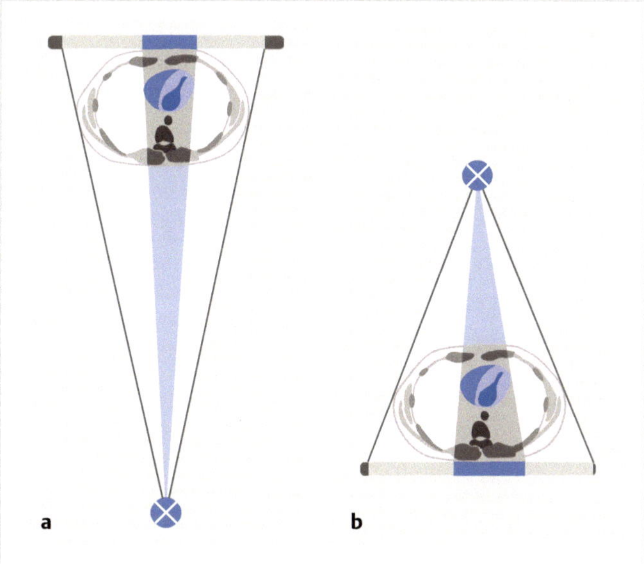

Fig. 1.2 Geometric distortion in standing and supine radiographs. Schematic diagram. **(a)** Standing PA radiograph with large focus detector distance: low magnification of cardiac opacity. **(b)** Supine AP radiograph with small focus detector distance: high magnification of cardiac opacity.

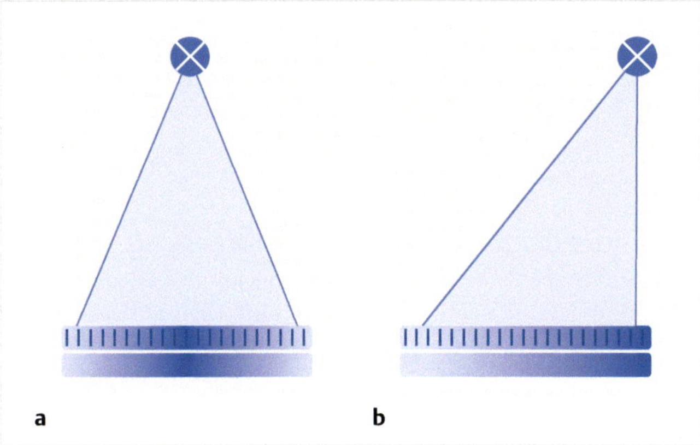

Fig. 1.3 Grid artifact because of decentered X-ray tube. Schematic diagram. **(a)** Normal image: symmetric radiolucency of both hemithoraces. **(b)** Grid artifact: the decentered tube causes right hemithorax opacity.

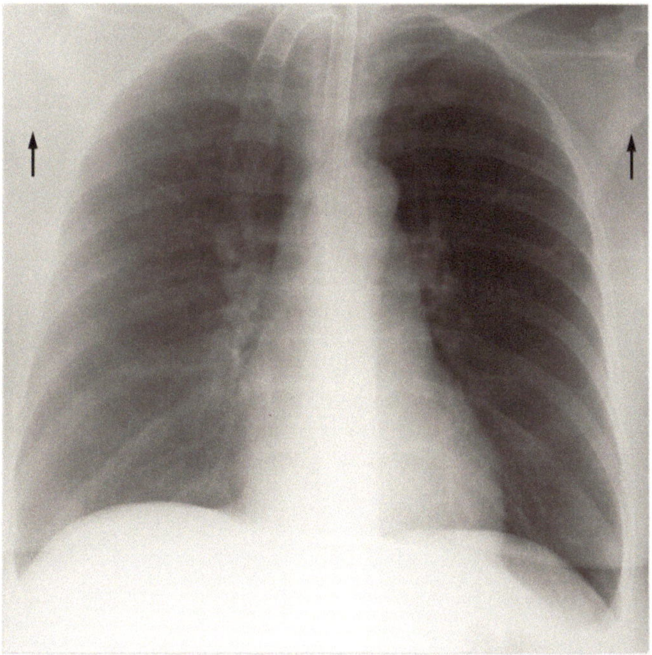

Fig. 1.4 Grid artifact. Radiograph (supine radiograph). Different radiolucency of both axillae (*arrows*) as distinguishing feature of that artifact.

obtained. The mobile detector is positioned beneath the thorax of the supine patient and the tube of the mobile radiography unit is placed above the patient. The focus detector distance should be 90 to 120 cm. For several reasons, supine radiographs have poorer image quality than standing or sitting radiographs:

- The reduced focus detector distance results in greater geometric distortion; the mediastinal width and heart size appear enlarged on the supine radiograph (▶Fig. 1.2); the heart is farther away from the detector, showing greater geometric enlargement.
- The diaphragm is higher, resulting in reduced inspiration depth.
- Lung perfusion has no gravity-mediated caudocranial gradient; it is not possible to diagnose pulmonary blood flow redistribution.
- Since the tube voltage used is lower, bone superimposition is more pronounced.
- The lower generator power of mobile radiography units results in a longer exposure time and is likely to cause motion blur due to breathing or heart pulsations.

Note

The imaging position (standing, sitting, supine) should be noted on the radiograph. Besides, for mechanically ventilated patients, information on the ventilation parameters is helpful for image interpretation, in particular on the positive end expiratory pressure (PEEP).

The use of an antiscatter grid can enhance the image quality for obese patients, albeit at the expense of higher radiation exposure. A characteristic artifact is observed if the X-ray tube is not positioned above the middle of the detector fitted with an antiscatter grid (▶Fig. 1.3). To distinguish this artifact from pathologic hemithorax opacity, it may be useful to compare radiolucency of both axillae (▶Fig. 1.4). Unequal radiolucency is suggestive of a *grid artifact.*

Skin folds on the patient's back result from placement of the X-ray detector between the bed and patient and can mimic pneumothorax (pseudo-pneumothorax).

1.2 Fluoroscopy

Chest fluoroscopy is mainly used for functional assessment of diaphragmatic movement. A standardized fluoroscopy examination procedure is described.[6]

Before commencing fluoroscopy examination, the patient practices deep breathing with the mouth open. In addition, the patient should repeat the sniff test around twice: the patient breathes deeply in and out with the mouth open, closes the mouth, and, again, with the mouth closed, breathes in deeply and strongly as fast as possible. The patient repeats this procedure once.

During examination, the patient stands against the vertically tilted fluoroscope. If the patient cannot be examined in a standing position because of their general condition, the patient sits on the footplate of the fluoroscope. The image section is centered vertically on the diaphragm and the image is collimated laterally as far as necessary. Next the patient breathes normally two to three times under fluoroscopic guidance, and then takes two to three forced breaths in and out. This is followed by conduct of the sniff test, also two to three times. The patient is then rotated by 90° and the examination sequence described is repeated in the lateral beam path.

The image documentation comprises the fluoroscopy video sequences of the PA and lateral fluoroscopy images which are digitally archived.

1.3 Computed Tomography

The enormous innovative boost experienced over the past two decades in computed tomography (CT) technology has greatly enhanced scanner performance. This, too, has led to increasing diversification of the technical features of CT equipment. Currently, scanners with a row count of between 1 and 640 are used for routine imaging. As such, standardization of examination protocols is virtually impossible. Various valuable internet sources of information provide vendor-specific CT examination protocols (e.g., www.ctisus.com). Below are listed some basic aspects to be considered in *CT examination protocols*:

- *Radiation exposure:* Tube voltage, tube current, and pitch should be adjusted such that the radiation exposure complies with the reference values specified for diagnostic imaging of patients of normal weight. Relevant reference values vary greatly among different countries.[7]
- *Tube voltage*: For most applications, a tube voltage of 110 to 120 kVp is suitable. For computed tomography angiography (CTA), the tube voltage may be reduced in certain circumstances to 80 to 100 kVp, in particular for pediatric or slim patients.[8,9]
- *Automatic tube current modulation*: Due to the major differences in the absorption profiles of the thorax in the craniocaudal and axial directions, the use of automatic tube current modulation has greatly contributed to dose reduction.[8] However, there is a risk of this automated facility preselecting a very high tube current for obese patients. It is therefore recommended to limit the maximum tube current in the scan parameters if this is technically possible. Other considerations apply for low-dose CT.
- *Slice thickness*: The detector configuration should provide for a reconstructed slice thickness of 1 to 1.5 mm. But that does not apply to CT scanners with a limited row count, for which a compromise has to be made between the minimum slice thickness possible and the scan duration. A limiting factor for the slice thickness in such cases is the maximum length of breath suspension that can be maintained before breathing artifacts degrade the image quality. There does not appear to be much benefit in selecting a slice thickness of substantially less than 1 mm in the thoracic region because of the ensuing rise in image noise; a reduced slice thickness is unlikely to confer any additional diagnostic insights of relevance.
- *Image reconstructions recommended for routine examinations*:
  - 5 mm axial for quick orientation also for the referring physician (soft-tissue and lung kernel).
  - Axial thin-slice reconstructions (1.5–3 mm) with soft-tissue kernel, in CTA possibly reduced slice thickness.
  - Axial thin-slice reconstructions (1–1.5 mm) with lung kernel to allow for volumetric measurements.
  - 3–5 mm coronal and sagittal.
- *Overlapping of thin-slice reconstructions*: To achieve a good image quality for 3D (three-dimensional) reformatting of image data and precise volumetry, overlapping reconstruction of the thin-slice series by at least 20% of slice thickness is recommended.
- *IV contrast*: If IV contrast administration is indicated, a fixed delay of 40 s may be used for most diagnostic purposes. Alternatively, a bolus tracking procedure could be employed. Here the arrival of the contrast bolus in the descending aorta triggers the scan. An additional delay of a few seconds is advisable, for example, to accentuate the contrast between a tumor and its surrounding tissues. The use of CTA for diagnostic exploration of pulmonary embolisms requires bolus tracking or a test bolus in the pulmonary trunk or right ventricle.
- *Scanning direction*: Examination is performed in deep inspiration. A caudocranial scanning direction helps to reduce breathing artifacts. First, the basal lung regions most susceptible to breathing artifacts are scanned, followed by the less susceptible apical regions. Furthermore, with appropriate contrast medium timing, beam hardening artifacts caused by highly concentrated contrast material in the superior vena cava and brachiocephalic veins can be reduced.

1.3.1 High-Resolution Computed Tomography

The term "high-resolution computed tomography" (HRCT) dates back to the early 1980s.[10] While that term has proved immutable over the past some 30 years, the underlying examination technology has undergone rapid development. Back then the body region to be scanned could only be visualized in sequential single slices, and acquisition of slices of 10-mm thickness represented the normal standard. Since each individual slice was acquisitioned in a separate breath-hold phase, imaging the entire lung took a lot of time.

Due to its low spatial resolution in the z-direction, the thick-slice CT was of limited value for differential diagnosis of diffuse lung parenchymal diseases. This differential diagnosis requires the assignment of pathologic changes to the structures of the pulmonary lobule, which is not possible with a 10-mm slice thickness. The key driver of HRCT was thus to generate thin slices of the lung parenchyma (slice thickness: around 1 mm) to improve such assignment. However, sequential 1-mm slices were not suitable for continuous imaging of the entire lung at that time. The only remedy here was therefore to acquisition discontiguous slices at greater distances apart (e.g., 10 mm). This inevitably results in incomplete visualization of the lung. For diagnosis of diffuse lung diseases, a number of representative slices suffice; however, thanks to the higher spatial resolution, it has been possible to achieve a diagnostic gain but there was a risk of focal changes being overlooked.

The term *HRCT* was thus normally understood as an examination technique which permits maximum spatial resolution[11]:

- Reduced slice thickness (maximum 1.5 mm) at greater distances apart (e.g., 10 mm).
- High radiation dose for the single slice (high tube voltage and high tube current).
- Edge-enhancing reconstruction kernel for maximum spatial resolution in the slice plane.
- Maximum image matrix (at least 512 × 512 pixels).

Since 1998, *multidetector CT* has been available providing for spiral imaging of the entire lung in 1-mm slices during a single-breath hold. This marked the advent of an alternative to the discontiguous thin single slices afforded by conventional HRCT. Its main advantage derives from the ability to display the entire lung in a slice thickness that hitherto had only been possible with HRCT. The problem of incomplete visualization of the lung parenchyma had now been resolved, albeit at the expense of higher radiation exposure and a minimally poorer image quality. Follow-up examinations became more precise since identical slice planes were always available for comparison of the previous and follow-up examinations. As such, in recent years thin-slice multidetector CT has just about fully supplanted the classic sequential HRCT.[12] Nowadays, sequential HRCT plays a limited role for follow-up examination of diffuse lung diseases in young patients[13] because of its lower radiation dose.

Note

Today, using modern scanners the entire lung can be imaged in continuous 1-mm slices in a few seconds. Hence, examination results of relatively good quality can be obtained even for severely dyspneic patients.

1.3.2 Low-Dose Computed Tomography

Many pathologic changes in the lung parenchyma contrast sharply with their surroundings. That means there is considerable potential for dose reduction in CT provided that the clinical issue of diagnostic interest is limited to detection or exclusion of high contrast objects. Typical examples of such clinical questions are early detection of lung cancer in the context of lung cancer screening, or detection of fungal pneumonia in immunocompromised patients. Both examinations are aimed at detection of foci of soft-tissue opacity in the aerated lung. Dose reduction causes considerably higher image noise (▶ Fig. 1.5) but this does not adversely affect detection of relevant findings.[14]

At a technical level, dose reduction in low-dose CT is generally achieved by *reducing the tube current.* To further reduce the dose (ultralow-dose CT), a lower tube voltage (80–100 kVp) is sometimes used.[15] The use of automatic exposure control is not generally recommended for low-dose CT.[16] Scanogram-adapted methods of tube current modulation are thought to be error-prone due to eccentric patient positioning. Online modulation of the tube current may be overregulated in the region of the shoulders and upper abdomen because of higher radiation

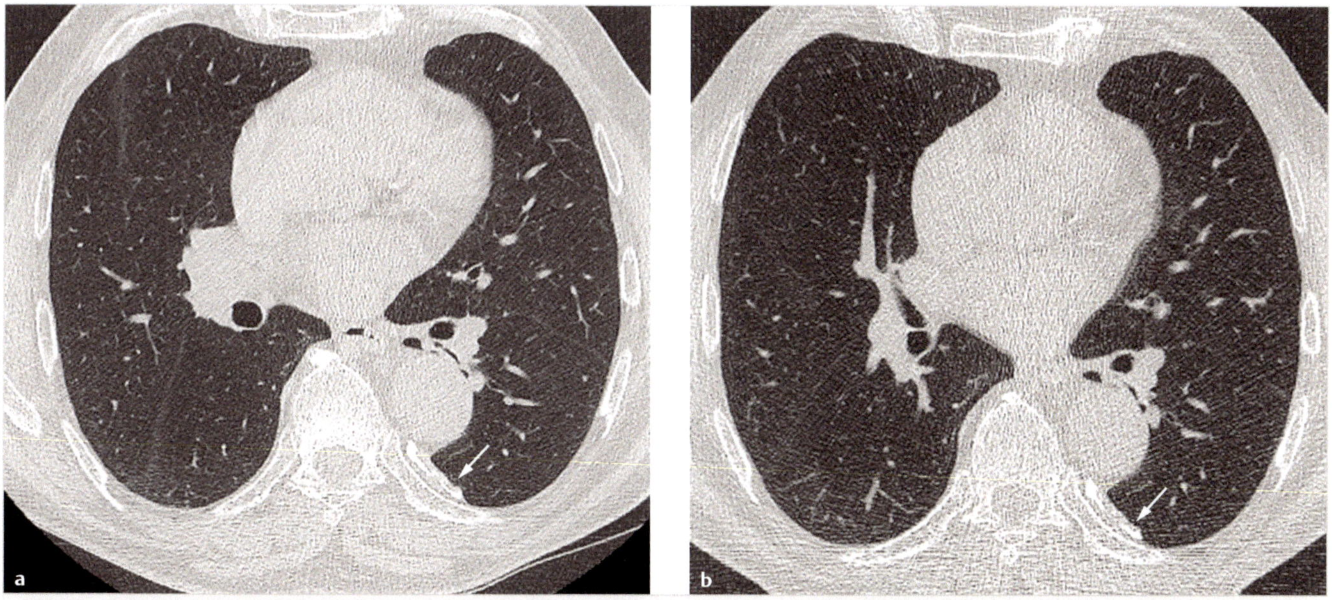

Fig. 1.5 Low-dose CT compared with standard CT. Higher image noise of low-dose CT, but good visualization of the pulmonary structures and of left posterior pleural plaque (*arrows*). **(a)** Standard CT with $CTDI_{Vol}$ of 6.5 mGy. **(b)** Low-dose CT with $CTDI_{Vol}$ of 1.5 mGy.

absorption. Both present a risk of unnecessarily high radiation exposure or inadequate image quality when the tube current is too low. A more robust approach entails the use of a weight-adapted, fixed tube current. Several lung cancer screening trials used a variety of low-dose CT protocols, which generally achieved an effective dose of approximately 1.5 mSv.[16,17] These provide for a dose saving of over 80% compared with standard CT; with ultralow-dose protocols, radiation exposure similar to a chest radiograph in two views can even be achieved.[15]

There are *limitations* with regard to the detection of subtle ground-glass opacities and early forms of pulmonary emphysema since these findings induce only minor changes of CT density compared to their surroundings.[18]

1.3.3 Special CT Examination Techniques

Expiratory CT scan

Many diseases of the small airways are associated with obstruction of the bronchioles. Standard CT inspiratory images may yield normal results. Only on an expiratory scan can the disease be detected through pronounced *air trapping* (▶Fig. 1.6).

Two examination techniques are available:

- *Sequential expiratory scans*: A few sequential expiratory scans, in addition to the inspiratory spiral scan, yield just slightly higher radiation exposure. Even severely dyspneic patients generally tolerate the very short breath-hold times for sequential expiratory scans. One drawback is the sampling error since only a small part of the lung parenchyma is displayed. Besides, interpretation of the findings with regard to air trapping may be difficult at times.
- *Expiratory volume acquisition*: In addition to an inspiratory spiral CT scan, a second expiratory spiral scan is obtained across the entire thorax. Its advantage is that it displays the whole of the lung and focal air trapping is not overlooked. But this involves higher radiation exposure, although the expiratory scan can be obtained in low-dose technique. Besides, patients cannot hold their breath in expiration for as long as in inspiration. If a very fast CT scanner is not available, a compromise must be reached between slice thickness and scan duration since otherwise breathing artifacts would adversely affect image interpretation.

Note

Visualization of the trachea on CT images helps to verify whether the image was obtained in expiration. In the latter case, the posterior wall of the trachea, the membranous part, will protrude anteriorly. This sign is particularly useful if there is massive diffuse air trapping and there is essentially no difference between the expiratory and inspiratory images. This shows whether air trapping was really present or whether the patient had not correctly implemented the breathing command. At times, such examination results are very difficult to interpret. Breathing dynamics imaging will help in cases of doubt (see below).

Expiratory CT in addition to an inspiratory CT scan is also recommended for differential diagnosis of lung fibrosis—in particular, for differentiation between usual interstitial pneumonia and chronic hypersensitivity pneumonitis.[19]

Dynamic CT of the Ventilation Cycle

Dynamic CT of the ventilation cycle is indicated if there are difficulties in interpreting the expiratory scans or because of suspected dynamic respiratory tract stenosis which cannot be identified in inspiration.[20,21]

The easiest approach for this examination is to use the *bolus tracking* feature implemented in many CT scanners and to set

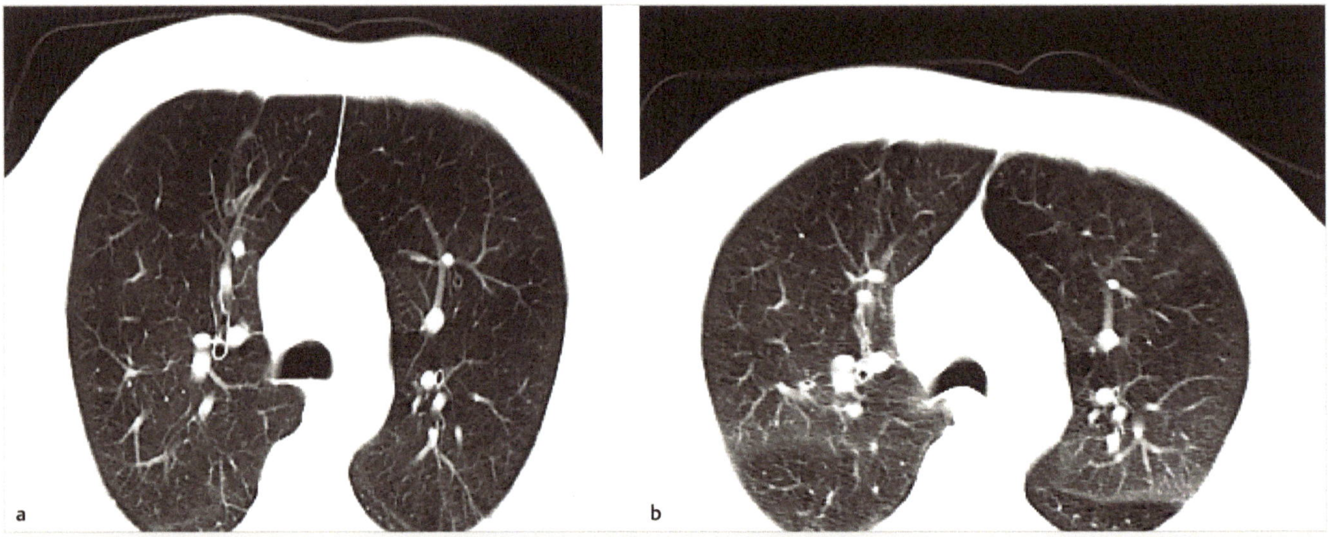

Fig. 1.6 Expiratory CT for visualization of small airway disease. (a) Hardly any abnormalities in inspiration. **(b)** In expiration greater evidence of air trapping (darker areas) in the diseased lung parenchyma.

the threshold value to start the scan high enough so that it is never reached. To begin with, the patient takes a few normal breaths under bolus tracking, followed by a few forced breaths. Eventually, the bolus tracking mode must be stopped manually. An imaging frequency of one image per second suffices for interpretation of the findings.

For *evaluation*, lung parenchymal opacity is measured at the same site on all images using a region of interest of several centimeters, thus demonstrating how lung density changes in the course of the breathing cycles. These values can be displayed as graphs with the evaluation software present in many CT scanners (▶Fig. 1.7). The measurements are to be performed in both lungs.

> **Note**
>
> It is advisable to acquisition dynamic CT scans in different lung levels; at least three measurements are recommended in the upper, middle, and lower field.

A change of at least 50 HU (Hounsfield units) in lung parenchymal density during a breathing cycle is normal. Lower values are interpreted as air trapping (see ▶Fig. 1.7). In the presence of severe unilateral respiratory tract stenosis, a paradoxical increase in the density of the diseased lung may be identified in inspiration.

Imaging in the Prone Position

Occasionally, *dependent opacities* in the posterior segments of the lower lobes may manifest as a diffuse increase in lung parenchymal density. They make it more difficult to evaluate the subpleural space and, at times, are misinterpreted as an early form of diffuse parenchymal lung disease. If differentiating physiologic dependent opacities from incipient parenchymal lung disease is of clinical relevance, this can be done by obtaining an additional CT scan with the patient in the prone position. Whereas lung parenchymal disease will persist, dependent opacities disappear in the prone position (▶Fig. 1.8). It is important to make this distinction, for

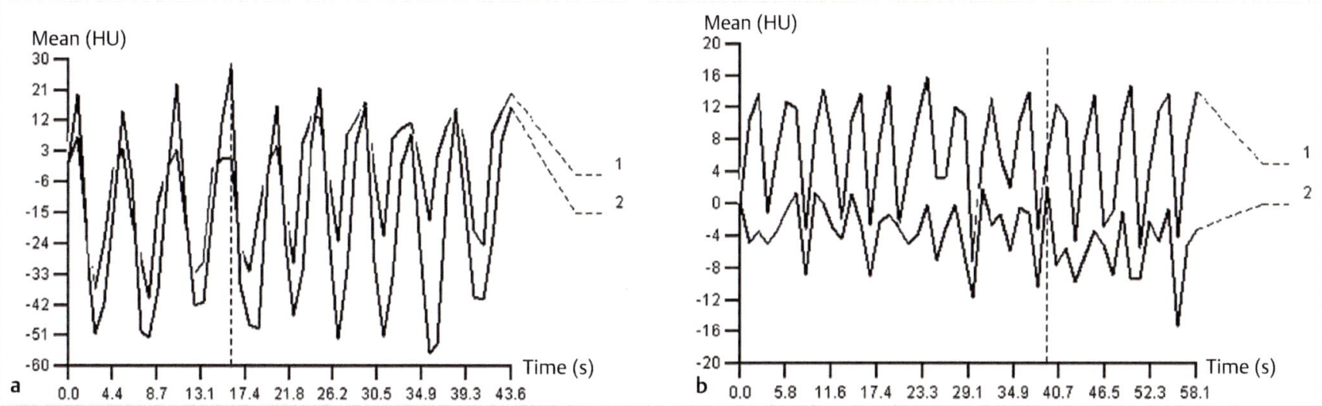

Fig. 1.7 Dynamic CT of the ventilation cycle. Visualization of lung density during several breathing cycles. Illustrated in each case are measurements in the right (curve 1) and in the left lung (curve 2). **(a)** Normal results for the left lung (2). Density changes in one breathing cycle of more than 50 HU (Hounsfield units). On the right (1), mild air trapping with lower density amplitude. **(b)** Extensive air trapping. Only minor changes in lung parenchymal density; in the left lung (2) more massive air trapping than on the right (1).

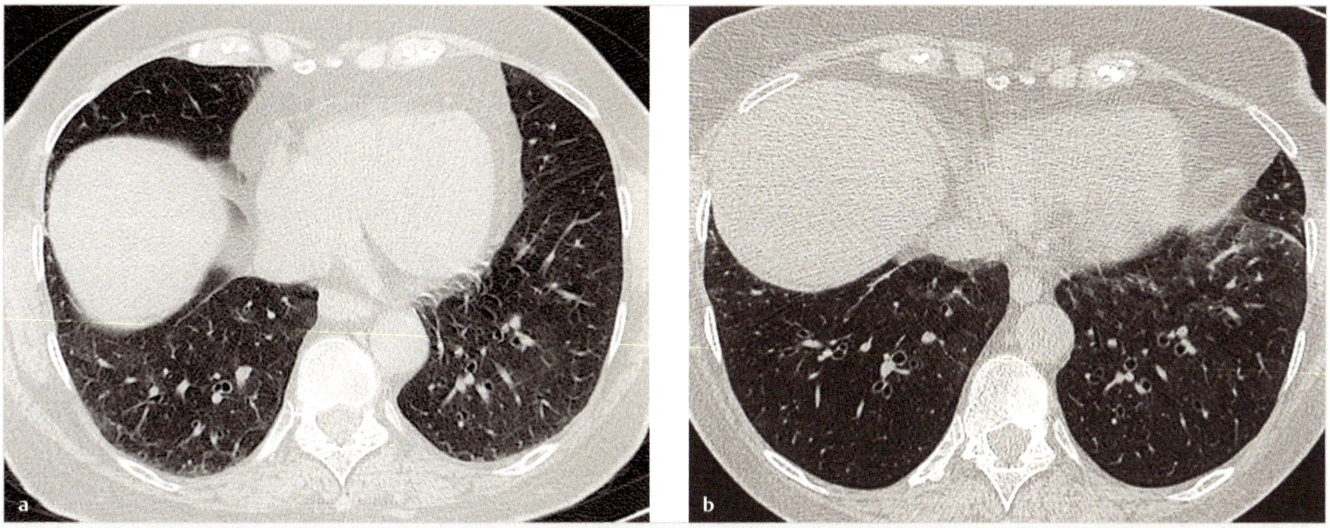

Fig. 1.8 Dependent opacities in both lungs. CT images. **(a)** In supine position: Subpleural densities in the posterior lower lobes. **(b)** In the prone position: complete resolution of findings (image rotated by 180°).

example, when evaluating occupational lung diseases (see Chapter 18).

A few sequential CT scans are generally sufficient for reliable differential diagnosis. There is no need for an additional spiral scan to display the lungs in their entirety.

Dynamic Contrast Enhancement

Dynamic contrast enhancement may be useful in differential diagnosis of pulmonary nodules (see Chapter 21) in certain clinical situations. This technique is based on the observation that the absence of contrast enhancement by a nodule makes its *malignancy* very unlikely. One advantage of this method is its high predictive value of benignity of around 96%.[22] But a drawback is its low specificity (58%) since, apart from malignant, many benign nodules also exhibit contrast enhancement.

First, a short unenhanced thin-slice spiral CT scan of the nodule is obtained. Then IV contrast is injected (110 mL with 3 mL/s flow rate) and the scan is repeated after 60, 120, 180, and 240 seconds. Nodule density is measured with a region of interest comprising around two-thirds of the nodule (▶ Fig. 1.9). An increase in density by less than 15 HU in all four spiral scans following contrast administration compared with unenhanced examination is considered predictive of benignity.[22] The procedure is suitable for nodules with at least 8 mm diameter.

1.3.4 Dual-Energy Computed Tomography

Dual-energy CT (DECT) scans the body region to be examined utilizing X-rays of two different energy levels. The usual practice is to use two energy levels of approximately 140 and 80 kVp. Depending on the CT scanner manufacturer and equipment features, different technical solutions are employed:

- One scan, synchronous imaging with two X-ray tubes, of different tube voltage, which are offset by approximately 90°.
- One scan, quasi-synchronous imaging using very fast voltage switching in one X-ray tube, thus providing for acquisition of alternating projections with high and low tube voltage.
- One scan, synchronous imaging using one X-ray tube and detectors of different spectral sensitivity.
- Two scans, asynchronous imaging with acquisition in rapid succession of two spiral scans with different tube voltages.

The data thus acquisitioned provide additional information and postprocessing possibilities beyond conventional CT imaging[23]:

- *Iodine maps*: Utilizing an algorithm for material decomposition the iodine content of each voxel is determined and displayed in a parametric image (▶ Fig. 1.10). This shows contrast enhancement, which can be used as a surrogate parameter for lung perfusion.
- *Spectral imaging*: From the DECT dataset, monoenergetic images with different virtual tube voltages can be calculated. The standard CT image acquisitioned with a tube voltage of 120 kVp corresponds to the image impression of a monoenergetic image at 70 kV. Monoenergetic images with a lower virtual tube voltage exhibit higher radiation absorption of the iodinated contrast material. Accordingly, for example, a CTA with poor vascular contrast can be subsequently improved when interpreting the monoenergetic images at lower virtual kV levels (e.g., 50 kV).
- *Virtual unenhanced imaging*: From the primary CT dataset acquisitioned with IV contrast, virtual unenhanced images can be calculated for better evaluation of contrast enhancement by pulmonary nodules. However, in certain cases there may not be reliable concordance between density measurement on virtual unenhanced CT images and the actual unenhanced CT density.
- *Xenon-enhanced ventilation visualization*: Pulmonary ventilation can be visualized with DECT by using inhaled xenon similarly as for the iodine maps described above.[24]

1.4 Magnetic Resonance Imaging

Jürgen Biederer

1.4.1 Introduction

Thanks to the latest developments in equipment and pulse sequence technology, magnetic resonance imaging (MRI) is set

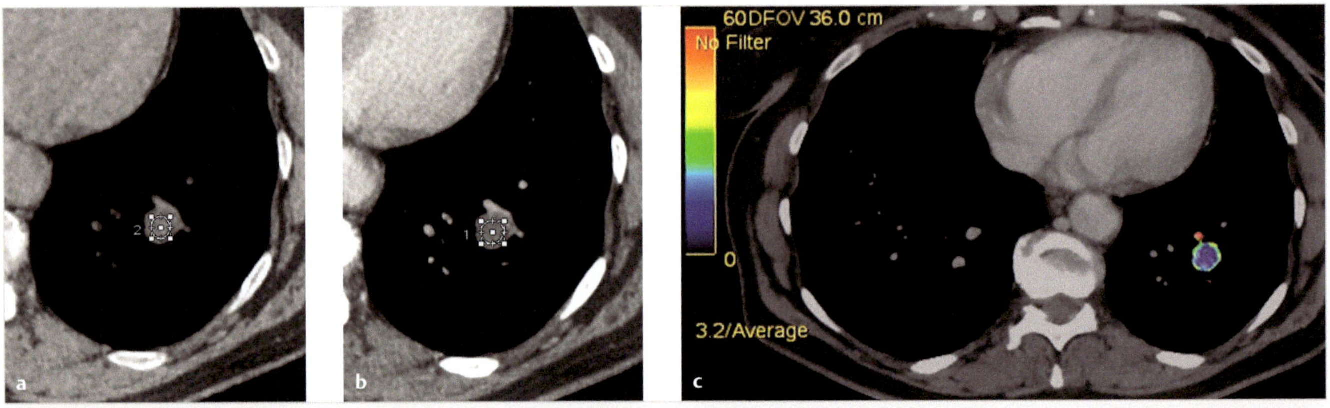

Fig. 1.9 Benign nodule in left lower lobe. Dynamic CT contrast enhancement. **(a)** Unenhanced CT: Mean nodule density on CT: 18 HU. **(b)** 60 s after IV contrast injection: No significant contrast enhancement (CT density: 26 HU). **(c)** Visualization of low contrast enhancement on parametric image.

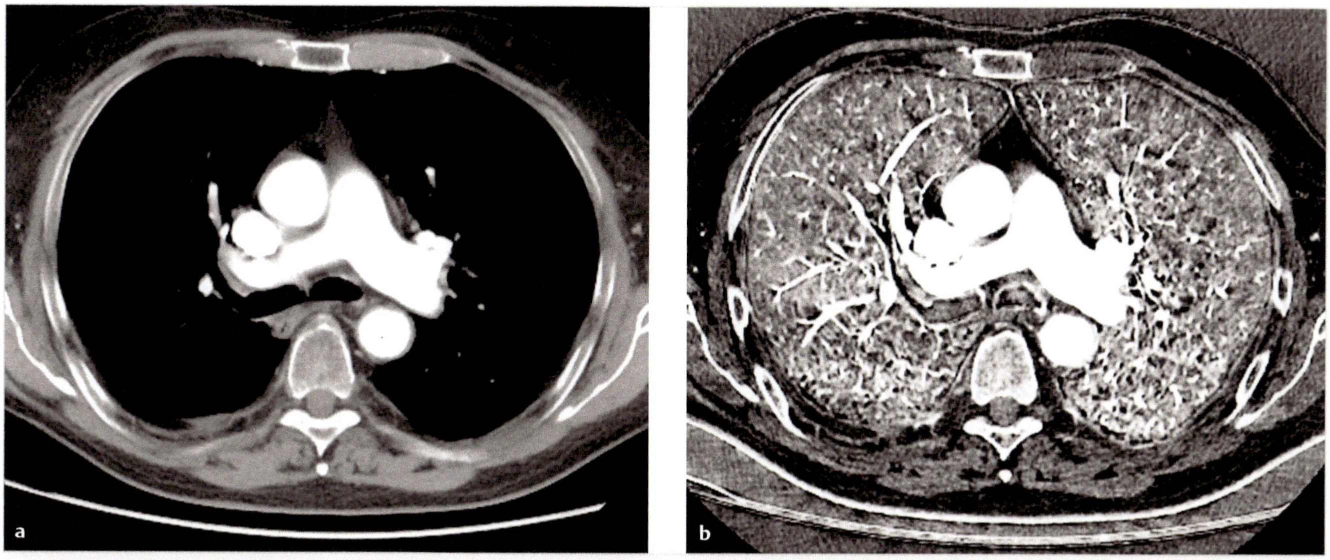

Fig. 1.10 **DECT for visualization of contrast enhancement. (a)** Parenchymal image. **(b)** Parametric image with visualization of iodine content of each voxel, "iodine map."

to become the third most important modality, together with radiography and CT, for diagnostic imaging of the lung. The state of the art permits its widespread deployment not just as a radiation-free alternative for young patients and pregnant women: more than any other imaging modality, MRI offers the combined advantage of insights into morphology and functional information (on lung perfusion, breathing mechanics) within a single examination. Notwithstanding the current state of the technology, many potential users continue to have reservations about utilizing lung MRI, mainly because of the widespread assumption that a reliable and reproducible image quality is difficult to achieve in the everyday routine setting. Essentially, there are two hurdles that reinforce these reservations:

- First, MRI is much more complex than other modalities. Trying to get to grips with this technology at one's own initiative using noncustomized product sequences can be tedious and disappointing. For a successful start, it is therefore recommended to use as far as possible standardized and preset sequence packets, as offered by some MRI scanner manufacturers.[25] The aim of this present section is to give an overview of the sequence techniques, diagnostic facilities, and sequence packets tailored to the most commonly encountered clinical problems.
- The second hurdle relates to the interpretation and evaluation of the images. Experienced thoracic radiologists are not often familiar with the contrasts and poorer spatial resolution of MRI compared with CT, and may need time to get used to the new modality. In addition to attending courses and studying the pertinent literature, new users are therefore advised to arrange guest visits to radiology institutes already using lung MRI.

Unlike radiography and CT, MRI is not based on ionizing radiation but rather on excitation of the rotating hydrogen nuclei in water and organic compounds. The specific anatomic and physiologic nature of the lung is therefore challenging for MRI: in the ventilated lung, the large organ volume contains only a small amount of tissue and fluids which, due to the low proton density, exhibits little signal, with an unfavorable signal-to-noise ratio. This is further compounded by magnetic field inhomogeneities at the air–water interfaces causing decay of the weak signal within milliseconds. Therefore, modern sequence techniques with short echo times are needed in order to at all be able to detect the low signal emitted by the lung tissue. Other interfering factors are the continuous, often irregular movements of the chest caused by breathing and heartbeat. Hence, the healthy, ventilated lung tissue exhibits no, or at most only low, signal which is at times obscured by pulsation artifacts. The majority of pathologic findings are now known to be associated with a higher density of tissue or fluid collections. As such, thanks to their characteristic high signal and good soft-tissue contrast, clinically relevant MRI findings can be distinguished from the intact, dark lung tissue (▸Fig. 1.11).[26]

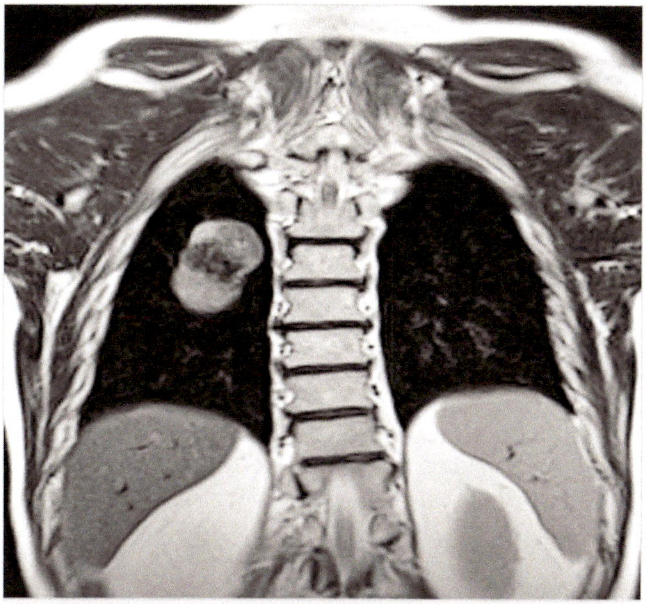

Fig. 1.11 Adenocarcinoma in posterior upper lung lobe. MR image. The tumor has areas of variable signal intensity, reflecting tumor portions with different histopathologic differentiation.

I

1.4.2 Equipment Technology

In principle, MRI of the lung can be performed at either low *field strengths* (1.0 T and lower) or also in high-field scanners at 3 T. Modern 1.5 T MRI scanners are equipped with gradient strengths of more than 40 mT/m and gradient rise times of more than 200 mT/(m × ms), permitting echo times of less than 1.5 ms. Therefore, thanks to superior magnetic field homogeneity, higher lung signal and less susceptibility to artifacts, low-field strength scanners tend to be more suitable than their high-field strength counterparts. However, modern 3 T MRI scanners are typically equipped with powerful gradient systems that offset the undesirable effects of higher field strengths coming into play in the lung (reduced lung signal, increased fluid artifacts in certain sequences). At the other side of the spectrum, low-field strength scanners have an altogether less powerful gradient system, which means that the potential benefits of lung MRI cannot be fully exploited at low-field strength.[26] The following recommendations for the sequence protocol are thus intended for 1.5 T scanners but can also be applied at 3 T.[27]

Multichannel coil systems and parallel imaging techniques play a crucial role in enhancing the performance of modern MRI scanners. In *parallel imaging*, the spatial arrangement of multiple coil elements is exploited to gain additional spatial information from the differences in the sensitivity profiles of the various elements. With parallel imaging, the imaging time can be shortened or, alternatively, a higher spatial resolution can be achieved in the same imaging time. Besides, parallel imaging at higher field strengths (e.g., 3 T) can help to reduce energy deposition in the patient and remain within the limits of the specific absorption rate.

Note

Since the gain in imaging speed or spatial resolution comes at the expense of slight signal loss, the acceleration factors should not exceed 2 or 3 for lung examination. Otherwise, there would be a marked increase in the noise level. Because of lung movement calibration of the sensitivity profile should be integrated into the sequence (e.g., GRAPPA, auto SENSE, FLEX). If that is not the case, there is a risk of interfering artifacts arising from the spatial incongruence between the sensitivity scan and the actual imaging phase.[26]

For routine practice, the use of dedicated *multielement body coils* in combination with the scanner's back or spinal coil has proved beneficial. To optimize image quality at the apex of the lung (superior thoracic aperture, brachial plexus), it can be helpful to use additionally at least the posterior element of the neck coil if that combination is possible.

There are various techniques available to control *motion artifacts*,[26] the easiest and most robust being fast images in the breath-hold technique. Where appropriate, lung imaging can be divided into several breath-hold phases (multi-breath-hold technique). This is the most practical and fastest technique for the clinical setting. For acquisition of high-resolution images or examination of patients who are unable to hold their breath long enough (in general several breath-hold phases of 15–20 s are needed), respiratory-triggered sequences can also be used. Here, the respiratory signal is generated either mechanically (by means of a pneumatic respiratory belt or a belt showing changes in electrical impedance) using the navigator technique or, alternatively, an MR-compatible spirometer.[28] In the navigator technique, a small examination volume is positioned on an element subject to respiratory motion, e.g., the dome of the diaphragm; movement of the contrasting structure is automatically analyzed in the breathing phase. In respiratory-triggered sequences, images are then acquisitioned only in the defined inspiratory or expiratory phases.

The main disadvantage of any *triggered technique* is the additional time needed.[25] Triggered images of the thorax can take as long as 3 to 5 min. If an extra triggering step is included after the cardiac phase (double-trigger technique), the imaging time is further increased by several minutes. Therefore, respiratory-triggered sequences play only a minor role in routine practices.

Currently, the most common protocol recommendations are based on *fast sequences in the breath-hold technique*. With these sequences, a routine examination of the chest without contrast medium administration can be executed in 15 min, and with contrast in 20 min.[25] Respiratory-triggered sequences are offered as an alternative to patients who are unable to hold their breath long enough, or as an option for children whose cooperation throughout the examination procedure cannot be expected.[29] Inclusion of additional fast sequences in free breathing will complete the protocol with information about the patient's impaired breathing mechanics and gross cardiac function.

In principle, the examination can be performed in the breath-hold technique in either inspiration or expiration. Image acquisition in *expiration* can be used to visualize the lung parenchymal signal since on expiratory images the proton density per volume fraction is higher and the signal yield greater.[26] However, for most diagnostic purposes the positive contrast of pathologic lung changes against the dark signal exhibited by the lung tissue is exploited, hence *inspiratory* images are suitable.

Note

Since other standard thoracic imaging techniques are predominantly conducted in inspiration (chest radiographs, CT), comparison of previous examination results with MRI is facilitated when using inspiratory scans.[25]

1.4.3 Pulse Sequences for Diagnostic Imaging

With parallel imaging, large volumes, such as the chest, can be imaged in high detail resolution, with high signal-to-noise ratio and in one breath hold. Typically, fast gradient-echo (GE) sequences, steady-state GE sequences, and fast spin-echo (SE) sequences are used for this purpose.

Fast Gradient-Echo Sequences

Fast GE sequences (FLASH, SPGR, FFE) are part of the standard protocol presets of modern MRI scanners and very robust in practice. With parallel imaging and slice volume interpolation (e.g., volumetric interpolated breath-hold acquisition), volume acquisition of the entire thorax with 5-mm slice thickness is possible in one breath-hold phase.[30] Whereas unenhanced images can typically be obtained without fat signal suppression (good delineation of the mediastinal lymph nodes against the unenhanced bright fatty tissue), fat signal suppression is routinely recommended after contrast medium administration since the contrast-enhanced lymph nodes stand out clearly against the dark background of the suppressed fatty tissue signal.[31]

Steady-State Gradient-Echo Sequences

Steady-state GE sequences (bSSFP, TrueFISP, FIESTA, BFE) are used to achieve very short scanning times; hence, they are commonly used for MRI of the heart but are also advantageous for imaging the lung. Flip angles of generally more than 50° provide for T2w/T1w (T2- to T1-weighted) image contrast and visualize fluids and blood with high signal intensity thanks to long T2 constants. Steady-state GE sequences are therefore suitable for examining the pulmonary vessels without application of contrast medium.[32]

Fast Spin-Echo Sequences

After initial excitation, fast spin-echo (FSE) sequences (RARE/HASTE, Turbo-FSE, TSE) utilize multiple 180° refocusing pulses to expedite signal readout. In extreme cases, a single excitation pulse after multiple refocusing pulses is enough to obtain information for a single slice (RARE sequence). Armed with the knowledge that the image information is contained in redundant form in the k-space (mirrored), the imaging time can be further shortened by performing only partial readout (partial or half-Fourier sequences, e.g., HASTE). Because of the 180° refocusing pulses, the acquisition times of FSE sequences are essentially longer than those of GE or steady-state GE sequences. At the same time, energy deposition is higher, hence the limits of the specific absorption rate are also reached more quickly. FSE sequences are typically acquired in the multislice 2D mode.[26] However, acquisition of single slices, e.g., with only half-Fourier readout (HASTE), can be so fast that heartbeat motion is fully compensated. Therefore, HASTE sequences are a good option if evaluating chest organs in proximity to the heart.[31]

FSE sequences offer an option where, instead of constant parallel orientation of all slices, by using *rotating phase encoding* (PROPELLER/BLADE) the impact exerted by heartbeat and blood flow artifacts in the phase encoding direction can be considerably reduced.[26]

Diffusion-weighted imaging (DWI) sequences are also performed with fat signal suppression. These comprise different basic SE sequences on which a signal is superimposed, making the signal emitted by fluid-containing images susceptible to restricted brownian motion of the water molecules (diffusibility). With low diffusion weighting, the image is like that of a fat-signal suppressed T2w SE sequence, whereas with higher diffusion weighting tumor tissue, in particular with greater cellularity, reduced extracellular space, large nuclei, dense intracellular protein deposition, and, in all cases, resulting restricted brownian molecular motion, is visualized with high signal intensity.[33,34] Furthermore, DWI sequences are particularly useful for the detection of mediastinal lymph nodes which are depicted with high signal intensity.

Contrast-Enhanced Sequences

For most clinical diagnostic purposes (e.g., tumor staging), basic *manual intravenous contrast injection*, followed by fat-saturated fast GE sequences, is sufficient (▸Fig. 1.12). Pulmonary angiograms with excellent image quality can be obtained using fast GE sequences and automated intravenous injection of a T1 time-shortening contrast agent (typically gadolinium chelates). Taking full advantage of a breath-hold time of around 20 s, an image quality on a par with that of CT can be achieved (▸Fig. 1.13).

As an alternative, modern scanners and sequence techniques also offer a *faster variant of contrast-enhanced MRA* (magnetic resonance angiography) for time-resolved 3D visualization of pulmonary circulation. At the expense of slightly poorer detail resolution, the volume data of the entire thorax can be acquired at an interval of 1 to 2 s. The time resolution of this 4D perfusion sequence is enough for separation of arterial, parenchymal, and venous phases.[28,35] The parenchymal phase is

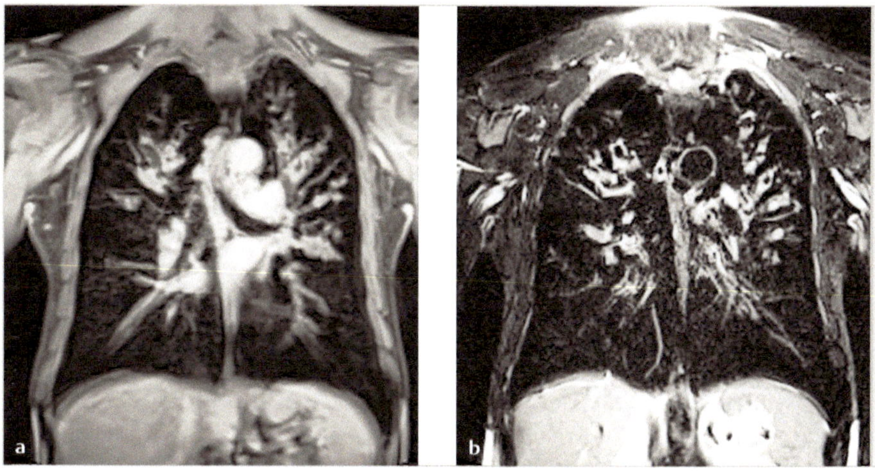

Fig. 1.12 Cystic fibrosis. MR images. Inflammatory thickening of bronchial walls, bronchiectasis and secretory retention, pronounced in bilateral upper lung lobes. **(a)** Coronal, fat-signal suppressed T1w GE sequence following contrast injection. **(b)** Fat-signal suppressed T2w FSE sequence.

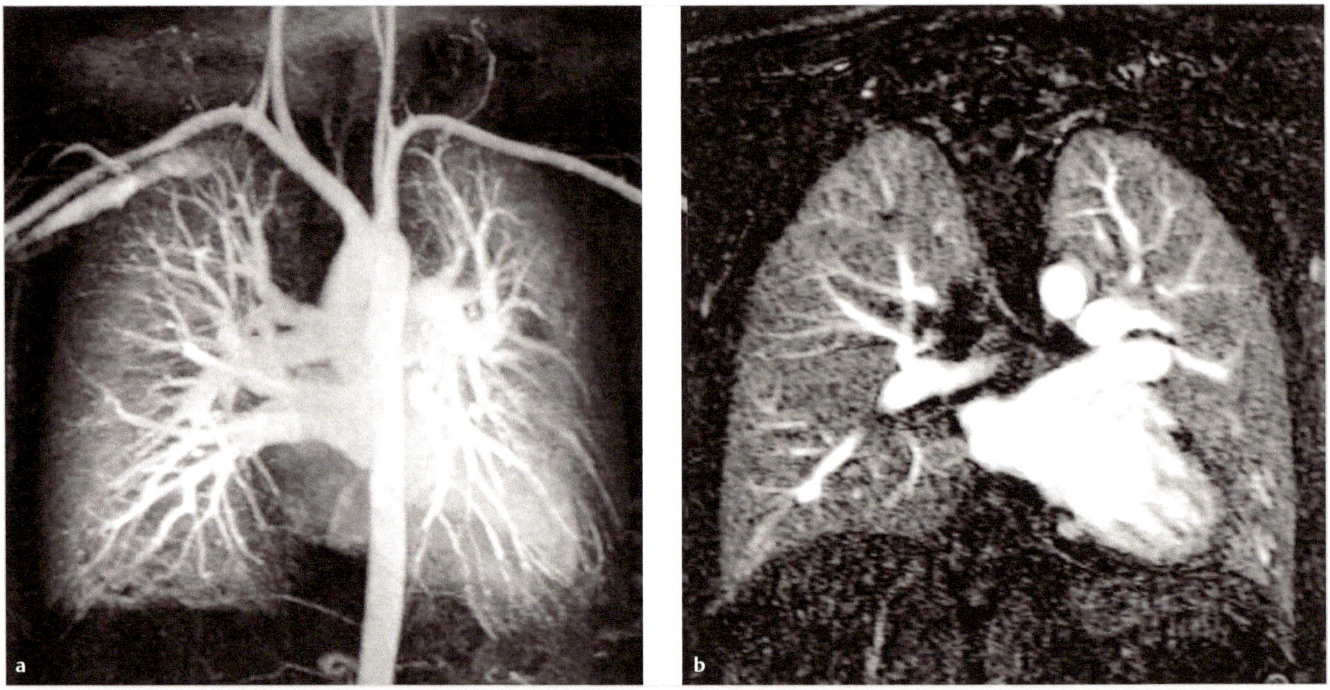

Fig. 1.13 **MRA (magnetic resonance angiography) optimized to parenchymal phase of the thorax for exclusion of pulmonary embolism. (a)** MIP (maximum intensity projection). **(b)** Coronal, single slice without any evidence of intravasal thrombi or parenchymal perfusion deficits.

particularly suitable for detection of discrete perfusion deficits or, with the aid of suitable software, for calculation of parameter maps of regional lung perfusion, regional blood volume, and transit times.

The most expedient approach for *combination of both techniques* may be to first perform a time-resolved perfusion sequence with a small amount of contrast medium. In addition to providing data on regional lung perfusion, this can also help identify the optimal time point for contrast medium injection (typically up to 0.2 mmol/kg body weight) for subsequent acquisition of high resolution MRA.[36,37]

Functional Magnetic Resonance Imaging of the Lung

More than any other modality used for diagnostic imaging of the thorax and lungs, MRI has the potential to combine morphologic and functional information. The best known techniques involve visualization of the *breathing mechanics* (movements of the chest wall, diaphragm, mediastinum, lung tissue, and airways; ▶Fig. 1.14) as well as contrast-enhanced diagnostic evaluation of lung perfusion with fast GE and steady-state free-precession sequences.

1.4.4 Recommendations for Examination Protocols

Protocol recommendations have been published that are able to match the different generic sequence designations to the various scanner configurations.[25] The following recommendations are tailored to that basic concept.

To gain acceptance in routine practice, a sequence protocol for MRI of the lung must be easy to apply, be robust, and endowed with reproducible image quality and high diagnostic power at the most commonly used field strength (1.5 T). More complex components such as an electrocardiogram, placement of a respiratory belt, or IV contrast administration should be avoided as far as possible. Practical solutions should be devised for common problems such as shortness of breath or for young children.

It is proposed to have one common basic protocol for all important clinical problems which permits modular supplementation for specific purposes, e.g., for tumor staging or evaluation of pathologies related to the pulmonary vessels and lung perfusion. For emergency situations, e.g., acute pulmonary artery embolism, fast and efficient procedures should be available which, when warranted, can also be incorporated into a tight routine MRI schedule or can be implemented by night on-call personnel with only limited MRI experience.

The modular design of the sequence protocols presented below should also enable users to put together customized packets, with additional sequences, for example, for heart MRI during cardiopulmonary imaging or for combination with modules for other applications.

Examination Requirements and Preparation

In view of the longer scanning times involved, the image quality in MRI is essentially more dependent on the patient's cooperation than in radiography or CT. A robustly designed examination protocol will thus allow for a certain amount of redundancy with regard to the clinical relevance of the different sequence

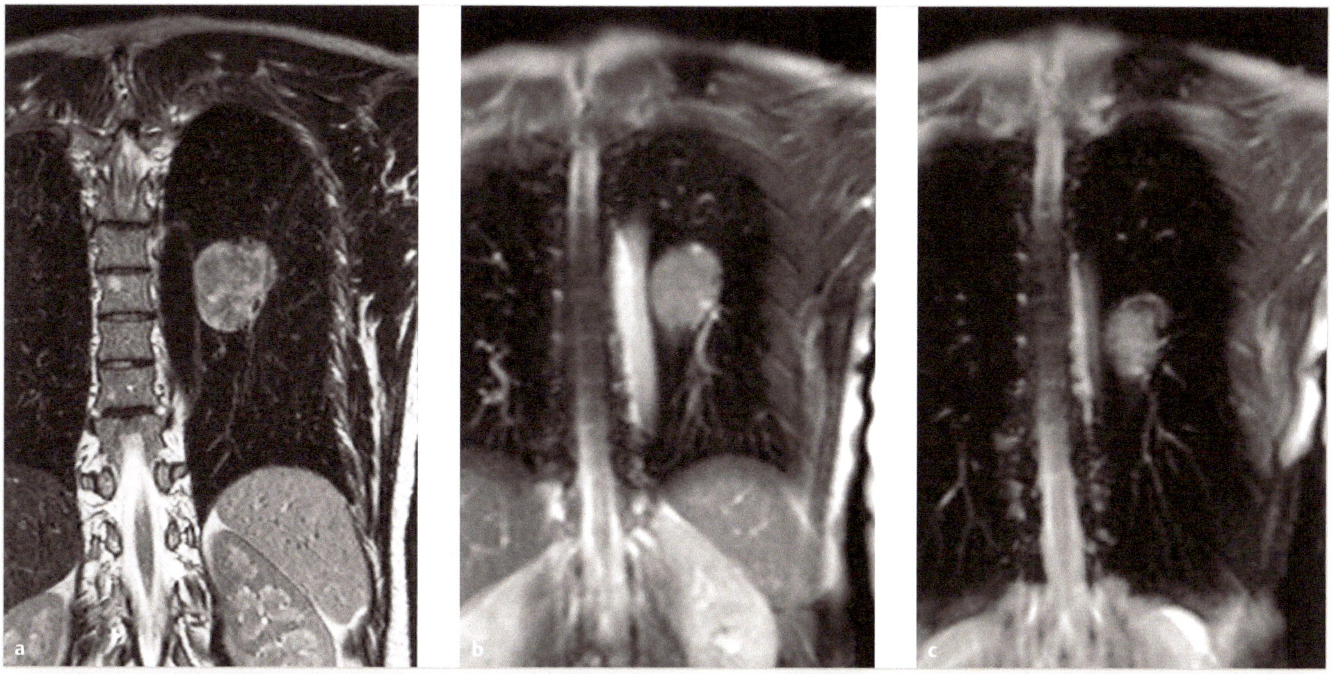

Fig. 1.14 Adenocarcinoma in left upper lobe. MRI of the breathing mechanics. **(a)** Expiratory, respiratory-triggered T2w FSE image. **(b)** The steady-state GE expiratory image shows the tumor in a similar position as in **a.** **(c)** In inspiration the steady-state GE image shows the diaphragm at a much lower level and the tumor somewhat displaced caudally.

components to compensate for the inadequate image quality of any of the acquisition results.[25] For T2w FSE sequences triggered versions are available, thus prolonging the examination time in the standard protocol by around 10 min. A respiratory belt helps to control the patient's respiratory motion also during the imaging phase.[31]

Fundamentals of a Basic Protocol for Lung Examination

From the sequence families presented above, pragmatic protocols are assembled in routine practice. The following overview is based on the generic designations of the sequences.

Note

Typical parameters for MRI of the lung (15 min):

- *Field of view*: coronal 450 to 500 mm, transverse 400 mm.
- *Matrix*: 256 to 384 pixels (gated/triggered up to 512).
- *Pixel size*: smaller than 2 × 2 mm.
- *Slice thickness:*
  - 2D sequences: 4 to 6 mm.
  - 3D sequences: 4 mm.
  - MRA: maximum 2 mm.

A synopsis can be consulted in the literature to reconcile these with the product designations used by the scanner manufacturers.[25] As a basic setting and depending on the patient's size, the field of view is typically set at 450 to 500 mm in the coronal and 400 mm in the transverse plane. The matrix size is 256 to 384 pixels (for triggered FSE sequences up to 512 pixels). Accordingly, the pixels' size is less than 2 × 2 mm. For 2D acquisitions, the slice thickness selected is 4 to 6 mm, for 3D acquisitions the slice thickness is 4 mm or less, and for MRA in a coronal orientation it is 2 mm or less.[38]

Choosing a Suitable Sequence

As a basic protocol for lung MRI, T1w GE sequences and T2w FSE sequences are typically combined.[25] It is suggested to acquire images in two planes, normally the coronal and transverse planes. To increase protocol sensitivity for mediastinal lymph nodes and bone findings (e.g., metastases), at least one of the T2w FSE sequences should be obtained using spectral fat saturation or an inversion pulse (STIR [short-tau inversion recovery]) with suppressed fat signal. Since rib fractures and metastases are easier to identify in transverse slices, it is recommended to use fat saturation at least for the transverse slices. Another obligatory component of a standard protocol is to perform a steady-state free-precession sequence in free breathing as this increases sensitivity for detection of a pulmonary artery embolism or gross cardiac dysfunction. Respiratory-belt or navigator-triggered T2w FSE sequences with high detailed resolution are recommended only as an optional component, since they are time consuming and lead to an overall examination time of more than 5 minutes. They greatly increase image resolution, especially of the chest wall, and are recommended, in particular, if detailed visualization of the brachial plexus or mediastinum is required.[36]

I

Note

MRI protocol of the lung:
- Basic protocol (15 min):
  - 3D-GE sequence (transverse, breath-hold technique).
  - Multislice 2D FSE sequences (T2w FSE; coronal and transverse [transverse fat saturated], multi-breath-hold technique).
  - Fast steady-state GE sequences (coronal, optional transverse; in free breathing).
- *Optional*: high-resolution T2w FSE sequences (coronal or transverse; respiratory-belt or navigator-triggered).

Depending on the initial findings obtained with this basic protocol, contrast-enhanced sequences can be added—likewise, using volume-interpolated 3D-GE sequences, but now with fat saturation to improve visualization of contrast-enhanced tissue and mediastinal lymph nodes. Accordingly, contrast-enhanced 3D-GE sequences in the coronal and transverse plane, in addition to the above-named basic protocol, are recommended as a tumor protocol. Since the in-plane resolution of 3D-GE sequences is superior to the resolution in the slice thickness, image acquisition should definitely be performed in two planes. This appears justifiable as images can be obtained in a single breath-hold phase. The use of DWI sequences is optional for a tumor protocol. The addition of contrast-enhanced sequences to the basic protocol prolongs the overall examination time by around 5 to 20 min.[25]

Note

Supplementary MRI protocol for masses added to the basic protocol (additional 5 min):
- DWI images (transverse; in multi-breath-hold technique or gated or triggered).
- 3D-GE sequence after contrast agent application (coronal and transverse, fat signal suppressed; breath-hold technique).

For a *basic protocol* tailored to pathologies of the *pulmonary vessels*, the combination of three available vascular sequences is recommended[29,36,39]:
- Unenhanced steady-state free-precession sequence.
- Real-time high-resolution, fast 3D-GE sequence for visualization of lung perfusion.
- High spatial resolution, angiographic 3D-GE sequence.

The real-time high-resolution sequence can be utilized to determine the optimal time point to inject contrast agent for the angiographic sequence. Lastly, a 3D-GE sequence should be performed in the transverse plane with fat saturation. If the previous sequences had been adversely affected by motion artifacts, the closing 3D-GE sequence can achieve good results to round off the examination with adequate vascular contrast.

Note

MRI protocol for diseases of the pulmonary vessels (15 min):
- Steady-state GE sequences (steady-state free-precession sequences; coronal and transverse; in free breathing).
- 3D-MRA time-resolved (4D-GE sequence; coronal; small contrast bolus; in shallow breathing).
- 3D-MRA high spatial resolution (3D-GE sequence; coronal; k-space-centered contrast bolus; in shallow breathing).
- 3D-MRA high spatial resolution (3D-GE sequence; coronal; k-space-centered contrast bolus; breath-hold technique).
- *Optional*: supplementary sequences from the basic protocol.

With the basic protocols described above, all important clinical questions related to the lung can be resolved. It is recommended to save the respective variations of the basic sequences as protocol presets on the scanner to serve as readily available standards for solving various diagnostic dilemmas when needed. In addition to the suggested standards, users are encouraged to use their own discretion in combining the different components and tailoring them to the respective clinical situation.

1.5 Ultrasonography

Ultrasonography has its place in diagnostic imaging of the thorax—in particular, for detection of pleural diseases. Its most common application is for diagnosis of pleural effusions and other pleural fluid collections as well as of pneumothorax.[40] Ultrasound can also be used for diagnostic exploration of a number of pulmonary diseases affecting the pleura or in the atelectatic lung.

In general, convex transducers with a frequency of 2 to 5 MHz, as also employed for abdominal diagnostic purposes, are used. Pleural effusions are best explored with the patient in the sitting position as this makes them more amenable to ultrasonographic detection than the supine position. To increase the distance between the ribs, the patient can be examined with the arms raised above the head. The supine position is suitable for diagnosis of pneumothorax since this causes the pleural air to rise anteriorly, facilitating its detection on ultrasound.

Pathologic processes of the chest wall are also displayed with high spatial resolution on ultrasound. Here, high-frequency linear transducers with at least 7.5 MHz are used since in general only a small penetration depth is needed and the high spatial resolution of these transducers yields excellent image quality.[41]

1.6 Positron Emission Tomography–Computed Tomography

Positron emission tomography–computed tomography (PET-CT) provides both anatomic and functional information. The PET-CT scanner combines a computed tomography (CT) scanner and a positron emission tomography (PET) scanner. The latter is used to trace radioactive pharmaceuticals in the body, while displaying their distribution in cross-sectional images. The glucose analog FDG (^{18}fludeoxyglucose /fluorodeoxyglucose) is used for diagnostic imaging of chest diseases. This is absorbed by the cells in the same way as glucose but, because of its molecular structure, it cannot be broken down by the cell like glucose for energy production. FDG therefore accumulates in the cells.

Tumor cells and inflammatory cells have a higher glucose metabolism and, accordingly, an increased glucose requirement. Besides, tumors are often oxygen-deficient and, as such, tumor cells must increasingly resort to anaerobic glycolysis to meet their energy needs. Anaerobic compared with aerobic glycolysis yields essentially less energy, in turn further increasing the glucose requirement of these cells. On FDG-PET, these processes are visualized as increased accumulation of FDG in malignant tumors and inflammatory tissue.

Examination is carried out in several substeps:

1. Intravenous administration of the radioactive FDG. This is followed by a resting phase of 1 h.
2. CT scan acquisition. There are two ways to do this:
   - Diagnostic CT: This is generally done, after IV contrast administration, as diagnostic whole-body CT. CT scan acquisition during breathing baseline assures optimal image fusion with PET. For oncologic indications acquisition of an additional low-dose CT scan of the lung parenchyma in deep inspiration will increase sensitivity for lung metastases.[42]
   - Low-dose CT: If whole-body CT is not clinically indicated, the low-dose CT scan is acquisitioned unenhanced. This provides data for attenuation correction of PET and, at the same time, for anatomic assignment of the PET findings.
3. PET scan acquisition.

Note

Typical applications of FDG-PET in thoracic radiology:

- Staging of malignant tumors, in particular detection of distant metastases, and of lymph node metastases.
- Differential diagnosis of pulmonary nodules.
- Primary tumor search in cancer of unknown primary (CUP) syndrome.
- Diagnosis of early aortitis.[43]

1.7 Image Reformatting

Modern workstations provide the radiologist with numerous options for image postprocessing, which can also be availed of for thoracic diagnostic purposes. This facility may be used by the radiologist when interpreting the imaging findings, explaining the findings of the primary diagnosis to the referring physicians, or for planning treatment. The significance of the various postprocessing procedures in thoracic diagnostics is presented in ▸Table 1.3. The availability of a suitable thin-slice CT dataset is a precondition for practical implementation of these methods.

1.8 Computer-Assisted Diagnosis

1.8.1 Computer-Assisted Detection

Commercial software is available for both computer-assisted diagnostic (CAD) interpretation of chest radiographs as well as of CT datasets.[47,48] Most software solutions are designed for detection of pulmonary nodules. Radiologists have only moderate sensitivity in this regard but that can be improved through the use of suitable software.

Table 1.3 Image reformatting procedures and their application in diagnostic imaging of the thorax[44,45,46]

Procedure	Applications	Importance		
		Diagnosis	Demonstration	Treatment planning
MIP	• Detection of lung nodules • Detection of pulmonary embolism	+ +	(+)	–
MinIP	• Detection of emphysema • Visualization of airway stenosis	++	+	+
MPR	• Visualization of vascular and bronchial structures • Intervention planning for bronchoscopy	+	+	+
VRT	• Visualization of complex findings (in particular demonstration of osseous and vascular structures and the position of implants)	(+)	++	(+)
Virtual endoscopy	• Interventional planning for bronchoscopic biopsies	-	+	+

Abbreviations: MinIP, minimum intensity projection; MIP, maximum intensity projection; MPR, multiplanar reformatting; VRT, volume rendering technique.

Depending on the software used, the imaging findings are evaluated immediately on calling up the function at the diagnostic workstation or the results will have already been preprocessed and stored. The latter systems can invest more computing time in analysis, thus making a positive contribution to diagnostic accuracy.

Note

A thin-slice CT dataset is required to assure a good diagnostic yield. Overlapping reconstructed slices of <2 mm slice thickness are a minimum requirement.

Deployment of such software can enhance the quality of CT diagnostic imaging in oncological settings and might shorten image reading time.[49] In addition, it is used for preoperative planning prior to resection of pulmonary metastases.[50]

1.8.2 Volumetry

Volumetry is now established as a standard diagnostic procedure for management of pulmonary nodules. As for other computer-assisted techniques, this, too, requires a thin-slice CT dataset with a slice thickness of less than 2 mm with overlapping reconstruction.

Volumetry software is commercially available as part of the standard software package of many CT scanners or of diagnostic workstations. After marking a nodule on a CT image, the software automatically calculates its volume. Depending on the particular type of software, the user has various options for manual correction of the results of automatic measurement, for example, for elimination of adjacent blood vessels from the automatically calculated nodule volume.

References

[1] Adler AM, Carlton RR, eds. Introduction to Radiologic & Imaging Sciences & Patient Care. 6th ed. St. Louis, MO: Elsevier Saunders; 2015

[2] Long BW, Rollins JH, Smith BJ. Merrill's Atlas of Radiographic Positioning & Procedures. St. Louis, MO: Mosby Inc.; 2015

[3] Bradley M, Williams C, Walshaw MJ. The value of routine expiratory chest films in the diagnosis of pneumothorax. Arch Emerg Med 1991;8(2):115–116

[4] Seow A, Kazerooni EA, Pernicano PG, Neary M. Comparison of upright inspiratory and expiratory chest radiographs for detecting pneumothoraces. AJR Am J Roentgenol 1996;166(2):313–316

[5] European Commission. European Guidelines on Quality Criteria for Diagnostic Radiographic Images. Luxembourg: Office for Official Publications of the European Communities; 1996

[6] Nason LK, Walker CM, McNeeley MF, Burivong W, Fligner CL, Godwin JD. Imaging of the diaphragm: anatomy and function. Radiographics 2012;32(2):E51–E70

[7] European Commission. Diagnostic reference levels in thirty-six European countries: Part 2/2 (22.12.2014). Available at: https://ec.europa.eu/energy/sites/ener/files/documents/RP180%20part2.pdf

[8] Kalra MK, Sodickson AD, Mayo-Smith WW. CT radiation: key concepts for gentle and wise use. Radiographics 2015;35(6):1706–1721

[9] Viteri-Ramírez G, García-Lallana A, Simón-Yarza I, et al. Low radiation and low-contrast dose pulmonary CT angiography: Comparison of 80 kVp/60 ml and 100 kVp/80 ml protocols. Clin Radiol 2012;67(9):833–839

[10] Todo G, Ito H, Nakano Y, et al. High resolution CT (HR-CT) for the evaluation of pulmonary peripheral disorders [in Japanese] Rinsho Hoshasen 1982;27(12):1319–1326

[11] Webb WR, Müller NL, Naidich DP. High-Resolution CT of the Lung. 4th ed. Philadelphia, PA: Wolters Kluwer/Lippincott Williams & Wilkins; 2009

[12] Sundaram B, Chughtai AR, Kazerooni EA. Multidetector high-resolution computed tomography of the lungs: protocols and applications. J Thorac Imaging 2010;25(2):125–141

[13] Garcia-Peña P, Lucaya J. HRCT in children: technique and indications. Eur Radiol 2004;14(Suppl 4):L13–L30

[14] Diederich S, Lenzen H, Windmann R, et al. Pulmonary nodules: experimental and clinical studies at low-dose CT. Radiology 1999;213(1):289–298

[15] Wang R, Sui X, Schoepf UJ, et al. Ultralow-radiation-dose chest CT: accuracy for lung densitometry and emphysema detection. AJR Am J Roentgenol 2015;204(4):743–749

[16] Chiles C. Lung cancer screening with low-dose computed tomography. Radiol Clin North Am 2014;52(1):27–46

[17] The Japanese Society of CT Screening Low-dose CT Lung Cancer Screening Guidelines for Pulmonary Nodules Management Version 2. Available at: http://www.jscts.org/pdf/guideline/NoduleManagement-v2.pdf. Accessed November 16, 2017

[18] Kim Y, Kim YK, Lee BE, et al. Ultra-low-dose CT of the thorax using iterative reconstruction: evaluation of image quality and radiation dose reduction. AJR Am J Roentgenol 2015;204(6):1197–1202

[19] Raghu G, Remy-Jardin M, Myers JL, et al; American Thoracic Society, European Respiratory Society, Japanese Respiratory Society, and Latin American Thoracic Society. Diagnosis of Idiopathic Pulmonary Fibrosis. An Official ATS/ERS/JRS/ALAT Clinical Practice Guideline. Am J Respir Crit Care Med 2018;198(5):e44–e68

[20] Helm E, Talakoub O, Grasso F, et al. Use of dynamic CT in acute respiratory distress syndrome (ARDS) with comparison of positive and negative pressure ventilation. Eur Radiol 2009;19(1):50–57

[21] Baroni RH, Ashiku S, Boiselle PM. Dynamic CT evaluation of the central airways in patients undergoing tracheoplasty for tracheobronchomalacia. AJR Am J Roentgenol 2005;184(5):1444–1449

[22] Swensen SJ, Viggiano RW, Midthun DE, et al. Lung nodule enhancement at CT: multicenter study. Radiology 2000;214(1):73–80

[23] Kang MJ, Park CM, Lee CH, Goo JM, Lee HJ. Dual-energy CT: clinical applications in various pulmonary diseases. Radiographics 2010;30(3):685–698

[24] Zhang LJ, Zhou CS, Schoepf UJ, et al. Dual-energy CT lung ventilation/perfusion imaging for diagnosing pulmonary embolism. Eur Radiol 2013;23(10):2666–2675

[25] Biederer J, Beer M, Hirsch W, et al. MRI of the lung (2/3). Why ... when ... how? Insights Imaging 2012;3(4):355–371

[26] Wild JM, Marshall H, Bock M, et al. MRI of the lung (1/3): methods. Insights Imaging 2012;3(4):345–353

[27] Fink C, Puderbach M, Biederer J, et al. Lung MRI at 1.5 and 3 Tesla: observer preference study and lesion contrast using five different pulse sequences. Invest Radiol 2007;42(6):377–383

[28] Eichinger M, Puderbach M, Fink C, et al. Contrast-enhanced 3D MRI of lung perfusion in children with cystic fibrosis--initial results. Eur Radiol 2006;16(10):2147–2152

[29] Biederer J, Mirsadraee S, Beer M, et al. MRI of the lung (3/3)-current applications and future perspectives. Insights Imaging 2012;3(4):373–386

[30] Biederer J, Both M, Graessner J, et al. Lung morphology: fast MR imaging assessment with a volumetric interpolated breath-hold technique: initial experience with patients. Radiology 2003;226(1):242–249

[31] Puderbach M, Hintze C, Ley S, Eichinger M, Kauczor HU, Biederer J. MR imaging of the chest: a practical approach at 1.5T. Eur J Radiol 2007;64(3):345–355

[32] Kluge A, Gerriets T, Müller C, et al. [Thoracic real-time MRI: experience from 2200 examinations in acute and ill-defined thoracic diseases] RoFo Fortschr Geb Rontgenstr Nuklearmed 2005;177(11):1513–1521

[33] Henzler T, Schmid-Bindert G, Schoenberg SO, Fink C. Diffusion and perfusion MRI of the lung and mediastinum. Eur J Radiol 2010;76(3):329–336

[34] Koyama H, Ohno Y, Aoyama N, et al. Comparison of STIR turbo SE imaging and diffusion-weighted imaging of the lung: capability for detection and subtype classification of pulmonary adenocarcinomas. Eur Radiol 2010;20(4):790–800

[35] Heidemann RM, Griswold MA, Kiefer B, et al. Resolution enhancement in lung 1H imaging using parallel imaging methods. Magn Reson Med 2003;49(2):391–394

[36] Biederer J, Bauman G, Hintze C, et al. Magnetresonanztomographie. Pneumologe 2011;8:234–242

[37] Puderbach M, Risse F, Biederer J, et al. In vivo Gd-DTPA concentration for MR lung perfusion measurements: assessment with computed tomography in a porcine model. Eur Radiol 2008;18(10):2102–2107

[38] Kauczor H. MRI of the Lung. Berlin: Springer; 2009

[39] Kluge A, Luboldt W, Bachmann G. Acute pulmonary embolism to the subsegmental level: diagnostic accuracy of three MRI techniques compared with 16-MDCT. AJR Am J Roentgenol 2006;187(1):W7–14

[40] Husain LF, Hagopian L, Wayman D, Baker WE, Carmody KA. Sonographic diagnosis of pneumothorax. J Emerg Trauma Shock 2012;5(1):76–81

[41] Koh DM, Burke S, Davies N, Padley SP. Transthoracic US of the chest: clinical uses and applications. Radiographics 2002;22(1):e1

[42] Juergens KU, Weckesser M, Stegger L, et al. Tumor staging using whole-body high-resolution 16-channel PET-CT: does additional low-dose chest CT in inspiration improve the detection of solitary pulmonary nodules? Eur Radiol 2006;16(5):1131–1137

[43] Bossert M, Prati C, Balblanc JC, Lohse A, Wendling D. Aortic involvement in giant cell arteritis: current data. Joint Bone Spine 2011;78(3):246–251

[44] Beigelman-Aubry C, Hill C, Guibal A, Savatovsky J, Grenier PA. Multi-detector row CT and postprocessing techniques in the assessment of diffuse lung disease. Radiographics 2005;25(6):1639–1652

[45] Fishman EK, Ney DR, Heath DG, Corl FM, Horton KM, Johnson PT. Volume rendering versus maximum intensity projection in CT angiography: what works best, when, and why. Radiographics 2006;26(3):905–922

[46] Nair A, Godoy MC, Holden EL, et al. Multidetector CT and postprocessing in planning and assisting in minimally invasive bronchoscopic airway interventions. Radiographics 2012;32(5):E201–E232

[47] Abe H, MacMahon H, Engelmann R, et al. Computer-aided diagnosis in chest radiography: results of large-scale observer tests at the 1996–2001 RSNA scientific assemblies. Radiographics 2003;23(1):255–265

[48] Girvin F, Ko JP. Pulmonary nodules: detection, assessment, and CAD. AJR Am J Roentgenol 2008;191(4):1057–1069

[49] Beyer F, Zierott L, Fallenberg EM, et al. Comparison of sensitivity and reading time for the use of computer-aided detection (CAD) of pulmonary nodules at MDCT as concurrent or second reader. Eur Radiol 2007;17(11):2941–2947

[50] Schramm A, Wormanns D, Leschber G, Merk J. Reliability of a computer-aided detection system in detecting lung metastases compared to manual palpation during surgery. Interact Cardiovasc Thorac Surg 2011;12(1):20–23

Chapter 2

Basic Anatomy

2 Basic Anatomy

Contrary to likely expectations, this present chapter does not give a comprehensive description of the anatomy of the chest organs. Rather, it highlights a number of anatomic landmarks of interest in routine radiology.

2.1 The Mediastinum

> **Note**
>
> The mediastinum is the space between left and right lung bordered anteriorly by the sternum, posteriorly by the spinal column, cranially by the superior thoracic aperture, caudally by the diaphragm, and laterally on both sides by the pleura.

The division of the mediastinum into compartments (▶Table 2.1) is of practical importance, in particular, for diagnostic radiology of mediastinal tumors. Differential diagnosis will vary greatly in accordance with tumor localization. The most common systems are the three-compartment model (anterior, middle, and posterior mediastinum) and the four-compartment model (like the three-compartment model, plus superior mediastinum).[1] There are other less well-known compartment systems.[2]

Since there is no rigid border between the described mediastinal compartments, pathologic processes can spread unchecked from one compartment to another.

2.1.1 The Vascular System

Aorta

The thoracic portion of the aorta is divided into three segments:

- *Ascending aorta*: Maximum width of 3.5 cm.
- *Aortic arch with the origins of the supra-aortic arteries*: The most common normal variant—bicarotid trunk (common origin of the brachiocephalic trunk and the left common carotid artery; ▶Fig. 2.1).
- *Descending aorta*: Maximum width distal to the aortic arch of 2.6 cm, where it passes the diaphragm maximum 2.4 cm.[3]

Table 2.1 Anatomic compartments of the mediastinum based on the three- and four-compartment model[2]

Compartments	Border
Three-compartment model	
Anterior mediastinum	Space extending from sternum to the anterior surface of the pericardium, ascending aorta, and brachiocephalic vessels
Middle mediastinum	Space between anterior and posterior mediastinum
Posterior mediastinum	Space between the posterior surface of the pericardium and the large vessels extending to the thoracic spine
Four-compartment model	
Plus: superior mediastinum	Space above the aortic arch

An *aortic aneurysm* is defined as dilation of the aorta by at least 1.5-fold its normal maximum diameter. The simplified limit values are 5 cm for the ascending aorta and 4.5 cm for the thoracic descending aorta.

Anomalies of the aortic arch are divided into five groups:

- *Duplicated aortic arch*: This can cause compression of the central airways.
- *Right-sided aortic arch with mirror-image vascular branching*: This should not be misinterpreted on radiographs as a mediastinal mass (▶Fig. 2.2).
- *Right-sided aortic arch with abnormal vascular branching.*
- *Left aortic arch with abnormal vascular branching*: The most common finding here is a lusoria artery, i.e., an aberrant right subclavian artery that branches as the last artery from the aortic arch and runs toward the right in a retroesophageal direction and may lead to impaired swallowing (▶Fig. 2.3).
- *Cervical aortic arch.*

The embryonic ductus Botalli (ductus arteriosus) is a connection between the aortic arch and pulmonary trunk that is obliterated after birth, giving rise to the *ligamentum arteriosum*, which at times can be identified on computed tomography (CT) as a connective tissue strand (▶Fig. 2.4). In addition to the aortic valve level and the diaphragmatic aortic hiatus, this constitutes the third fixation point for the thoracic aorta. Therefore, this site is particularly susceptible to aortic rupture secondarily to chest injuries (see Chapter 15).

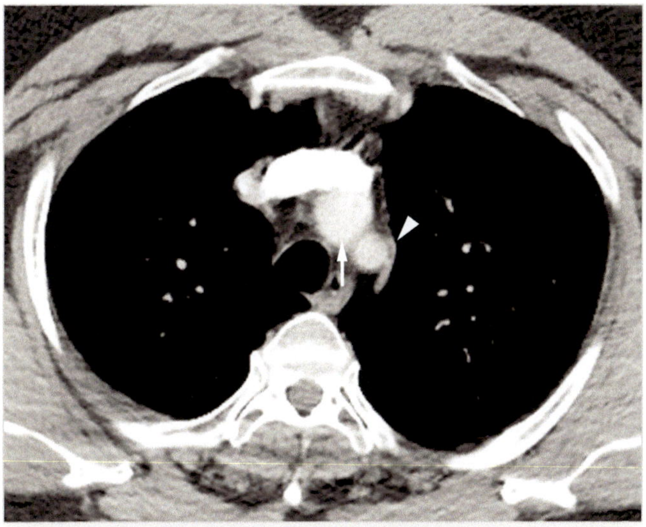

Fig. 2.1 Bicarotid trunk. CT image. Cranial to the aortic arch, there are only two arterial vessels: the bicarotid trunk (*arrow*) and the left subclavian artery (*arrowhead*).

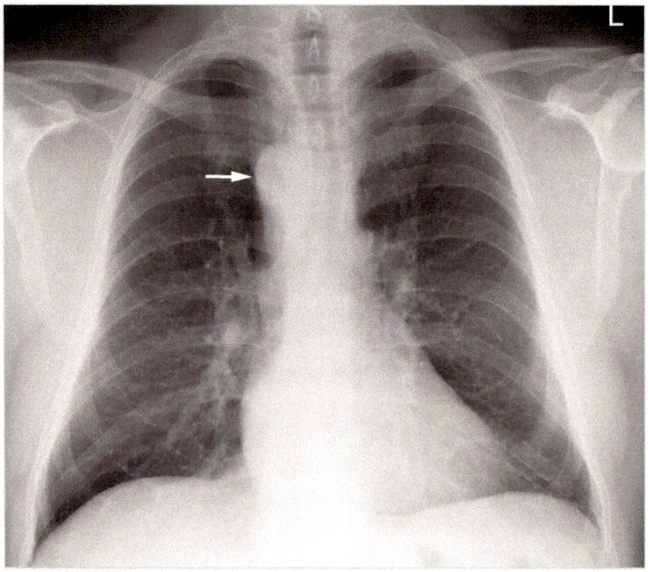

Fig. 2.2 Right-sided aortic arch (*arrow*). Radiograph.

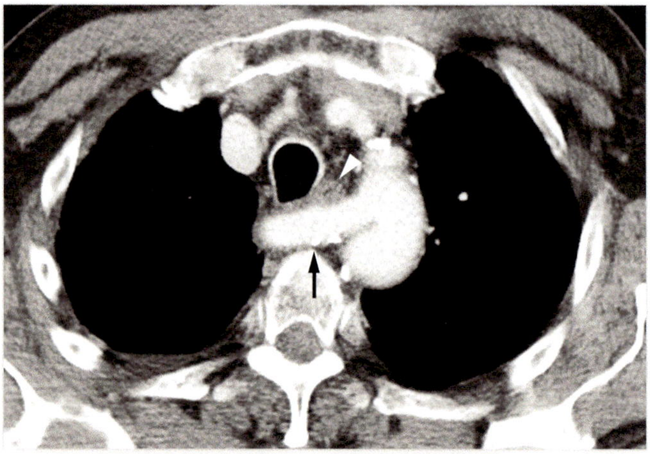

Fig. 2.3 Lusoria artery (*arrow*). CT image. Right subclavian artery running posterior to the esophagus (*arrowhead*).

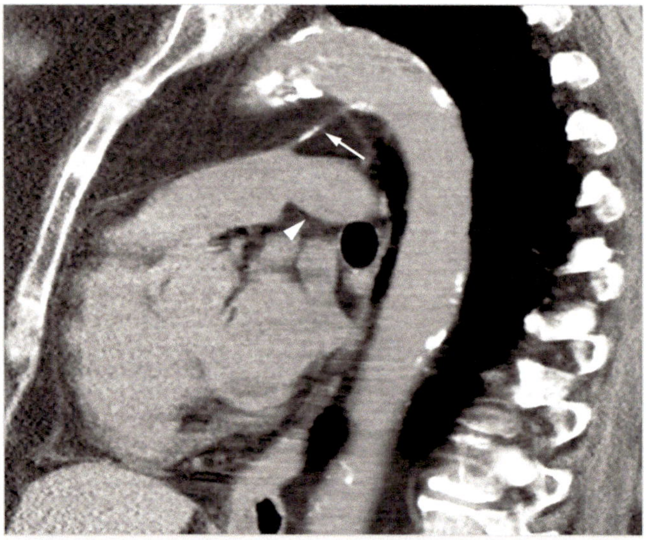

Fig. 2.4 Partially calcified ligamentum arteriosum (*arrow*). Caudal to it, pulmonary trunk (*arrowhead*), cranial the aortic arch. CT image, parasagittal MPR (multiplanar reformation).

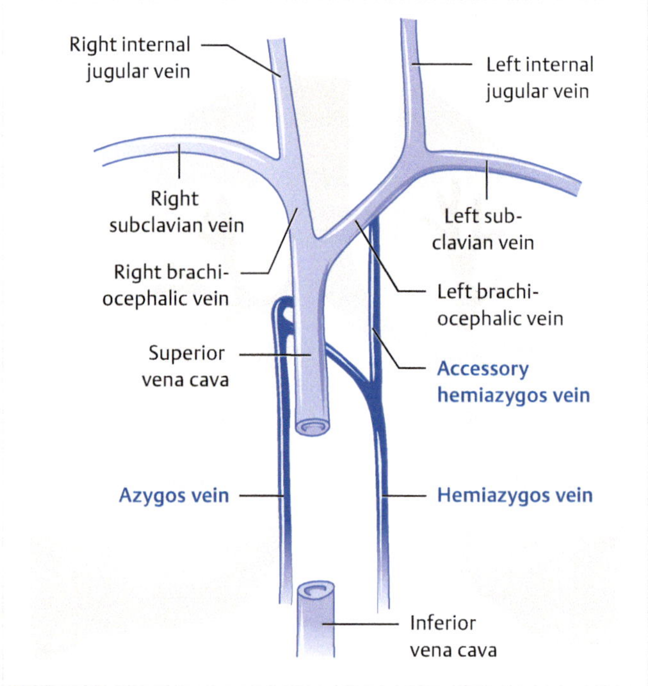

Fig. 2.5 Central veins in thorax. Schematic diagram.

Pulmonary Arteries

Like the aorta, the central pulmonary arteries are elastic-type arteries, while the peripheral pulmonary arteries distal to the segmental arteries are of the muscular type. This is why, following a rise in pressure the central, but not the peripheral, pulmonary arteries appear dilated. On radiographs, *amputated hila are seen*, in particular, in the presence of underlying chronic obstructive lung disease.

Bronchial Arteries

The lungs have duplicate blood supply: via the large-caliber pulmonary arteries, accounting for the entire cardiac output, and via the small-caliber systemic bronchial arteries supplying the lungs. Their origin is variable but the majority of the left-sided bronchial arteries arise directly from the thoracic aorta, while their right-sided counterparts originate from the third right intercostal artery.[4] They course along the bronchi to the periphery.

Bronchial arteries of normal width can be visualized on angiography but rarely on CT. Dilated bronchial arteries can also be identified on CT (see ▶Fig. 14.5) and are seen, in particular, in the presence of bronchiectasis and chronic thromboembolic pulmonary hypertension.

Central Veins

The central thoracic veins are illustrated in ▶Fig. 2.5. The anatomy of the venous system of the chest organs is often brought to the attention of the radiologist following malpositioning of a central venous catheter.

One important anatomic variant is *persistent left superior vena cava* (▶Fig. 2.6), mainly draining into the coronary sinus. Identification on the radiograph, at the left mediastinal border, of a central venous catheter or pacemaker that had been inserted from the left and now runs caudally is suggestive of such a venous anomaly. Infrequently, it drains into the left atrium or into a pulmonary vein, thus giving rise to a right-left shunt.[5]

Conspicuous dilation of the azygos vein points to an obstruction or the absence of vasculature in the flow region of the inferior vena cava, often involving agenesis of segments of the inferior vena cava (▶Fig. 2.7).

Pulmonary Veins

Each of the two lungs is drained by two pulmonary veins that terminate in the left atrium. The right lower lobe and middle lobe share a common venous drainage system. ▶Fig. 2.8 shows the course of the central pulmonary veins on CT.

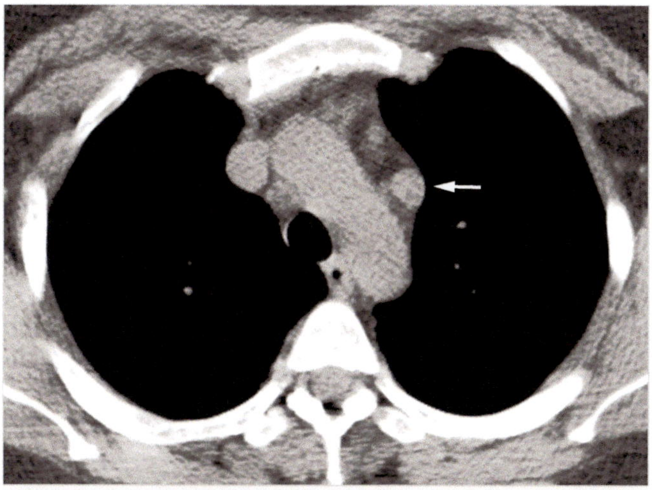

Fig. 2.6 Persistent left superior vena cava. CT image. Large-caliber venous vessel on the left, lateral to the aortic arch (*arrow*).

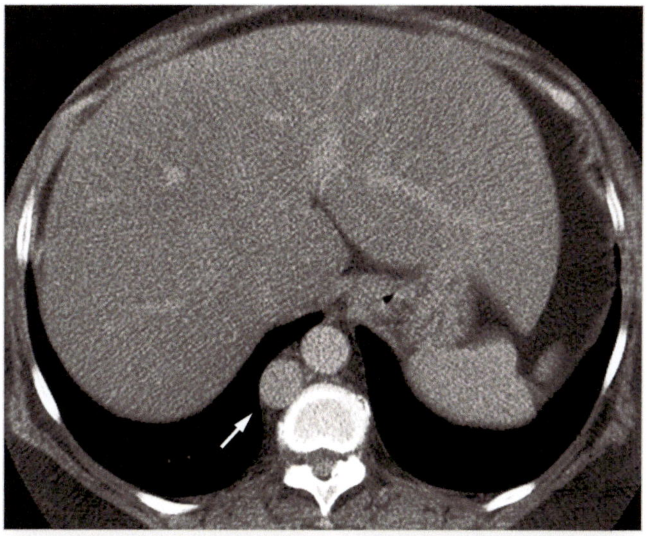

Fig. 2.7 Agenesis of the intrahepatic segment of the inferior vena cava. CT image. Extensively dilated azygos vein (*arrow*) on the right, beside the aorta.

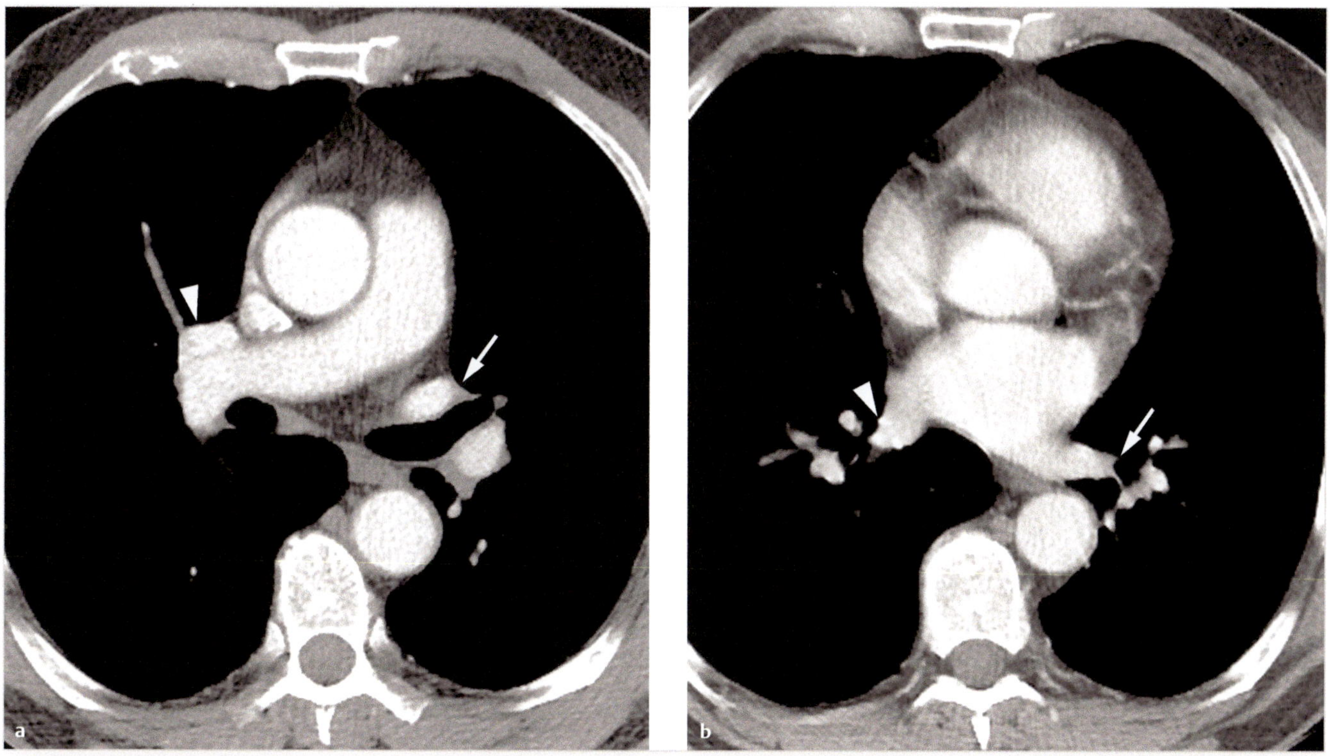

Fig. 2.8 Course of the pulmonary veins. CT image. **(a)** Section somewhat caudal to the tracheal bifurcation: left (*arrow*) and right superior pulmonary vein (*arrowhead*). **(b)** Section at the level of the left atrium: left (*arrow*) and right inferior pulmonary vein (*arrowhead*).

Details of partial anomalous termination of pulmonary veins in systemic veins, resulting in a left-right shunt, are given in Section 19.[5].

2.1.2 The Lymphatic System

Conversancy with the lymphatic drainage system of the lungs is paramount in thoracic oncology. Both lungs drain via hilar and mediastinal lymph nodes into the thoracic duct. The latter is generally not identifiable on imaging, apart from the cisterna chyli which can sometimes be seen on CT or MRI between the diaphragmatic crura as a cystic structure measuring several millimeters. The thoracic duct terminates in the left venous angle, i.e., at the confluence of the left internal jugular vein and the subclavian vein.

The IASLC (International Association for the Study of Lung Cancer) nomenclature should be used for naming mediastinal and hilar *lymph node stations* in the examination reports (▶Table 2.2 and ▶Fig. 2.9).[6]

> **Note**
>
> Since the 7th revised version of the IASLC nomenclature (entered into force in 2010), borders of paratracheal lymph node stations differ from earlier nomenclature versions.6 Henceforth, the left border of the trachea serves as the border between the right and left paratracheal lymph node stations (▶Fig. 2.10); formerly, this had been the midline of the trachea.

Peripheral intrapulmonary lymph nodes often manifest as smoothly marginated, intrapulmonary nodules, typically located at a maximum subpleural distance of 10 mm, with a longitudinal oval, less commonly rounded, shape (see ▶Fig. 21.7).

Their size may change over time, becoming larger and then smaller again.

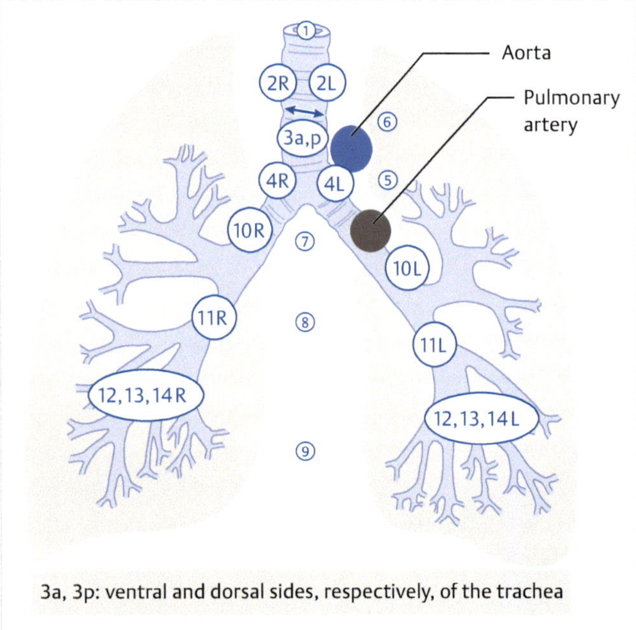

Fig. 2.9 Mediastinal and hilar lymph node stations based on the IASLC nomenclature. Schematic diagram. Lymph node stations 3a and 3p are located anterior and posterior, respectively, to the trachea.

2.1.3 The Trachea and Bronchi

Around 16 to 20 horseshoe-shaped cartilage clasps form and stabilize the anterior and lateral walls of the trachea (cartilaginous part). There are no cartilage clasps in the posterior wall of the trachea (membranous part); instead, this contains smooth muscle. Accordingly, this region is more susceptible to injury.

The carina is the structure at the tracheal bifurcation, at the distal end of the trachea. Here it merges with the two mainstem

Table 2.2 Mediastinal and hilar lymph node stations[6]

Station	Side	Designation
1		Low cervical, supraclavicular, and sternal notch nodes
2	2L, 2R	Upper paratracheal
3a		Prevascular
3p		Retrotracheal
4	4L, 4R	Lower paratracheal
5		Subaortic
6		Para-aortic (ascending aorta or phrenic)
7		Subcarinal
8		Paraesophageal (below carina)
9		Pulmonary ligament
10	10L, 10R	Hilar
11	11L, 11R	Interlobar
12	12L, 12R	Lobar
13	13L, 13R	Segmental
14	14L, 14R	Subsegmental

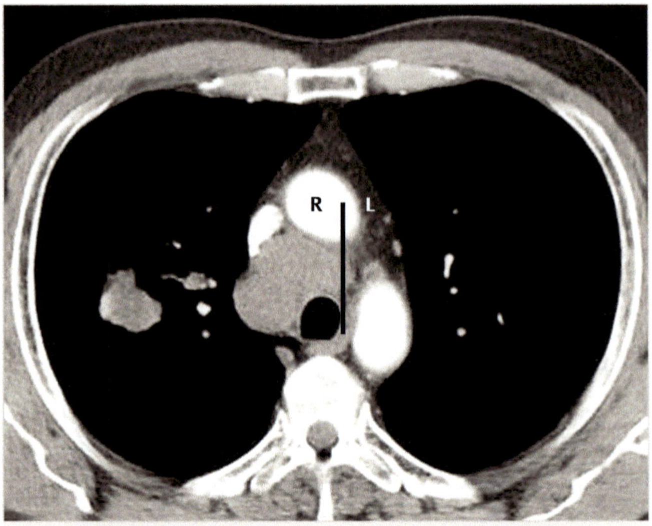

Fig. 2.10 Border between the right paratracheal (R) and left paratracheal (L) lymph node station (line). In addition, peripheral lung carcinoma in right upper lobe. CT image.

bronchi, with the right bronchus exhibiting a steeper caudal course than the left. The central bronchi, unlike the peripheral small bronchi, also contain cartilage clasps. At times, radiologists can identify these clasps in older patients due to their calcification.

Occasionally, *variants* are observed in the structure of the bronchial tree, of which the most common is a right apical upper lobe segmental bronchus branching directly from the trachea (▶Fig. 2.11).

2.1.4 The Thymus

In young children, the thymus is a large parenchymatous organ in the anterior mediastinum. During childhood and adolescence, it undergoes, in individual cases highly variable, involution, with increasing conversion of the thymic parenchyma to fatty tissue (▶Fig. 2.12).[7] On MRI, the thymus generally appears somewhat larger than on CT. This may be due to better visualization on MRI of the converted fatty thymic tissue.[8] The size of the thymus as measured in studies on CT was 1.1 ± 0.4 cm in 6- to 19-year-olds and 0.5 ± 0.3 cm in the over 50-year-olds; the maximum size was 1.8 cm in persons younger than 20 years and later 1.3 cm.[8,9] A larger thymus size of 15 to 20 mm has been seen in adults on MRI.[10]

Various external causes result in thymic enlargement, known as thymic rebound, especially in young adolescents.

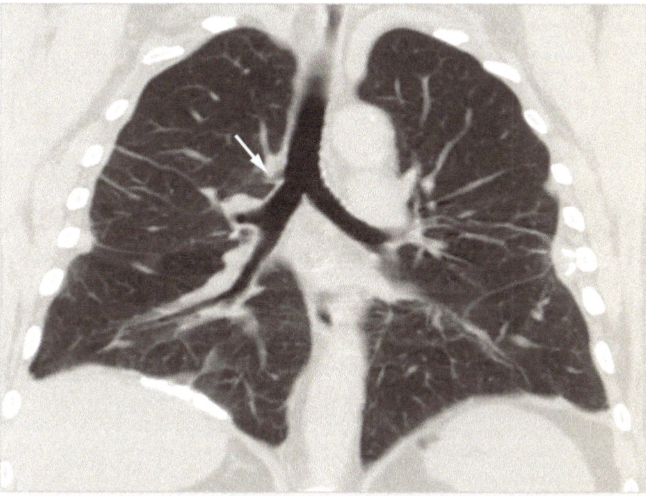

Fig. 2.11 Origin of the right apical upper lobe segmental bronchus arising directly from the trachea (*arrow*). In addition, bilateral pleural plaques. CT image, coronal MinIP (minimum intensity projection).

2.2 The Heart and Pericardium

Already back in the 1920s one radiology textbook described 20 different heart configurations.[11] With the advent of echocardiography for routine cardiology diagnosis, considerably less importance was ascribed to heart size and heart configuration when interpreting radiographic findings. Ultrasound thus obviated the need to look for indirect signs of enlargement of the heart cavities. Nonetheless, radiologists should be conversant with a few basic signs which, with only moderate accuracy, point to *pathologic heart size on radiographs* (▶Fig. 2.13):

- When the ratio of the transverse cardiac diameter to the transverse thoracic diameter (cardiothoracic index) in the posteroanterior (PA) radiograph is more than 0.5.[12,13]
- When the right border of heart is more than 2 cm away from the right border of the spine in the PA radiograph.
- When the anterior heart border in the lateral image abuts the sternum by more than one-third of its length.
- When in the lateral image the contrast-enhanced esophagus is displaced posteriorly.[14]

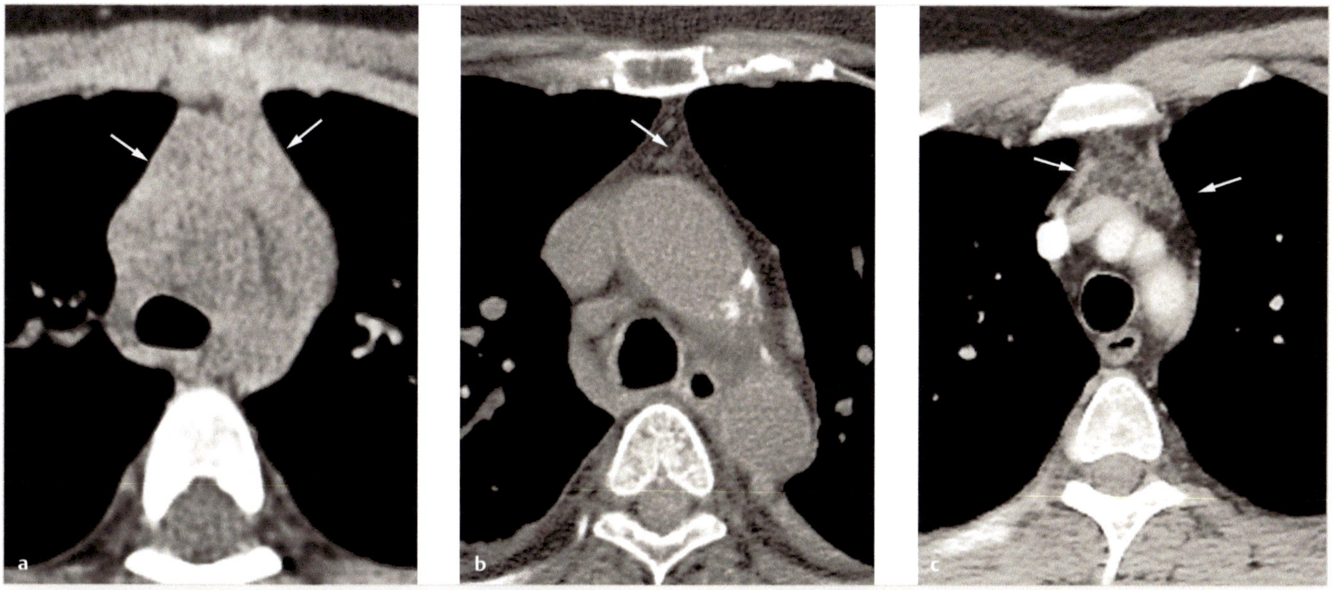

Fig. 2.12 Physiologic thymic involution. Widespread interindividual variability. **(a)** Thymus of 9-year-old boy: large, soft-tissue dense thymus (*arrows*). **(b)** Thymus of 14-year-old boy: extensive thymic involution (*arrow*). **(c)** Thymus of 18-year-old boy: still large fatty thymic remnants (*arrows*).

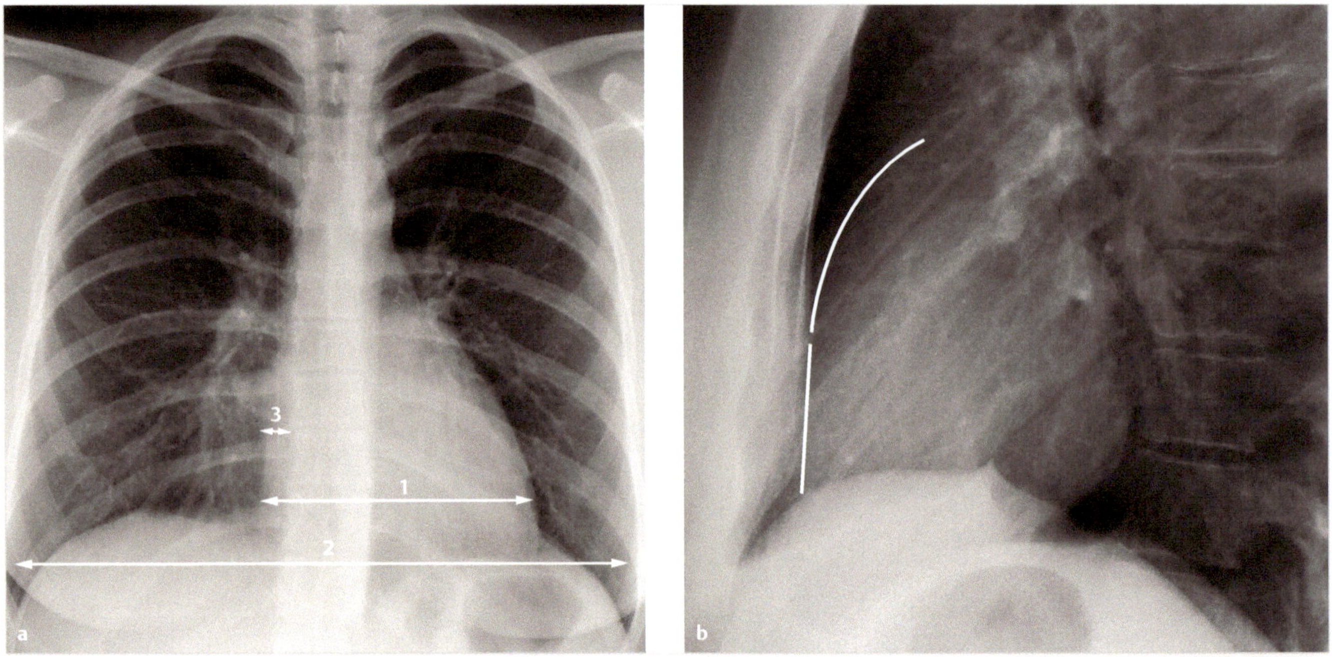

Fig. 2.13 Radiologic signs of heart enlargement on radiograph. (a) PA radiograph: cardiothoracic index (1/2), distance between the right border of heart from the thoracic spine (3). **(b)** Lateral image: sternal contact surface of heart.

Other radiologic signs, such as the vena cava triangle in the lateral image,[15] are poorly correlated with the size of the heart cavities.[14]

The pericardium is the sac, composed of rigid connective tissue, enclosing the heart. The inner mobile part consists of two serosal layers: the *visceral layer of pericardium*, surrounding the heart, and the *parietal layer of pericardium* fused with the pericardium (epicardium).

Normally, around 10-mL fluid is present in the intervening capillary space. The term *pericardial effusion* is used to denote a significant increase in that fluid amount.

The pericardium extends cranially to the aortic arch. Often, the superior pericardial reflection can be seen on CT anterior to the tracheal bifurcation. A small amount of *pericardial fluid* in this region should not be misinterpreted as lymphadenopathy (▸Fig. 2.14).

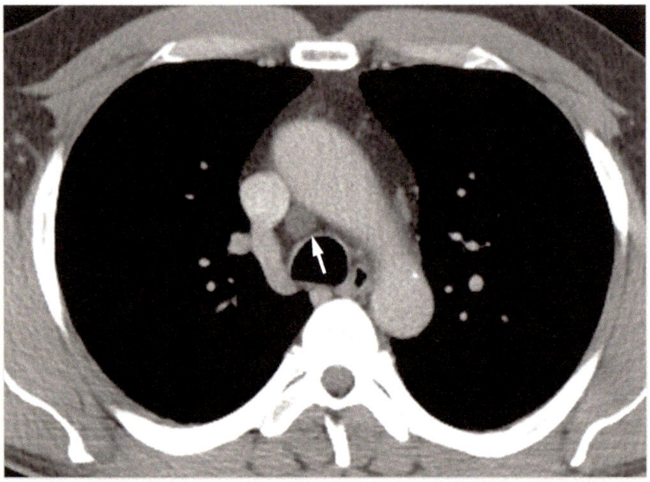

Fig. 2.14 Fluid in the superior pericardial reflection (*arrow*). CT image.

2.3 The Lung

2.3.1 Hilar Structures

The hilum of lung (plural: hila of lungs) is the indentation in the medial surface of the lung through which the systemic and pulmonary arteries and veins as well as the bronchi, lymph vessels, and nerves enter and exit the lung. In addition, several lymph nodes are present in this anatomic region. All these structures are shown on the radiograph.[2]

2.3.2 The Lobes and Segments of the Lung

Each lung is composed of lobes, the right of an upper, middle, and lower lobe, and the left of only an upper and lower lobe. Instead of a middle lobe, the caudal portion of the left upper lobe is formed by the lingula. The lobes are, often incompletely, covered with visceral pleura. Each lung lobe contains two to five segments (▸Table 2.3 and ▸Fig. 2.15). The left lung has two special features:

- Segments 1 and 2 of the left lung have a common bronchial origin; many classification systems list these as a single segment, the apicoposterior segment of the upper lobe (1/2). In practice, surgeons and bronchoscopists generally make a distinction between segments 1 and 2 despite their common origin.
- Segment 7 is usually absent in the left lung. Additional lung lobes may be found, in particular, in the right lung, mainly the right cranial *azygos vein lobe* (▸Fig. 2.16), and, less

Table 2.3 Lung segments

Number, right	Designation, right	Designation, left	Number, left
1R	Apical UL segment	Apicoposterior UL segment	1/2L
2R	Posterior UL segment		
3R	Anterior UL segment	Anterior UL segment	3L
4R	Lateral ML segment	Superior lingular segment	4L
5R	Medial ML segment	Inferior lingular segment	5L
6R	Apical LL segment	Apical LL segment	6L
7R	Mediobasal LL segment		
8R	Anterobasal LL segment	Anterobasal LL segment	8L
9R	Laterobasal LL segment	Laterobasal LL segment	9L
10R	Posterobasal LL segment	Posterobasal LL segment	10L

Abbreviations: LL, lower lobe; ML, middle lobe; UL upper lobe.

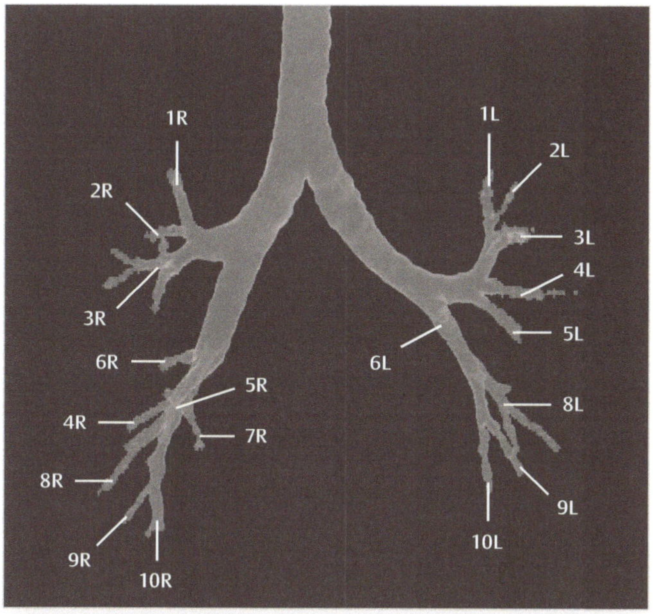

Fig. 2.15 Lung segments. CT image, VRT (volume rendering technique) of the bronchial system. For segment designations, see ▶Table 2.3.

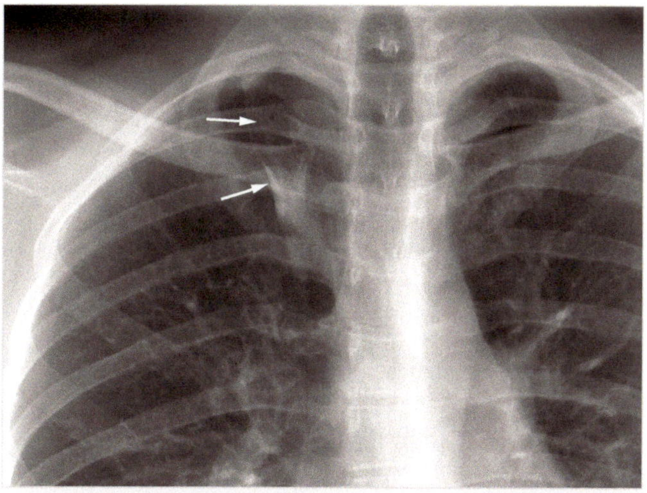

Fig. 2.16 Azygos vein lobe (*arrows*). Radiograph, magnified section.

commonly, the *cardiac lobe* situated in the right paracardiac region.

2.3.3 Connective Tissue Compartments

Weibel has described a model of the lung where the connective tissue is composed of three compartments (▶Fig. 2.17)[16]:

- The axial connective tissue encloses the bronchi and pulmonary arteries, has an arborized structure arising from the hilum, and comprises two components: The central peribronchovascular connective tissue extends peripherally into the centrilobular connective tissue.
- The peripheral connective tissue arises from the visceral pleura where it forms the subpleural connective tissue, from which the interlobular septa continue into the lung, giving rise to the soft tissue "container" of the lobules.
- Within the lobule, the centrilobular and peripheral connective tissue merges with the intralobular connective tissue, which is a fine network of connective tissue fibers in the alveolar walls.

2.3.4 The Lobule

The lobule, also referred to as the secondary pulmonary lobule,[2] is a polygonal structure with an edge length of around 1 to 2 cm, and is the smallest structural unit of the lung enclosed in connective tissue. It is the lobules that confer this apparent polygonal pattern on the lung surface. The bronchiole and associated pulmonary artery are located at the center of each lobule. Pulmonary veins and lymph vessels are embedded in the interlobular septa at the periphery of the lobule (▶Fig. 2.18).[17]

Despite its high spatial resolution, high-resolution CT (HRCT) is unable to visualize thin structures measuring around 100 µm. By contrast, structures with a diameter of around 0.5 mm are routinely demonstrated. As such, the bronchiolar wall and interlobular septum cannot be visualized on HRCT, unlike the pulmonary arteries, at the center, and the veins at

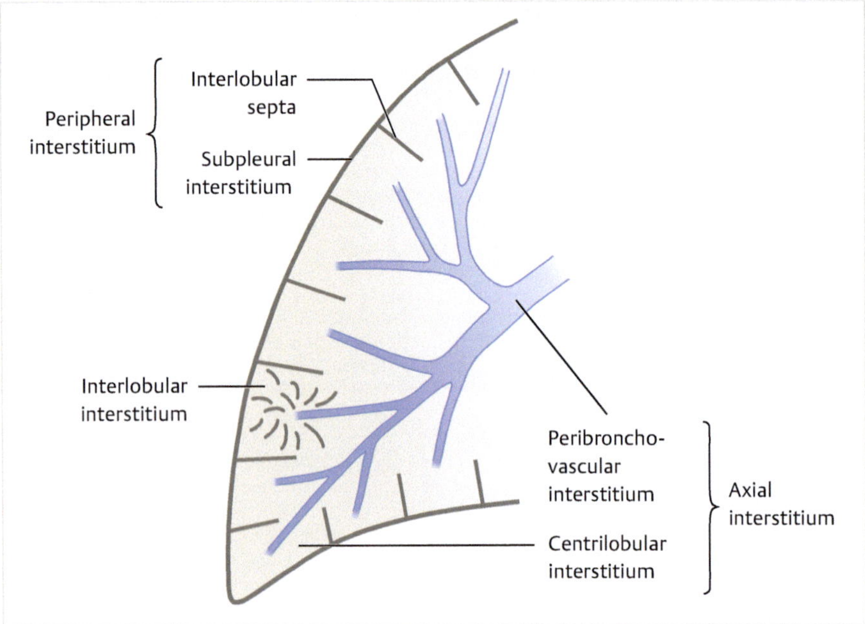

Fig. 2.17 Pulmonary connective tissue compartments after Weibel. Schematic diagram.

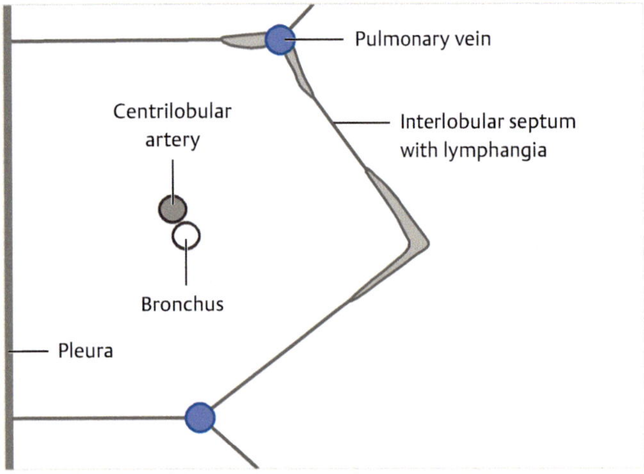

Fig. 2.18 Lung lobule. Schematic diagram.

the periphery of the lobule. If interlobular septa are identifiable on HRCT, this is generally because of pathologic thickening as seen, for example, in interstitial pulmonary edema. An exception to that rule is the anterior portion of the lower lobes (especially segment 8), of the middle lobe, and lingula in which isolated interlobular septa can be recognized, even in healthy people.[18]

2.4 The Pleura

Two pleural layers, the parietal and the visceral pleura, line the chest cavity. They form a serous membrane and a mobile layer that covers the lungs versus the chest wall. In the region of the hila of lungs, the parietal pleura merges with the viscera pleura. The parietal pleura consists of three parts: the costal, diaphragmatic, and mediastinal pleura. Each has a separate lymph drainage system; this determines the typical localization of lymph node metastases originating from malignant tumors of the pleura (▸Table 2.4).[19] Conversely, the visceral pleura drain together with the lung parenchyma into the hilar and mediastinal lymph nodes.

Table 2.4 Lymph drainage system of the parietal pleura[19]

Regions	Lymph drainage system
Costal parietal pleura	Intercostal lymph nodes, in cranially located pathologies also axillary lymph nodes
Diaphragmatic parietal pleura	Phrenic lymph nodes
Mediastinal parietal pleura	Parasternal lymph nodes

2.5 The Diaphragm

The diaphragm serves as a caudal barrier for the chest cavity and is the most important respiratory muscle. Normally, the diaphragm is situated one thoracic vertebra higher on the right compared with the left. Viewed on radiographs in deep inspiration, it projects on the right at the level of the 11th thoracic vertebra, on the left at the level of the 12th thoracic vertebra. A bilateral high-riding diaphragm is observed in obese patients because of their physical constitution. This must be differentiated from diaphragmatic paresis, which also causes a high-riding diaphragm. Section 13.4 describes functional disorders of the diaphragm.[20]

References

[1] Fraser RS, Paré PD. Fraser and Paré's Diagnosis of Diseases of the Chest. 4th ed. Philadelphia, PA: W.B. Saunders; 1999

[2] Hansell DM, Bankier AA, MacMahon H, McLoud TC, Müller NL, Remy J. Fleischner Society: glossary of terms for thoracic imaging. Radiology 2008;246(3):697–722

[3] Posniak HV, Olson MC, Demos TC, Benjoya RA, Marsan RE. CT of thoracic aortic aneurysms. Radiographics 1990;10(5):839–855

[4] Leonhardt H, Rauber A, Kopsch F. Anatomie des Menschen: Textbuch und Atlas. Stuttgart: Thieme; 1987/1988

[5] Tahir E, Karul M, Yamamura J. Persistent left superior vena cava with connection to the left superior lung vein: imaging and clinical implications RoFo Fortschr Geb Rontgenstr Nuklearmed 2014;186(11):1037–1038

[6] Rusch VW, Asamura H, Watanabe H, Giroux DJ, Rami-Porta R, Goldstraw P; Members of IASLC Staging Committee. The IASLC lung cancer staging project: a proposal for a new international lymph node map in the forthcoming seventh edition of the TNM classification for lung cancer. J Thorac Oncol 2009;4(5):568–577

[7] Moore AV, Korobkin M, Olanow W, et al. Age-related changes in the thymus gland: CT-pathologic correlation. AJR Am J Roentgenol 1983;141(2):241–246

[8] Nishino M, Ashiku SK, Kocher ON, Thurer RL, Boiselle PM, Hatabu H. The thymus: a comprehensive review. Radiographics 2006;26(2):335–348

[9] Baron RL, Lee JK, Sagel SS, Peterson RR. Computed tomography of the normal thymus. Radiology 1982;142(1):121–125

[10] de Geer G, Webb WR, Gamsu G. Normal thymus: assessment with MR and CT. Radiology 1986;158(2):313–317

[11] Schittenhelm A. Textbuch der Röntgendiagnostik. Berlin: Julius Springer; 1924

[12] Browne RFJ, O'Reilly G, McInerney D. Extraction of the two-dimensional cardiothoracic ratio from digital PA chest radiographs: correlation with cardiac function and the traditional cardiothoracic ratio. J Digit Imaging 2004;17(2):120–123

[13] Danzer C. The cardiothoracic ratio: an index of cardiac enlargement. Am J Med Sci 1919;157:513–521

[14] Glover L, Baxley WA, Dodge HT. A quantitative evaluation of heart size measurements from chest roentgenograms. Circulation 1973;47(6):1289–1296

[15] Keats TE, Rudhe U, Foo GW. Inferior vena caval position in the differential diagnosis of atrial and ventricular septal defects. Radiology 1964;83:616–621

[16] Weibel ER. Fleischner Lecture. Looking into the lung: what can it tell us? AJR Am J Roentgenol 1979;133(6):1021–1031

[17] Reuter M, Biederer J. Identification of lung architecture using HRCT [in German] Radiologe 2009;49(2):159–172

[18] Zerhouni E. Computed tomography of the pulmonary parenchyma. An overview. Chest 1989;95(4):901–907

[19] Jeong YJ, Kim S, Kwak SW, et al. Neoplastic and nonneoplastic conditions of serosal membrane origin: CT findings. Radiographics 2008;28(3):801–817, discussion 817–818, quiz 912

[20] Nason LK, Walker CM, McNeeley MF, Burivong W, Fligner CL, Godwin JD. Imaging of the diaphragm: anatomy and function. Radiographics 2012;32(2):E51–E70

Chapter 3

General Symptomatology

3 General Symptomatology

3.1 Projection Radiography

3.1.1 Generic Signs

The Fleischner Society has incorporated a number of generally accepted radiologic signs into its *Glossary of Terms for Thoracic Imaging* (see Chapter 25). Examples of these signs include the following:

- Air bronchogram.
- Air crescent sign.
- Silhouette sign.

Knowledge of other general signs not featured in the glossary can at times be useful in radiologic differential diagnosis, e.g.[1]:

- *Cervicothoracic sign*: An intrathoracic mass whose cranial border is seen to project on posteroanterior (PA) radiographs superior to the clavicles must be located dorsally since the posterior portions of the lung apices extend farther cranially than their anterior counterparts.
- *Extrapleural sign*: A mass arising from the chest wall, pleura or mediastinum which on a radiograph exhibits a blurred, ill-defined border with tapered margins and an obtuse angle, whereas an intrapulmonary lesion has a more defined border and acute angle. For more information, please consult Section 11.5 and ▶Fig. 11.9.
- *Gloved finger sign*: Dilated, mucoid-impacted bronchi that on radiographs manifest as gloved fingers. This sign is typically observed in allergic bronchopulmonary aspergillosis and mucoviscidosis. But it can also present concomitantly with myriad other diseases secondary to longstanding central bronchial obstruction.
- Golden S sign: This refers to the lateral bulging of a central tumor secondary to lobe atelectasis; see ▶Fig. 9.15. The resultant reverse S shape was initially used by R. Golden only to describe the external contour of the atelectatic area of the right upper lobe,[2] but this can also be applied to other lobes.
- Deep sulcus sign: This refers to the abnormal increase in radiolucency seen on supine radiographs, originating from a costophrenic angle (sulcus) and extending into the lateral portions of the adjacent upper abdominal quadrant. This sign is indicative of anterior pneumothorax.

3.1.2 Unilateral Changes in Radiolucency

There are several causes for increased or decreased radiolucent hemithorax. Important causes as well as tips on differential diagnosis are presented in ▶Table 3.1; two examples are illustrated in ▶Fig. 3.1 and ▶Fig. 3.2.

> **Note**
>
> For supine radiographs with antiscatter grid, one should first establish whether this is a genuine change in radiolucency or a grid artefact. That distinction can be made more easily through analysis of the axillary radiolucency: equal radiolucency of both axillae is suggestive of a genuine radiolucency change.

3.1.3 Atelectasis

The term *atelectasis* is used to denote hypoventilation of the lung parenchyma, often caused by bronchial obstruction. This and other causes are listed in ▶Table 3.2.

Table 3.1 Causes of unilateral changes in thoracic radiolucency on radiograph

Maximum decrease in unilateral radiolucency: "white-out hemithorax"	Large pleural effusion (see ▶Fig. 3.1)	Volume increase
	Total atelectasis (see ▶Fig. 3.2)	Volume reduction
	Pneumonectomy	Volume reduction, possibly surgical clips in mediastinum and hilum
Unilateral decrease in radiolucency	Pleural effusion (in particular, posterior on supine images)	Ultrasound
	Pneumonia	Inflammatory biomarkers
	Lung carcinoma	Volume increase
	Pleural carcinosis	Volume increase
	Pleural mesothelioma	Volume reduction
	Thoracoplasty	Calcifications, thoracic deformity
Unilateral increase in radiolucency	Congenital lobar emphysema	Massive hyperventilation of the deceased lung lobe
	Swyer–James syndrome	Vascular rarefaction
	Foreign body	Air trapping due to valve mechanism
	Central lung carcinoma	Rarely, air trapping due to valve mechanism, more commonly atelectasis

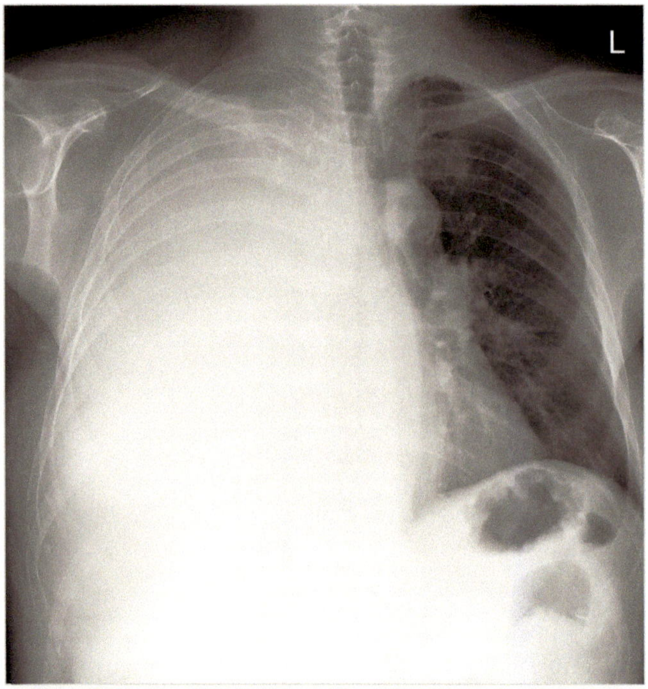

Fig. 3.1 Large right-sided pleural effusion. Radiograph. Mediastinal displacement to the left. Total compression atelectasis of the right lung.

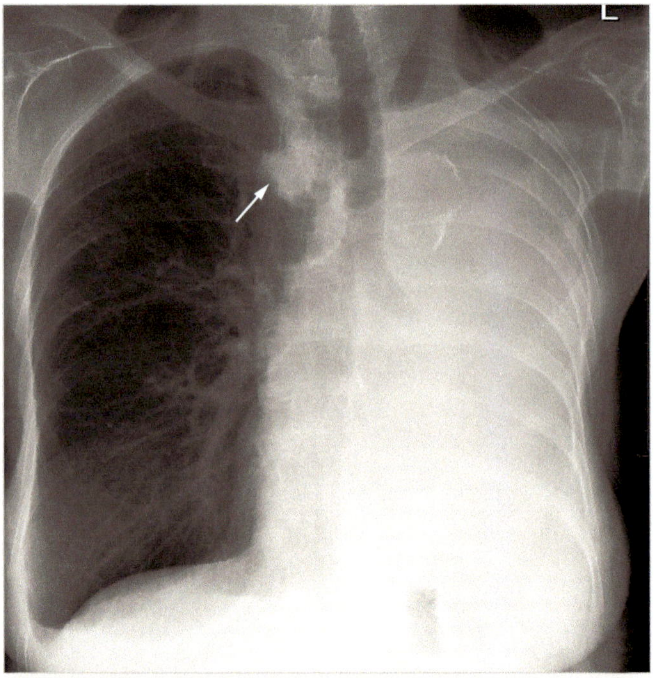

Fig. 3.2 Total atelectasis of the left lung secondary to central lung carcinoma. Radiograph. Lung metastasis in right upper lobe (*arrow*).

Table 3.2 Causes of atelectasis

Causes	Examples
Bronchial obstruction	Central tumor
	Inflammation (mucoid impaction)
	Foreign body
	Lymphadenopathy
Relaxation atelectasis	Pneumothorax (atelectasis secondary to intrinsic lung elasticity)
Compression atelectasis	Pleural effusion
	Large tumors of mediastinum, pleura and chest wall
	Diaphragmatic hernias
Surfactant deficiency	Adult respiratory distress syndrome

Atelectasis of an entire lung gives rise to the image of a "white-out hemithorax" (for differential diagnosis, see above). Atelectasis of individual lung lobes has a characteristic appearance specific to the implicated lobe:

- *Right upper lobe atelectasis* (▸Fig. 3.3): The right upper lobe collapses in a cranial and mediastinal direction. This, in turn, causes cranial displacement of the minor (horizontal) fissure, in particular, of the lateral portion. It also results in a high-riding diaphragm on the right. If atelectasis is caused by a central tumor, the tumor can at times be identified as bulging of the external contour of the atelectatic area, known as the Golden S sign.
- *Middle lobe atelectasis* (▸Fig. 3.4): The middle lobe collapses in an inferoposterior direction. On PA radiographs, this is seen as an upward directed, smoothly marginated opacity, whereas on lateral views it manifests as anterobasal triangular opacity.
- *Right lower lobe atelectasis* (▸Fig. 3.5): The right lower lobe collapses in a medioinferior direction. On PA radiographs, it causes right paracardiac and smoothly marginated lateral opacity. If this is misinterpreted as the right heart border, right-sided lower lobe atelectasis can be overlooked.

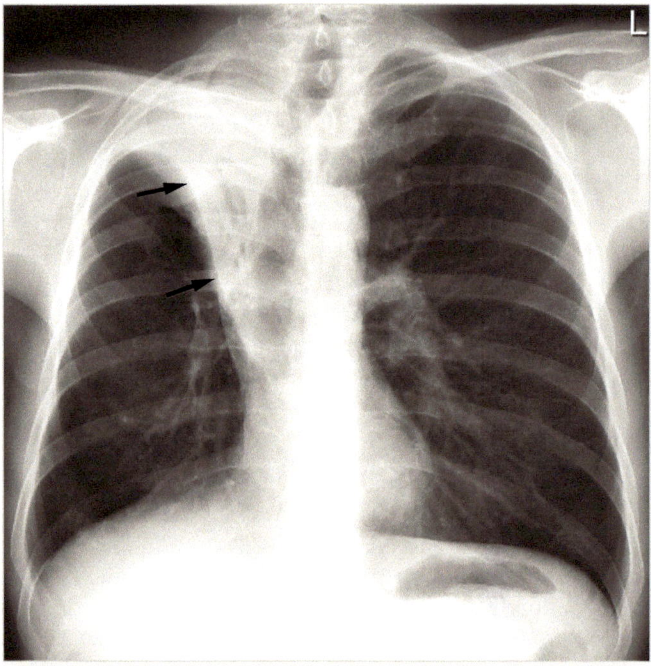

Fig. 3.3 Right upper lobe atelectasis. Radiograph. Atelectasis can be clearly identified on the PA radiograph (*arrows*).

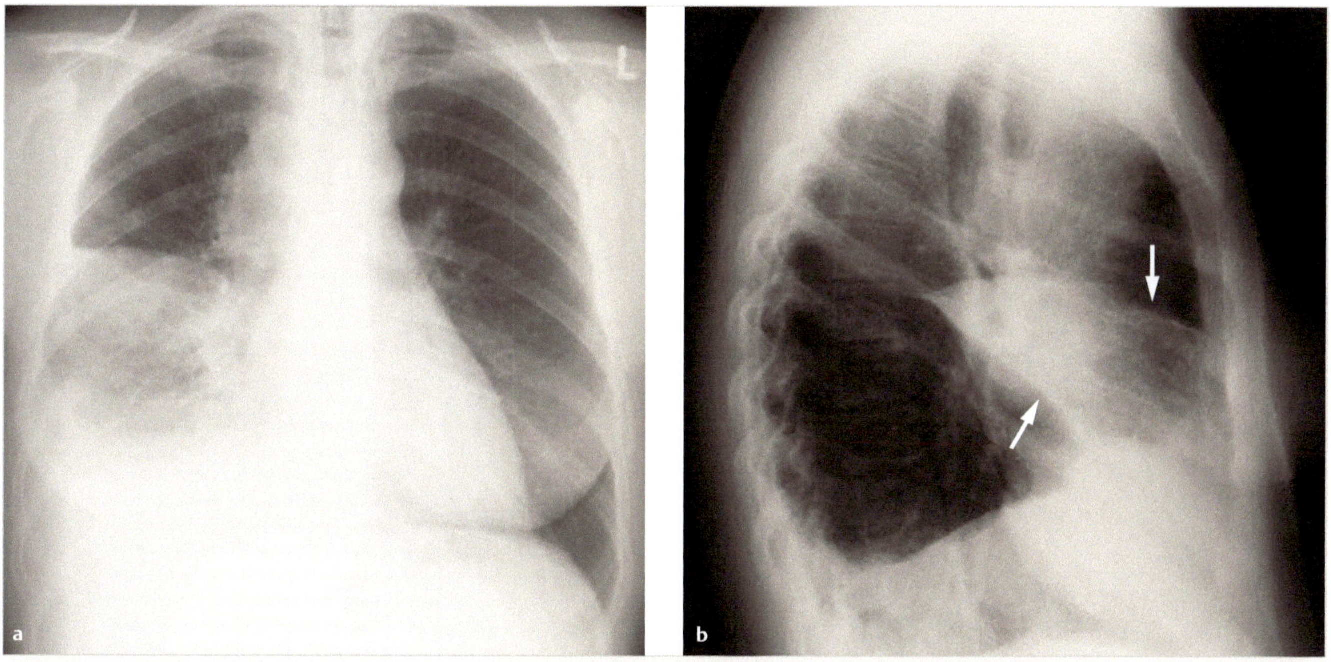

Fig. 3.4 **Middle lobe atelectasis.** Radiographs. Atelectasis can be clearly identified on the lateral view (**b,** *arrows*). **(a)** PA image. **(b)** Lateral view.

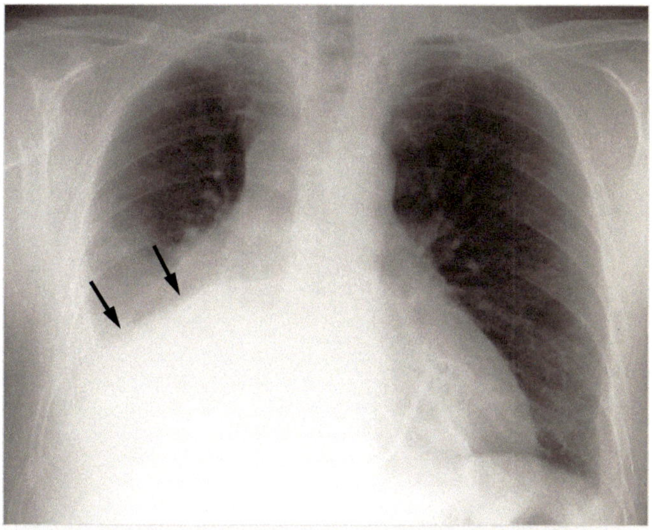

Fig. 3.5 **Right lower lobe atelectasis.** Radiograph. Atelectasis can be clearly seen on the PA radiograph (*arrows*).

- *Left upper lobe atelectasis* (▶ Fig. 3.6): The left upper lobe collapses in an anterosuperior direction. On PA radiographs, poorly marginated, paramediastinal opacity can be identified in the upper and middle fields. Upper lobe atelectasis is easier to diagnose on lateral views, where the compact opacity of the upper lobe can be seen before the anteriorly displaced fissure. Left-sided upper lobe atelectasis is often caused by malignant tumors.
- *Left lower lobe atelectasis* (▶ Fig. 3.7): The left lower lobe collapses medially, giving rise to paramediastinal triangular opacity in the retrocardiac region. Left lower lobe atelectasis is easily missed and misinterpreted as aortic elongation, especially on the supine radiographs of patients in the intensive care setting where it commonly presents.

3.2 Computed Tomography

3.2.1 Linear and Reticular Opacities

Linear and reticular opacities are caused by pathologic changes in the various connective tissue compartments:

- In the peripheral connective tissue: interlobular septal thickening.
- In the intralobular connective tissue: intralobular lines, honeycombing.
- In the axial connective tissue: thickening of the peribronchovascular connective tissue.

The reticular pattern is a collective term subsuming interlobular septal thickening, intralobular lines, and honeycombing.

Interlobular Septal Thickening

Isolated thickening of interlobular septa is seen, in particular, in hydrostatic pulmonary edema and lymphangitic carcinomatosis (▶ Fig. 3.8). Whereas *pulmonary edema* causes fluid displacement from the capillaries into the interstitium, in turn resulting in thickening of the interlobular septa, *lymphangitic carcinomatosis* leads to reduced lymph drainage of the lung parenchyma because of tumor thrombi in the lymphatic vessels.[3] Nodular thickening of the interlobular septa (*beaded septum sign*) can at times serve as a distinguishing criterion for lymphangitic carcinomatosis.

Interlobular septal thickening is also caused by numerous other diseases, for example, by usual interstitial pneumonia, sarcoidosis, pulmonary alveolar proteinosis, silicosis, and asbestosis as well as chronic extrinsic allergic alveolitis. In these diseases, the thickened interlobular septa are neither the most predominant nor the only patterns seen on imaging.

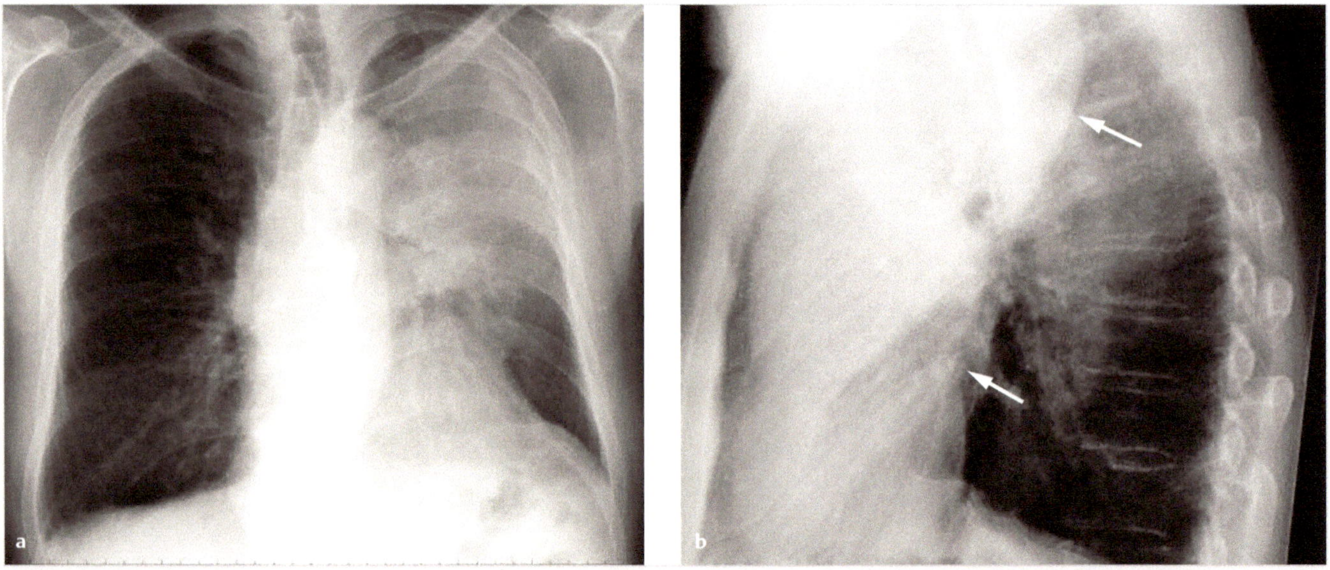

Fig. 3.6 **Left upper lobe atelectasis.** Radiographs. Atelectasis can be clearly identified on the lateral view. **(a)** On the PA radiograph, diffuse opacity of the left upper and middle fields. **(b)** Atelectasis is easier to identify on the lateral view (*arrows*).

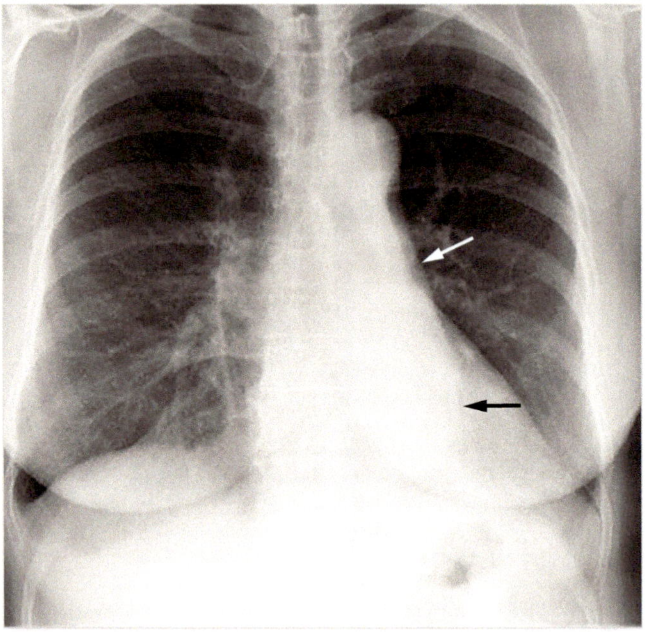

Fig. 3.7 **Left lower lobe atelectasis.** Radiograph. On the PA radiograph, apparent retrocardiac opacity (*arrows*).

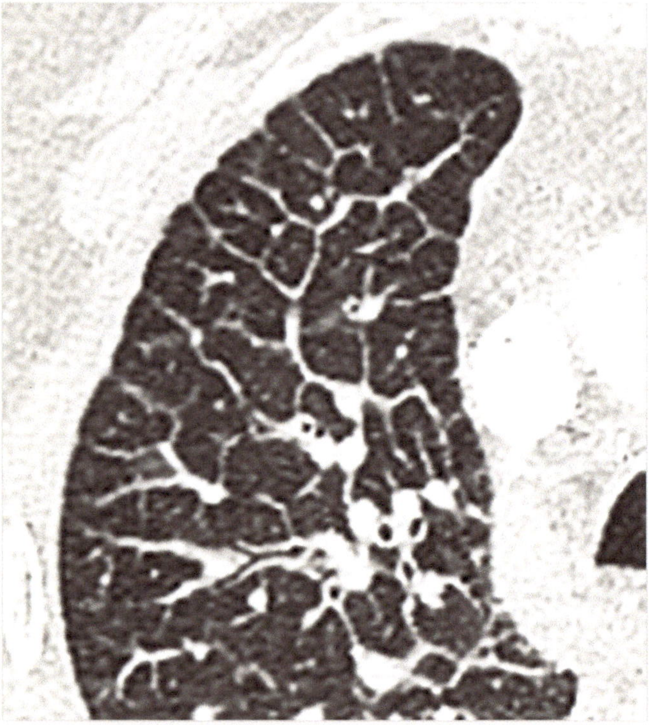

Fig. 3.8 **Interlobular septal thickening.** CT image.

Intralobular Lines

Thickening of the intralobular connective tissue is a characteristic feature of fibrotic lung diseases,[4,5] but is also observed in many other diseases. On CT, it manifests as a fine-meshed, reticular pattern (▶Fig. 3.9), bestowing a serrated appearance on the normally smooth interfaces between the lung parenchyma and vasculature or pleura (interface sign).

These findings are similar to those of honeycombing, which also has a reticular structure. In honeycombing, the network meshes are formed by the walls of air-containing cysts of very low opacity. Conversely, lung tissue of normal or increased opacity is found between the network meshes in the setting of intralobular lines.

Honeycombing

Honeycombing develops secondarily to cystic destruction of the lung parenchyma, mainly in the subpleural space. Its characteristic appearance derives from the polygonal subpleural opacities surrounding the cystically destroyed lung tissue. The resultant image is similar to that of a honeycomb (▶Fig. 3.10).

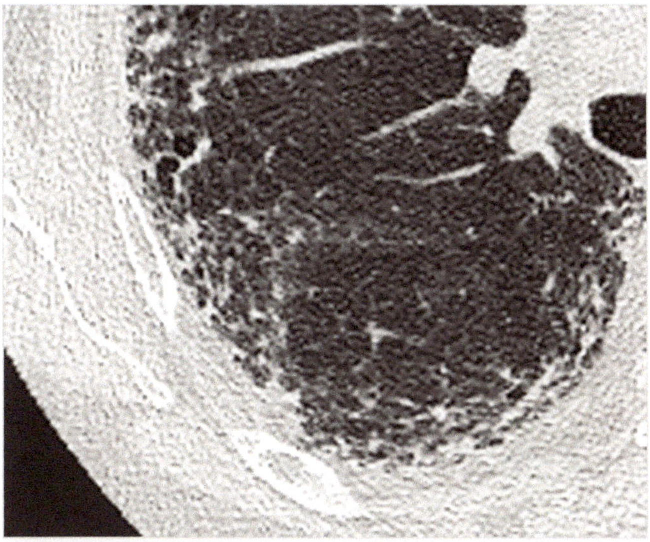

Fig. 3.9 **Intralobular lines.** CT image.

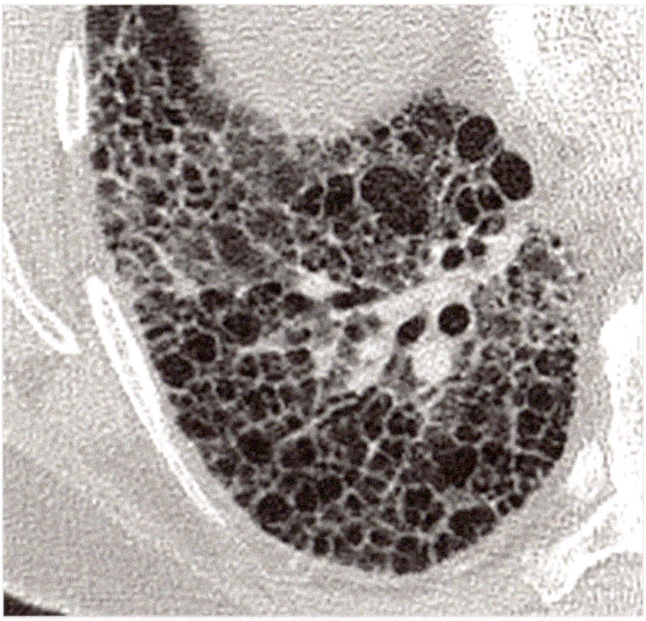

Fig. 3.10 **Honeycombing.** CT image.

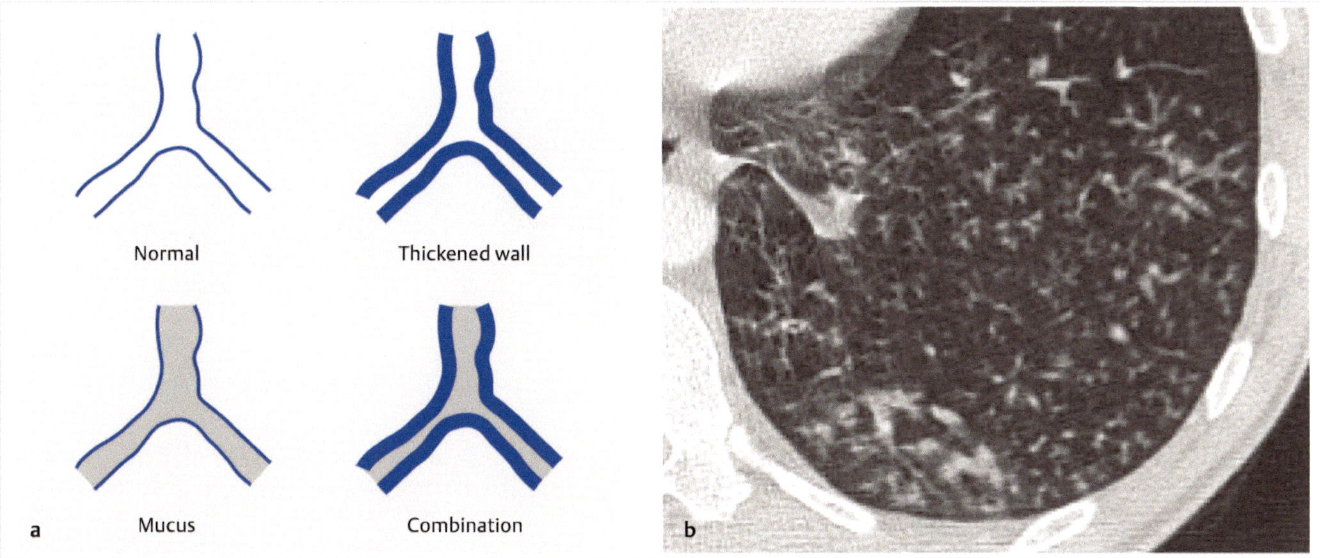

Fig. 3.11 **Tree-in-bud pattern. (a)** Schematic diagram of the small bronchi with wall thickening and mucoid impaction. **(b)** CT image with tree-in-bud pattern.

Unlike intralobular lines, honeycombing is not reversible on treatment.

Axial Connective Tissue

Thickening of the peribronchovascular connective tissue is caused by fluid collection, e.g., as seen in interstitial pulmonary edema, or by a pathologic process such as fibrosis or inflammation. Pathologic changes in the centrilobular connective tissue manifest as centrilobular nodules and as a tree-in-bud pattern.

The *tree-in-bud pattern* (▸Fig. 3.11) derives its name from the associated arborized structure of centrilobular opacities with discrete terminal thickening.[6] This pattern is due to thickening of the bronchial wall, fluid collection, e.g., with mucus, within the bronchial lumen, or a combination of both abnormalities. The tree-in-bud pattern is generally indicative of bronchiolitis. It is often seen in tuberculosis as a sign of disease activity but can also present in inactive tuberculosis and in other infections.[7]

3.2.2 Nodular Opacities

HRCT is ideal for differential diagnosis of nodular patterns since nodules can be identified in relation to the structures of the lobule.[8] Three types of multiple nodule distribution are distinguished (▸Fig. 3.12). Based on nodular morphology, a further distinction is made between interstitial and airspace nodules: interstitial nodules are small, sharply marginated opacities of soft-tissue density, whereas airspace nodules have an

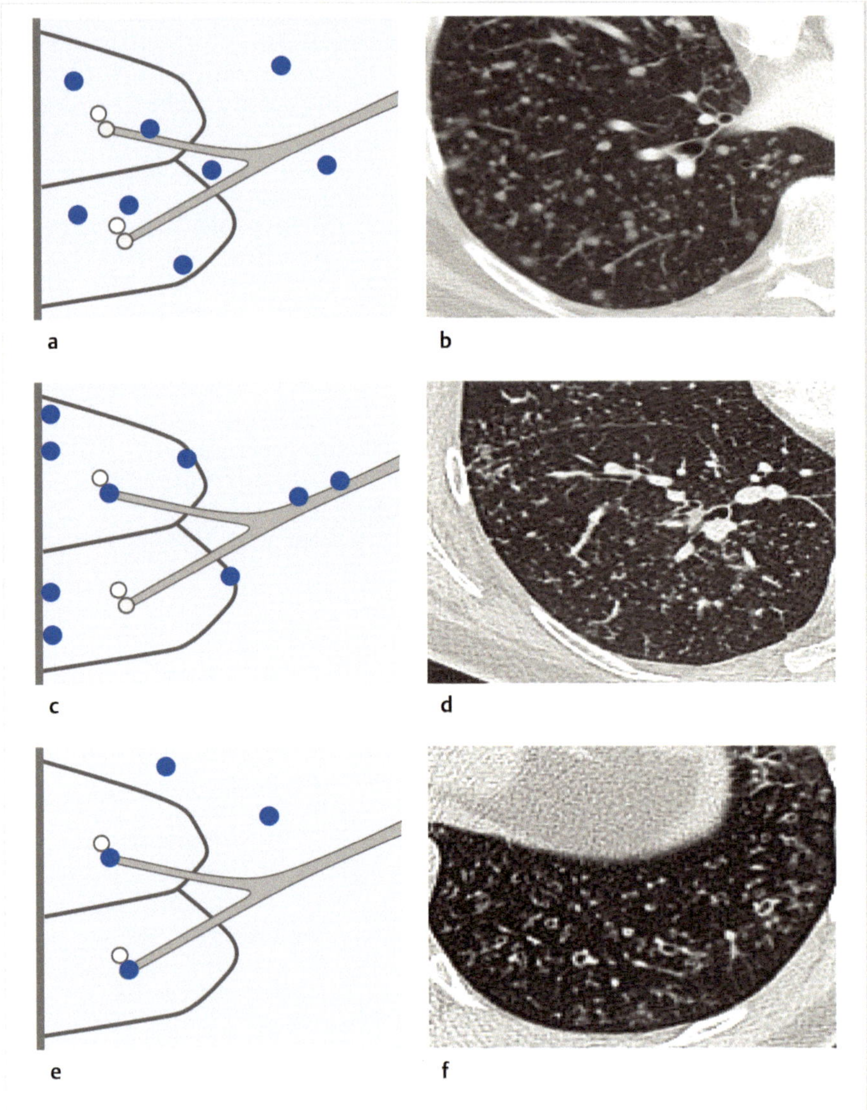

Fig. 3.12 Nodular pattern. (a) Random distribution (schematic diagram). **(b)** Random distribution (CT). **(c)** Perilymphatic distribution (schematic diagram). **(d)** Perilymphatic distribution (CT). **(e)** Centrilobular distribution (schematic diagram). **(f)** Centrilobular distribution (CT).

ill-defined margin and ground-glass opacity. That distinction can be useful, especially for centrilobular nodules.

Random Distribution

Random distribution is caused by disease processes that hematogenously spread to the lung. This is why the nodules are seen randomly distributed in the lung parenchyma. No correlation can be established between the individual nodules and the centrilobular structures or interlobular septa. Diseases typically implicated in hematogenous dissemination are miliary tuberculosis, certain types of fungal pneumonia (e.g., *Candida* pneumonia) and hematogenous lung metastases from tumors that tend to give rise to diffuse small nodular lung metastases.

Perilymphatic Distribution

This constellation of findings derives from intrapulmonary disease spread along the lymphatic vessels. At the lung periphery, nodules are seen in the interlobular septa and subpleural area, while in the lung core they are found in the peribronchovascular connective tissue. The extent of involvement of these locations varies according to the specific diseases. Perilymphatic distribution is the most common pulmonary manifestation in sarcoidosis and silicosis.[9] Lymphangitic carcinomatosis, too, exhibits perilymphatic distribution but this is more widespread than in the other two diseases and is also accompanied by interlobular septal thickening.

Centrilobular Distribution

Centrilobular distribution includes broader differential diagnosis compared with the two aforementioned distribution patterns[10] since many centrilobular structures may exhibit pathologic changes. The disease often originates in the bronchioles, less commonly in the vasculature or centrilobular connective tissue.

Centrilobular nodules are seen in association with bronchiolitis and bronchopneumonia but noninfectious diseases of the bronchioles also give rise to centrilobular nodules, e.g., cryptogenic organizing pneumonia and respiratory bronchiolitis.[11] Subacute extrinsic allergic alveolitis is accompanied by numerous centrilobular ground-glass nodules which, when seen together with extensive, mosaic-like or diffuse ground-glass opacity, produce quite a pathognomonic CT image (see ▶Fig. 7.7).[12] Vasculitis may also arise from the centrilobular arterioles. Likewise, tumors, especially lepidic adenocarcinomas, give rise to centrilobular nodules.

Clinical data and other concomitant image patterns seen on HRCT help streamline differential diagnosis or even arrive at a specific diagnosis.

3.2.3 Increased Lung Opacity

Increased lung opacity is caused by infiltrative changes in the lung parenchyma.[13] These may be of inflammatory (e.g., pneumonia) or tumorous genesis (e.g., adenocarcinoma). Infiltrates are differentiated into consolidation and ground-glass opacity:

- *Consolidation*: This refers to pathologic changes in the lung parenchyma which completely replace the alveolar air with inflammatory or tumorous infiltrates. On HRCT, the normal lung architecture can no longer be delineated from these pathologic changes. Consolidation is always caused by an alveolar pathologic process.
- *Ground-glass opacity*: This presents a more ambiguous differential diagnostic spectrum. While parenchymal opacity of the implicated lung areas is increased, the magnitude of the increase is not such that the lung architecture is obscured. The pulmonary vessels can still be identified within the areas of ground-glass opacity. Ground-glass opacity may be caused by an alveolar process which, like consolidation, displaces air from the alveolar spaces. Notwithstanding, at microscopic level aerated alveoli are seen adjacent to areas of consolidation. The etiologic spectrum of implicated conditions ranges from wallpaper-like (lepidic) tumor growth along the alveolar walls (e.g., in adenocarcinoma) through pneumonia-associated infiltrates to pulmonary hemorrhage with partial filling of the alveolar spaces. Alternatively, ground-glass opacity may have its origin in an interstitial process causing connective tissue hypertrophy at microscopic level, in turn resulting in increased parenchymal lung opacity. This involves a florid process as seen in interstitial pneumonia or interalveolar septal fibrosis.

Note

In general, ground-glass opacity is viewed as a florid process that is in principle reversible. However, it can also be caused by irreversible interalveolar septal fibrosis.[14]

3.2.4 Decreased Lung Opacity

Decreased lung opacity occurs in settings of reversible and irreversible hyperventilation of the lung parenchyma, in particular in obstructive lung diseases. In *acute bronchial asthma*, diffuse decreased parenchymal lung opacity can be observed secondary to reversible hyperventilation of the lung.

In *pulmonary emphysema*, the characteristic morphology can be identified on CT depending on the nature of emphysema:

- In *centrilobular emphysema*, well-defined rounded, centrilobular areas of decreased lung opacity can be identified.
- In *paraseptal emphysema*, more or fewer large bullae are seen on the surface of the lungs.
- Diagnosis of *panlobular pulmonary emphysema* may be a challenge. Diffuse decreased lung opacity is observed on HRCT but this is much less conspicuous than in the case of other types of emphysema.

Even in patients with severe functional impairment, it may not be possible to find hardly any evidence of the corresponding morphology on CT.

Following lung and bone marrow transplantation, *bronchiolitis obliterans* is of major clinical importance, leading to chronic rejection after lung transplant or manifesting as graft versus host disease (GvHD) after stem cell transplant. In both cases, diffuse decreased parenchymal opacity is seen in the lung areas concerned.[15]

3.2.5 Cysts

Cystic lung diseases are relatively rare. There are two important entities giving rise to the typical constellation of findings seen on HRCT[16]:

- Detection of closely approximated small nodules and cysts in a young patient or older smoker is suggestive of *Langerhans cell histiocytosis*.[17]
- Only women of reproducible age very occasionally experience diffuse cystic destruction of the lung parenchyma, suggestive of lymphangioleiomyomatosis.

3.2.6 Radiologic Signs of Fibrosis

Fibrotic tissue remodeling leads to cystic destruction of the lung parenchyma, in particular, in the subpleural space. On radiology, this manifests as honeycombing. In addition, shrinkage of the diseased lung areas triggers traction phenomena in adjacent structures, such as traction bronchiectasis and traction bronchiolectasis. The architecture of the entire lung undergoes fibrotic changes, causing displacement of the interlobar fissures and bundled-like bronchial structures. These traction phenomena are seen as a reliable radiologic sign of fibrosis, implying irreversible fibrotic lung destruction. Other image patterns are essentially reversible.[18,19,20]

Note

Reliable signs of fibrosis on CT:

- Honeycombing.
- Traction bronchiectasis and traction bronchiolectasis.
- Displacement of lung fissures.
- Bundling of bronchial structures.

References

[1] Algın O, Gökalp G, Topal U. Signs in chest imaging. Diagn Interv Radiol 2011;17(1):18–29

[2] Golden R. The effect of bronchostenosis upon the roentgen ray shadow in carcinoma of the bronchus. AJR Am J Roentgenol 1925;13:21–30

[3] Rehbock B, Hieckel HG. Diagnostic imaging of pulmonary lymphangiosis carcinomatosis [in German] Radiologe 2004;44(5):465–471

[4] Gotway MB, Freemer MM, King TE Jr. Challenges in pulmonary fibrosis. 1: Use of high resolution CT scanning of the lung for the evaluation of patients with idiopathic interstitial pneumonias. Thorax 2007;62(6):546–553

[5] Souza CA, Müller NL, Flint J, Wright JL, Churg A. Idiopathic pulmonary fibrosis: spectrum of high-resolution CT findings. AJR Am J Roentgenol 2005;185(6):1531–1539

[6] Waitches GM, Stern EJ. High-resolution CT of peripheral airways diseases. Radiol Clin North Am 2002;40(1):21–29

[7] Lee KS, Hwang JW, Chung MP, Kim H, Kwon OJ. Utility of CT in the evaluation of pulmonary tuberculosis in patients without AIDS. Chest 1996;110(4):977–984

[8] Patti A, Tognini G, Spaggiari E, Bnà C, Zompatori M. Diffuse, micronodular lung disease. The high-resolution CT approach. A pictorial essay [in Italian] Radiol Med (Torino) 2004;107(3):139–144

[9] Lynch JP III, Kazerooni EA, Gay SE. Pulmonary sarcoidosis. Clin Chest Med 1997;18(4):755–785

[10] Sharma V, Shaaban AM, Berges G, Gosselin M. The radiological spectrum of small-airway diseases. Semin Ultrasound CT MR 2002;23(4):339–351

[11] Marten K. Smoking-related interstitial lung diseases [in German] RoFo Fortschr Geb Rontgenstr Nuklearmed 2007;179(3):268–275

[12] Glazer CS, Rose CS, Lynch DA. Clinical and radiologic manifestations of hypersensitivity pneumonitis. J Thorac Imaging 2002;17(4):261–272

[13] Lee KS, Kim EA. High-resolution CT of alveolar filling disorders. Radiol Clin North Am 2001;39(6):1211–1230

[14] Nowers K, Rasband JD, Berges G, Gosselin M. Approach to ground-glass opacification of the lung. Semin Ultrasound CT MR 2002;23(4):302–323

[15] Chan A, Allen R. Bronchiolitis obliterans: an update. Curr Opin Pulm Med 2004;10(2):133–141

[16] Hartman TE. CT of cystic diseases of the lung. Radiol Clin North Am 2001;39(6):1231–1244

[17] Tazi A. Adult pulmonary Langerhans' cell histiocytosis. Eur Respir J 2006;27(6):1272–1285

[18] Ellis SM, Hansell DM. Idiopathic interstitial pneumonias: imaging-pathology correlation. Eur Radiol 2002;12(3):610–626

[19] Pipavath S, Godwin JD. Imaging of interstitial lung disease. Clin Chest Med 2004;25(3):455–465, v-vi

[20] Raoof S, Raoof S, Naidich DP. Imaging of unusual diffuse lung diseases. Curr Opin Pulm Med 2004;10(5):383–389

Chapter 4

Indications

4 Indications

This chapter summarizes fundamental indications for diagnostic radiologic imaging for various diseases. The indications listed in the following tables are intended as a guide and are not a substitute for individual assessment of an appropriate diagnostic test in a specific case (▶Table 4.1, ▶Table 4.2, ▶Table 4.3).[1–20]

Table 4.1 Indications for radiography of the chest organs

Examinations	Indications/contraindications
Primary examination	• Asthma—controversial: for primary diagnosis, on hospital admission, before mechanical ventilation, if poor response to treatment • Clinically suspected pneumonia or tuberculosis • Hemoptysis • Suspected diffuse parenchymal lung disease • Dyspnea • Chronic cough • Chronic obstructive lung disease: for primary diagnosis or if change in symptoms • Suspected occupational lung disease (silicosis, coal workers' pneumoconiosis, asbestosis) • Hemodynamically unstable polytrauma • Screening for pulmonary metastases in patients with extrathoracic malignancy • Intensive care patient: • Admission to intensive care unit • Deterioration of clinical condition • After placement of catheters or chest tubes • Possibly, after chest tube removal • Preoperatively: • Advanced age (particularly >70 years) • Increased risk (patient- or procedure-related)
Not indicated	• Suspected pulmonary embolism (primary CTA) • Routine diagnosis in intensive care unit in stable clinical condition

Abbreviation: CTA, computed tomography angiography.

Table 4.2 Indications for CT of the chest organs

Examinations	Indications/contraindications
Primary examination	• Suspected pulmonary embolism • Hemodynamically stable polytrauma • Suspected acute aortic syndrome
Follow-up examination	• Pneumonia: – For progressive pneumonia – For delayed response to treatment – For lung abscess – For immunosuppressed patients und suspected opportunistic infection • For suspected tuberculosis if chest radiography is equivocal • Differential diagnosis of diffuse parenchymal lung disease • Suspected thoracic tumor, staging thoracic tumors • Chronic obstructive lung disease: diagnosis of pulmonary emphysema, suspected bronchiectasis • Hemoptysis • Pleural effusion of unknown origin • Recurrent spontaneous pneumothorax • Pulmonary hypertension • Suspected occupational lung disease (silicosis, coal workers' pneumoconiosis, asbestosis) • Screening for pulmonary metastases in patients with extrathoracic malignancy • Atypical presentation of asthma
Not indicated	Uncomplicated community-acquired pneumonia

Table 4.3 Indications for other imaging modalities

Imaging modality	
Thoracic MRI	• Pancoast tumor (superior sulcus tumor) • Mediastinal tumor or mediastinal infiltration by lung carcinoma • Diseases of the chest wall • Suspected pulmonary embolism in pregnant women or if CT contrast agent is contraindicated • Follow-up of mucoviscidosis
Thoracic ultrasound	• Diseases of the chest wall • Pleural fluid collections • Pulmonary diseases originating in the pleura
PET-CT	• Staging thoracic tumors • Differential diagnosis of pulmonary nodule • Restaging of lymphomas in certain clinical settings • Primary diagnostic exploration of CUP syndrome

Abbreviations: CT, computed tomography; CUP, cancer of unknown primary; MRI, magnetic resonance imaging; PET-CT, positron emission tomography/computed tomography.

References

[1] American College of Radiology. ACR Appropriateness Criteria: acute respiratory illness in immunocompetent patients. Available at: https://acsearch.acr.org/docs/69446/Narrative/. Accessed November 9, 2017

[2] American College of Radiology. ACR Appropriateness Criteria: acute respiratory illness in immunocompromised patients. Available at: https://acsearch.acr.org/docs/69447/Narrative/. Accessed November 10, 2017

[3] American College of Radiology. ACR Appropriateness Criteria: blunt chest trauma. Available at: https://acsearch.acr.org/docs/3082590/Narrative/. Accessed November 10, 2017

[4] American College of Radiology. ACR Appropriateness Criteria: imaging of possible tuberculosis. Available at: https://acsearch.acr.org/docs/3099187/Narrative/. Accessed November 10, 2017

[5] American College of Radiology. ACR appropriateness criteria: non-invasive clinical staging of bronchogenic carcinoma. Available at: https://acsearch.acr.org/docs/69456/Narrative/. Accessed November 10, 2017

[6] American College of Radiology. ACR Appropriateness Criteria: nontraumatic aortic disease. Available at: https://acsearch.acr.org/docs/3082597/Narrative/. Accessed November 10, 2017

[7] American College of Radiology. ACR Appropriateness Criteria: occupational lung diseases. Available at: https://acsearch.acr.org/docs/3091680/Narrative/. Accessed November 10, 2017

[8] American College of Radiology. ACR Appropriateness Criteria: radiographically detected solitary pulmonary nodule. Available at: https://acsearch.acr.org/docs/69455/Narrative/. Accessed November 10, 2017

[9] American College of Radiology. ACR Appropriateness Criteria: routine chest radiography. Available at: https://acsearch.acr.org/docs/69451/Narrative/. Accessed November 10, 2017

[10] American College of Radiology. ACR Appropriateness Criteria: screening for pulmonary metastases. Available at: https://acsearch.acr.org/docs/69454/Narrative/. Accessed November 10, 2017

[11] American College of Radiology. ACR Appropriateness Criteria: suspected pulmonary hypertension. Available at: https://acsearch.acr.org/docs/71095/Narrative/. Accessed November 10, 2017

[12] American College of Radiology. ACR Appropriateness Criteria: chronic dyspnea-suspected pulmonary origin. Available at: https://acsearch.acr.org/docs/69448/Narrative/. Accessed November 10, 2017

[13] American College of Radiology. ACR Appropriateness Criteria: intensive care unit patients. Available at: https://acsearch.acr.org/docs/69452/Narrative/. Accessed November 10, 2017

[14] Chung KF, Wenzel SE, Brozek JL, et al. International ERS/ATS guidelines on definition, evaluation and treatment of severe asthma. Eur Respir J 2014;43(2):343–373

[15] Galiè N, Humbert M, Vachiery J-L, et al. 2015 ESC/ERS Guidelines for the diagnosis and treatment of pulmonary hypertension: The Joint Task Force for the Diagnosis and Treatment of Pulmonary Hypertension of the European Society of Cardiology (ESC) and the European Respiratory Society (ERS): Endorsed by: Association for European Paediatric and Congenital Cardiology (AEPC), International Society for Heart and Lung Transplantation (ISHLT). Eur Respir J 2015;46(4):903–975

[16] Konstantinides SV, Torbicki A, Agnelli G, et al; Task Force for the Diagnosis and Management of Acute Pulmonary Embolism of the European Society of Cardiology (ESC). 2014 ESC guidelines on the diagnosis and management of acute pulmonary embolism. Eur Heart J 2014;35(43):3033–3069, 3069a–3069k

[17] Mandell LA, Wunderink RG, Anzueto A, et al; Infectious Diseases Society of America. American Thoracic Society. Infectious Diseases Society of America/American Thoracic Society consensus guidelines on the management of community-acquired pneumonia in adults. Clin Infect Dis 2007;44(Suppl 2):S27–S72

[18] Galiè N, Humbert M, Vachiery JL, et al. ESC/ERS Guidelines for the diagnosis and treatment of pulmonary hypertension. Eur Respir J 2015;46(4):903–975

[19] National Institute for Health and Care Excellence (NICE). Lung Cancer: Diagnosis and Management [NG122]. London, March 2019

[20] Torres A, Niederman MS, Chastre J, et al. International ERS/ESICM/ESCMID/ALAT guidelines for the management of hospital-acquired pneumonia and ventilator-associated pneumonia: Guidelines for the management of hospital-acquired pneumonia (HAP)/ventilator-associated pneumonia (VAP) of the European Respiratory Society (ERS), European Society of Intensive Care Medicine (ESICM), European Society of Clinical Microbiology and Infectious Diseases (ESCMID) and Asociación Latinoamericana del Tórax (ALAT). Eur Respir J 2017;50(3):1700582

Part II

Diseases of the Chest and Special Findings

II

Chapter 5

Pneumonia

5 Pneumonia

> **Note**
>
> In pathology, the term *pneumonia* is used to denote any inflammatory reaction of the lung. In clinical terms, a distinction is made between microbially induced inflammation, i.e., pneumonia, and an inflammatory reaction caused by physical or chemical noxae, known as pneumonitis.

Like all inflammatory processes, when pneumonia resolves it either results in restoration to the original state (*restitutio ad integrum*) without any perceptible morphologic damage to the lung parenchyma or gives rise to impaired healing (*restitution cum defectu*). Radiologically, the latter manifests as *carnified pneumonia* in which the original lung tissue is replaced by nonfunctional scar tissue.

Several pathologic *types* are distinguished, each with its own specific radiologic correlate:

- *Alveolar pneumonia*: the inflammatory reaction is primarily confined to the airspaces and has three different manifestations:
  - Lobar pneumonia: one entire lung lobe is evenly affected, attesting to microbial spread via the bronchial system and pores of Kohn. Lobar pneumonia follows a sequence of congestion → red hepatization → gray hepatization → yellow hepatization → resolution. Extensive consolidation of the affected lobe of lung is seen radiologically (▶Fig. 5.1).
  - Bronchopneumonia: bronchogenic microbial spread results in inflammation of the peribronchial lung parenchyma, where there is less extensive spread than that seen in lobar pneumonia. This is the most common type of pneumonia. Imaging shows peribronchial ground-glass opacity and consolidation, which again are less extensive compared with lobar pneumonia. These opacities are not found throughout the entire lobe; often, they are seen simultaneously in several lobes (▶Fig. 5.2).
  - Focal pneumonia: this manifests as a local focus of inflammation that does not spread further within the lung parenchyma. Often, focal pneumonia is asymptomatic or oligosymptomatic, making it difficult on differential diagnosis to distinguish this from lung carcinoma since both conditions manifest as consolidation or focal ground-glass opacity (▶Fig. 5.3).

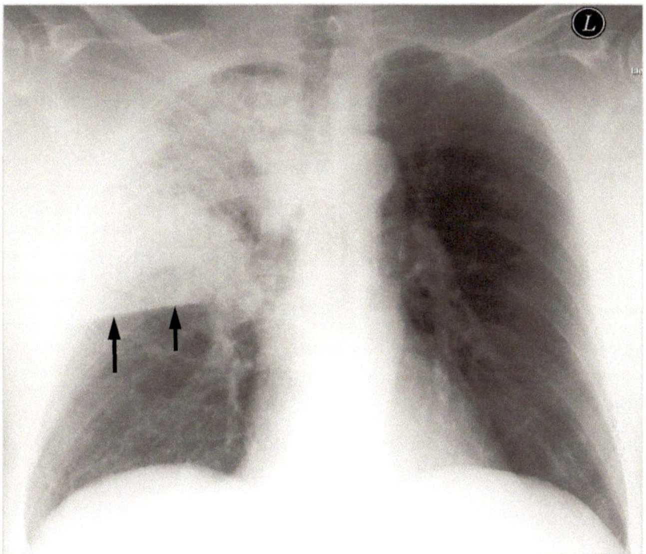

Fig. 5.1 Lobar pneumonia in the right upper lobe. Radiograph. The inferior margin of the consolidation is sharply bounded by the minor fissure (*arrows*); the middle lobe is not affected.

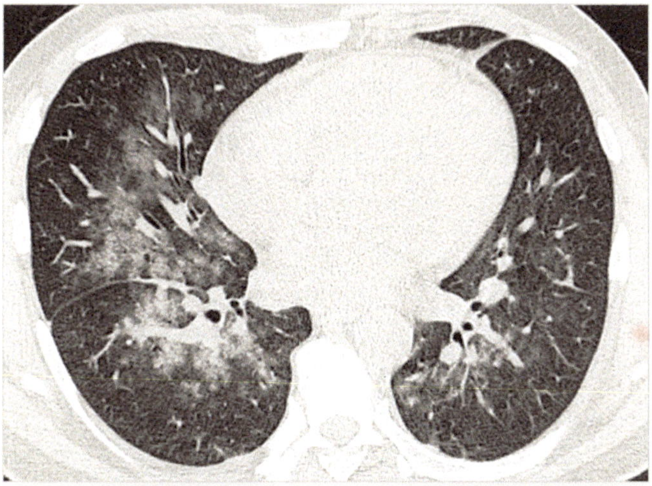

Fig. 5.2 Bronchopneumonia in the middle lobe and in both lower lobes. CT image.

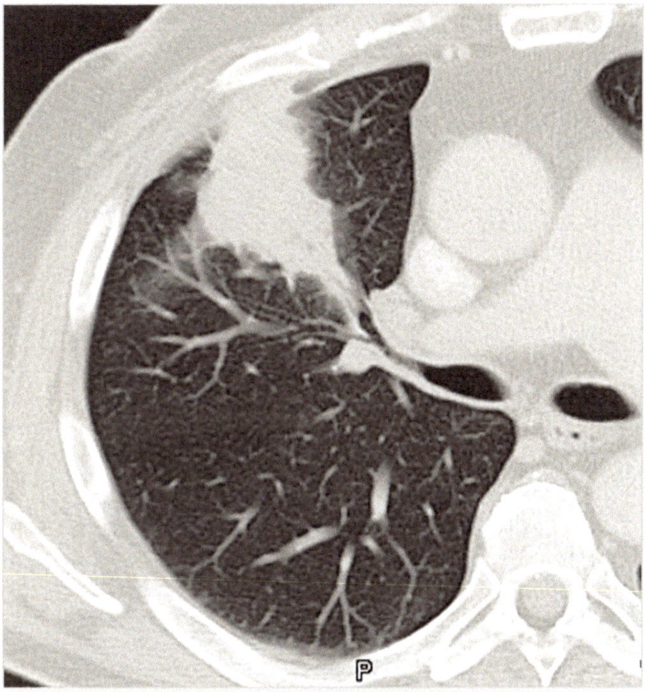

Fig. 5.3 Focal pneumonia in the right upper lobe. CT image.

- *Interstitial pneumonia*: the inflammatory reaction unfolds primarily in the lung interstitium, as characteristically observed for intracellular pathogens (e.g., viruses, chlamydiae). The predominant radiologic finding is ground-glass opacity (▶Fig. 5.4).

Depending on the number and virulence of the *pathogens* as well as on the patient's immunocompetence status, the very same pathogen can cause different types of pneumonia (e.g., pneumococci: lobar pneumonia or focal pneumonia). Conversely, various pathogens give rise to identical radiologic findings; e.g., bronchopneumonia can be caused by, for example, *Staphylococcus aureus*, *Klebsiella*, *Proteus*, or *Pseudomonas*. It is not possible radiologically to pinpoint the causative organism. However, in general, the type of microorganism implicated in pneumonia can be identified (bacteria, viruses, or fungi). On the basis of characteristic findings, the presence of mycobacteriosis or pneumocystis pneumonia may at least be suspected. From other typical imaging patterns, limited conclusions can be drawn on the suspected microbial spectrum (▶Table 5.1 and ▶Fig. 5.5, ▶Fig. 5.6, ▶Fig. 5.7, ▶Fig. 5.8, ▶Fig. 5.9, ▶Fig. 5.10).

Complications arising in association with pneumonia can result in delayed, or no, clinical improvement during antibiotic treatment or lead to relapse after initial successful treatment. The most common complications include:

- Pleural empyema: pleural empyema generally manifests as a rather large pleural effusion that is often multiloculated rather than free-flowing. It is not possible radiologically to make a reliable distinction between parapneumonic pleural empyema and noninfected, sympathetic pleural

Table 5.1 Characteristic findings in pneumonia and typical microbial spectrum[11]

Radiomorphology	Typical pathogens
Lobar consolidation (see ▶Fig. 5.1)	Mainly pneumococci
	Occasionally, *Klebsiella* (then often with increased volume of affected lung lobe)
	Staphylococcus aureus
	Legionella pneumophila
	Mycobacteria
Consolidation with cavitation (see ▶Fig. 5.5)	Staphylococcus aureus
	Gram-negative bacteria
	Klebsiella
	Proteus
	Pseudomonas
	Anaerobes
	Mycobacteria
	Small mycoplasma or viruses
Abscess (see ▶Fig. 5.6)	Mainly anaerobes
Focal pneumonia (see ▶Fig. 5.7)	Pneumococci
	Legionellae
	Coxiella burnetii
	As opportunistic infection: fungi
	Multiple nodules in hematogenous dissemination: *Staphylococcus aureus*
Reticulonodular pattern (see ▶Fig. 5.8)	Viruses
	Mycoplasma
Miliary pattern (see ▶Fig. 5.9)	Tuberculosis
	Candida pneumonia
Pneumatoceles/cysts (see ▶Fig. 5.10)	*Staphylococcus aureus*
	Pneumococci
	Klebsiella
	Pneumocystis jirovecii

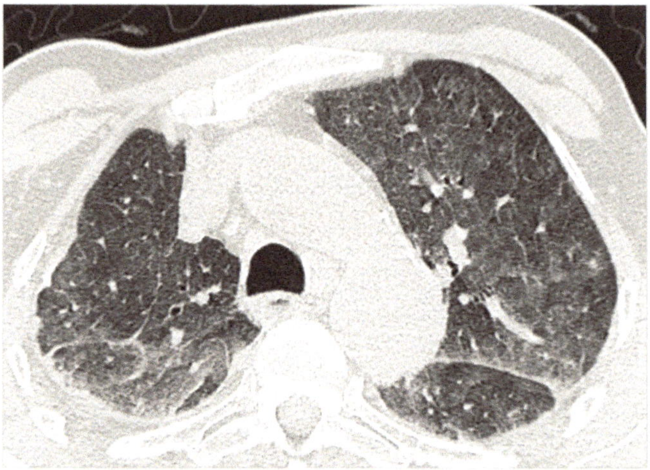

Fig. 5.4 Interstitial pneumonia. CT image. Diffuse, bilateral ground-glass opacity.

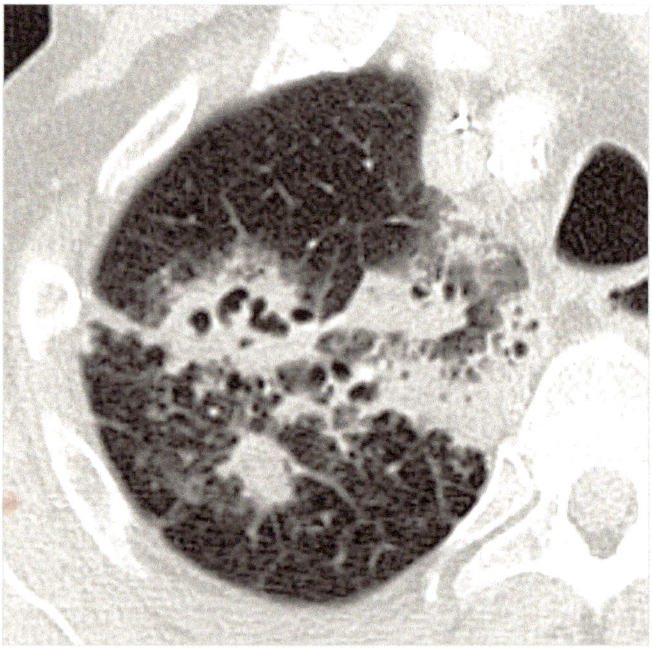

Fig. 5.5 Pneumonia in the right upper lobe. CT image. Central cavitation in consolidations.

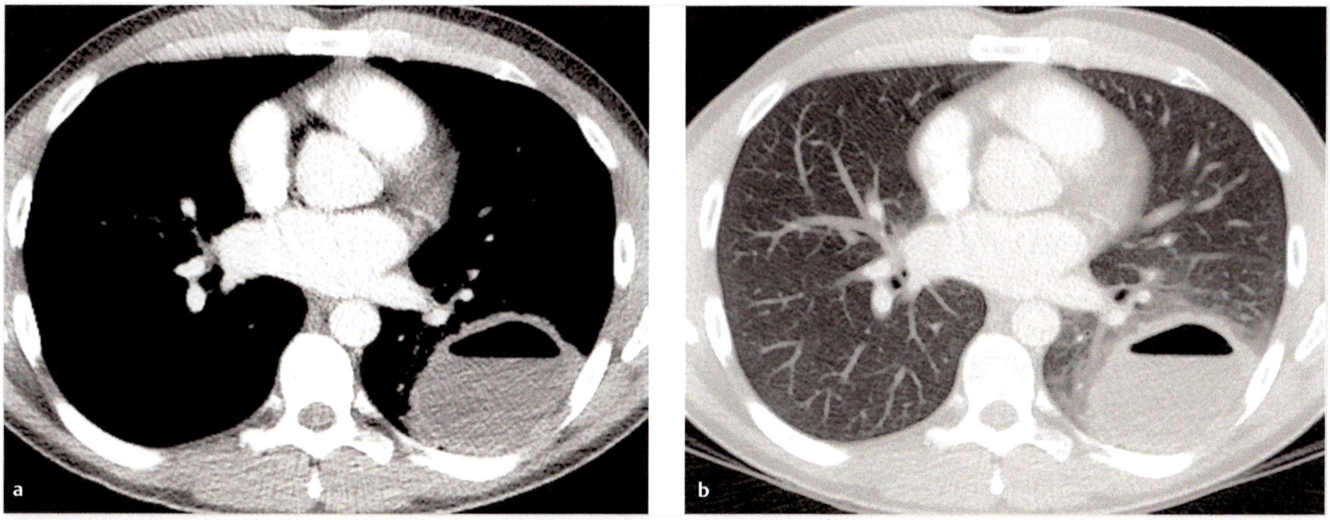

Fig. 5.6 Lung abscess in the left lower lobe. CT images. **(a)** Soft-tissue window: relatively thin-walled cavitation. **(b)** Lung window: air–fluid level in abscess.

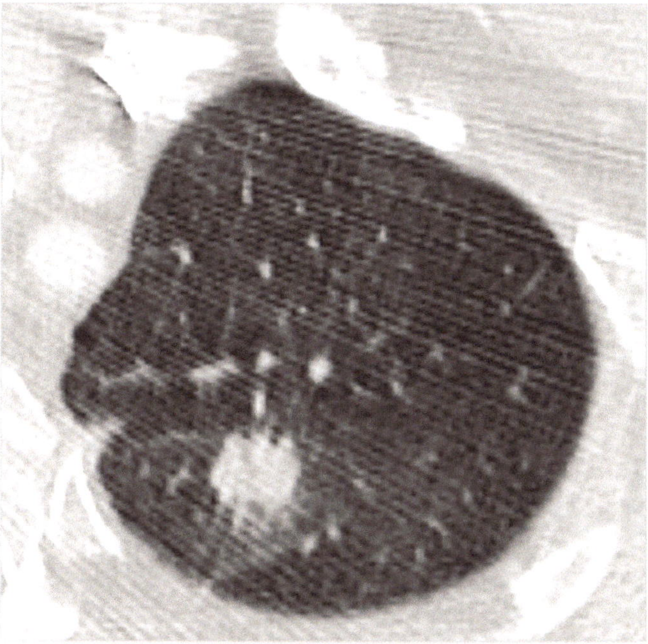

Fig. 5.7 Focal pneumonia in the left upper lobe. CT image

effusion (see criteria below suggestive of pleural empyema). In cases of justified clinical suspicion (no improvement, deterioration of general condition, or persistently high inflammatory laboratory results), differentiation can be made between pleural empyema and noninfected pleural effusion through thoracocentesis. This procedure is recommended for hospitalized patients whose lateral upright chest radiograph shows a pleural effusion of more than 5 cm.[1]

- *Abscess formation*: early abscess formation is seen on CT as rounded, largely water-isodense areas in lung regions affected by pneumonia. Later, following bronchial drainage of the liquid portions, abscess formation can be identified as cavitation on radiographs, too (see ▶Fig. 5.5). That antibiotics rarely penetrate into the inside of

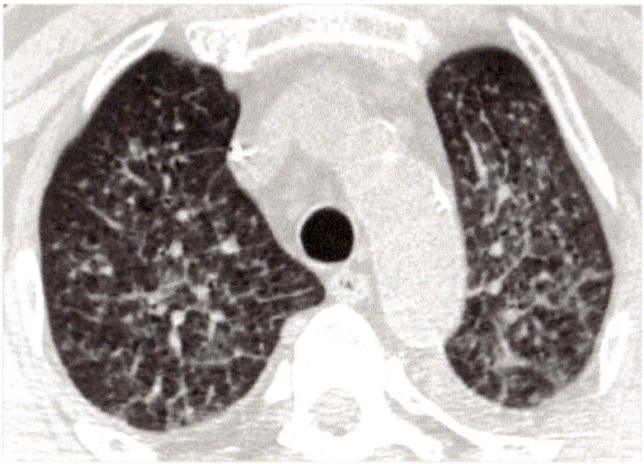

Fig. 5.8 Bilateral reticulonodular pattern in viral pneumonia. CT image.

abscesses gives rise to a delayed treatment response and the need for a prolonged treatment course. CT examination is indicated if a lung abscess is suspected[1] to rule out any mass, foreign body, infarction pneumonia, or superinfection caused by bronchial obstruction. If conservative antibiotic treatment fails, CT- or fluoroscopy-guided drainage may be useful.[2]

Note

Characteristic features of parapneumonic pleural empyema:

- Large, possibly multiloculated pleural effusion.
- Delayed onset in relation to the underlying pneumonia.
- Echogenic appearance on ultrasonography.
- On CT, thickening and contrast enhancement of the parietal and visceral pleura (split pleura sign).
- Persistently high or rising titers of inflammatory laboratory results despite regressing pneumonia.

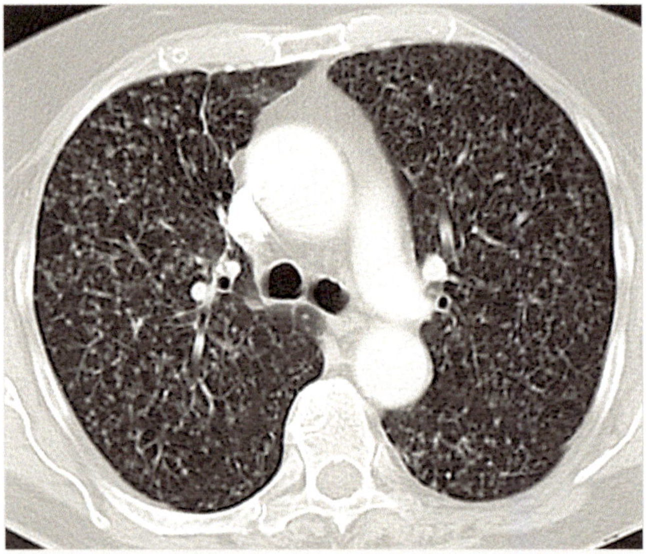

Fig. 5.9 **Miliary pattern in miliary tuberculosis.** CT image.

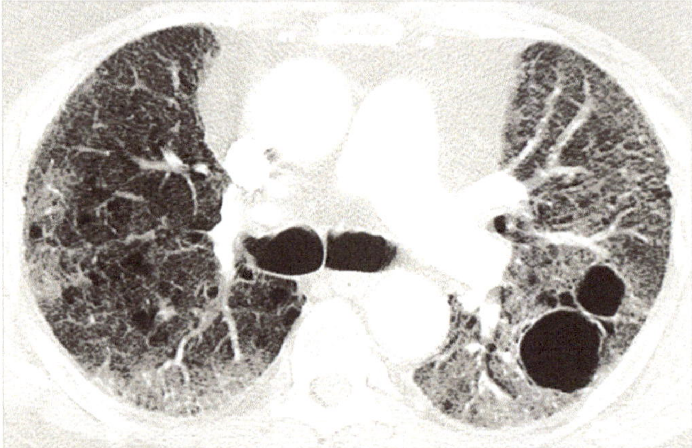

Fig. 5.10 **Cysts and ground-glass opacities in *Pneumocystis jirovecii* pneumonia.** CT image.

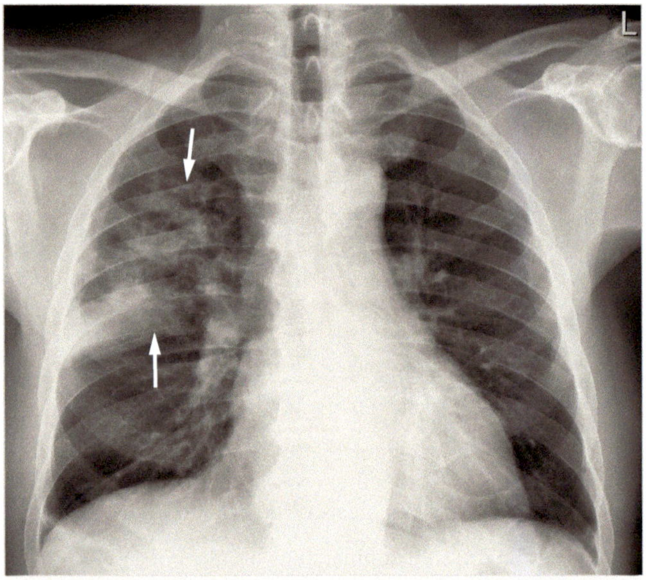

Fig. 5.11 **Community-acquired pneumonia in the right upper lobe (*arrows*).** Radiograph.

5.1 Community-Acquired Pneumonia

Community-acquired pneumonia is defined as acute infection of the lower respiratory tract with evidence of pulmonary opacity on radiographs, even in the absence of auscultation findings (▶Fig. 5.11).[1]

In clinical terms, a distinction is generally made between *typical and atypical pneumonia*, each involving a different spectrum of microorganisms. This distinction is illustrated in ▶Table 5.2 and can also be inferred from the radiologic image of pneumonia.

Community-acquired atypical pneumonia includes *viral pneumonia* which regularly causes epidemic outbreaks. In addition to seasonal influenza epidemics caused by influenza A and B viruses, in the recent past viral severe acute respiratory syndrome (SARS) as well as bird and swine flu has drawn attention. The radiologic findings for the various types of viral pneumonia are so similar as to preclude identification of the causative virus.

Note

Typical radiologic findings of viral pneumonia[3]:

- Bilateral ground-glass opacity.
- Bilateral, poorly marginated nodules.
- Bilateral, in the later course confluent, consolidation.
- Reticular opacity.
- Small centrilobular nodules.
- Hyperinflation of the lung parenchyma.
- Pleural effusion.
- Hilar lymphadenopathy (in children).

Risk stratification to determine the necessity for admission to the hospital or, possibly, for intensive medical therapy can be decided on the basis of the following clinical criteria (*CRB-65 index*[4]):

- *Respiratory rate*: at least 30/min.
- *Diastolic blood pressure*: maximum 60 mm Hg.
- *Systolic blood pressure*: maximum 90 mm Hg.
- *Clouding of consciousness*: present.
- *Age:* at least 65 years.

One point is assigned for each criterion met; the CRB-65 index is the sum of all points.

This determines the scope of diagnosis as presented in ▶Table 5.3. Radiography examination should in principle be performed in two planes at the time of diagnosis. There is no good evidence to support the use of follow-up X-ray examination on completion of treatment. It may be considered for risk patients at the earliest 2 weeks after ending treatment. CT examination is not indicated at the time of diagnosis.

Table 5.2 Characteristics of typical and atypical pneumonia

Parameters	Typical pneumonia	Atypical pneumonia
Microbial spectrum	Bacteria: • Pneumococci • Staphylococci	Obligate intracellular bacteria: • Chlamydiae • Mycoplasma • Legionellae Viruses
Clinical presentation	Acute picture: • Fever • Shaking chills • Cough • Purulent sputum • Reduced general state	Less acute picture: • Moderate fever • Headache • Joint pain
Inflammation site	Alveolar spaces	Interstitium
Radiologic image	Consolidation	Ground-glass opacity

Table 5.3 Risk stratification and diagnostic scope for community-acquired pneumonia[1]

Treatment	CRB-65 index	Radiograph needed for diagnosis	Radiograph for follow-up examination
Outpatient	0–1 No risk factors[a]	Recommended	Optional in the presence of risk factors for tumor disease At the earliest, 2 weeks after ending treatment
	0–1 With risk factors[a]	Obligatory	
Normal hospital ward or outpatient setting[b]	2	Obligatory	Recommended for active smokers
Intensive care unit	≥3	Obligatory	Age >65 years, severe concomitant diseases, at the earliest 2 weeks after ending treatment

[a]Risk factors:

- Antibiotic treatment in past 3 months.
- Residents of care homes.
- Severe concomitant diseases (congestive heart failure, liver cirrhosis, end-stage kidney disease, stroke with neurologic deficits).

[b]The CRB-65 index is intended merely as a guide and is not a substitute for clinical decision-making in a particular case.

> **Note**
>
> CT indications which may apply in the course of treatment of community-acquired pneumonia[1]:
> - Treatment failure:
>   - Progressive pneumonia:
>   - Deterioration of clinical state (respiratory insufficiency, severe sepsis, or septic shock).
>   - Radiologic progression seen only coincident with clinical deterioration.
>   - Delayed-response pneumonia: no clinical stability observed within 72 h of starting treatment (stability criteria: heart rate, maximum 100/min; respiratory rate, maximum 24/min; systolic blood pressure, at least 90 mm Hg; body temperature, maximum 37.8°C; oxygen partial pressure, at least 60 mm Hg; and oxygen saturation, at least 90%).
> - Suspected lung abscess.

Treatment failure can manifest as progressive pneumonia or as nonprogressive, delayed-response pneumonia:

- *Progressive pneumonia*: any increase in pulmonary opacities seen on radiographs within the first 72 h may be interpreted as progressive pneumonia only in the setting of coincident clinical deterioration.
- *Delayed-response pneumonia*: if there is no evidence of clinical stability within 72 h, other causes, also nonmicrobial, for the pulmonary opacities must be considered.

In both situations, a CT examination is usually indicated.[5,6]

5.2 Hospital-Acquired/Nosocomial Pneumonia

Hospital-acquired (nosocomial) pneumonia is defined as pneumonia presenting at least 48 h after the patient's admission to the hospital and which was not incubating at the time of admission.[7] It is the second most common hospital-acquired infection and causes considerable morbidity and mortality, in particular, in intensive care units. It often constitutes a limiting factor in immunosuppressant therapies, for example, in chemotherapy. The types of hospital-acquired pneumonia presenting during such treatment courses are caused by opportunistic pathogens and will be discussed in Section 5.3.

The *microbial spectrum* of hospital-acquired pneumonia differs from that implicated in community-acquired pneumonia. In the case of intensive care patients on long-term ventilation, infection is mainly attributed to hospital-specific bacterial pathogens. Due to the myriad forms of bacterial resistance, together with new types emerging during treatment, the clinical and radiologic course is more challenging compared with community-acquired pneumonia. Multifocal infiltrates and changing courses alternating between regressive and progressive findings are common (▶Fig. 5.12).

Differential diagnosis of hospital-acquired pneumonia from other pulmonary opacities is difficult, in particular, in ventilated patients. A summary of the various underlying causes is given in ▶Table 5.4. The suggestive effect of clinical data can make it harder to reach a correct diagnosis. For example, purulent sputum or tracheal secretion is often caused by infection of the upper airways, while elevated inflammatory laboratory results can have many causes in intensive care patients. It is therefore important to conduct meticulous image analysis and have access to comprehensive information on the clinical course. Ideally, the radiologic findings should be discussed with the treating clinicians.

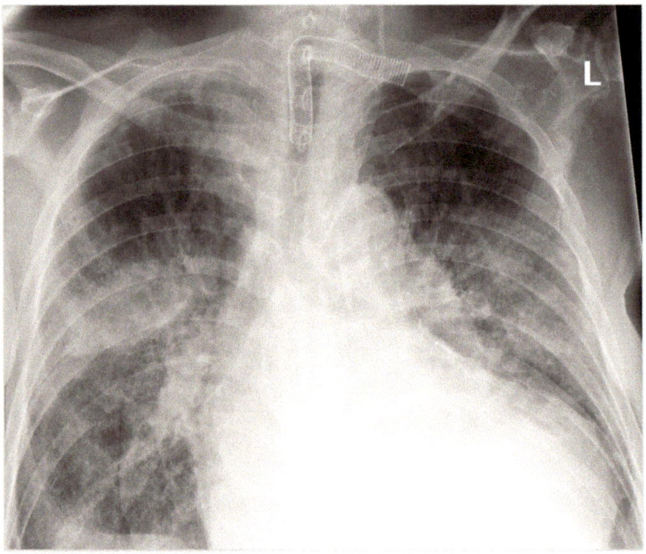

Fig. 5.12 Hospital-acquired pneumonia. Radiograph, supine position. Bilateral pulmonary opacities. Besides, cardiomegaly. Tracheal cannula, central venous catheter with catheter tip relatively peripherally in the left brachiocephalic vein.

5.3 Opportunistic Pneumonia

Opportunistic pneumonias are pulmonary infections that may arise because of the patient's compromised immune system. The microbial spectrum implicated in opportunistic pneumonia differs from that identified for community-acquired pneumonia as well as for other common forms of hospital-acquired pneumonia in immunocompetent patients. ▶Table 5.5 gives a summary of the various mechanisms of the immune system, typical diseases or forms of immunosuppressant treatment, and the resultant typical spectrum of opportunistic pathogens.

A number of typical clinical constellations can be identified[9]:

- *Aplasia*: this is defined as a decline in the neutrophil count to below 500/µL or in the leukocyte count to below 1,000/µL, often secondary to aplasiogenic chemo- or radiotherapy. This leads to diminished phagocytosis. The lung infections presenting during the initial days of onset of aplasia are often imputed to gram-positive cocci, especially *S. aureus*, and gram-negative bacteria, such as *Pseudomonas aeruginosa*. If aplasia persists for at least 5 days, fungal infections are identified additionally. In Europe, these are typically caused by *Aspergillus* and *Candida* species.[9]
- *AIDS* (acquired immunodeficiency syndrome): this leads to a reduction in the T helper cells (CD4-positive T lymphocytes) and, in turn, to reduced specific cellular immunity. The most common pulmonary infection is *Pneumocystis jirovecii* pneumonia, which is frequently the first manifestation of AIDS disease. Less commonly, tuberculosis and pulmonary toxoplasmosis are observed.[9]
- *Organ transplantations*: organ transplant results in reduced lymphocyte function due to immunosuppression, putting patients at risk for pneumonia caused by intracellular pathogens, such as *Legionella pneumophila*, and viruses (especially cytomegalovirus), as well as for mycobacteriosis, nocardiosis, and aspergillosis. *Aspergillus* and *Nocardia* account for two-thirds of infections in heart transplant patients. Lung transplant recipients are at higher risk for cytomegalovirus infection.[9]
- *Stem cell transplant*: in the conditioning phase, the patient's diseased bone marrow is destroyed by means of high-dose

Table 5.4 Differential diagnosis of hospital-acquired (nosocomial) pneumonia in intensive care patients with pulmonary opacity on radiograph[8]

Differential diagnosis	Remarks
Atelectasis	Common, displacement of other anatomic structures indicates loss of lung volume
Pleural effusion	Basal predominant homogenous grading increase of opacity on supine image, possibly lateral pleural fluid layer
Pulmonary edema	Mainly symmetrical, possibly cardiomegaly suggestive of congestive heart failure or clinical signs of another cause (e.g., kidney failure, sepsis)
Lung infarction	As sequela of pulmonary embolism; pleural-based triangular opacity (so-called Hampton hump), may be multiple
Adult respiratory distress syndrome	Diffuse bilateral opacities; no laboratory results suggestive of bacterial inflammation, severe respiratory insufficiency
Alveolar hemorrhage	Treatment-induced (drug toxicity) or caused by an underlying disease
Drug toxicity	This should also be taken into consideration in case of persistent bilateral pulmonary opacities; no pathognomonic radiologic findings for drug-induced lung disease; at times, the temporal coincidence between radiologic findings and administration or discontinuation of certain drugs can afford insights
Postoperative changes	Secondary to thoracic surgery: intrapulmonary hematomas, impaired lymph drainage, impaired pulmonary venous drainage

Table 5.5 Immune system mechanisms, disease-mediated deficiencies, and resultant opportunistic pneumonia[11,12]

Immune mechanism	Mediators	Damage	Spectrum of opportunistic microorganisms
Adaptive cellular response	T cell system	• Organ transplant • Stem cell transplant • Cortisone treatment • AIDS • Hodgkin lymphoma • Chronic lymphatic leukemia	• *Pneumocystis jirovecii* • Viruses (cytomegalovirus, herpes simplex virus) • Mycobacteria • Legionellae
Adaptive humoral response	Immunoglobulins	• Chemotherapy • Malignant melanoma • Chronic lymphatic leukemia • AIDS • Hypogammaglobulinemia	• Pneumococci • Gram-negative bacteria • Mycobacteria • Candida • *Pneumocystis jirovecii* • Viruses (cytomegalovirus, herpes simplex virus)
Innate cellular response	Macrophages/monocytes Granulocytes NK cells	• Chemotherapy • Radiotherapy • Stem cell transplant • Blood system disease • Bone marrow carcinosis (e.g., small cell lung carcinoma)	Staphylococcus aureus • Gram-negative bacteria • Fungi
Innate humoral response	Complement system Properdin system Monokines/lymphokines	• Multiple myeloma • Non-Hodgkin lymphoma • Chronic lymphatic leukemia	• *Streptococcus pneumoniae* • *Haemophilus influenzae*

Abbreviations: AIDS, acquired immunodeficiency syndrome; NK cells, natural killer cells.

chemotherapy and whole-body irradiation, making the patient particularly susceptible to pneumococcal pneumonia during this phase. In the wake of conditioning and stem cell transplant, the risk of opportunistic pneumonia is similar to that faced by aplastic patients.

- *High-dose corticosteroid treatment*: this results in impairment of granulocyte function, thus compromising chemotactic activity. Patients are at increased risk for *P. jirovecii* pneumonia. Preexisting tuberculosis may be reactivated.[9]

Radiographic images of opportunistic infections may be normal or show only uncharacteristic changes.[10] CT is indicated if opportunistic pneumonia is suspected but no evidence of pneumonia is seen on the radiograph. Aplastic patients with certain risk constellations, e.g., receiving aplasiogenic chemotherapy or following stem cell transplant, often become febrile. In such settings, there is virtually always an indication for CT. It is precisely for this cohort of patients that all efforts must be made to exploit the CT dose reduction potentials and opt for low-dose CT scans.

5.3.1 Fungal Pneumonia

By virtue of their ubiquitous nature, *Aspergillus* and *Candida* are the main opportunistic causal agents of fungal pneumonia.

Aspergillus spp. are molds that give rise to infections with extremely varied characteristics depending on their invasiveness. A distinction is made between noninvasive aspergillomas, invasive pulmonary aspergillosis, and semi-invasive chronic necrotizing aspergillosis.[13] Another disease caused by *Aspergillus* spp., allergic bronchopulmonary aspergillosis, is discussed in the section on allergic pulmonary diseases.

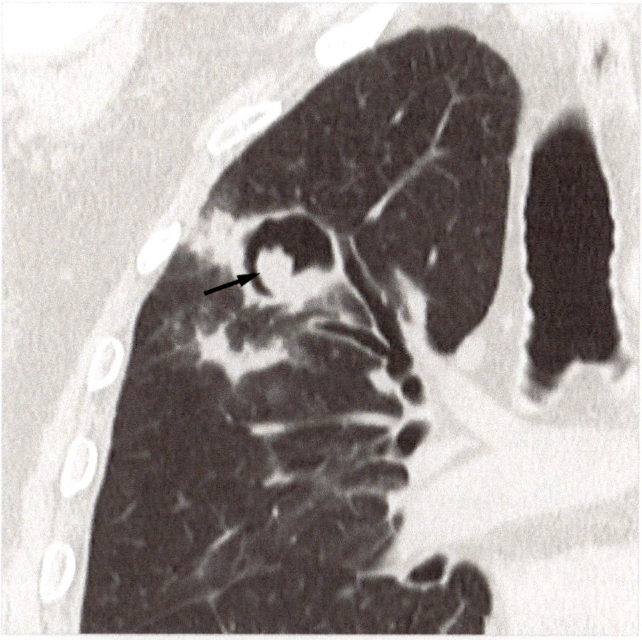

Fig. 5.13 Aspergilloma (*arrow*) in a preformed cavity in the right upper lobe. CT image, coronal.

Aspergilloma

Aspergilloma is a mycetoma composed of *Aspergillus* hyphae; in other words, it is like a round fungus ball. This grows in a preformed cavern, often in association with longstanding tuberculosis or sarcoidosis (▶Fig. 5.13). When the patient changes position, the fungus ball can move within the cavern in line with the force of gravity and this can serve as a diagnostic criterion. At times, the aspergilloma may fill the entire cavern and can no longer be distinguished from the cavern wall; instead, the entire lesion appears as a relatively homogeneous area of consolidation (▶Fig. 5.14). Noninvasive aspergilloma can progress to an invasive form of *Aspergillus* infection in immunocompromised patients.

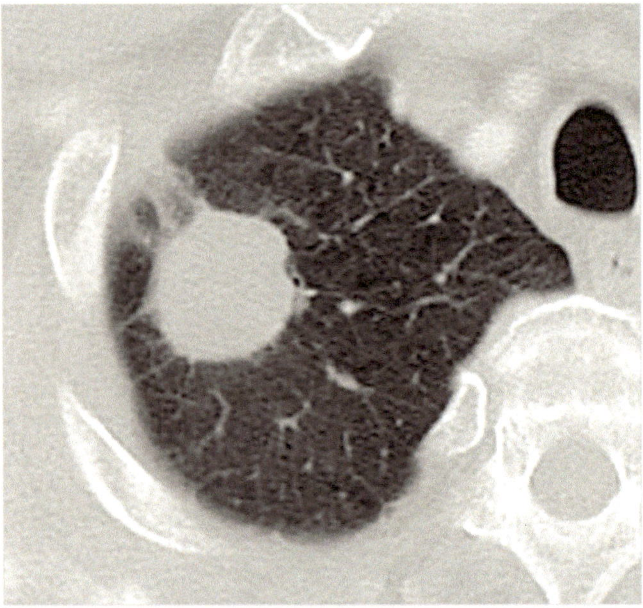

Fig. 5.14 Aspergilloma in the right upper lobe. CT image. The fungus ball cannot be distinguished from the cavern wall; the entire lesion manifests as a homogeneous nodule.

Invasive Pulmonary Aspergillosis

Patients who have become aplastic secondary to malignant hematologic diseases and ensuing treatment often develop life-threatening invasive pulmonary aspergillosis. This is rarely seen in patients without diagnosed severe immunoincompetence.[10]

An airborne infection route is implicated here. Molds generally result in *angioinvasive aspergillosis*, giving rise to bleeding and infarction of the lung parenchyma.[14] Typical radiologic findings are (▶Table 5.6):

- *Relatively few, largish nodules with halo sign* (ground-glass opacity surrounding the lesion [▶Fig. 5.15], reflecting areas of perifocal hemorrhage[15]).

Table 5.6 Characteristic CT morphology of invasive pulmonary aspergillosis[13,18]

Angioinvasive pulmonary aspergillosis	Acute respiratory tract invasive aspergillosis
• Few largish nodules with halo sign • Triangular consolidations with or without halo sign • Angiotropic localization of nodules • Intralesional open bronchi (open bronchus sign) • Late signs: air crescent sign	• Peribronchial consolidation • Centrilobular nodules (<5 mm) • Tree-in-bud pattern • Ground-glass opacity • Segmental consolidation

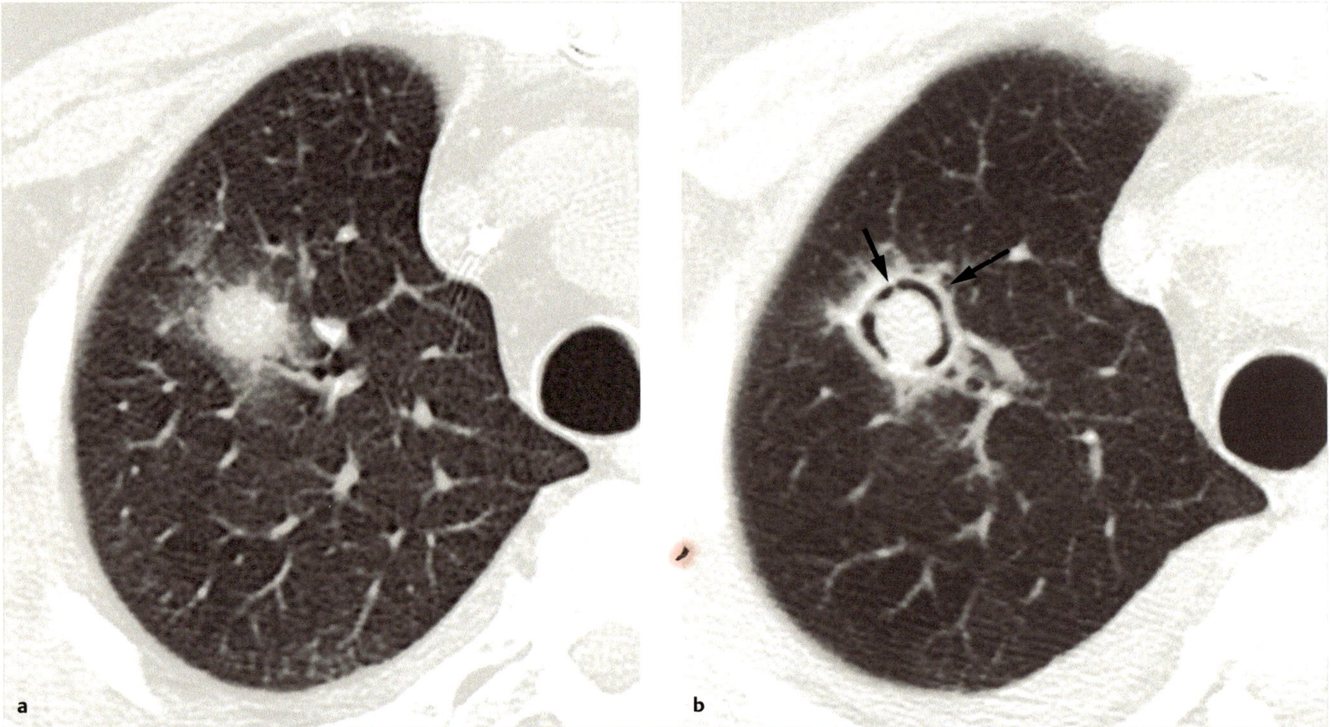

Fig. 5.15 Invasive pulmonary aspergillosis in the right upper lobe. CT images. Course over 2 weeks. **(a)** Baseline findings in aplastic patient: rounded consolidation in the right upper lobe, surrounded by ground-glass opacity, i.e., halo sign. **(b)** Two weeks later, patient is no longer aplastic: newly emerged air crescent sign (*arrows*), slight increase in nodule size.

- *Peripheral triangular consolidations with or without halo sign* (▶Fig. 5.16): in general, the nodules exhibit an angiotropic pattern.

The characteristic *air crescent sign* results from recovery of leukocyte function with absorption of necrotic tissue secondary to lung infarction and necrotic shrinkage.[16] This late sign of invasive pulmonary aspergillosis is observed in around half of all cases.[17]

> **Note**
>
> An increase in the size of *Aspergillus* nodules may also reflect recovery of the patient's immune response, with rising leukocyte counts (see ▶Fig. 5.15). Therefore, in the absence of further clinical information, it must not be interpreted as progression of invasive pulmonary aspergillosis.

In fewer than one-third of cases, the *Aspergillus* hyphae invade the bronchial wall causing *acute respiratory tract invasive aspergillosis* (▶Fig. 5.17).[14] Depending on localization, this gives rise to acute tracheobronchitis, exudative bronchiolitis, or bronchopneumonia.[13] The main findings in radiographs are consolidation with basal predominance and poorly marginated nodules. CT morphology is summarized in ▶Table 5.6.[18]

On rare occasions, respiratory tract invasive aspergillosis exhibits a chronic course involving a relatively indolent infection known as *chronic-necrotizing aspergillosis*. It starts as focal consolidation, going on to form a cavern through central colliquation (liquefaction). Its final appearance is similar to that of an aspergilloma; however, its pathogenesis is variable.[19–21]

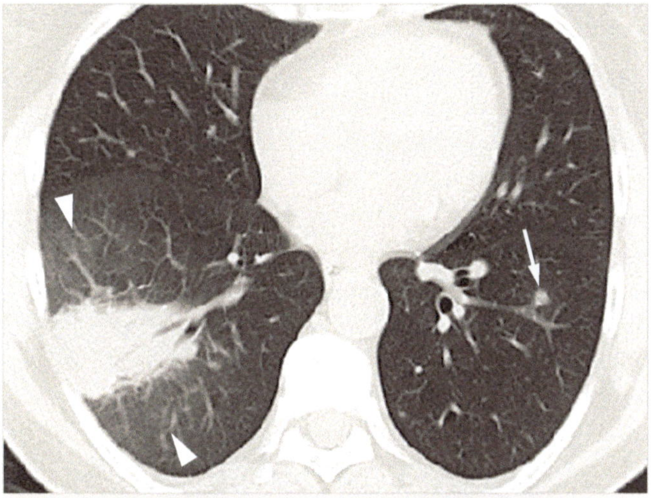

Fig. 5.16 Invasive pulmonary aspergillosis. CT image. Large triangular, peripheral consolidation in the right lower lobe, with pronounced halo sign (*arrowheads*); another smaller aspergillosis nodule in the left lower lobe (*arrow*).

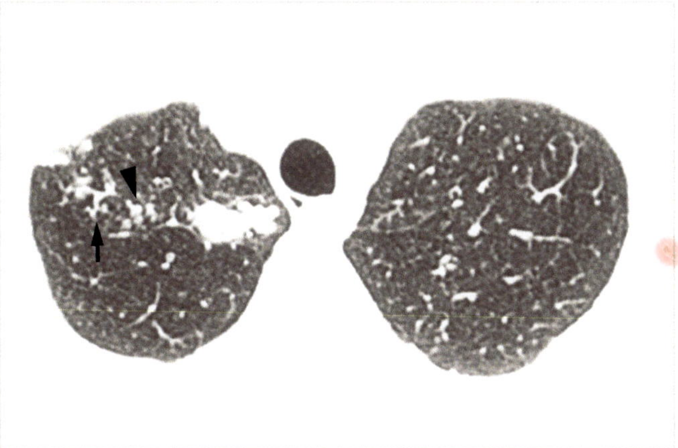

Fig. 5.17 Acute respiratory tract invasive aspergillosis. CT image. Consolidation in the right upper lobe, centrilobular nodules (*arrowheads*) and tree-in-bud pattern (*arrow*).

Candida Pneumonia

Candida spp. are yeasts, normally found in the gastrointestinal tract. If they manage to breach the intestinal barrier following a reduced immune response, the ensuing septicemia can lead to the spread of *Candida* yeasts to the lungs through hematogenous dissemination. The resultant radiologic image typically shows several small inflammatory foci in the lung. These manifest as numerous, mainly small nodules. On CT images, random distribution giving rise to a miliary pattern can be detected (▶Fig. 5.18).[11] Furthermore, ground-glass opacity and small areas of consolidation are often seen.

> **Note**
>
> Radiologic findings of *Candida* pneumonia:
> - Miliary pattern (multiple randomly distributed small nodules).
> - Ground-glass opacity.
> - Small areas of consolidation.

Pneumocystis jirovecii Pneumonia

This pathogen is classified as an ascomycete (sac fungus) belonging to the genus *Pneumocystis* and had formerly been assigned to the protozoa. The grammatically correct alternative notation *Pneumocystis jiroveci*[22] is no longer used; this *Pneumocystis* sp. was first characterized by Otto Jirovec.[23] Formerly, the pulmonary infection of humans with *Pneumocystis* was erroneously

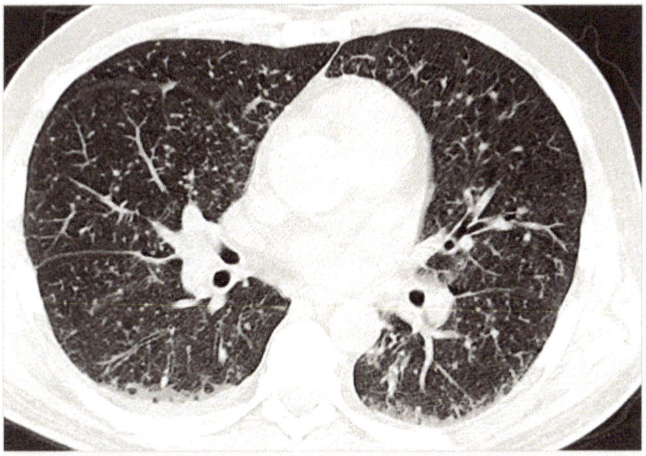

Fig. 5.18 *Candida* pneumonia. CT image. Multiple small, bilateral nodules with random distribution.

referred to as *Pneumocystis carinii* pneumonia, which is another subspecies of *Pneumocystis*.

P. jirovecii pneumonia is often the first manifestation of AIDS disease and affects two-thirds of AIDS patients in the course of disease. In clinical terms, it presents as progressive dyspnea, tachypnea, tachycardia, and low-grade fever, but with generally normal auscultation results.[24]

Imaging reveals characteristic bilateral perihilar opacities that become increasingly more diffuse and homogeneous as infection progresses (▶Fig. 5.19).[25] Localized infiltrates, multiple nodules, pneumatoceles, or a reticular pattern are seen less frequently.[24,25] At times the radiograph is normal, thus in marked contrast with the patient's considerable dyspnea. The corresponding CT image shows extensive ground-glass opacity (▶Fig. 5.20).[26] ▶Table 5.7 gives a summary of typical radiologic findings.[27] The eponymous cystic changes (see ▶Fig. 5.10) are rarely observed in non-AIDS patients.[28,29] Often, atypical manifestations of *P. jirovecii* pneumonia are seen radiologically. Therefore, in such cases the suspected diagnosis of *P. jirovecii* pneumonia cannot, as such, be inferred from this constellation of radiologic findings (▶Fig. 5.21).

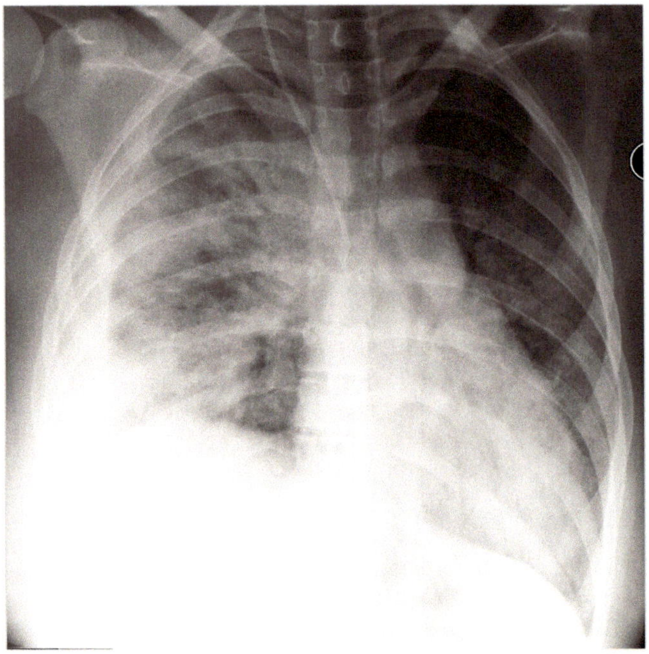

Fig. 5.19 ***Pneumocystis jirovecii*** **pneumonia.** Radiograph. Bilateral, diffuse ground-glass opacities as well as right pleural effusion.

Table 5.7 Radiologic findings in *Pneumocystis jirovecii* pneumonia

Diagnostic imaging modalities	Findings
Radiograph	• Perihilar bilateral opacities • Diffuse bilateral opacities • Localized opacities • Multiple nodular opacities • Cysts • Reticular pattern • Pneumothorax
CT	• Irregular or diffuse bilateral ground-glass opacities, with relative subpleural sparing • Interlobular septal thickening • Intralobular lines • Consolidation • Cysts • Pneumothorax

5.3.2 Viral Pneumonia

Viral pneumonia not just presents as an opportunistic infection but also affects immunocompetent patients. It is caused by a limited number of viruses and is discussed in the section on community-acquired pneumonia. Opportunistic viral pneumonia causes considerable morbidity and mortality in immunocompromised patients, and occasionally rare opportunistic pathogens are identified.[30]

Respiratory syncytial virus is the main cause of severe pneumonia in stem-cell and organ-transplant recipients.[31,32] Other typical opportunistic pathogens causing viral pneumonia are:

- Cytomegalovirus in organ-transplant and AIDS patients (▶Fig. 5.22).
- Herpes simplex virus in AIDS patients and intensive care patients with adult respiratory distress syndrome (▶Fig. 5.23).
- Varicella zoster virus.

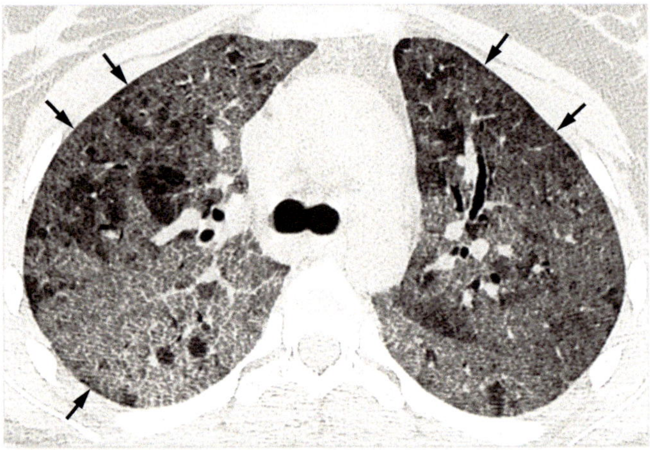

Fig. 5.20 ***Pneumocystis jirovecii*** **pneumonia.** CT image. Bilateral, diffuse ground-glass opacities, partially sparing the anterior subpleural space (*arrows*).

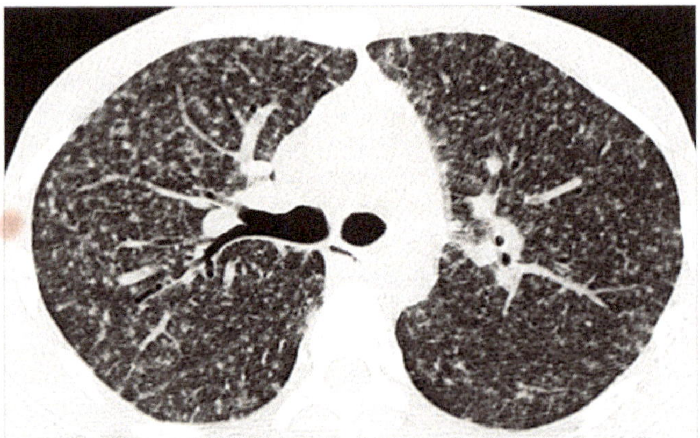

Fig. 5.21 ***Pneumocystis jirovecii*** **pneumonia with atypical appearance.** CT image. Diffuse, bilateral centrilobular nodules and slight diffuse ground-glass opacities.

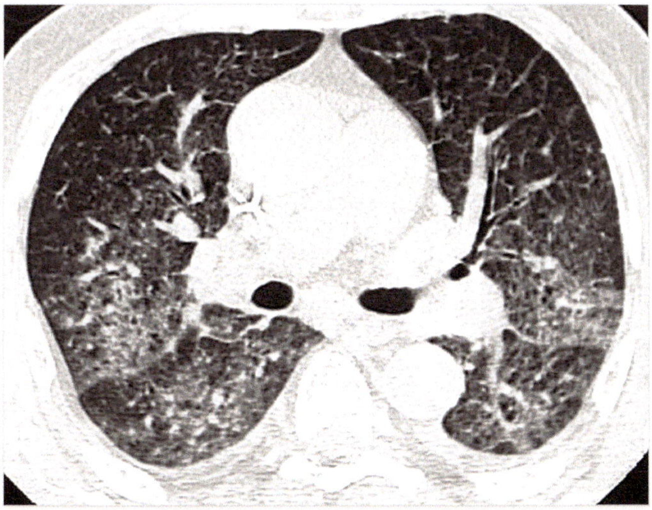

Fig. 5.22 Cytomegalovirus pneumonia. CT image. Bilateral ground-glass opacities and intralobular lines.

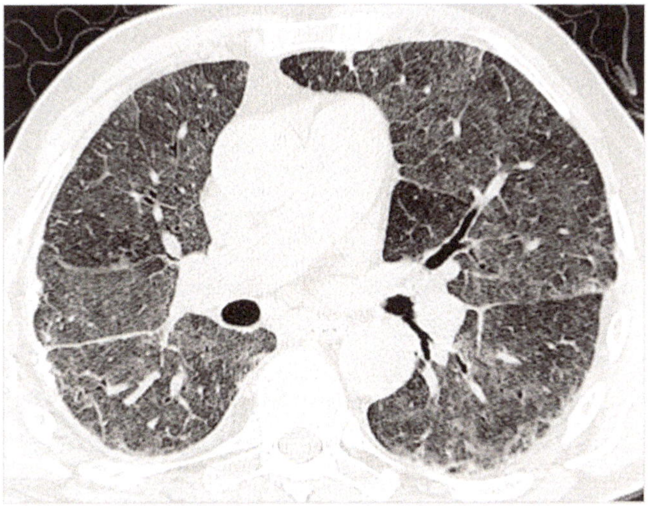

Fig. 5.23 Herpes simplex virus pneumonia. CT image. Diffuse, bilateral ground-glass opacities.

The radiographic findings are similar to those seen for viral pneumonia in immunocompetent patients. In addition, varicella zoster virus pneumonia exhibits characteristic, randomly distributed, nodules measuring 1 to 10 mm.[3,11]

> **Note**
>
> The most important insight afforded by imaging in opportunistic viral pneumonia is exclusion of a typical bacterial pneumonia that would necessitate antibiotic treatment.

Identification of the causative organism is important for differential diagnosis and treatment; this is usually based on serology. In the presence of bilateral ground-glass opacity, *P. jirovecii* pneumonia must be included in differential diagnosis and is ruled out through bronchoscopy and bronchoalveolar lavage. The various types of viral pneumonia cannot be reliably distinguished radiologically.

5.4 Mycobacteriosis

Mycobacteriosis, pneumonia caused by mycobacteria, is relatively rare in developed countries. The causative organism of tuberculosis is *Mycobacterium tuberculosis*. Atypical mycobacteriosis is caused by mycobacteria other than *M. tuberculosis* and *Mycobacterium leprae* and are known as "mycobacteria other than tuberculosis" (MOTT). All mycobacterial pathogens implicated in mycobacteriosis exhibit extreme stability both in and outside the human body.

5.4.1 Tuberculosis

Together with HIV (human immunodeficiency virus) and malaria, tuberculosis is one of the most prevalent infectious diseases worldwide. While it is relatively uncommon in developed countries, it is likely that this incidence will increase for various reasons in the coming years. Multidrug-resistant tuberculosis (MDR-TB), resistant to conventional tuberculostatic agents, is becoming increasingly more widespread. Besides, isolated cases of extensively drug-resistant tuberculosis (XDR-TB), which first emerged in 2006 in South Africa, have been detected in the meantime in Europe. These pathogens are extremely difficult to treat since they exhibit multiple resistances to all known classes of tuberculostatics.[33] Due to migration from regions with a high prevalence of resistant tuberculosis (especially sub-Saharan Africa and Central Asia), drug-resistant mycobacteria are also increasingly spreading to developed countries. Newly emerging genotypes (Beijing genotypes) have greatly increased the contagiousness and virulence of mycobacteria.[34] Exposure to an infected person in confined spaces poses a risk of infection to others even within a few minutes. Conversely, for spread of conventional tuberculosis genotypes, continuous exposure for several hours is needed.

Pathogenesis

Mycobacteria are almost always inhaled as aerosols and thus spread through an airborne route to the lung. Here, they elicit a local inflammatory reaction and undergo phagocytosis in the alveolar spaces by the alveolar macrophages. However, the macrophages are unable to kill the mycobacteria. Instead, they grow within the macrophages, and when these rupture, they are released again. They then spread along the lymphatic drainage vessels and first come into contact with the specific (adaptive) immune system in the regional lymph nodes, resulting in sensitization of the T lymphocytes. The ensuing specific immune response leads to containment of the inflammatory foci through granuloma formation. Within the granuloma, the mycobacteria are enclosed by a wall composed of epithelioid cells, Langerhans giant cells, and lymphocytes (tuberculoma). A central area of caseous necrosis is then formed. While the mycobacteria are now contained within the granuloma, they can survive for decades within these granulomas and, in the event of any decline in the patient's immune response, trigger reactivation of tuberculosis. Mycobacterial *transmission* unfolds:

- Per continuitatem.
- Via the lymphatic drainage vessels.

- Via the bloodstream.
- Endobronchially.

The various transmission routes are exploited at various times and to different degrees for spread of mycobacteria within the body. The clinical symptoms and radiographic findings vary accordingly (► Fig. 5.24).

Primary Infection

Primary infection first manifests as discrete inflammation of the lung parenchyma, giving rise to focal pneumonia known as a *Ghon focus*. Immunologic reactions in locoregional lymph nodes cause ipsilateral hilar lymphadenopathy. This combination of Ghon focus, lymphangitis toward the hilum, and hilar lymphadenopathy is known as the *Ranke complex* or primary complex. A lung infiltrate is seen more often than hilar lymphadenopathy in adults (► Fig. 5.25), whereas the converse is observed in children. This process is generally asymptomatic or exhibits clinical signs of mild infection. It generally resolves with granuloma formation. The caseous necrosis in the Ghon focus and affected hilar lymph nodes can calcify, thus persisting for decades as a visible remnant of the resolved primary infection (► Fig. 5.26). Ghon foci can also persist as nodules

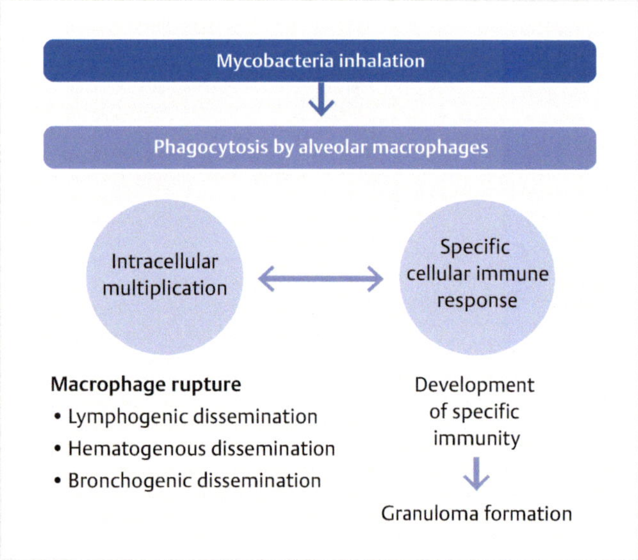

Fig. 5.24 Pathogenesis of pulmonary tuberculosis. Schematic diagram.

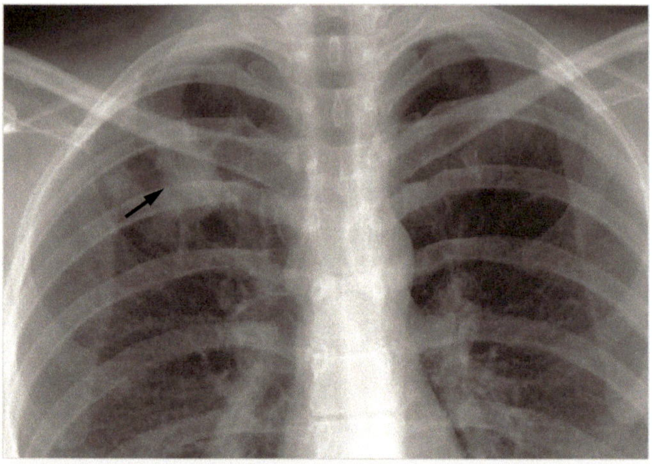

Fig. 5.25 Tuberculosis primary infection. Magnified section of radiograph. Primary pulmonary opacity or Ghon focus in the right upper lobe (*arrow*). No evidence of hilar lymphadenopathy on radiograph.

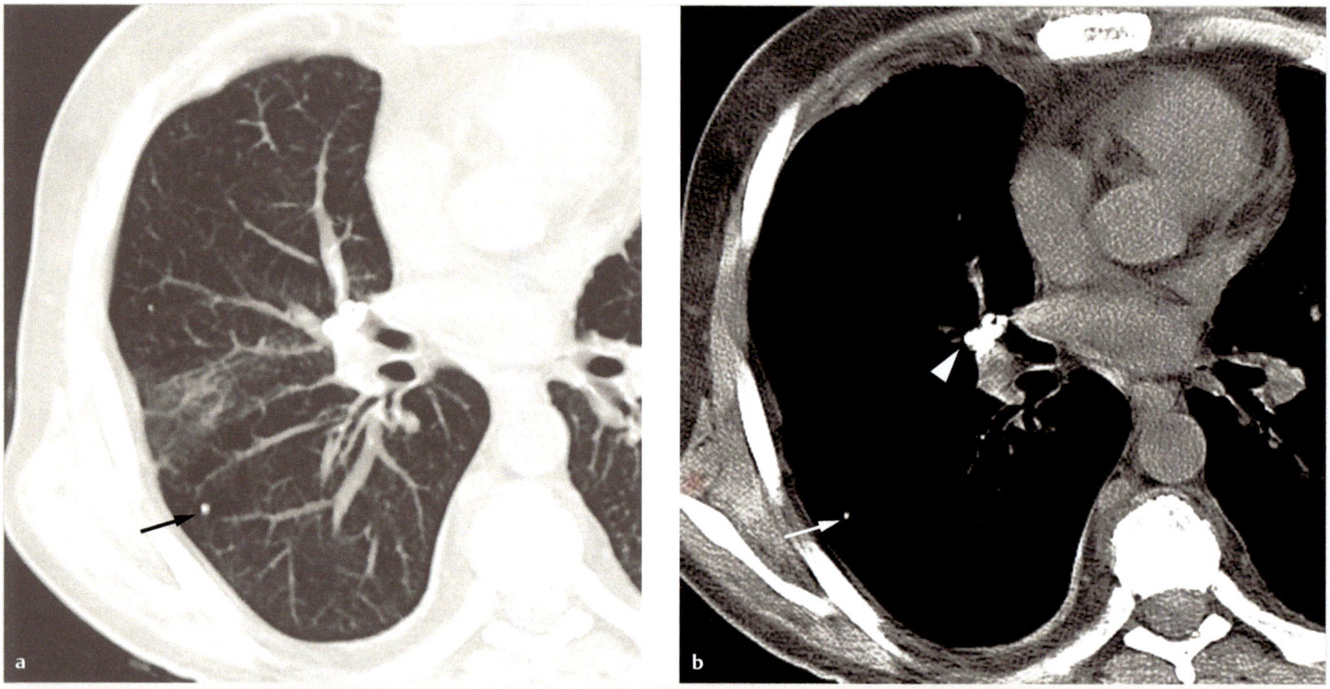

Fig. 5.26 Remnants of Ranke complex. CT images. Ghon focus **(a, b,** *arrows*) and calcified right hilar lymph nodes **(b,** *arrowheads*). **(a)** Lung window. **(b)** Soft-tissue window.

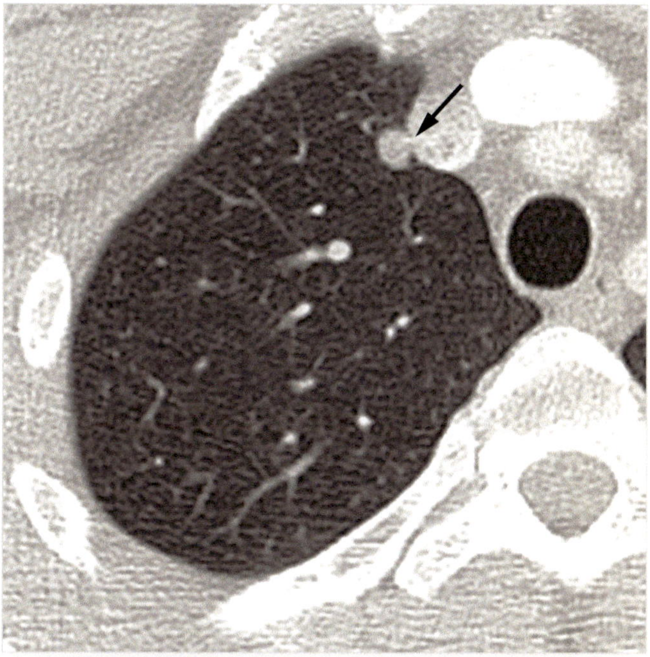

Fig. 5.27 Tuberculoma in the right upper lobe (*arrow*). CT image. Remnants of primary tuberculosis.

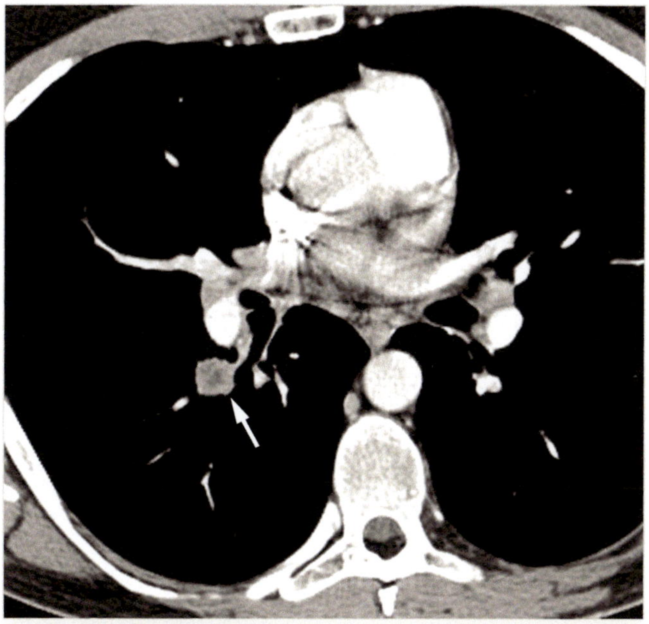

Fig. 5.28 Tuberculous lymphadenitis. CT image. Characteristic central necrosis in enlarged lymph nodes (*arrow*).

of soft-tissue density (tuberculomas) and are one differential diagnosis for solitary pulmonary nodules (▶Fig. 5.27). These residual reservoirs are of relevance in the event of any immunosuppressant treatment (e.g., administration of tumor necrosis factor-α inhibitors), since they can give rise to reactivation of previously inactive tuberculosis.

Progressive Primary Infection

In around 5% of cases, primary infection does not resolve, going on instead to progressive primary infection. Symptoms (cough, expectoration, hemoptysis, dyspnea, weight loss, fever, night sweats, lethargy, later cachexia) may now be exhibited, in particular in the presence of a high number of, or highly virulent, mycobacteria or a diminished immune response and be expressed differently:

- *Tuberculous lymphadenitis* (▶Fig. 5.28): As infection progresses in the affected hilar lymph nodes, it can then spread to the mediastinal lymph nodes. At CT, characteristic hypodense areas of central necrosis can be found in affected lymph nodes. Children have softer bronchial walls and are thus more susceptible to atelectasis secondary to the pressure exerted by the enlarged lymph nodes on the bronchi. Less frequently, this gives rise to hyperinflation by means of a valve mechanism.
- *Progressive Ghon focus* (▶Fig. 5.29): If the immune system is not able to contain the infection within the primary site of infection (Ghon focus), the infection may spread per continuitatem into larger areas of the lung, thus resulting in large consolidations and progressive destruction of the involved lung.

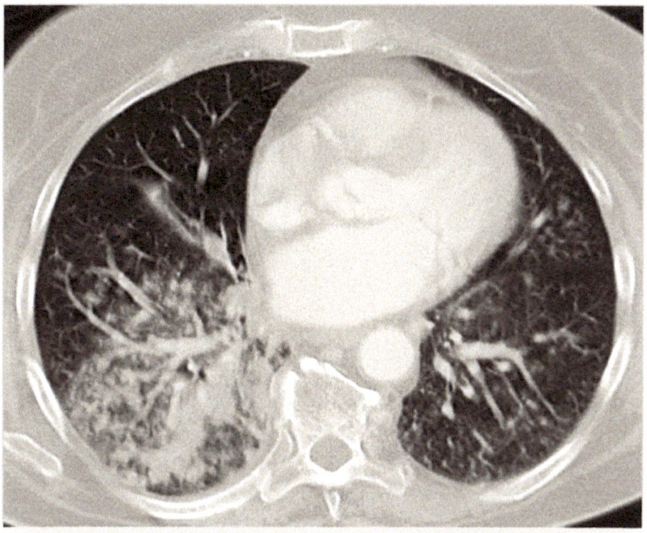

Fig. 5.29 Progressive Ghon focus. CT image. Extensive consolidation and ground-glass opacity in the right lower lobe.

Postprimary Tuberculosis

Progressive primary tuberculosis evolves to postprimary infection, with mycobacteria spreading increasingly in the lung and other organs. Postprimary pulmonary tuberculosis comprises two phases:

- *Generalization beyond the primary site of infection*: Generalization occurs predominantly through hematogenous dissemination, mainly via the lymphatic drainage vessels and the thoracic duct into the venous bloodstream. Once in the bloodstream, the mycobacteria are distributed once again in the lung. Bronchogenic spread is also possible once the mycobacteria have gained access to the bronchial system.
- *Organ stage*: This unfolds with increasing spread in the lung parenchyma and progressive lung destruction.

Generalization

Depending on the number of mycobacteria in the bloodstream and their virulence, different courses of generalization are possible:

- *Less extensive hematogenous transmission* usually occurs bilaterally, in particular, in segments 1, 2, and 6. Depending on the patient's immune response, the hematogenous foci result in either exudative inflammation (▶Fig. 5.30) or granuloma formation with possible subsequent calcification (Simon foci; ▶Fig. 5.31).
- *Miliary tuberculosis* (▶Fig. 5.32): Hematogenous spread of large numbers of mycobacteria causes diffuse lung disease in the regions where the blood-borne bacteria form small inflammatory foci of the size of a millet seed in the lungs. This is known as miliary tuberculosis (Latin: milium = millet), which on CT exhibits a randomly distributed pattern of small pulmonary nodules (miliary pattern).
- *Septicemia*: In the setting of an anergic immune response, acute mycobacterial sepsis is often fatal, even with no evidence of the radiographic findings of tuberculosis. However, the generic radiologic findings associated with sepsis may be observed.
- *Tuberculous pleurisy* (▶Fig. 5.33): In 5% of cases, a lymphocytic pleural effusion is the sole manifestation of tuberculosis infection[35]; in 20% of those cases, mycobacteria can be isolated with thoracocentesis. In the long-term course, the thickened pleural layers may undergo massive calcification, which persists over decades. This can cause considerable shrinkage of the affected hemithorax (▶Fig. 5.34).

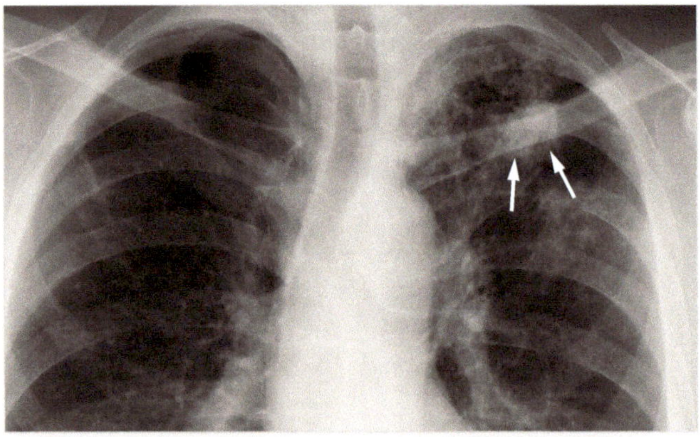

Fig. 5.30 Exudative consolidation in tuberculosis. Magnified section of radiograph. Area of ill-defined, retroclavicular consolidation in the left upper lobe (*arrows*).

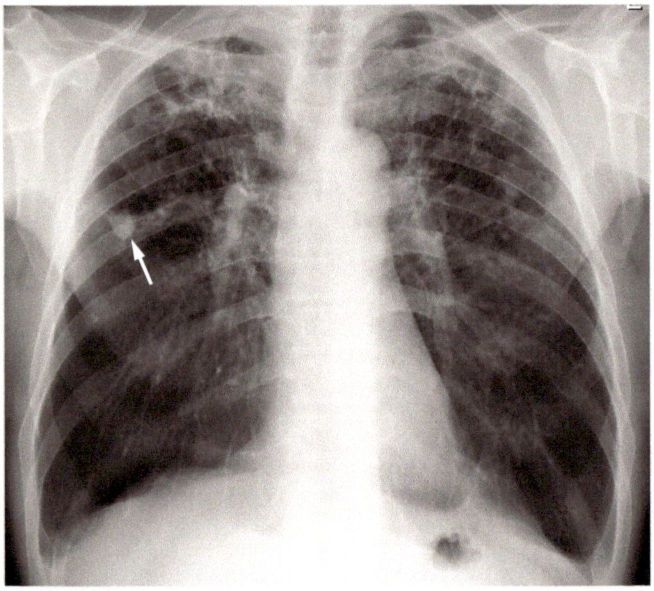

Fig. 5.31 Simon foci in both upper lobes in tuberculosis. Radiograph. Sharply marginated nodular opacity in both apices of lung; also Ghon focus in the right middle zone (*arrow*).

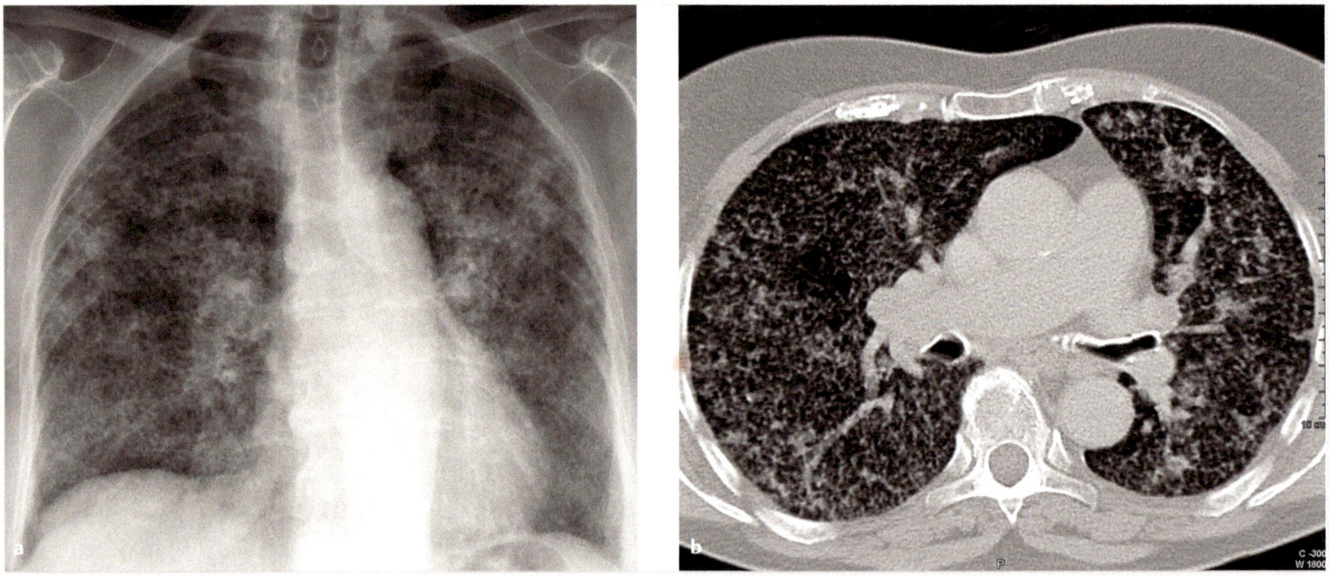

Fig. 5.32 Miliary tuberculosis with miliary pattern. (a) Radiograph: diffuse, bilateral micronodular pattern. **(b)** CT image: numerous, sharply marginated, randomly distributed micronodular nodules.

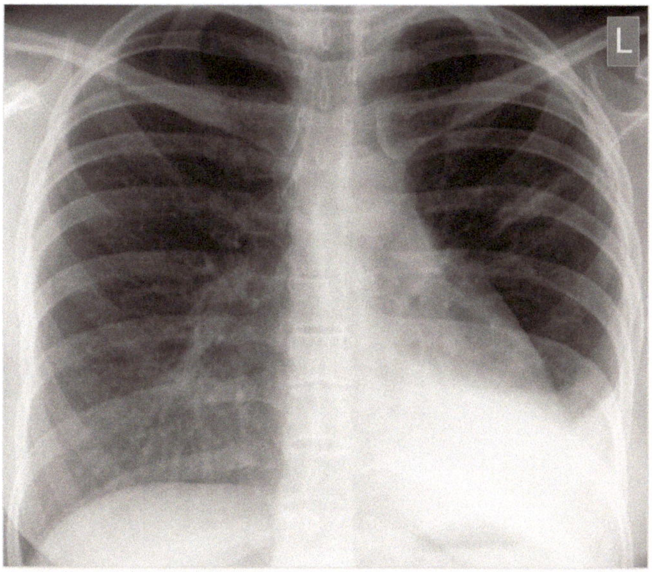

Fig. 5.33 Tuberculous pleurisy. Radiograph. Left pleural effusion, as sole evidence on radiograph of tuberculosis infection.

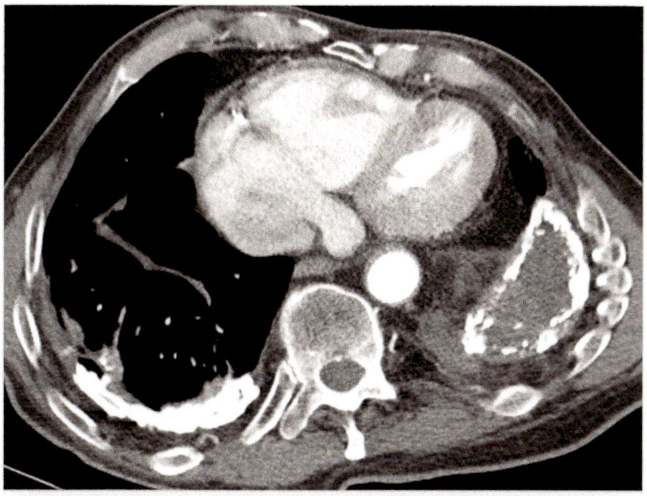

Fig. 5.34 Calcified tuberculous pleurisy. CT image. Extensive bilateral calcification of parietal and visceral pleura. Massive shrinkage of left hemithorax.

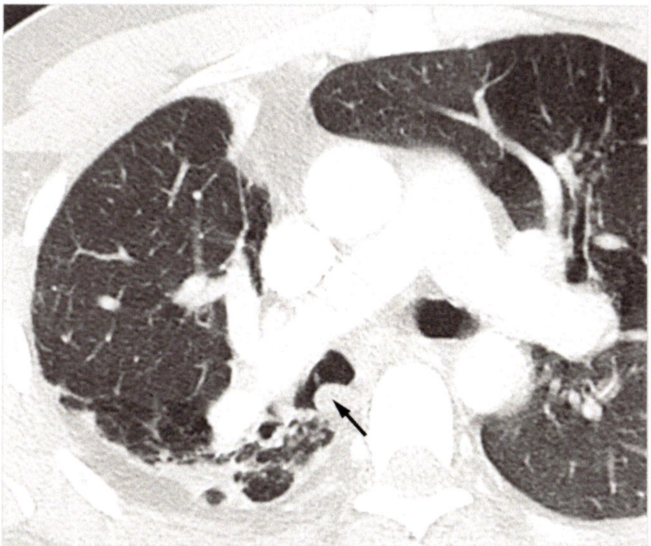

Fig. 5.35 Bronchogenic dissemination of tuberculosis. CT image. Invasion of right mainstem bronchus by an enlarged tuberculous lymph node (*arrow*). The right lung is smaller due to fibrocirrhotic tuberculosis.

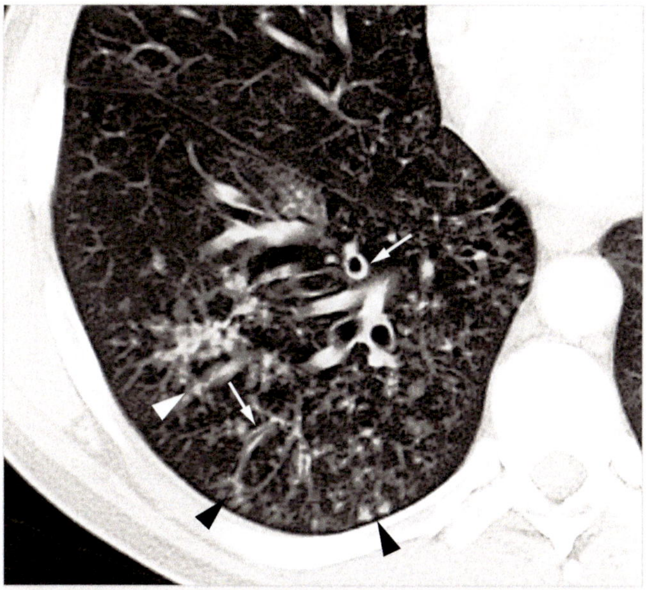

Fig. 5.36 Bronchogenic dissemination of tuberculosis. CT image. Caseous bronchitis with thickening of bronchial walls (*arrows*) and pronounced tree-in-bud pattern in the right lower lobe indicating inflammation of small bronchi and bronchioles (*arrowheads*).

In the subsequent course of infection, the disease spreads, as described above, in two ways:

- *Late hematogenous generalization*: Mycobacteria can now be carried in the bloodstream from lung regions with manifest tuberculosis or from the infected hilar or mediastinal lymph nodes via the thoracic duct. Embarking on such a route, tuberculosis infection can be spread to other organs (preferentially the thoracic and lumbar vertebral column, less frequently to other bones, meninges, the liver, kidneys, adrenal glands, urinary tract, genital tract). Besides, massive bacteremia can give rise to miliary tuberculosis (see above).
- *Late bronchogenic generalization*: Mycobacteria can gain access to the bronchi via perforation of necrosis into the bronchial system, where they cause inflammatory changes (caseous bronchitis). Also, infected hilar lymph nodes may infiltrate the bronchial system (▸Fig. 5.35) and cause bronchogenic spread of bacteria from the lymph nodes. Radiographic signs of endobronchial spread include wall thickening of the major bronchi (▸Fig. 5.36) and tree-in-bud pattern due to involvement of the minor bronchi and bronchioles.

Organ Stage

Advanced organ stage of pulmonary tuberculosis generally reflects a mixture of the aforementioned transmission routes. Four, also coexisting, types can merge into each other:

- *Exudative pulmonary tuberculosis*: Failure to contain infection in granulomas will result in caseous pneumonia with, in some cases, extensive consolidation and ground-glass opacities (▸Fig. 5.37).

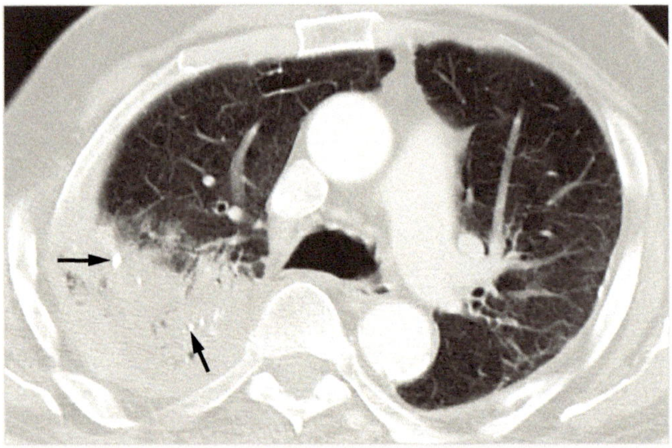

Fig. 5.37 Exudative tuberculosis. CT image. Extensive consolidation in the right lower lobe. Small calcified granulomas within the consolidation (*arrows*).

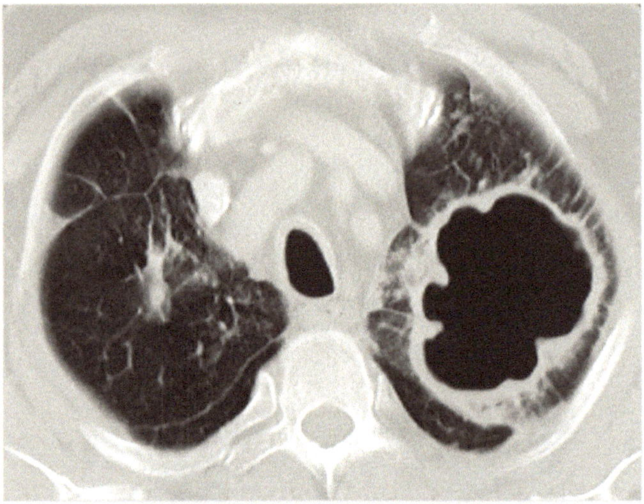

Fig. 5.39 Cavitary tuberculosis. CT image. Extensive cavitation in the left upper lobe.

- *Productive pulmonary tuberculosis*: An intact immune system is usually able to contain the infection foci in granulomas (tuberculomas), thus "producing" tuberculomas. Radiologically, these are seen as multiple, sharply marginated nodules (▶ Fig. 5.38).
- *Cavitary pulmonary tuberculosis*: Extension of colliquative necroses into the bronchial system leads to cavitation, with cavities measuring up to several centimeters (▶ Fig. 5.39). At the same time, dissemination of the cavity content gives rise to bronchogenic distribution of the mycobacteria.
- *Fibrocirrhotic pulmonary tuberculosis*: Chronic inflammation causes coarse fibrotic changes which, in turn, lead to shrinkage of the affected lung regions (▶ Fig. 5.40). Scar emphysema and bronchiectasis are typical concomitant findings.

Reactivation and Reinfection

Mycobacteria can survive for years to decades inside granulomas without ever causing clinically manifest disease. Impairment of the patient's immune response even after a very

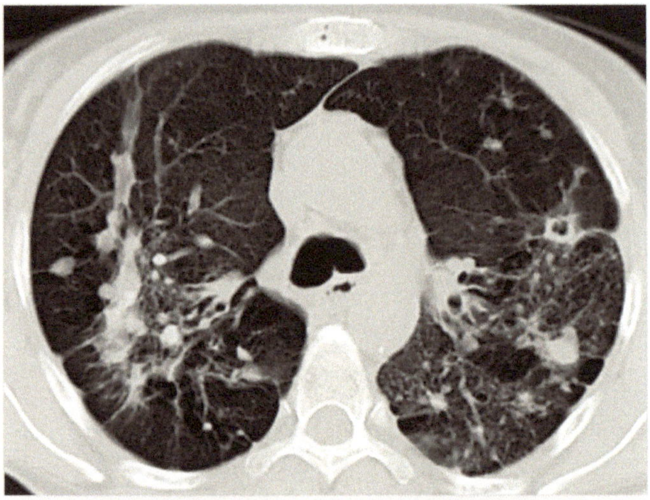

Fig. 5.38 Productive tuberculosis. CT image. Sharply marginated nodules in both upper lobes.

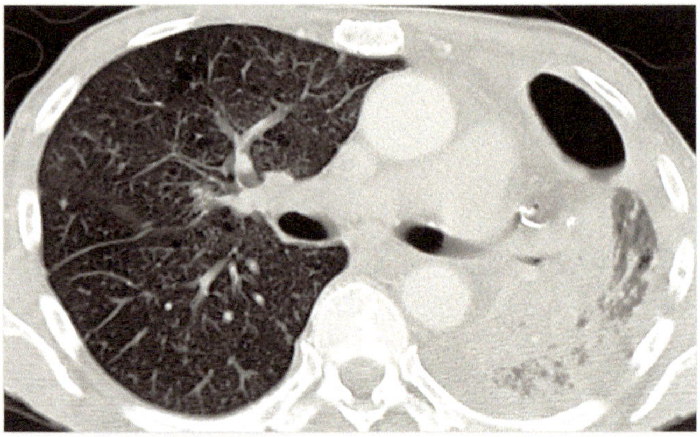

Fig. 5.40 Fibrocirrhotic tuberculosis. CT image. Cirrhotic shrinkage of the left lung with consolidation and mediastinal displacement toward the left.

long time can trigger reactivation of tuberculosis. *Endogenous reactivation* of previous primary tuberculosis represents the most common form of postprimary tuberculosis in the native population in most developed countries. By contrast, younger patients from tuberculosis-endemic regions undergo *exogenous reinfection*.

Patients without AIDS disease and AIDS patients with preserved cellular immunity show some special features of postprimary pulmonary tuberculosis compared with primary infection:

- Lymphadenopathy is rare and seen only in around 5% of cases.[36]
- Tuberculosis infiltrates are typically localized in the apical and posterior upper lobe segments as well as in the apical lower lobe segments (▶ Fig. 5.41).[37]
- Cavitation is more prevalent in postprimary (50%) than in primary infection (less than 30%).[36]

AIDS patients with reduced cellular immune responses have virtually no immunologic memory. This means that lymphadenopathy does not regress in the course of infection but often persists in the postprimary phase (▶ Fig. 5.42). Cavitation is rare in these patients.

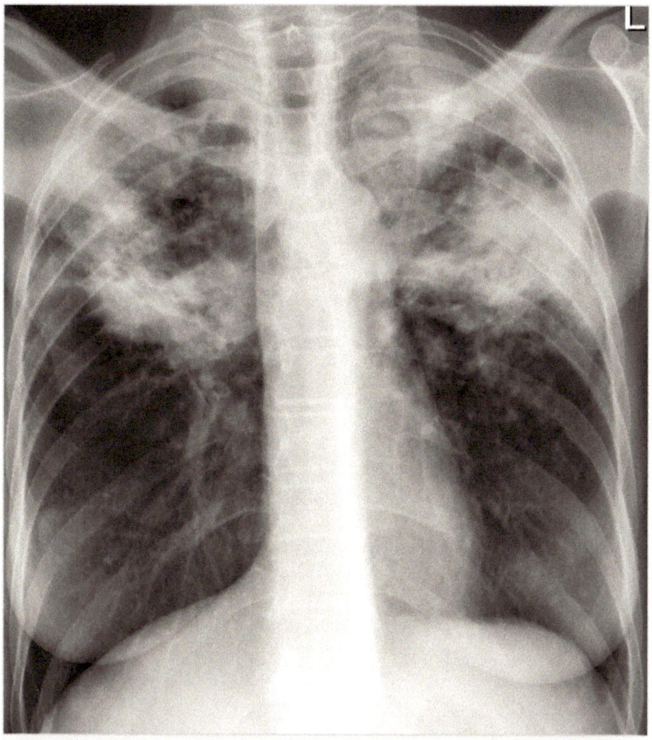

Fig. 5.41 **Postprimary tuberculosis.** Radiograph. Consolidations in both upper lobes, in particular in segments 1 and 2.

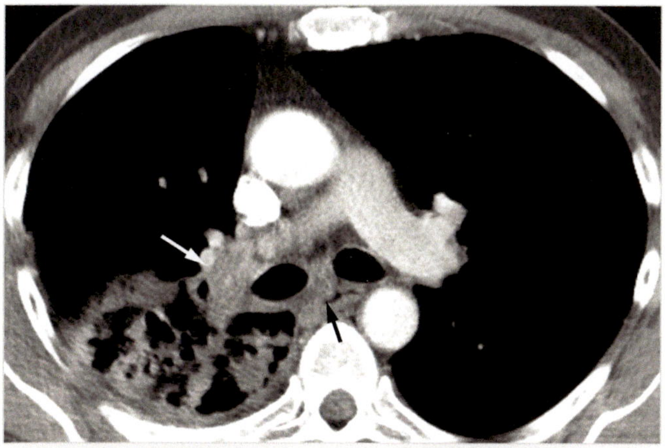

Fig. 5.42 **Postprimary tuberculous lymphadenopathy in AIDS patient.** CT image. Right hilar and subcarinal lymphadenopathy (*arrows*). Extensive consolidation in the right upper lobe.

Active and Open Tuberculosis

Active tuberculosis is present if mycobacterial infection causes disease symptoms (cough, hemoptysis, fever, night sweats, or weight loss). If tuberculostatic treatment has not yet been initiated, mycobacteria can be found in sputum, tracheal and bronchial secretions, or gastric juice at the time of diagnosis. The most sensitive detection method is bacteriologic culture, which is the gold standard for diagnosis of active tuberculosis. However, the culture results are available only after 2 to 6 weeks. While mycobacteria can be rapidly identified in body fluids on microscopy, this method is much less sensitive than bacteriologic culture. The tuberculin skin test and γ-interferon test (interferon-γ release assay, IGRA) are two indirect immunologic assays that yield results within hours to a few days. But their sensitivity and specificity are lower than those of culture isolation techniques.

If mycobacteria are found in the patient's body fluids in such high numbers as to be detectable already on microscopy, the infection is classified as *open tuberculosis*. The patient has to be considered as potentially highly infective since pathogens spread in droplets into the ambient air can survive in an infectious state for several hours. As such, the term *open tuberculosis* is clinically defined. Open tuberculosis can be suspected from the imaging results if cavitation is seen in untreated tuberculosis. The cavity content harbors mycobacteria which, if there is extension into the bronchial system, can be coughed up into the environment. Normally, within 3 weeks of starting treatment, open tuberculosis will have evolved to closed tuberculosis, which is no longer highly infectious.

Tuberculosis activity is difficult to assess radiographically. ▸Table 5.8 (left column) gives a summary of the radiologic signs that in a well-defined clinical condition (e.g., as part of an environmental investigation) can serve as criteria for active tuberculosis yielding a sensitivity of 87% and specificity of 89%. If the signs of active or inactive tuberculosis listed in ▸Table 5.8 (right column) are taken into account additionally, sensitivity rises to 98% but at the expense of specificity, which drops to just 75%.[38] Stability of the imaging findings over at least 4 to 6 months is considered a reliable sign of inactivity.[37,39,40] In exceptional cases, disease can still be active if the radiographic findings remain unchanged over an even longer period of time.[37]

Note

Characteristic signs of active tuberculosis on CT[37,41]:

- Centrilobular, branching opacities.
- Lobular consolidation.
- Centrilobular nodules.
- Tree-in-bud pattern.
- Cavitation.
- Ground-glass opacities.

Unfortunately, these findings are also seen in a relevant proportion of inactive tuberculosis cases, making it impossible to reliably distinguish active from inactive disease radiologically; instead, identification of mycobacteria in clinical specimen (e.g., sputum) is required.[37]

Table 5.8 Findings on radiograph indicative of active tuberculosis (left column) or of active or inactive tuberculosis (right column).

Radiographic signs of active tuberculosis	Radiographic signs of active or inactive tuberculosis
• Consolidation • Ground-glass opacity • Cavitation • Poorly marginated nodules • Pleural effusion • Hilar or mediastinal lymphadenopathy • Miliary pattern	• Noncalcified nodules • Linear opacities (fibrotic scars) • Volume loss and retraction • Bronchiectasis in the upper lobes • Calcified nodules[a]

[a]Calcified nodules can be deemed as definitively inactive; their transition to active tuberculosis is not expected.

Complications

As a sequela of fungal colonization, aspergillomas can grow in old tuberculosis cavities or, less frequently, in areas of bronchiectasis. These attract clinical attention through hemoptysis, which is fatal in 5% of cases.[37,42]

Cavitation can erode pulmonary arteries, giving rise to *pseudoaneurysms* called Rasmussen aneurysms (▶ Fig. 5.43). Aneurysmatic rupture can at times cause life-threatening hemoptysis.[37,43,44]

Cavitation-mediated pleural erosion causes spontaneous pneumothorax, resulting in turn in a *bronchopleural fistula* (▶ Fig. 5.44).

Extensive tuberculous destruction of the lung causes rarefaction of the pulmonary capillary bed. This leads to pulmonary hypertension and onset of *chronic pulmonary heart disease.*

Invasion of the chest wall by pleural empyema can result in extensive suppurative inflammation known as *empyema necessitatis* (or *empyema necessitans*) (▶ Fig. 5.45).[45,46]

Assessment of Treatment Response

Whether patients with an initial *positive sputum test* have responded to treatment is best clinically determined by repeat sputum analysis; a negative sputum test is interpreted as a sign of successful treatment. Conversely, radiologic follow-up during treatment is less useful. However, obtaining radiographic evidence on completion of treatment is advisable as this documents what has been achieved with treatment and serves as a baseline for future assessment to diagnose reactivation of tuberculosis.[37,47]

If the *sputum test is initially negative*, radiologic follow-up scans and the clinical condition are the most important parameters for ongoing assessment of treatment response. Radiographic deterioration of pulmonary opacities and progressive lymphadenopathy within the first 3 months is seen in one-third of pediatric patients[48] and occasionally in adult patients. Overall, regression of radiographic findings is slow. After 3 months, lack of improvement of imaging results can be interpreted as treatment failure in adults and is suggestive of tuberculostatic resistance or an intervening pathologic process, e.g., a superinfection.[37] Regression of the radiologic findings takes up to 2 years; lymphadenopathy may persist for even longer.[37,48]

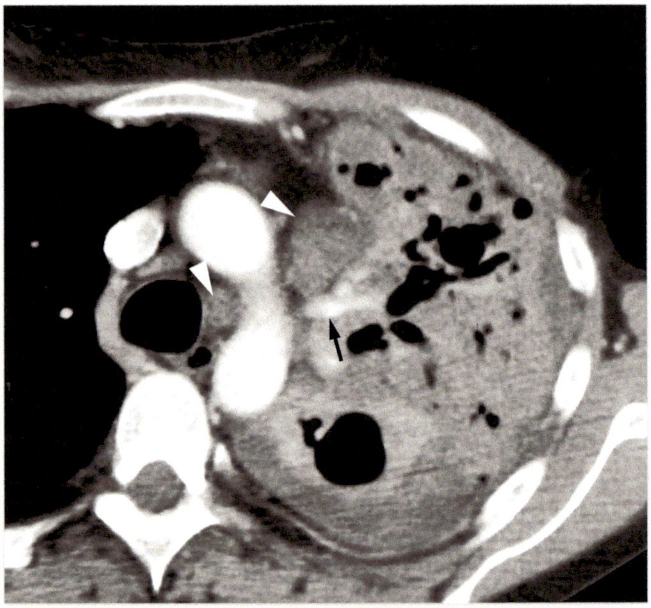

Fig. 5.43 Pulmonary artery pseudoaneurysm (*arrow*) in the left upper lobe, showing tuberculous destruction and extensive cavitation. CT image. Besides, mediastinal lymphadenopathy (*arrowheads*).

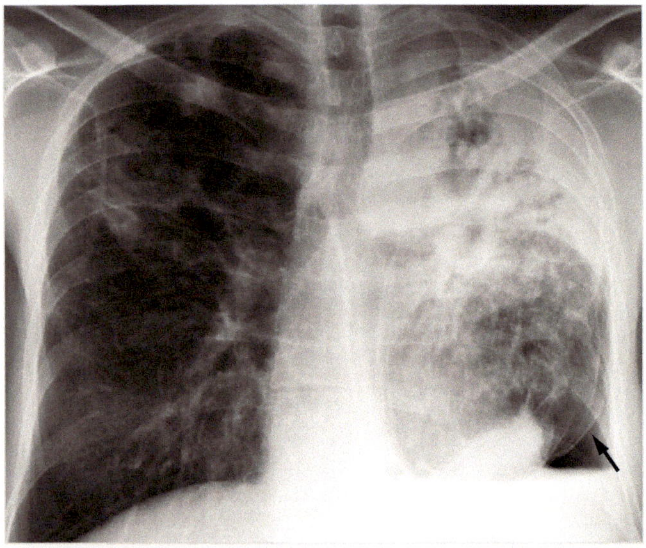

Fig. 5.44 Spontaneous pneumothorax (*arrow*) secondary to a bronchopleural fistula in the left upper lobe, showing tuberculous destruction. Radiograph.

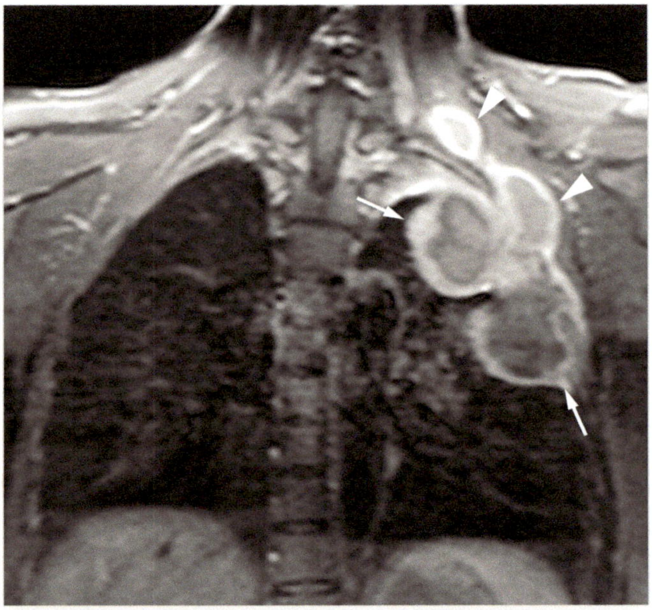

Fig. 5.45 Chest wall abscesses (*arrowheads*) secondary to tuberculous pleural empyema (*arrows*). Coronal T1w contrast-enhanced MR image. Marked contrast medium uptake by the abscess walls and the region of pleural empyema.

Findings Related to Old Treatment Methods

Tuberculostatics have been available since the mid-1940s. Prior to that, efforts were made to heal the diseased lung by bringing the infection to a halt. The sequelae of such therapeutic measures can still be seen today; hence, they are briefly addressed below:

- *Plombage* (▸Fig. 5.46): Subpleural deposition of large quantities of paraffin compressed the diseased lung and it was hoped that this would halt infection.
- *Thoracoplasty* (▸Fig. 5.47): Surgical rib resection was performed to reduce the size of the affected hemithorax and thus halt infection in the diseased lung. Marked volume reduction of one hemithorax and multiple rib resections can be identified radiologically.

Often, these findings are interspersed with the residual findings of coexisting tuberculosis.

5.4.2 Atypical Mycobacteriosis

Atypical mycobacteriosis is caused by mycobacteria that are different from those that cause tuberculosis and leprosy. These are known as mycobacteria other than tuberculosis (MOTT). MOTT mycobacteria are ubiquitous and most are saprophytes. Lung infection is predominantly caused by *Mycobacterium kansasii* or by mycobacteria belonging to the *Mycobacterium avium intracellulare* complex (MAC).[49–52] Infection is transmitted via the airborne route from the ambient environment. Unlike tuberculosis, person-to-person transmission has no role apart from in AIDS patients in whom the lung can become infected from the gastrointestinal tract through bacteremia.[50,52]

Nonpathogenic colonization is common, in particular, in association with bronchiectasis and pulmonary emphysema. Therefore, a positive microbial test result is not sufficient grounds for initiating treatment.

> **Note**
>
> The American Thoracic Society has defined the following criteria for MOTT infection[51,53]:
>
> - *Pulmonary opacities with cavitation*: Two or more sputums or bronchial washings that are acid-fast bacilli smear positive or produce moderate-to-heavy growth on culture.
> - *Pulmonary opacities without cavitation*: Two or more sputums or bronchial washings that are acid-fast bacilli smear positive or produce moderate to heavy growth on culture and the isolate is *M. kansasii* or a MAC species and cannot be cleared from the sputum with either bronchial hygiene or 2-week drug therapy.
> - Mycobacterial isolation from lung biopsy.[50,53]

Immunocompetent patients exhibit two different characteristic clinical and radiologic *disease patterns* (▸Table 5.9). Their symptoms are similar, mainly with cough and hemoptysis of insidious onset[50–54]:

- *Classic MOTT infection* (▸Fig. 5.48): This infection mimics findings of tuberculosis. It mainly affects patients between the ages of 50 and 70 years who have underlying pulmonary diseases (chronic obstructive lung disease) or other risk factors (smoking, alcoholism). Fever and weight loss are observed. Diffuse hematogenous dissemination as seen in miliary tuberculosis is rare.

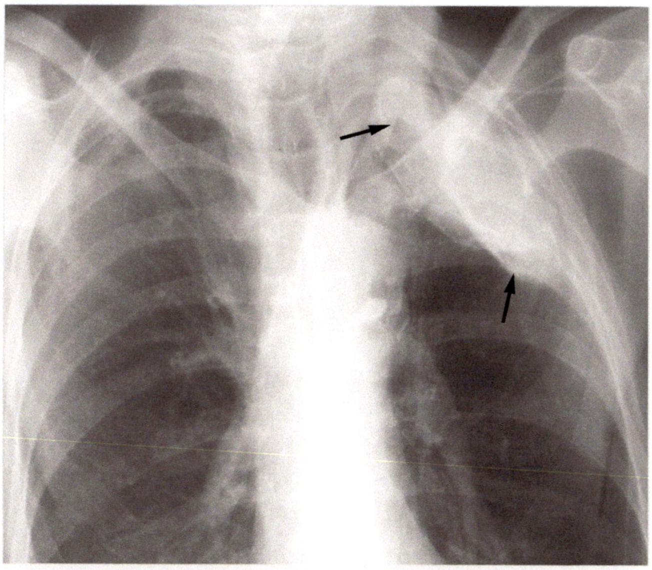

Fig. 5.46 Plombage (*arrows*) for compression of the left upper lobe. Magnified section of radiograph. Smoothly marginated lateral opacity in the left upper zone.

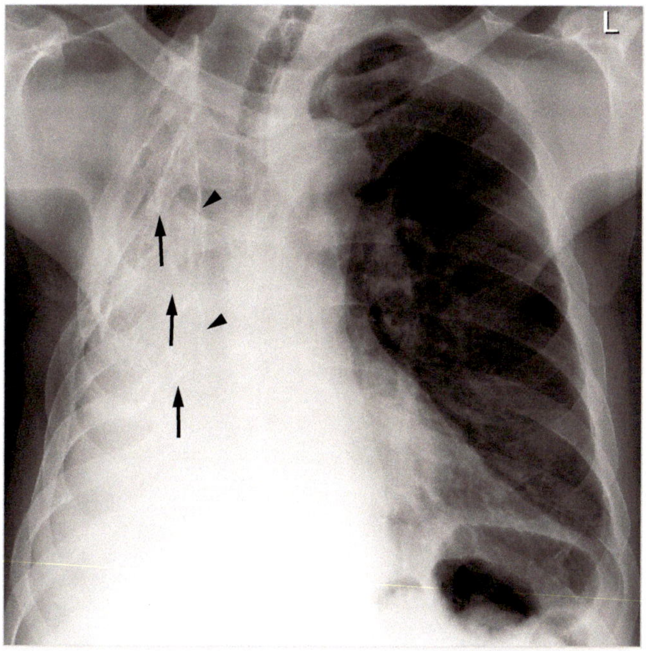

Fig. 5.47 Thoracoplasty of the right hemithorax. Radiograph. Posterolateral resected rib segments identifiable (*arrows*); besides, calcified pleurisy as remnant of tuberculosis (*arrowheads*).

II

Table 5.9 Radiologic findings of atypical mycobacteriosis in the case of immunocompetent patients[50–55]

Classic MOTT infection	Nonclassic MOTT infection
• Apical consolidation and nodules • Apical scars • Cavitation • Pleural thickening • Endobronchial dissemination (tree-in-bud pattern, centrilobular nodules) • Occasionally, pleural effusion and lymphadenopathy	• Multiple bilateral, poorly marginated, randomly distributed nodules • No apical predominance • Bronchiectasis, especially in the middle lobe and lingula

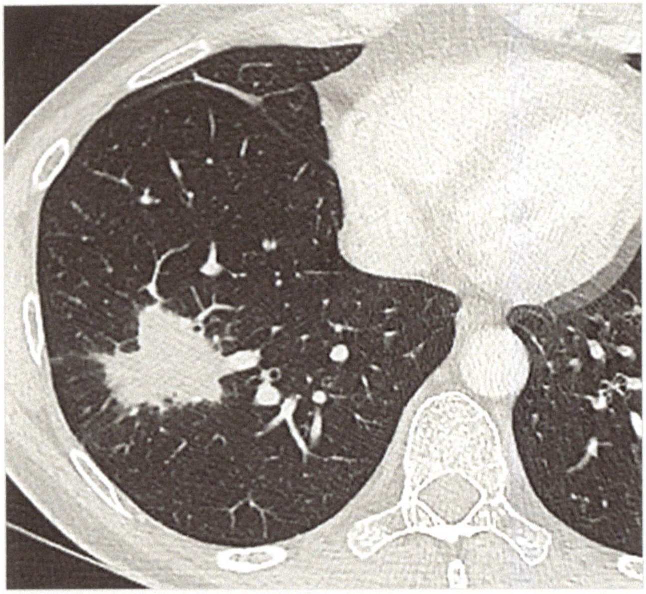

Fig. 5.48 Atypical mycobacteriosis. CT image. Classic MOTT infection with area of consolidation, as seen in primary tuberculosis, in the right lower lobe.

- *Nonclassic MOTT infection* (▶ Fig. 5.49): In 20 to 30% of cases, no predisposing diseases are present. This disease type is observed predominantly in women aged around 70 years. Fever is rare. This disease is typically caused by MAC pathogens.

The disease findings seen radiologically for immunosuppressed patients, in particular *AIDS patients*, are similar to those of primary tuberculosis. A proportion of MAC infections originate from the gastrointestinal tract. Hence, a miliary pattern, as in miliary tuberculosis, is seen in cases of diffuse hematogenous dissemination.

5.5 Summary

Pneumonia is a disease involving microbial inflammation of the lung parenchyma. It heals without any sequelae (*restitutio ad integrum*) or results in the lung parenchyma being replaced by nonfunctional scar tissue (*restitutio cum defectu*, carnified pneumonia). Depending on its origin, a distinction is made between community-acquired, hospital-acquired, and opportunistic pneumonia:

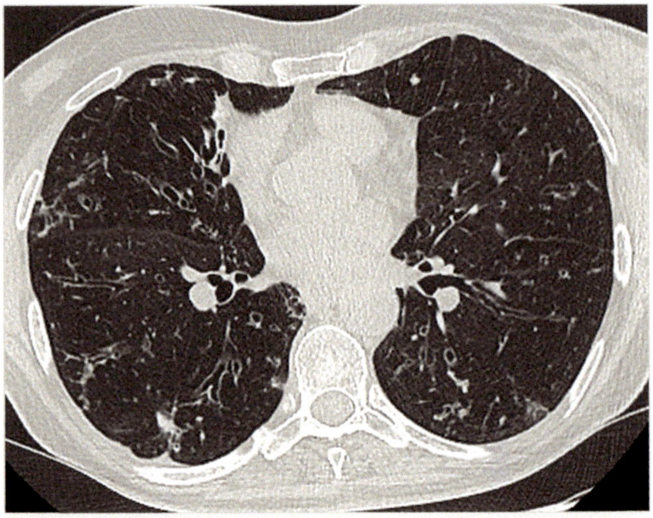

Fig. 5.49 Atypical mycobacteriosis. CT image. Nonclassic MOTT infection with bronchiectasis, tree-in-bud pattern, and multiple small nodules.

- *Community-acquired pneumonia*: This is usually classified as either typical or atypical pneumonia. Typical pneumonia exhibits the classic clinical picture of pneumonia (fever with shaking chills, cough, purulent sputum, reduced general condition). The implicated pathogens are generally bacteria (pneumococci, staphylococci). Atypical pneumonia presents with flu-like symptoms and only moderate fever and the main causative pathogens are obligate intracellular bacteria (chlamydiae, mycoplasma, legionellae) or viruses (in particular influenza viruses A and B). Pneumonia diagnosis requires evidence of a pulmonary opacity on a chest radiograph in two views. Radiologic follow-up examination may be considered at the earliest 2 weeks after ending treatment, except for milder courses of disease. CT has a diagnostic role only in the event of complications (progressive pneumonia, delayed-response pneumonia, and suspected lung abscess). Thoracocentesis is needed for large pleural effusions. Treatment-refractory lung abscesses can be drained with imaging guidance (CT or fluoroscopy).
- *Hospital-acquired (nosocomial) pneumonia*: This presents at least 48 hours after the patient's admission to the hospital. It is particularly prevalent in intensive care units as a complication of mechanical ventilation. The microbial spectrum of hospital-acquired pneumonia differs from that implicated in community-acquired pneumonia. Hospital-acquired pneumonia is mainly attributed to hospital-specific, often multidrug resistant, bacterial pathogens. Differential diagnosis from pulmonary opacities of other genesis is difficult, in particular in intensive care patients (see ▶ Table 5.4). Access to clinical and laboratory data is useful for differential diagnosis. Discussion of the radiologic findings with the referring clinician will make it easier to achieve a correct diagnosis.
- *Opportunistic pneumonia*: This affects immunosuppressed patients. The spectrum of opportunistic pathogens differs in accordance with the underlying cause of immunosuppression (e.g., AIDS, treatment-related in the wake of chemotherapy, radiotherapy, or high-dose cortisone treatment, after stem cell and organ transplantations), and is also a function of the nature of the ensuing immunodeficiency.

Identification of rare types of pathogens is also common.
Typical disease manifestations:
- Fungal pneumonia in aplastic patients (especially invasive pulmonary aspergillosis and *Candida* pneumonia).
- *P. jirovecii* pneumonia is often the first manifestation of AIDS disease.
- Viral pneumonia in transplant patients.

Mycobacteriosis is found worldwide, and together with malaria and AIDS, tuberculosis is the most common infectious disease. However, in developed countries there are few new cases of tuberculosis. The disease course consists of three stages:

- *Primary tuberculosis*: This presents as a pulmonary opacity with concomitant lymphadenopathy (primary complex). In 95% of cases, it heals after an almost asymptomatic course. In 5% of cases, it evolves to progressive primary infection, manifesting as hilar lymph node tuberculosis or progressive infection of the primary focus.
- *Generalization*: Generalization initially takes place hematogenously, typically bilaterally into the lung segments 1, 2, and 6, and is at times diffuse (miliary tuberculosis). Other organs may also be affected. Later, the disease is spread via the bronchi (bronchogenic dissemination).
- *Organ stage*: During this stage, tuberculosis continues to spread in the lungs, generally exhibiting a mixed pattern of hematogenous, lymphogenic, bronchogenic, and continuous spread. It is mainly only at this stage that tuberculosis is diagnosed.

The last two stages are collectively known as "postprimary tuberculosis." Lymphadenopathy is now much less frequent but cavitation is more common than in primary tuberculosis.

Identification of the remnants of old tuberculosis is a common incidental finding on radiographs, especially manifesting as calcified primary complex or calcified pleural thickening. The disease can be reactivated at any time from these residual repositories if there is a decline in immune defense.

Atypical mycobacteriosis embarks on two courses in immunocompetent patients: one is similar to tuberculosis (classic) and the other is characterized by nodules and bronchiectasis (nonclassic). Immunocompromised patients exhibit a disease pattern similar to that of primary tuberculosis.

References

[1] Mandell LA, Wunderink RG, Anzueto A, et al; Infectious Diseases Society of America. American Thoracic Society. Infectious Diseases Society of America/American Thoracic Society consensus guidelines on the management of community-acquired pneumonia in adults. Clin Infect Dis 2007;44(Suppl 2):S27–S72

[2] van Sonnenberg E, D'Agostino HB, Casola G, Wittich GR, Varney RR, Harker C. Lung abscess: CT-guided drainage. Radiology 1991;178(2):347–351

[3] Kim EA, Lee KS, Primack SL, et al. Viral pneumonias in adults: radiologic and pathologic findings. Radiographics 2002;22(Spec No):S137–S149

[4] Lim WS, van der Eerden MM, Laing R, et al. Defining community acquired pneumonia severity on presentation to hospital: an international derivation and validation study. Thorax 2003;58(5):377–382

[5] Franquet T. Imaging of pneumonia: trends and algorithms. Eur Respir J 2001;18(1):196–208

[6] Tomiyama N, Müller NL, Johkoh T, et al. Acute parenchymal lung disease in immunocompetent patients: diagnostic accuracy of high-resolution CT. AJR Am J Roentgenol 2000;174(6):1745–1750

[7] Torres A, Niederman MS, Chastre J, et al. International ERS/ESICM/ESCMID/ALAT guidelines for the management of hospital-acquired pneumonia and ventilator-associated pneumonia: Guidelines for the management of hospital-acquired pneumonia (HAP)/ventilator-associated pneumonia (VAP) of the European Respiratory Society (ERS), European Society of Intensive Care Medicine (ESICM), European Society of Clinical Microbiology and Infectious Diseases (ESCMID) and Asociación Latinoamericana del Tórax (ALAT). Eur Respir J 2017;50(3):1700582

[8] Wormanns D. Chest radiography: performance, indications and interpretation. In: Barr RG, Parr D, Vogel-Claussen J, eds. Imaging (ERS Monograph). Sheffield: European Respiratory Society; 2015

[9] Beigelman-Aubry C, Godet C, Caumes E. Lung infections: the radiologist's perspective. Diagn Interv Imaging 2012;93(6):431–440

[10] Herbert PA, Bayer AS. Fungal pneumonia (Part 4): invasive pulmonary aspergillosis. Chest 1981;80(2):220–225

[11] Beyer F, Wormanns D. Imaging of pneumonia Radiologe 2011;51(5):405–416, quiz 417–418

[12] Tuengerthal S. The radiology of opportunistic pneumonias. I: Epidemiological, laboratory and clinical background Radiologe 2005;45(4):373–383, quiz 384

[13] Buckingham SJ, Hansell DM. Aspergillus in the lung: diverse and coincident forms. Eur Radiol 2003;13(8):1786–1800

[14] Orr DP, Myerowitz RL, Dubois PJ. Patho-radiologic correlation of invasive pulmonary aspergillosis in the compromised host. Cancer 1978;41(5):2028–2039

[15] Kuhlman JE, Fishman EK, Siegelman SS. Invasive pulmonary aspergillosis in acute leukemia: characteristic findings on CT, the CT halo sign, and the role of CT in early diagnosis. Radiology 1985;157(3):611–614

[16] Albelda SM, Talbot GH, Gerson SL, Miller WT, Cassileth PA. Pulmonary cavitation and massive hemoptysis in invasive pulmonary aspergillosis. Influence of bone marrow recovery in patients with acute leukemia. Am Rev Respir Dis 1985;131(1):115–120

[17] Kim MJ, Lee KS, Kim J, Jung KJ, Lee HG, Kim TS. Crescent sign in invasive pulmonary aspergillosis: frequency and related CT and clinical factors. J Comput Assist Tomogr 2001;25(2):305–310

[18] Logan PM, Primack SL, Miller RR, Müller NL. Invasive aspergillosis of the airways: radiographic, CT, and pathologic findings. Radiology 1994;193(2):383–388

[19] Binder RE, Faling LJ, Pugatch RD, Mahasaen C, Snider GL. Chronic necrotizing pulmonary aspergillosis: a discrete clinical entity. Medicine (Baltimore) 1982;61(2):109–124

[20] Franquet T, Müller NL, Giménez A, Domingo P, Plaza V, Bordes R. Semi-invasive pulmonary aspergillosis in chronic obstructive pulmonary disease: radiologic and pathologic findings in nine patients. AJR Am J Roentgenol 2000;174(1):51–56

[21] Gefter WB, Weingrad TR, Epstein DM, Ochs RH, Miller WT. "Semi-invasive" pulmonary aspergillosis: a new look at the spectrum of aspergillus infections of the lung. Radiology 1981;140(2):313–321

[22] Frenkel JK. Pneumocystis jiroveci n. sp. from man: morphology, physiology, and immunology in relation to pathology. Natl Cancer Inst Monogr 1976;43:13–30

[23] Vanek J, Jirovec O. Parasitäre Pneumonie. Interstitielle Plasmazellenpneumonie der Frühgeborenen, verursacht durch Pneumodystis Carinii. Zentralbl Bakteriol Orig 1952;158(1)(-)(2):120–127

[24] Thomas CF Jr, Limper AH. Pneumocystis pneumonia. N Engl J Med 2004;350(24):2487–2498

[25] DeLorenzo LJ, Huang CT, Maguire GP, Stone DJ. Roentgenographic patterns of Pneumocystis carinii pneumonia in 104 patients with AIDS. Chest 1987;91(3):323–327

[26] Gruden JF, Huang L, Turner J, et al. High-resolution CT in the evaluation of clinically suspected Pneumocystis carinii pneumonia in AIDS patients with normal, equivocal, or nonspecific radiographic findings. AJR Am J Roentgenol 1997;169(4):967–975

[27] Kanne JP, Yandow DR, Meyer CA. Pneumocystis jiroveci pneumonia: high-resolution CT findings in patients with and without HIV infection. AJR Am J Roentgenol 2012;198(6):W555–61

[28] Hardak E, Brook O, Yigla M. Radiological features of Pneumocystis jirovecii Pneumonia in immunocompromised patients with and without AIDS. Hai 2010;188(2):159–163

[29] Kovacs JA, Hiemenz JW, Macher AM, et al. Pneumocystis carinii pneumonia: a comparison between patients with the acquired immunodeficiency syndrome and patients with other immunodeficiencies. Ann Intern Med 1984;100(5):663–671

[30] Rohmann K, Drömann D. Viruspneumonie bei immuninkompetenten Patienten. Pneumologe 2013;10:335–340

[31] Boeckh M. The challenge of respiratory virus infections in hematopoietic cell transplant recipients. Br J Haematol 2008;143(4):455–467

[32] Ison MG, Hayden FG. Viral infections in immunocompromised patients: what's new with respiratory viruses? Curr Opin Infect Dis 2002;15(4):355–367

[33] Mitnick CD, Shin SS, Seung KJ, et al. Comprehensive treatment of extensively drug-resistant tuberculosis. N Engl J Med 2008;359(6):563–574

[34] Lillebaek T, Andersen AB, Dirksen A, Glynn JR, Kremer K. Mycobacterium tuberculosis Beijing genotype. Emerg Infect Dis 2003;9(12):1553–1557

[35] Choyke PL, Sostman HD, Curtis AM, et al. Adult-onset pulmonary tuberculosis. Radiology 1983;148(2):357–362

[36] Woodring JH, Vandiviere HM, Fried AM, Dillon ML, Williams TD, Melvin IG. Update: the radiographic features of pulmonary tuberculosis. AJR Am J Roentgenol 1986;146(3):497–506

[37] Leung AN. Pulmonary tuberculosis: the essentials. Radiology 1999; 210(2):307–322

[38] World Health Organization. Systematic Screening for Active Tuberculosis: Principles and Recommendations. Geneva: World Health Organization; 2013

[39] American Thoracic Society. American Thoracic Society. Diagnostic standards and classification of tuberculosis. Am Rev Respir Dis 1990;142(3):725–735

[40] Miller WT, MacGregor RR. Tuberculosis: frequency of unusual radiographic findings. AJR Am J Roentgenol 1978;130(5):867–875

[41] Lee KS, Hwang JW, Chung MP, Kim H, Kwon OJ. Utility of CT in the evaluation of pulmonary tuberculosis in patients without AIDS. Chest 1996;110(4):977–984

[42] Fraser RS. Pulmonary aspergillosis: pathologic and pathogenetic features. Pathol Annu 1993;28(Pt 1):231–277

[43] Ramakantan R, Bandekar VG, Gandhi MS, Aulakh BG, Deshmukh HL. Massive hemoptysis due to pulmonary tuberculosis: control with bronchial artery embolization. Radiology 1996;200(3):691–694

[44] van den Heuvel MM, van Rensburg JJ. Images in clinical medicine. Rasmussen's aneurysm. N Engl J Med 2006;355(16):e17

[45] Kellie SP. Empyema necessitatis. Chest 2010;138:39A

[46] Lee WS, Jean SS, Bai KJ, Lam C, Hsu CW, Chen RJ. Empyema necessitatis due to Mycobacterium tuberculosis. J Microbiol Immunol Infect 2015;48(4):461–462

[47] Bass JB Jr, Farer LS, Hopewell PC, et al; American Thoracic Society and The Centers for Disease Control and Prevention. Treatment of tuberculosis and tuberculosis infection in adults and children. Am J Respir Crit Care Med 1994;149(5):1359–1374

[48] Leung AN, Müller NL, Pineda PR, FitzGerald JM. Primary tuberculosis in childhood: radiographic manifestations. Radiology 1992;182(1):87–91

[49] Haque AK. The pathology and pathophysiology of mycobacterial infections. J Thorac Imaging 1990;5(2):8–16

[50] Miller WT Jr. Spectrum of pulmonary nontuberculous mycobacterial infection. Radiology 1994;191(2):343–350

[51] Webb WR, Müller NL, Naidich DP. High-Resolution CT of the Lung. 4 ed. Philadelphia, PA: Wolters Kluwer/Lippincott Williams & Wilkins; 2009

[52] Woodring JH, Vandiviere HM. Pulmonary disease caused by nontuberculous mycobacteria. J Thorac Imaging 1990;5(2):64–76

[53] Wallace RJ, O'Brien R, Glassroth J, et al. Diagnosis and treatment of disease caused by nontuberculous mycobacteria. Am Rev Respir Dis 1990;142(4):940–953

[54] Christensen EE, Dietz GW, Ahn CH, et al. Pulmonary manifestations of Mycobacterium intracellularis. AJR Am J Roentgenol 1979; 133(1):59–66

[55] Christensen EE, Dietz GW, Ahn CH, Chapman JS, Murry RC, Hurst GA. Radiographic manifestations of pulmonary Mycobacterium kansasii infections. AJR Am J Roentgenol 1978;131(6):985–993

Chapter 6

Diffuse Parenchymal Lung Diseases

6 Diffuse Parenchymal Lung Diseases

A systematic approach to differential diagnosis of diffuse parenchymal lung diseases based on the radiologic findings is given in Chapter 24.

Diffuse parenchymal lung diseases are divided into four groups[1]:

- Parenchymal lung diseases of known origin: These include myriad diseases linked to environmental, occupational, and drug-induced causes as well as pulmonary manifestations of systemic diseases, such as collagen vascular diseases.
- Idiopathic interstitial pneumonias (IIPs): On histology, these are characterized by interstitial inflammation or fibrosis of lung parenchyma. They may exhibit the same histologic pattern as the first group of diseases but their cause is unknown. The most recent IIP classification dates back to 2012 and comprises a structured system with three groups of common IIP, rare IIPs, and unclassifiable IIPs (▶Fig. 6.1). Furthermore, 2 to 20% of IIPs are genetically mediated and are classified as familial IIP.
- Granulomatous diseases: The most prominent disease in this group is sarcoidosis, which is also of unknown origin. Its most salient feature is the formation of granulomas.
- Other forms of diffuse parenchymal lung diseases: These include pulmonary Langerhans cell histiocytosis, lymphangioleiomyomatosis, pulmonary alveolar proteinosis, diffuse types of eosinophilic pneumonia, and various types of vasculitis with pulmonary involvement.

6.1 Idiopathic Interstitial Pneumonias

IIPs are a heterogeneous group of rare, noninfectious inflammatory lung diseases of unknown origin. They are typically associated with a pathologic process of the lung interstitium. These diseases are classified in accordance with their histologic findings and are of highly variable prognosis. The main clinical manifestation is gradually progressive dyspnea.

The *IIP classification* of 2012 by the American Thoracic Society and European Respiratory Society divides the various clinical disease manifestations, including those exhibiting different histologic patterns, into a structured system of several groups:

- Common IIP:
  - Chronic fibrosing *IIP*:
    - Idiopathic pulmonary fibrosis (IPF).
    - Idiopathic nonspecific interstitial pneumonia (NSIP).
  - Acute or subacute fibrosing idiopathic interstitial pneumonia:
    - Acute interstitial pneumonia (AIP).
    - Cryptogenic organizing pneumonia (COP).
  - Smoking-related idiopathic interstitial pneumonia:
    - Respiratory bronchiolitis-interstitial lung disease (RB-ILD).
    - Desquamative interstitial pneumonia (DIP).

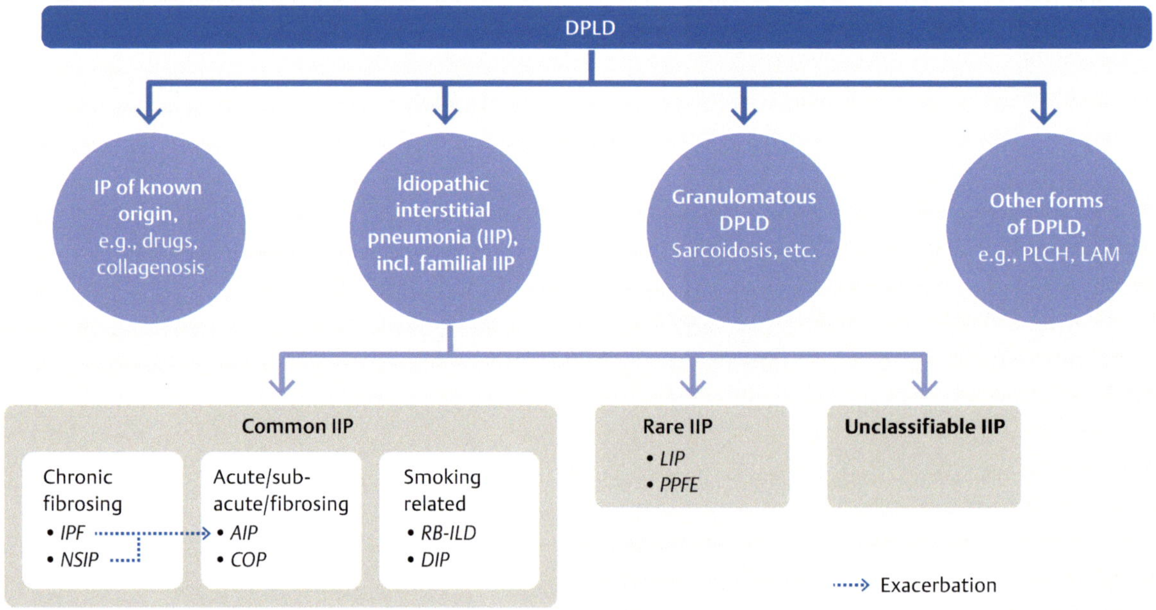

Fig. 6.1 Classification of diffuse parenchymal lung diseases. AIP, acute interstitial pneumonia; COP, cryptogenic organizing pneumonia; DIP, desquamative interstitial pneumonia; DPLD, diffuse parenchymal lung disease; IIP, idiopathic interstitial pneumonias; IP, interstitial pneumonia; IPF, idiopathic pulmonary fibrosis; LAM, lymphangioleiomyomatosis; LIP, lymphoid interstitial pneumonia; NSIP, nonspecific interstitial pneumonia; PLCH, pulmonary Langerhans cell histiocytosis; PPFE, pleuropulmonary fibroelastosis, RB-ILD, respiratory bronchiolitis-interstitial lung disease.

- Rare idiopathic interstitial pneumonia:
  - Idiopathic lymphoid interstitial pneumonia (LIP).
  - Idiopathic pleuroparenchymal fibroelastosis (PPFE).
- Unclassifiable idiopathic interstitial pneumonia.
- Familial idiopathic interstitial pneumonia.

Classification based on the histologic pattern results in ambiguous assignment of clinical disease entities. For example, usual interstitial pneumonia (UIP) is the underlying histologic pattern of idiopathic pulmonary fibrosis. Furthermore, UIP pattern is found in pulmonary manifestations of collagen vascular diseases, especially in rheumatoid arthritis. Therefore, detection of UIP pattern is not sufficient for diagnosis of idiopathic pulmonary fibrosis; differential diagnosis must exclude other causes of usual interstitial pneumonia. Conversely, a clinically defined disease can produce various histological patterns: in rheumatoid arthritis, for example, the patterns of both usual and nonspecific interstitial pneumonia may occur.

▶Table 6.1 summarizes the histological patterns of the common idiopathic interstitial pneumonias and their corresponding clinical disease entities.

Note

In this classification system, radiology is closely related to pathology since both specialties describe finding patterns rather than disease entities. CT findings may be virtually pathognomonic of a histological pattern in some diseases. Additional clinical information is always needed to link a histologic and a radiologic pattern to a specific disease.

6.1.1 The Role of Radiology

An abnormal *chest radiograph* together with a pathologic pulmonary function test usually raises the suspicion of an idiopathic interstitial pneumonia. *CT* is a key component in diagnosis of diffuse parenchymal lung diseases and thus obligatory. The most important contribution of CT is to identify UIP pattern; in this case, lung biopsy is not required to establish the diagnosis. CT is also able to reach a reliable diagnosis for some other diffuse parenchymal lung diseases, such as lymphangioleiomyomatosis.

In the remaining cases, *lung biopsy* is usually necessary for a confident clinic-pathologic diagnosis because CT findings alone do not narrow the differential diagnosis to a single entity.[1] In general, bronchoalveolar lavage makes little contribution to diagnosis but can be useful for differential diagnosis; at times, transbronchial biopsy yields enough lung tissue for histologic diagnosis, especially when performed as cryobiopsy. The advantage of this bronchoscopic procedure is its ability to rule out alternative diagnoses, e.g., sarcoidosis, infection, or malignant disease.[2] Video-assisted thoracoscopic wedge resection is regarded as the standard technique for lung biopsy in idiopathic interstitial pneumonia since it is associated with considerably lower morbidity and mortality compared with open surgical lung biopsy.[3] However, all surgical procedures carry the risk of exacerbating the disease to be diagnosed, especially in pulmonary fibrosis. CT imaging is indispensable for definition of suitable target zones for biopsy. Histology specimens should be obtained from regions with active disease; it is hardly possible to determine the underlying disease from areas with advanced lung fibrosis.

Diagnostic exploration of diffuse parenchymal lung disease is a dynamic process requiring *multidisciplinary discussion* between pneumologists, radiologists, and pathologists (▶Fig. 6.2). At times, the diagnosis may need to be reevaluated in the light of new clinical aspects or histologic findings in the course of disease.

6

6.1.2 Idiopathic Pulmonary Fibrosis

Idiopathic pulmonary fibrosis (IPF) is characterized by the histologic pattern of usual interstitial pneumonia (UIP): architectural destruction, fibrosis often with honeycombing, scattered fibroblastic foci, patchy distribution, and involvement of the periphery of the lobule.[1] It predominantly affects patients above the age of 50 years; the median age at time of diagnosis is above 60 years. Idiopathic pulmonary fibrosis can be diagnosed by excluding any known cause of usual interstitial pneumonia. The disease generally progresses in stages and is quite refractory to treatment. Of all idiopathic interstitial pneumonias, after acute interstitial pneumonia, it has the second worst prognosis with a 5-year survival rate of between 20 and 40%.

In around half of cases, the findings on high-resolution CT (HRCT) are so characteristic that they are regarded as pathognomonic of usual interstitial pneumonia. That image pattern is termed in the following as "UIP pattern."

Table 6.1 Pathologic and clinical classification of common idiopathic interstitial pneumonias[1]

Pathologic pattern	Clinical disease manifestations
Usual interstitial pneumonia	Idiopathic pulmonary fibrosis
Nonspecific interstitial pneumonia	Idiopathic nonspecific interstitial pneumonia
Organizing pneumonia	Cryptogenic organizing pneumonia (formerly bronchiolitis obliterans with organizing pneumonia, BOOP)
Diffuse alveolar damage	Acute interstitial pneumonia
Respiratory bronchiolitis	Respiratory bronchiolitis-interstitial lung disease
Desquamative interstitial pneumonia	Desquamative interstitial pneumonia

II

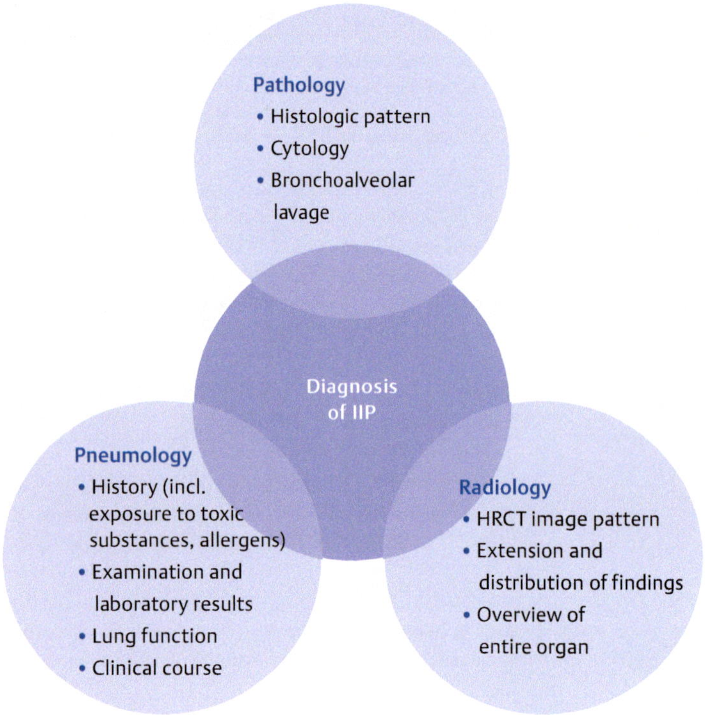

Fig. 6.2 Multidisciplinary discussion between pneumologist, radiologist, and pathologist for diagnosis of idiopathic interstitial pneumonias. This is also termed "CRP" diagnosis: clinician + radiologist + pathologist. HRCT, high-resolution CT; IIP, idiopathic interstitial pneumonia.

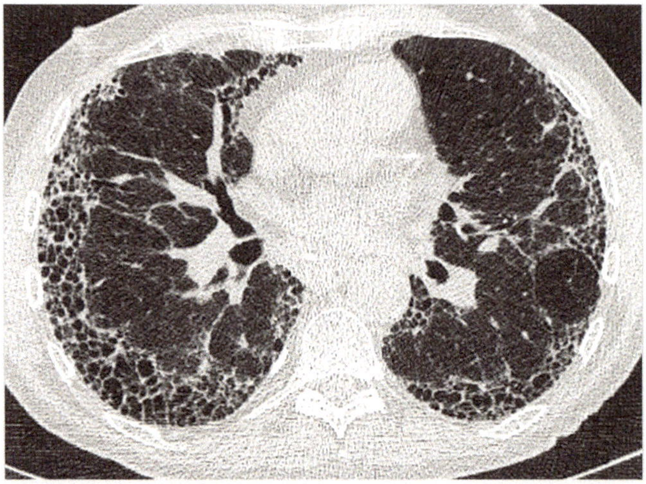

Fig. 6.3 Usual interstitial pneumonia. CT image. Small-cystic lung destruction resulting in extensive honeycombing, in particular in the subpleural space of both lower lobes.

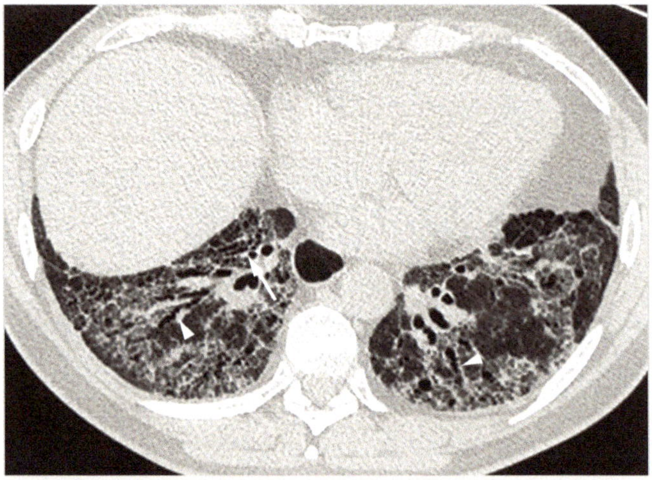

Fig. 6.4 Usual interstitial pneumonia. CT image. Ground-glass opacities and intralobular lines, traction bronchiectasis in both lower lobes (*arrowheads*) and mild honeycombing in the right lower lobe (*arrow*).

Note

CT findings of usual interstitial pneumonia[4,5]:

- Bilateral small cystic lung destruction, honeycombing (▶ Fig. 6.3).
- Predominantly, intralobular lines (▶ Fig. 6.4).
- Ground-glass opacities that are less pronounced than intralobular lines (see ▶ Fig. 6.4).
- Subpleural, basal predominance.
- Traction bronchiectasis and traction bronchiolectasis (see ▶ Fig. 6.4).
- Parenchymal distortion with bundling of bronchial structures and distortion of lobar fissures.

HRCT is sufficiently reliable to identify usual interstitial pneumonia through its pathognomonic CT pattern as presented in ▶ Table 6.2. Lung biopsy is not recommended for confirmation of diagnosis in these cases.[6] The other HRCT patterns of lung fibrosis (probable UIP, indeterminate, and alternative diagnosis) are less likely to unlikely (in descending order) to be associated with usual interstitial pneumonia. Therefore, to establish the appropriate diagnosis in the presence of these HRCT patterns, lung biopsy is recommended by the American Thoracic Society, and endorsed by the European Respiratory Society and the Japanese Respiratory Society and the Latin American Thoracic Society.[6] Contrarily, the Fleischner Society does not recommend lung biopsy in the presence of probable UIP pattern on HRCT.[7]

Table 6.2 HRCT scanning patterns of lung fibrosis[6]

UIP pattern	Probable UIP pattern	Indeterminate for UIP	Findings suggestive of alternative diagnosis
• Subpleural and basal predominant; distribution is often heterogeneous (variants of distribution: occasionally diffuse, may be asymmetrical) • Honeycombing with or without peripheral traction bronchiectasis or bronchiolectasis[a]	• Subpleural and basal predominant; distribution is often heterogeneous • Reticular pattern with peripheral traction bronchiectasis or bronchiolectasis • May have mild GGO	• Subpleural and basal predominant • Subtle reticulation; may have mild GGO or distortion ("early UIP pattern") • CT features and/or distribution of lung fibrosis that do not suggest any specific etiology ("truly indeterminate")	*CT features*: • Cysts • Marked mosaic attenuation • Predominant GGO • Profuse micronodules • Centrilobular nodules • Nodules • Consolidation *Predominant distribution*: • Peribronchovascular • Perilymphatic • Upper or mid-lung *Other*: • Pleural plaques (consider asbestosis) • Dilated esophagus (consider CTD) • Distal clavicular erosions (consider RA) • Extensive lymph node enlargement (consider other etiologies) • Pleural effusions, pleural thickening (consider CTD/drugs)

Abbreviations: CT, computed tomography; CTD, connective tissue disease; GGO, ground-glass opacities; RA, rheumatoid arthritis; UIP, usual interstitial pneumonia.
[a]Superimposed CT features: mild GGO, reticular pattern, pulmonary ossification.

Table 6.3 Radiologic differential diagnosis of usual interstitial pneumonia

Differential diagnosis	Distinguishing features of usual interstitial pneumonia
Nonspecific interstitial pneumonia	• Less ground-glass opacities • More honeycombing and less traction bronchiectasis • Mainly seen in subpleural space
Asbestosis (asbestos dust disease)	No pleural plaques or pleural calcification
Chronic hypersensitivity pneumonitis	• Basal and peripheral predominance • More honeycombing • No air trapping
Stage IV sarcoidosis	• No micronodules • No large bullae

Differential Diagnosis

Important differential diagnoses include nonspecific interstitial pneumonia, chronic hypersensitivity pneumonitis, asbestosis, and stage IV sarcoidosis. The most helpful differential diagnostic features are listed in ▸Table 6.3. Distinction between usual interstitial pneumonia and fibrotic nonspecific interstitial pneumonia may be difficult; relative subpleural sparing, predominant traction bronchiolectasis without obvious honeycombing, and pronounced ground-glass opacities suggest nonspecific interstitial pneumonia. One study reported the relatively rare finding of dendriform subpleural calcifications, which are occasionally observed in usual interstitial pneumonia but not in nonspecific interstitial pneumonia.[4] Chronic hypersensitivity pneumonitis often shows an apical predominance of fibrosis, and air trapping is a frequent finding. Stage IV sarcoidosis usually has a coarser fibrosis with adjacent emphysematous areas. Occasionally, it is not possible to distinguish between idiopathic pulmonary fibrosis and asbestos dust-induced lung disease (asbestosis). However, asbestosis without concomitant findings of asbestos-induced pleural disease (pleural plaques, pleural calcification) is rare.[8]

6.1.3 Idiopathic Nonspecific Interstitial Pneumonia

Nonspecific interstitial pneumonia (NSIP), like usual interstitial pneumonia, is defined on the basis of its histologic presentation. Two types are distinguished:

- *Cellular type*: This involves mild to moderate chronic interstitial inflammation with type II pneumocyte hyperplasia in the affected areas.
- *Fibrotic type*: This is associated with relatively homogeneous interstitial fibrosis.

Mixed pictures of both types are not uncommon. This *pattern of nonspecific interstitial pneumonia* is seen in collagen vascular disease, hypersensitivity pneumonitis, and in drug-induced lung disease as well as in infections and immunodeficiency settings (e.g., in HIV infections).[1,9] If no cause can be found, the clinical disease manifestation is regarded as idiopathic nonspecific interstitial pneumonia. It is thought that a proportion of the cases diagnosed as idiopathic disease are attributable to underlying, hitherto clinically inapparent, undifferentiated collagenosis.[10,11] Such cases do not really constitute idiopathic entities but are pulmonary manifestations of subclinical collagen vascular disease.

The clinical course of nonspecific interstitial pneumonia is very variable. The cellular type responds better to treatment than the fibrotic type does and thus has a better prognosis. The mean age of disease onset is around 50 years,[12,13] but nonspecific interstitial pneumonia is found even in children.[14] The most common response to treatment is an unchanging or improved condition; even virtually complete regression may be observed and relapse of the disease is not uncommon.[12] Progression with a fatal outcome is also possible–in particular, in fibrotic NSIP.[1]

Chest radiography typically shows foci of irregular bilateral, basal reticular opacities.[14] On *CT*, characteristic findings are observed:

Note

CT findings of nonspecific interstitial pneumonia[12,15]:

- Intralobular lines (▶Fig. 6.5).
- Traction bronchiectasis in areas with reticular opacities (▶Fig. 6.6).
- Symmetrical, bilateral ground-glass opacities with basal and peripheral predominance is the only finding in one-third of cases (see ▶Fig. 6.6).
- The subpleural region may be relatively spared.
- Small areas of consolidation (▶Fig. 6.7).
- Honeycombing.

Ground-glass opacity is a reflection of either active inflammation or fine interstitial fibrosis. Identification of traction bronchiectasis in these areas is consistent with the latter.

CT imaging does not allow for a reliable diagnosis of nonspecific interstitial pneumonia since there is widespread overlap with the CT features of other diseases. Therefore, biopsy should be considered for a definite diagnosis.

Differential Diagnosis

Differential diagnosis of nonspecific interstitial pneumonia is complex due to the wide range of CT features and their overlap with findings of other diseases (see ▶Fig. 6.7). The most common differential diagnoses and useful features for discrimination are illustrated in ▶Table 6.4. If only ground-glass opacity is visualized, radiological discrimination from desquamative interstitial pneumonia is difficult. Honeycombing presenting in association with fibrotic-type NSIP is difficult to distinguish from usual interstitial pneumonia. Chronic hypersensitivity pneumonitis can give rise to an identical radiologic and histologic picture and, occasionally, can be differentiated from idiopathic nonspecific interstitial pneumonia only on the basis of its clinical presentation. The same applies for collagen vascular disease with lung involvement.

6.1.4 Cryptogenic Organizing Pneumonia

Organizing pneumonia is a common reaction pattern of the lung parenchyma to different pathologic conditions, such as infections or tumors as well as the most diverse physical and chemical stimuli. Lung involvement of different diseases (e.g., collagen vascular diseases and inflammatory bowel diseases) may present as organizing pneumonia.[18] Defective healing

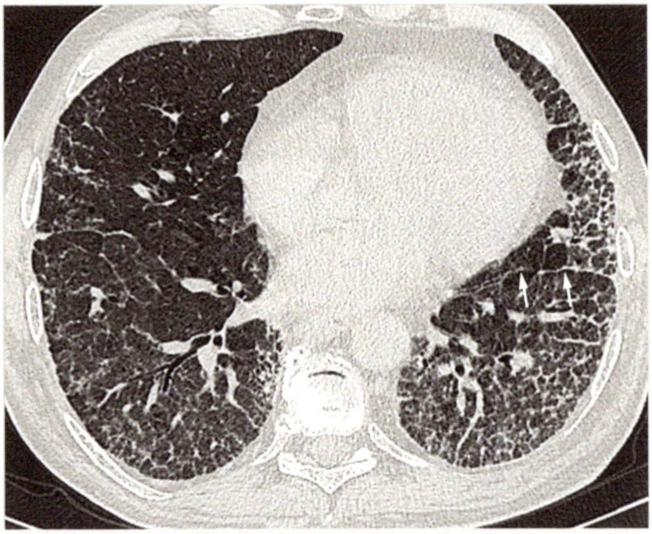

Fig. 6.5 Nonspecific interstitial pneumonia. CT image. Extensive reticular opacities and ground-glass opacities but no honeycombing and only slight parenchymal distortion (distortion of the left interlobular region: *arrows*).

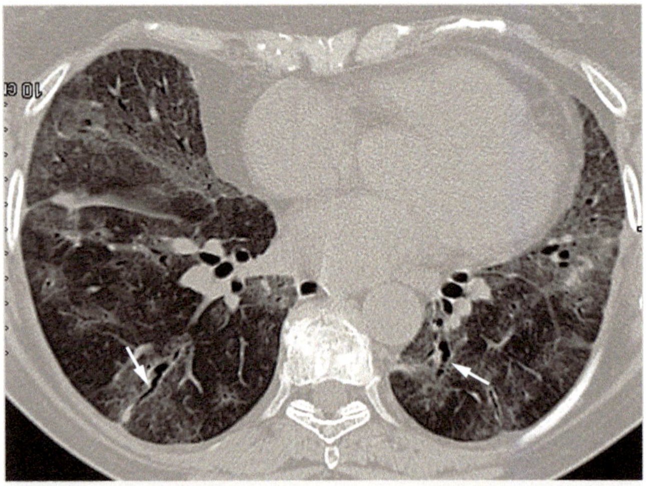

Fig. 6.6 Nonspecific interstitial pneumonia. CT image. Extensive bilateral ground-glass opacities associated with traction bronchiectasis (*arrows*).

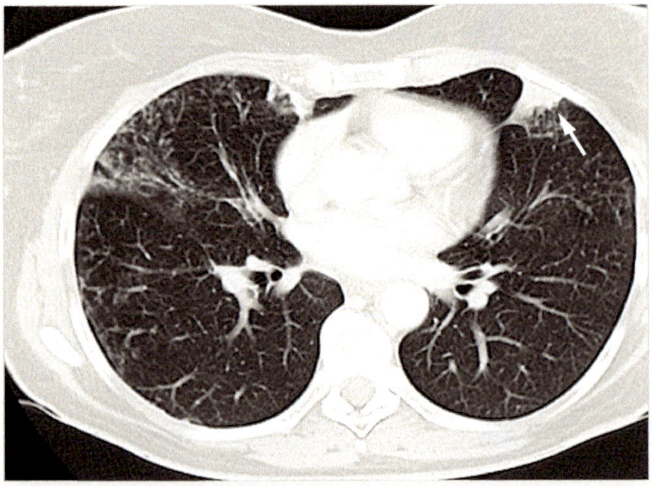

Fig. 6.7 Nonspecific interstitial pneumonia, cellular type. CT image. Ground-glass opacities, mild intralobular lines, and peripheral consolidation (*arrows*).

secondary to abscesses or in association with granulomatous polyangiitis or Wegener granulomatosis also manifests as organizing pneumonia.[1] Cryptogenic organizing pneumonia (COP), like other forms of idiopathic interstitial pneumonia, is present in settings where no known cause can be identified to explain the histologic pattern of organizing pneumonia.

> **Note**
>
> The use of the former, synonymous term "bronchiolitis obliterans with organizing pneumonia" (BOOP) is no longer recommended.

Typical age of disease onset is around 60 years. The disease course to diagnosis is rather short, usually less than 3 months and is associated with cough and dyspnea to varying degrees. Often, a low respiratory tract infection is initially suspected and unsuccessfully treated with several antibiotics. Diagnostic efforts are continued in the light of persistent pulmonary opacities and ultimately lead to diagnosis of cryptogenic organizing pneumonia. The disease generally has a good prognosis and completely regresses within a few weeks in most patients receiving oral steroids. However, recurrences are common during the first 3 months of discontinuing or reducing steroid medication. Life-threatening disease progression is only very rarely observed.[1]

Table 6.4 Differential diagnosis of nonspecific interstitial pneumonia[16,17]

Differential diagnosis	Distinguishing features of nonspecific interstitial pneumonia
Usual interstitial pneumonia	More ground-glass opacities, younger patients
Chronic hypersensitivity pneumonitis	No apical predominance
Cryptogenic organizing pneumonia	Not only consolidation
Desquamative interstitial pneumonia	Not only ground-glass opacities

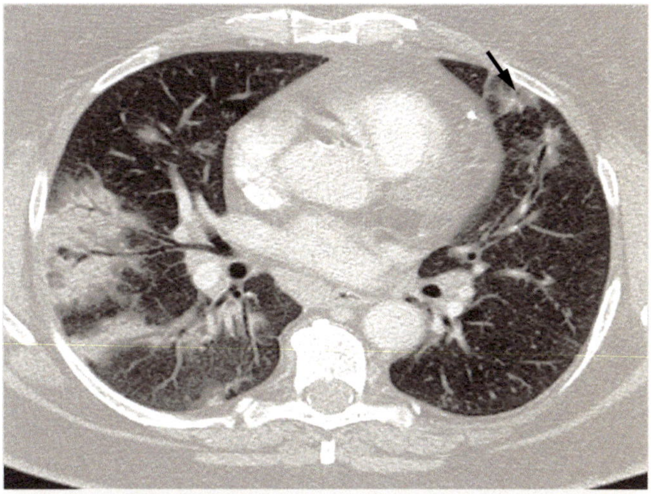

Fig. 6.8 Cryptogenic organizing pneumonia. CT image. Bilateral peripheral consolidation and, to a lesser extent, also ground-glass opacities (*arrow*).

Left untreated, the infiltrates occasionally disappear but are frequently replaced by new infiltrates at other sites.

Chest radiography typically reveals areas of unilateral or bilateral, occasionally also solitary, consolidation. Their location may change over the course of several weeks. In some cases, focal lesions are observed.[1] Less common is a reticulonodular pattern, which is associated with a poorer response to steroids and increased risk of progression to lung fibrosis.[19]

While cryptogenic organizing pneumonia is not associated with any specific *CT findings*, characteristic constellations of findings are common.[20,21,22]

> **Note**
>
> CT findings in cryptogenic organizing pneumonia:
> - Consolidation, mainly bilateral, either in peripheral or peribronchovascular regions.
> - Poorly marginated nodules, in some cases with air bronchogram.
> - Cylindrical bronchiectasis within consolidations.
> - Rare but suggestive signs are a perilobular distribution and the reversed halo sign.

Unilateral or bilateral consolidation is identified in 90% of cases, in some cases with air bronchogram. Ground-glass opacities are seen mainly in the peripheral regions of consolidations (▸Fig. 6.8). Most consolidations have irregular margins but only few show spicules.[23] Occasionally, they contain areas of mild cylindrical bronchiectasis. Two distribution patterns can be identified: a peripheral or subpleural pattern (see ▸Fig. 6.8) and a peribronchial pattern (▸Fig. 6.9). In 10% of cases, only a single consolidation is found (▸Fig. 6.10). Small bronchus-associated nodules are seen in half of cases. Around 15% of patients have multiple large nodules with irregular margins, often with air bronchogram.[23]

The combination of a characteristic clinical course with progressive pulmonary opacities over several weeks despite antibiotics and a characteristic CT pattern with bilateral subpleural or peribronchial consolidation is highly suggestive of cryptogenic organizing pneumonia. Nonetheless, a definite diagnosis cannot be made with imaging; in two-thirds of cases,

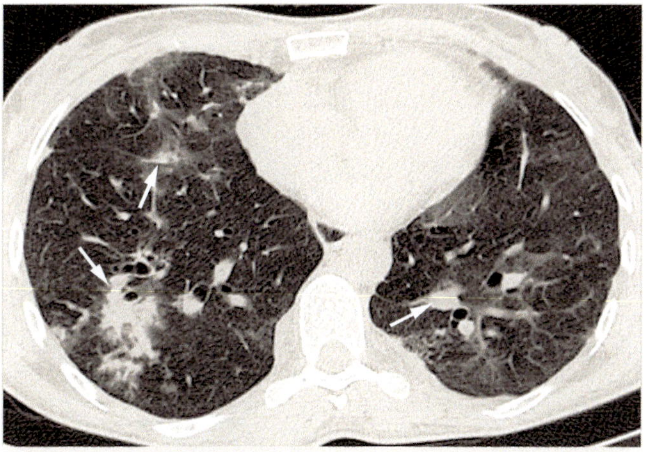

Fig. 6.9 Cryptogenic organizing pneumonia. CT image. Bilateral peribronchovascular opacities (*arrows*).

II

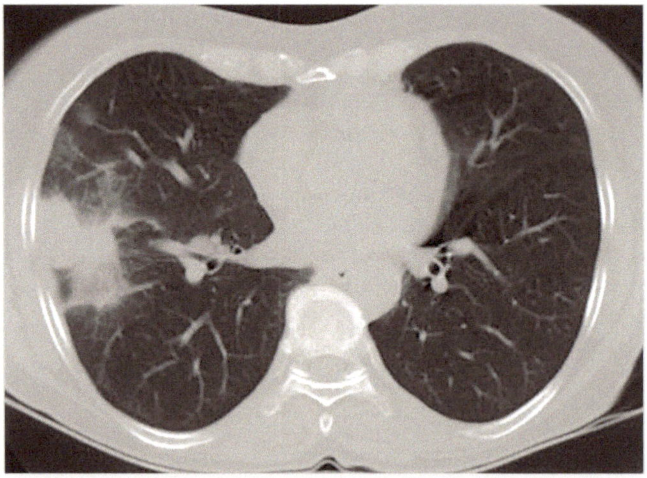

Fig. 6.10 Cryptogenic organizing pneumonia. CT image. Solitary consolidation surrounded by ground-glass opacity. On CT, no evidence of other lesions.

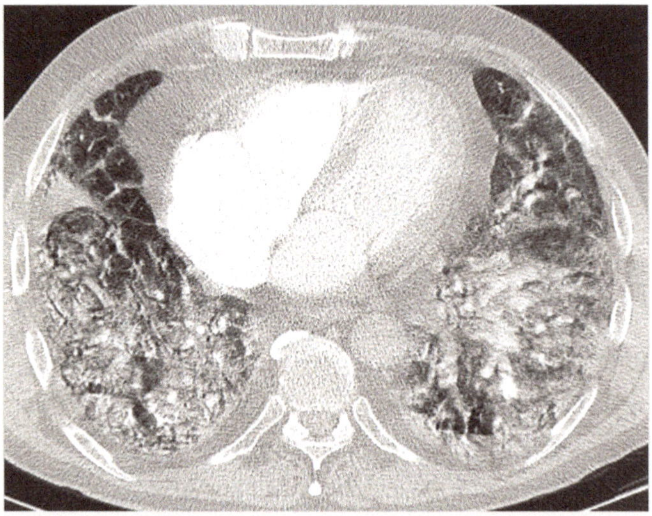

Fig. 6.11 Acute interstitial pneumonia. CT image. Extensive bilateral consolidation and ground-glass opacities.

the diagnosis can be confirmed following histologic examination of the transbronchial *biopsy* specimen taken during bronchoscopy, which is indispensable in any case. Otherwise, an additional transthoracic or surgical lung biopsy may be necessary.

Differential Diagnosis

The differential diagnosis of antibiotic-refractory pulmonary opacities is described in detail in Chapter 23; it depends on the CT finding pattern in each individual case. For a solitary consolidation, differential diagnosis includes tumors (lung carcinoma, in particular adenocarcinoma, lymphoma); infectious pneumonia, including septic embolism; infarction pneumonia as well as chronic eosinophilic pneumonia. For multiple consolidations, the spectrum of differential diagnoses additionally includes vasculitis and sarcoidosis. In the presence of multiple nodules, lung metastases must also be considered.[1] Many of these potential differential diagnoses can be excluded on the basis of the clinical or laboratory findings—otherwise, with transbronchial biopsy.

6.1.5 Acute Interstitial Pneumonia

Acute interstitial pneumonia (AIP) is a severe disease with the worst prognosis of all diffuse parenchymal lung diseases. It involves rapidly progressive, diffuse interstitial pneumonia, which presents on histology as diffuse alveolar damage (DAD).[24,25,26] As in the case of other types of idiopathic interstitial pneumonia, the findings associated with diffuse alveolar damage are designated as acute interstitial pneumonia if no underlying cause has been identified. The early exudative phase is characterized by diffusely distributed edema, formation of hyaline membranes, and acute interstitial inflammation. In the ensuing organizing phase, loose fibrosis develops, in particular, in the alveolar septa and type II pneumocyte hyperplasia.[25] This is followed by either disease resolution as ***restitutio ad integrum*** or development of lung fibrosis. This histologic pattern is indistinguishable from adult respiratory distress syndrome (ARDS). It is likely that many of the cases described in 1944 as Hamman–Rich syndrome were, in fact, cases of acute interstitial pneumonia.[25,27]

Acute interstitial pneumonia predominantly affects patients around the age of 60 years. It shows no gender prevalence and is not associated with smoking. Viral respiratory tract infection symptoms emerge in a few days as severe exertional dyspnea, and AIP is generally diagnosed within a few weeks. The majority of patients exhibit the clinical picture of adult respiratory distress syndrome and require mechanical ventilation. There is no known effective causal treatment and the mortality rate is at least 50%, with most deaths occurring within the first or second month after disease onset.[24] If the patient survives the disease, lung fibrosis may develop; disease relapse may occur.[1,28,29]

Chest radiography shows bilateral, patchily distributed opacities with positive air bronchogram.[30] Often the costophrenic angles remain spared. There are no signs of heart failure; pleural effusion is rare. Diffuse consolidation of both lungs increases over time. Later, consolidation resolves as the exudative phase progresses to the organizing phase, with reticular opacity now manifested.[1]

> **Note**
>
> The *CT findings* of acute interstitial pneumonia (▶ Fig. 6.11) are similar to those of adult respiratory distress syndrome[1,30,31]:
>
> - Extensive bilateral, patchily distributed ground-glass opacities with variable predominance; individual lobules may be spared, resulting in a geographic pattern appearance.
> - Consolidation in the dependent lung.
> - In the organizing phase: intralobular lines, traction bronchiectasis, parenchymal distortion, and honeycombing.

Ground-glass opacity develops during the exudative phase.[32] The appearance of traction bronchiectasis and parenchymal distortion marks the transition to the ensuing organizing phase.

> **Note**
>
> Idiopathic lung fibrosis as well as nonspecific interstitial pneumonia may acutely exacerbate in acute interstitial pneumonia.

Differential Diagnosis

The findings associated with acute interstitial pneumonia resemble those of adult respiratory distress syndrome, but the latter tends to exhibit a symmetrical distribution pattern and basal predominance.[33] The failure to find a cause for adult respiratory distress syndrome facilitates clinical differentiation. Extensive, bilateral ground-glass opacities in conjunction with respiratory insufficiency, often necessitating mechanical ventilation, is also found in pulmonary infections, in particular in *Pneumocystis jirovecii* pneumonia. Diffuse pulmonary hemorrhage has a similar appearance on CT. Both can be excluded on bronchoscopy. Desquamative interstitial pneumonia also exhibits bilateral ground-glass opacity but has a milder clinical course. In hydrostatic edema, additional findings such as cardiomegaly, pleural effusion, and thickening of the peribronchovascular interstitium as well as interlobular septal thickening are present or other clinical conditions causing hydrostatic edema such as renal failure exist. Pulmonary alveolar proteinosis is typically associated with a "crazy-paving" pattern, i.e., superimposition of interlobular septal thickening and intralobular lines in areas of ground-glass opacity. An advanced bilateral lung cancer, in particular, a multifocal adenocarcinoma, may exhibit a similar CT pattern but embarks on a more protracted clinical course.[1]

6.1.6 Respiratory Bronchiolitis-Interstitial Lung Disease

Respiratory bronchiolitis (RB) as well as respiratory bronchiolitis-interstitial lung disease (RB-ILD) are found only in smokers.

Often, *respiratory bronchiolitis* is diagnosed as an incidental finding on biopsy. It is thought to be present to varying degrees in all active smokers.[34] Histology reveals pigmented macrophages in the first- and second-order respiratory bronchioles.

In general, respiratory bronchiolitis does not cause any symptoms.[35] Only rarely are gradually increasing dyspnea, cough, and restrictive lung function present. Exclusively these symptomatic cases are designated as *respiratory bronchiolitis-interstitial lung disease*. Respiratory bronchiolitis-interstitial lung disease affects active smokers with at least 30 pack years (number of cigarette packs per day multiplied by the number of years smoked) predominantly between the ages of 40 and 50 years. Smoking cessation often improves symptoms; the disease also responds to steroids. However, progression of disease may occur despite smoking cessation in a minority of cases. Respiratory bronchiolitis-interstitial lung disease does not progress to lung fibrosis. The incidence of transition to desquamative interstitial pneumonia is unclear.

Chest radiography appears normal in certain cases. The most common finding in three-quarters of cases is bronchial wall thickening. Ground-glass opacity is found in around two-thirds of cases.[1,36]

The most salient features on CT are signs of bronchiolitis (▶ Fig. 6.12).

> **Note**
>
> CT findings of respiratory bronchiolitis, also respiratory bronchiolitis-interstitial lung disease[34,37,38]:
>
> - Centrilobular nodules, often ground-glass nodules.
> - Thickening of the central and peripheral bronchial walls.
> - Patchy ground-glass opacity.
> - Air trapping with areas of reduced lung density.
> - Often, normal findings.

The CT signs can regress on cessation of cigarette smoking or on treatment. Besides, there is often centrilobular emphysema, especially in apical regions.[36,39] It remains unclear if this is a coexistent finding as a sequela of smoking.[34]

Differential Diagnosis

Because of the histologic continuum from RB-ILD to desquamative interstitial pneumonia (see below), there is widespread overlapping between the radiologic findings of these two entities.[36] However, centrilobular nodules are not typical of desquamative interstitial pneumonia. In nonspecific interstitial pneumonia, ground-glass opacity may also be the most salient feature. Centrilobular ground-glass nodules exhibit a pattern similar to that seen in subacute hypersensitivity pneumonitis.[1]

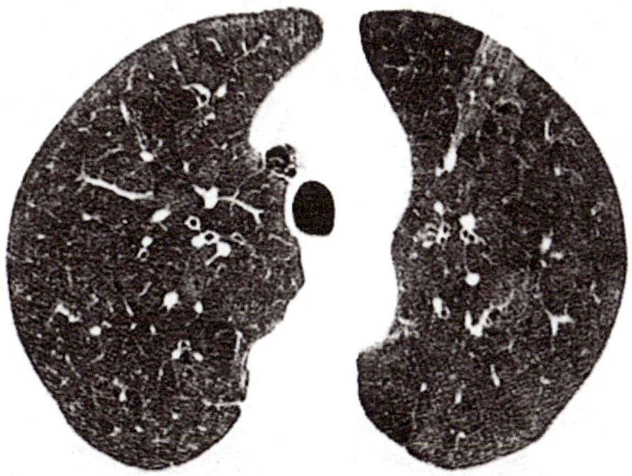

Fig. 6.12 Respiratory bronchiolitis-interstitial lung disease. CT image. Diffuse ground-glass opacities and subtle centrilobular ground-glass nodules.

6

II

6.1.7 Desquamative Interstitial Pneumonia

Desquamative interstitial pneumonia (DIP) is also associated with cigarette smoking but not as exclusively as respiratory bronchiolitis. Up to 20% of affected patients are nonsmokers. Histology shows an accumulation of pigmented macrophages in the alveoli. It was originally thought that the intra-alveolar cells were desquamated epithelial cells. That explains the misleading disease name, which has also been retained in the new classifications of idiopathic interstitial pneumonias. Macrophage accumulation is more pronounced than in respiratory bronchiolitis where this is confined to the respiratory bronchioles. The disease regresses in a large proportion of cases on cessation of smoking. Nonetheless, it progresses in one-quarter of patients even on treatment.[40,41,42]

Chest radiography is not able to reliably visualize desquamative interstitial pneumonia; no pathologic findings are identified in almost one-quarter of diseases diagnosed on biopsy.[1,40,43,44] Otherwise, the predominant findings are patchily distributed, bilateral ground-glass opacities with basal predominance.

CT depicts the characteristic findings of macrophage accumulation, leading to incomplete obliteration of the alveolar lumen and thus to increased parenchymal lung density on CT (▸Fig. 6.13). As such, ground-glass opacity is invariably the most salient feature.[45] These changes are found in three-quarters of cases to have basal predominance, in half of cases to have peripheral predominance, and in one-quarter of cases to be irregularly distributed.[1] Intralobular lines are often seen but less pronounced than ground-glass opacities; they are thought to reflect discrete lung fibrosis. Honeycombing is rarely found and when seen is of limited extent.

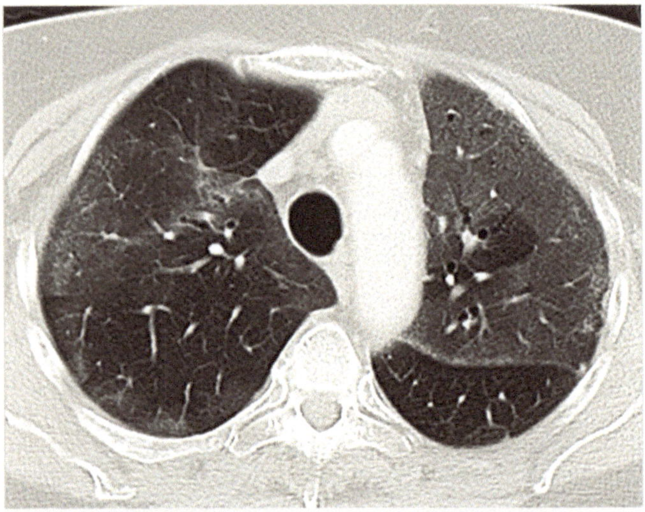

Fig. 6.13 Desquamative interstitial pneumonia. CT image. Diffuse bilateral ground-glass opacities.

Note

CT findings of desquamative interstitial pneumonia:
- Bilateral ground-glass opacities, mainly with basal predominance.
- Mosaic attenuation pattern.
- Intralobular lines.
- Rarely, subtle honeycombing.

Differential Diagnosis

At times, radiologic findings cannot be distinguished from that of respiratory bronchiolitis. Differential diagnosis should include other diseases showing predominantly ground-glass opacity, such as subacute hypersensitivity pneumonitis, sarcoidosis, and infections, e.g., *P. jirovecii* pneumonia[1] or viral pneumonia.

6.1.8 Rare Idiopathic Interstitial Pneumonias

Lymphoid interstitial pneumonia (LIP) is a lymphoproliferative disease characterized by diffuse pulmonary lymphoid hyperplasia. It may be difficult to distinguish from a pulmonary lymphoma on histology. It generally affects patients with immune deficiencies and is also seen in association with several systemic and autoimmune diseases[1]:
- AIDS.
- Rheumatoid arthritis.
- Sjögren syndrome.
- Systemic lupus erythematosus.
- Hashimoto thyroiditis.
- Pernicious anemia.
- Hemolytic anemia.
- Hypogammaglobulinemia.
- Chronic active hepatitis.
- Primary biliary cirrhosis.
- Myasthenia gravis.

Chest radiography is not useful in differential diagnosis. CT often depicts characteristic but not pathognomonic findings (▸Fig. 6.14).

Note

CT findings in lymphoid interstitial pneumonia[1,46]:
- Ground-glass opacities as the most predominant finding.
- Peribronchovascular cysts and peribronchovascular honeycombing.
- Intralobular lines.
- Predominantly, centrilobular lung nodules.
- Consolidation.

Pleuroparenchymal fibroelastosis (PPFE) is another pathologically defined rare idiopathic interstitial pneumonia; to date, there is a paucity of studies on the radiographic or CT morphology of this disease. Subpleural consolidation and nodules with apical predominance have been described (▶Fig. 6.15).[47]

There are other described histologic patterns that were not regarded as distinct entities of idiopathic interstitial pneumonias in the latest classification; they are suspected rather to represent variants of known idiopathic interstitial pneumonias or other diseases of known origin like collagen vascular diseases, hypersensitivity pneumonitis, or drug-induced lung disease.[22] A common feature of these rare diseases is the absence of pathognomonic imaging findings. They are diagnosed through histologic examination of biopsy specimens.

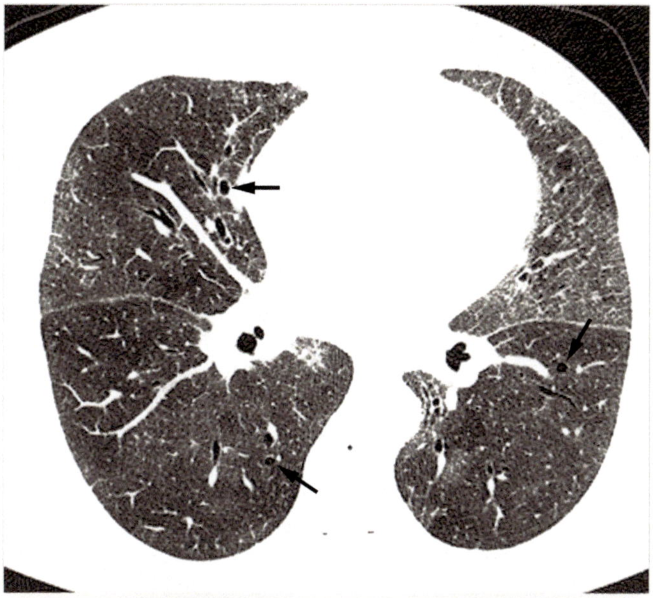

Fig. 6.14 Lymphoid interstitial pneumonia. CT image. Ground-glass opacities, isolated peribronchovascular cysts (*arrows*), and subtle intralobular lines in the lingula.

6.1.9 Familial Idiopathic Interstitial Pneumonia

Up to 20% of idiopathic interstitial pneumonias present as family clusters. The responsible genetic defects are known in around one-fifth of cases. Idiopathic lung fibrosis is more common than the other types of idiopathic interstitial pneumonia (▶Fig. 6.16).

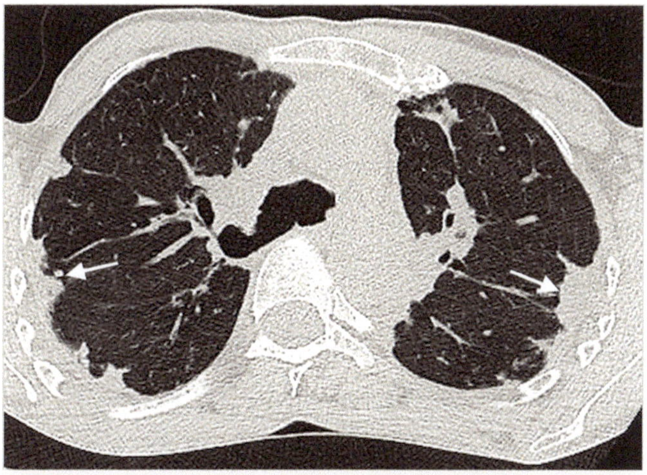

Fig. 6.15 Pleuroparenchymal fibroelastosis. CT image. Subpleural consolidation in the left upper lobe (*arrows*).

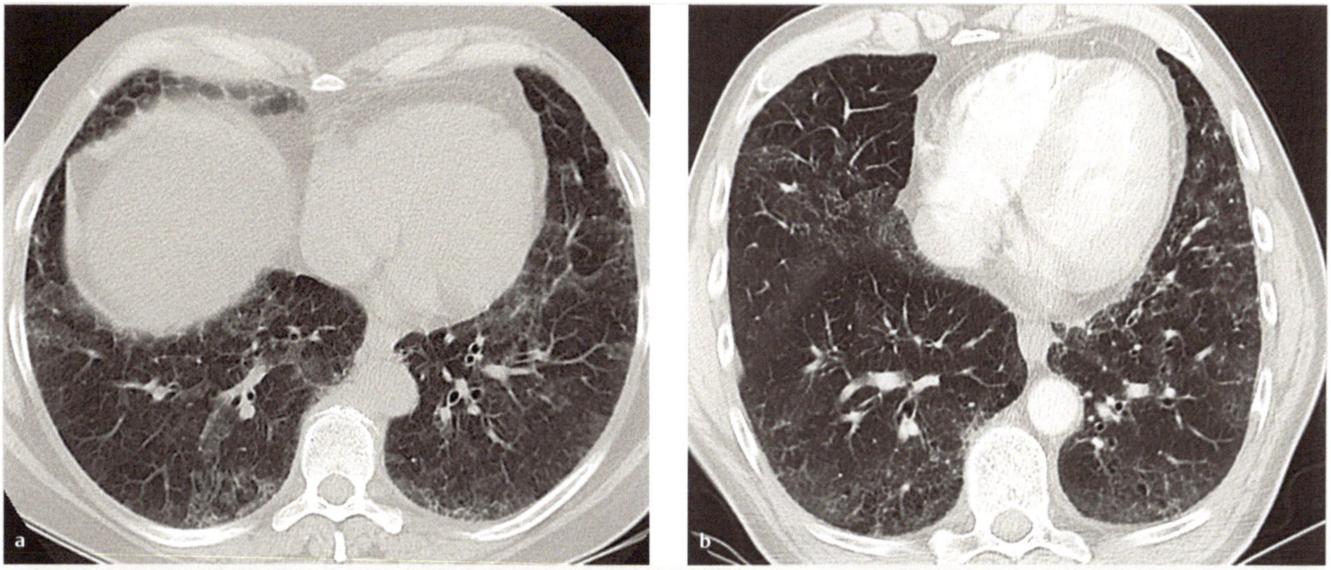

Fig. 6.16 Familial idiopathic interstitial pneumonia. CT images. Radiologic pattern of nonspecific interstitial pneumonia with predominant bilateral, basal ground-glass opacities, and intralobular lines, in siblings. **(a)** 61-year-old sister. **(b)** 59-year-old brother.

For that reason, a relevant family history should be taken from all patients with suspected idiopathic interstitial pneumonia.[22]

6.1.10 Unclassifiable Idiopathic Interstitial Pneumonias

In around 10% of idiopathic interstitial pneumonias, a definite diagnosis cannot be assigned, even after extensive multidisciplinary discussion, due to inconsistent clinical, radiologic, and pathologic findings. Cases that are unclassifiable because of an overlap of histologic patterns are often related to collagen vascular diseases or drug-induced lung diseases rather than being truly idiopathic.[22] In the future, it is probable that from a subset of hitherto unclassifiable cases, new disease entities of rare idiopathic interstitial pneumonia will emerge.

This heterogeneous group of diseases does not have uniform imaging features.

Unclassifiable idiopathic interstitial pneumonias are managed pragmatically in line with the most probable diagnosis reached after multidisciplinary discussion. The most probable disease entity gives an estimate of the likely clinical course of disease and determines the intensity of the treatment (▶Table 6.5).[48]

6.2 Diffuse Parenchymal Lung Diseases of Known Origin

6.2.1 Lung Involvement in Systemic Autoimmune Diseases

Myriad systemic diseases can present in the lung. Of the autoimmune-related diseases, collagen vascular diseases have the highest incidence of lung involvement. The histologic patterns of these lung diseases are identical to those seen in idiopathic interstitial pneumonia. ▶Table 6.6 gives an overview of the interstitial pneumonias found in collagen vascular diseases.

In some cases, clinical and laboratory findings are suggestive of but not definitive for a collagen vascular disease. Lung involvement in these cases often presents as interstitial pneumonia. If the radiological findings are consistent with interstitial pneumonia, and if certain clinical or serological features are present, the resulting diffuse parenchymal lung disease is called interstitial pneumonia with autoimmune features (IPAF).[49] The complex definition of IPAF is summarized in ▶Table 6.7.

Rheumatoid Arthritis

Lung involvement arises in one-fifth of rheumatoid arthritis patients. This is generally seen within the first 5 years of diagnosis.[10] Sometimes, lung disease occurs years before the clinical signs of rheumatoid arthritis. There are three types of pulmonary findings:

- *Diffuse parenchymatous lung disease*: Most commonly this reflects the pattern of usual interstitial pneumonia (UIP pattern, ▶Fig. 6.17), and less commonly the pattern of nonspecific interstitial pneumonia (NSIP pattern), organizing pneumonia, or lymphoid interstitial pneumonia.[10,64,65] Other entities such as diffuse alveolar damage, desquamative interstitial pneumonia, and pulmonary alveolar proteinosis have occasionally been identified on histology.[51] Prognosis

Table 6.5 Pragmatic classification of idiopathic interstitial pneumonias[22]

Disease course	Examples of known idiopathic interstitial pneumonias
Reversible and self-limited	Respiratory bronchiolitis-interstitial lung disease
Reversible with risk of progression	• Cellular and some fibrotic nonspecific interstitial pneumonias • Desquamative interstitial pneumonia • Cryptogenic organizing pneumonia
Stable with residual disease	Some fibrotic nonspecific interstitial pneumonias
Progressive, irreversible disease with potential for stabilization	Some fibrotic nonspecific interstitial pneumonias
Progressive, irreversible disease despite therapy	• Idiopathic pulmonary fibrosis • Some fibrotic nonspecific interstitial pneumonias

Table 6.6 Histologic pulmonary reaction pattern of diffuse parenchymal lung disease in systemic autoimmune diseases,[10,50] with incidence

Diseases	Histologic pattern							Literature
	UIP	NSIP	DAD	OP	RB	DIP	LIP	
Rheumatoid arthritis	+++	++	(+)	+		(+)	(+)	10,50,51,52,53,54,55
Systemic sclerosis	+	+++		(+)	(+)			50,56,57,58
Polymyositis-dermatomyositis	(+)	+++	+	+			+	50,54,59,60,61
Sjögren syndrome	+	+++		+		+	+	50,54,62,63
Lupus erythematosus	+	++	+			+	+	10
Undifferentiated collagenosis		++++						11,50

Abbreviations: DAD, diffuse alveolar damage; DIP, desquamative interstitial pneumonia; LIP, lymphoid interstitial pneumonia; NSIP, nonspecific interstitial pneumonia; OP, organizing pneumonia; RB, respiratory bronchiolitis; UIP, usual interstitial pneumonia.
Note: ++++, almost exclusively; +++, over 50%; ++, over 25%; +, over 10%;
(+), less than 10% or isolated cases.

Table 6.7 Criteria defining interstitial pneumonia with autoimmune features (IPAF)[49]

1. **Presence of interstitial pneumonia at CT or surgical lung biopsy** *and*
2. **Exclusion of alternative etiologies** *and*
3. **Does not meet criteria of a defined connective tissue disease** *and*
4. **At least one feature from at least two of these domains:**
   A. Clinical domain
   B. Serologic domain
   C. Morphologic domain

A. Clinical domain

1. Distal digital fissuring (i.e., "mechanic hands")
2. Distal digital tip ulceration
3. Inflammatory arthritis or polyarticular morning joint stiffness ≥60 min
4. Palmar telangiectasia
5. Raynaud phenomenon
6. Unexplained digital edema
7. Unexplained fixed rash on the digital extensor surfaces (Gottron sign)

B. Serologic domain

1. ANA ≥1:320 titer, diffuse, speckled, homogeneous patterns *or*
   a. ANA nucleolar pattern (any titer) *or*
   b. ANA centromere pattern (any titer)
2. Rheumatoid factor ≥2× upper limit of normal
3. Anti-CCP
4. Anti-dsDNA
5. Anti-Ro (SS-A)
6. Anti-La (SS-B)
7. Anti-ribonucleoprotein
8. Anti-Smith
9. Anti-topoisomerase (Scl-70)
10. Anti-tRNA synthetase (e.g., Jo-1, PL-7, PL-12; others are: EJ, OJ, KS, Zo, tRS)
11. Anti-PM-Scl
12. Anti-MDA-5

C. Morphologic domain

1. Suggestive radiology patterns by HRCT (see text for descriptions):
   a. NSIP
   b. OP
   c. NSIP with OP overlap
   d. LIP
2. Histopathology patterns or features by surgical lung biopsy:
   a. NSIP
   b. OP
   c. NSIP with OP overlap
   d. LIP
   e. Interstitial lymphoid aggregates with germinal centers
   f. Diffuse lymphoplasmacytic infiltration (with or without lymphoid follicles)
3. Multi-compartment involvement (in addition to interstitial pneumonia):
   a. Unexplained pleural effusion or thickening
   b. Unexplained pericardial effusion or thickening
   c. Unexplained intrinsic airways disease (by PFT, imaging or pathology)
   d. Unexplained pulmonary vasculopathy

Abbreviations: ANA, antinuclear antibody; LIP, lymphoid interstitial pneumonia; NSIP, nonspecific interstitial pneumonia; OP, organizing pneumonia; PFT, pulmonary function testing.

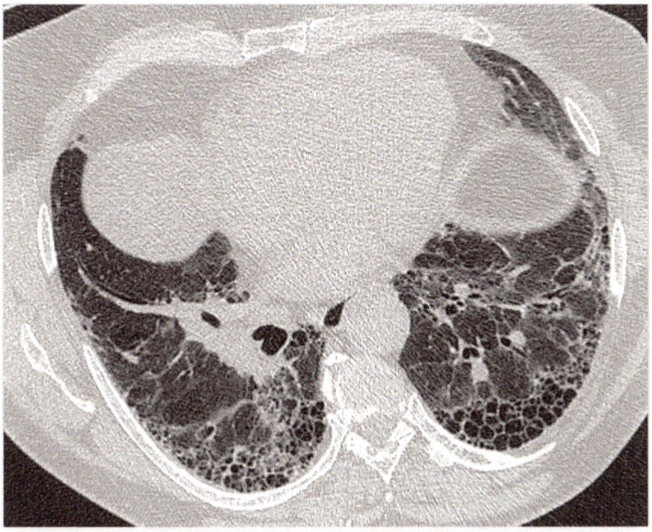

Fig. 6.17 Lung involvement in rheumatoid arthritis. CT image. Usual interstitial pneumonia pattern with peripheral intralobular lines and honeycombing.

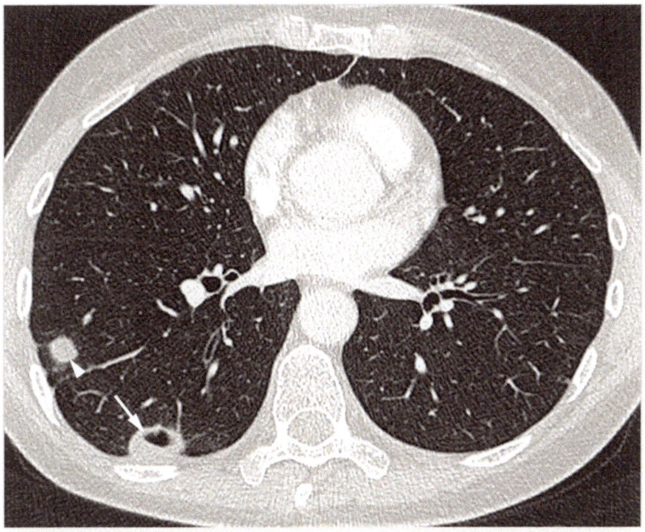

Fig. 6.18 Lung involvement in rheumatoid arthritis. CT image. Rheumatoid nodules. A solid (*arrowhead*) and a cavitating nodule (*arrow*) in the right lower lobe.

for the UIP pattern is poorer than for the NSIP pattern[50,66] but is better than for idiopathic cases of usual interstitial pneumonia (idiopathic pulmonary fibrosis).[10]

- *Diseases of the small airways*: In particular, bronchiolitis obliterans and lymphocytic bronchiolitis.[51] These are characterized by centrilobular micronodules with no clear localization predominance, tree-in-bud pattern, and at times, widespread air trapping. Cylindrical bronchiectases are also observed.
- *Rheumatoid nodules* (▶ Fig. 6.18): On histology, these are difficult to distinguish from granulomatous infections or granulomatous polyangiitis (Wegener granulomatosis).

However, the clinical context of known rheumatoid arthritis in patients with multiple, central necrotic, or cavitating nodules suggests the diagnosis.[10] Central necrosis can often be identified at CT after contrast injection.

II

If patients with rheumatoid arthritis exhibit new pulmonary symptoms or an existing lung involvement deteriorates, differential diagnosis should also consider:

- Opportunistic infections.
- Drug-induced lung disease, in particular due to methotrexate and infliximab.[10]

Systemic Sclerosis

Two courses of systemic sclerosis (SSc) are distinguished: a self-limiting type with subcutaneous calcification, Raynaud phenomenon, impaired esophageal motility, sclerodactyly, and telangiectasia as well as a more rare diffuse type with additional concomitant skin manifestations.[10]*Lung involvement* is common in both courses of disease and generally manifests as interstitial pneumonia. NSIP pattern (▶ Fig. 6.19) constitutes the most predominant histologic finding,[56] followed by UIP pattern.

Vascular involvement resulting in pulmonary hypertension is responsible for most deaths related to systemic sclerosis.[67] This is seen, in particular, in the self-limiting type of systemic sclerosis.[10]

Esophageal involvement is common. On CT, an air-filled dilated esophageal lumen is often visible (see ▶ Fig. 6.19). Esophageal barium swallow test shows reduced motility and lumen dilation, especially of the lower part of the esophagus.

Sjögren Syndrome

Sjögren syndrome, involving lymphocytic infiltration of the exocrine glands, causes sicca syndrome through impaired glandular function. A primary type (primary Sjögren syndrome) is differentiated from a secondary type associated with other diseases like rheumatoid arthritis, systemic lupus erythematosus, or systemic sclerosis.[10] The reports on the proportion of patients with lung involvement vary greatly in the literature between 9 and 75%.[10,62,68,69,70] The broad spectrum of pulmonary manifestations comprises interstitial pneumonias (in particular, nonspecific interstitial pneumonia, less commonly usual interstitial pneumonia, organizing pneumonia, or lymphoid interstitial pneumonia), primary pulmonary lymphoma, diffuse interstitial amyloidosis (▶ Fig. 6.20), and small airways diseases.[10,71]

CT demonstrates the underlying interstitial pneumonia—in particular, ground-glass opacities and reticular opacities in nonspecific interstitial pneumonia as well as centrilobular nodules, consolidation, ground-glass opacities, and perivascular cysts in lymphoproliferative disease (lymphoid interstitial pneumonia).

Polymyositis-Dermatomyositis

In polymyositis-dermatomyositis, two-thirds of all affected patients experience lung involvement early in the course of the disease, often even before or coincident with the skin and muscle symptoms.[10,72,73,74,75] Lung involvement frequently gives rise to life-threatening complications that limit the prognosis, especially in the acute forms of polymyositis-dermatomyositis.

NSIP pattern is the most common pulmonary manifestation (▶ Fig. 6.21), and is often associated with organizing pneumonia, less commonly also with usual interstitial pneumonia or lymphoid interstitial pneumonia. Besides, disease courses with diffuse alveolar damage refractory to corticosteroid treatment have a high mortality.[10]

The radiologic findings are consistent with the associated histologic patterns of mainly nonspecific interstitial pneumonia. In addition, consolidations are present in over 50% of patients[59,76,77] and probably due to organizing pneumonia. Pleural effusions are found in around 20% of cases.[10,59] Honeycombing does not occur.[10]

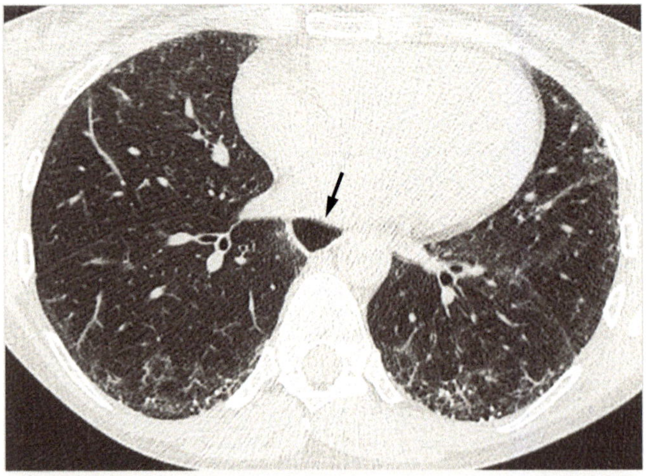

Fig. 6.19 Lung involvement in systemic sclerosis. CT image. Nonspecific interstitial pneumonia pattern with bilateral subpleural, intralobular lines and ground-glass opacities. Markedly dilated esophagus as a sign of its involvement in systemic sclerosis (*arrow*).

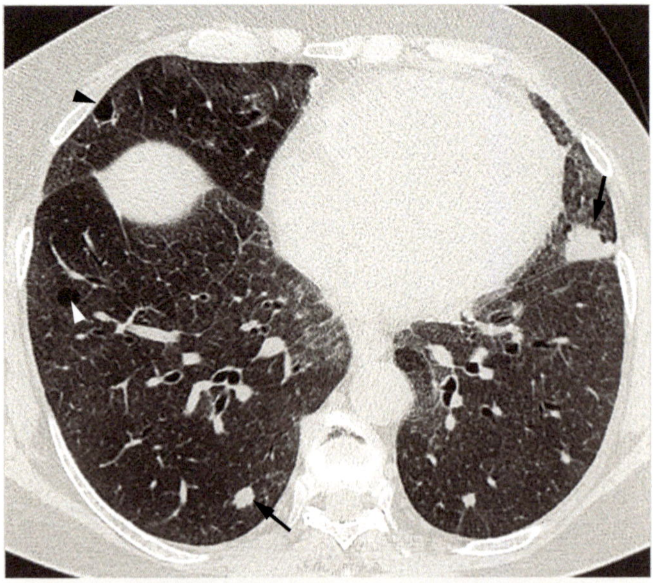

Fig. 6.20 Lung involvement in Sjögren syndrome. CT image. Nodules (*arrows*), confirmed on histology as amyloidosis, as well as cysts (*arrowheads*) and ground-glass opacities as findings of lymphoid interstitial pneumonia.

Systemic Lupus Erythematosus

Clinically relevant lung involvement in systemic lupus erythematosus (SLE) is less common than in other forms of collagenosis. However, severe pulmonary complications can determine the prognosis. Lung involvement is very variable.

Diffuse parenchymatous lung diseases (▶Fig. 6.22) are identified on CT in around one-third of systemic lupus erythematosus cases[78,79]; these are mainly asymptomatic with mild pathologic changes. In general, the radiologic findings are consistent with nonspecific interstitial pneumonia.[80]

Uncommon, but severe *complications* include:

- *Acute lupus pneumonitis* occurs in up to 4% of patients. On histology and radiology, it manifests as diffuse alveolar damage with extensive bilateral consolidation and ground-glass opacities (▶Fig. 6.23).
- *Diffuse alveolar hemorrhage* presents as a sequela of neutrophilic capillaritis in 2% of patients. It has a poor prognosis with a lethality of up to 90%. The radiological findings are similar to that of hemorrhage in acute lupus pneumonitis.[10]
- *Antiphospholipid syndrome* also has a very poor prognosis. It presents as adult respiratory distress syndrome, with pulmonary embolism, thrombosis of the pulmonary arteries, in situ microthrombi, and alveolar hemorrhage (▶Fig. 6.24).[81]

Shrinking lung syndrome is a very rare complication of collagen vascular diseases, primarily described in systemic lupus erythematosus,[82,83] but it has been also observed in Sjögren syndrome,[84] systemic sclerosis, undifferentiated collagenosis, and rheumatoid arthritis.[85] Bilateral weakness of the diaphragm causes a high-riding diaphragm, often associated with basal atelectasis. Its cause is unknown but is thought to be linked to myopathy of the diaphragm or intercostal muscles.[83,86,87] It does not involve diffuse parenchymal lung disease.

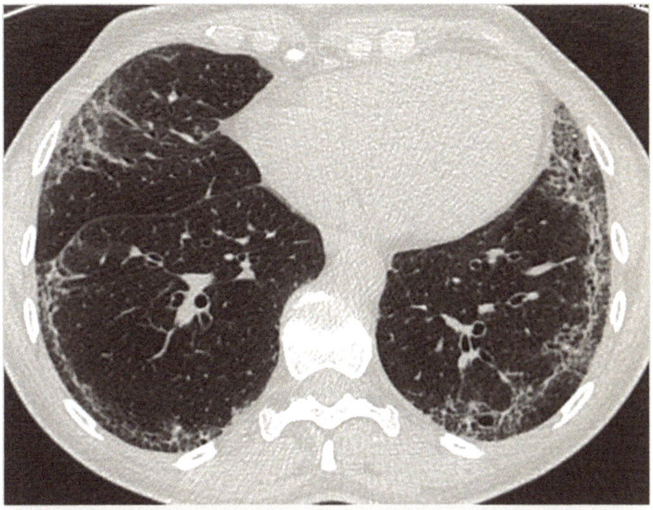

Fig. 6.21 Lung involvement in polymyositis-dermatomyositis. CT image. Nonspecific interstitial pneumonia pattern with subpleural ground-glass opacities and intralobular lines.

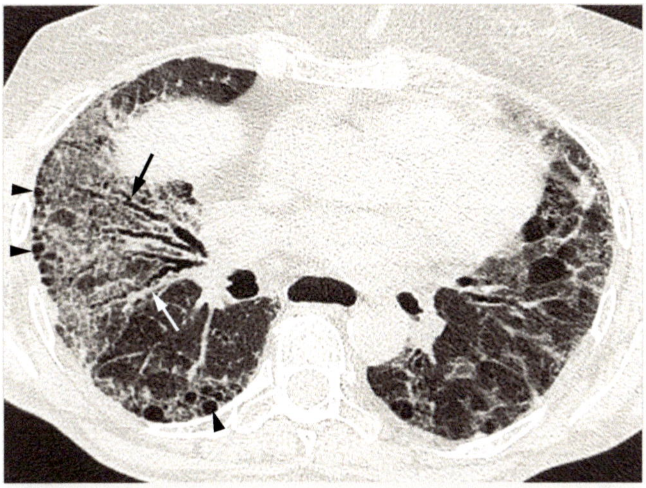

Fig. 6.22 Lung involvement in systemic lupus erythematous. CT image. Nonspecific interstitial pneumonia pattern with extensive bilateral ground-glass opacities, intralobular lines, and mild traction bronchiectasis (*arrows*). Subtle subpleural honeycombing is present, especially in the subpleural region of the right lower lobe (*arrowheads*).

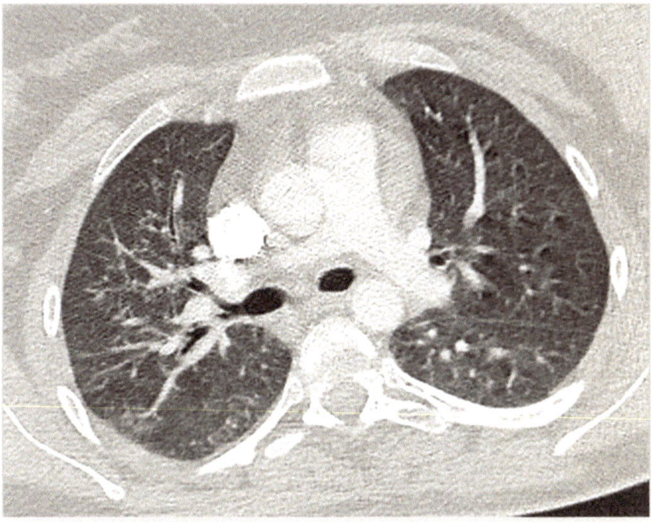

Fig. 6.23 Lung involvement in systemic lupus erythematous. CT image. Lupus pneumonitis. Bilateral diffuse ground-glass opacities.

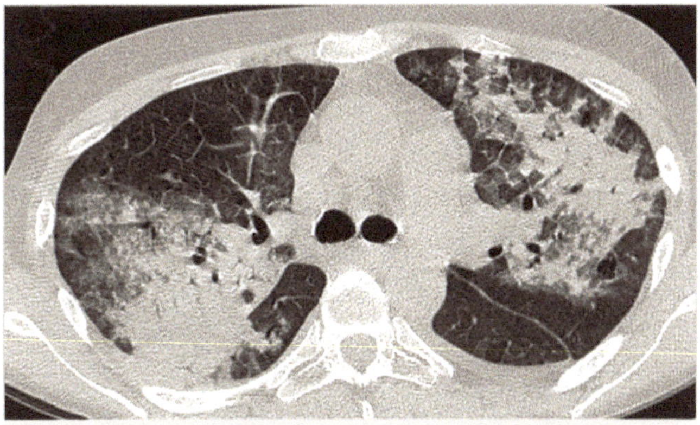

Fig. 6.24 Lung involvement in systemic lupus erythematous. CT image. Diffuse alveolar hemorrhage in anti-phospholipid syndrome. The subpleural space remains mostly spared.

Other appearances of systemic lupus erythematosus include pulmonary vasculitis, bronchiolitis obliterans, and pulmonary artery hypertension.[87,88]

Mixed Connective Tissue Disease

Mixed connective tissue disease (MCTD) combines the features of systemic sclerosis, systemic lupus erythematosus, and polymyositis-dermatomyositis. Lung involvement is extremely common (80% of patients).[89] In addition to diffuse parenchymal lung diseases, pleural effusion is found in half of cases and pulmonary hypertension in 4%[10] as well as several other conditions, e.g., vasculitis, pulmonary thromboembolisms, pulmonary hemorrhage, nodules, pulmonary cysts, lymphadenopathy, and impaired diaphragmatic motility.[10,90] The leading lung-related causes of death are pulmonary hypertension and respiratory insufficiency secondary to lung fibrosis.[10]

To date, there is a paucity of studies on the radiologic findings of mixed connective tissue disease. Imaging features were mainly determined by the underlying interstitial pneumonia, most frequently nonspecific or usual interstitial pneumonia.

6.2.2 Drug-Induced Lung Disease

Many drugs have the potential to induce lung diseases.[91] A distinction can be made between pulmonary complications related to the desired drug effect (e.g., pulmonary hemorrhage secondary to anticoagulant medication) and pulmonary toxicity as an adverse drug effect. The latter is more common and is caused by numerous drugs. In general, drugs can trigger various types of interstitial pneumonia in their idiopathic forms, as described in Section 6.1, right up to acute diffuse alveolar damage (▶ Fig. 6.25). The most common types of drug-induced interstitial pneumonia are nonspecific interstitial pneumonia and organizing pneumonia (▶ Fig. 6.26). Other conditions triggered as adverse drug effects include eosinophilic pneumonia, pulmonary hemorrhage, bronchiolitis obliterans, pulmonary edema, pulmonary veno-occlusive disease, and pulmonary hypertension.[91] Methotrexate has also been reported to cause lymphadenopathy.[92,93,94,95]

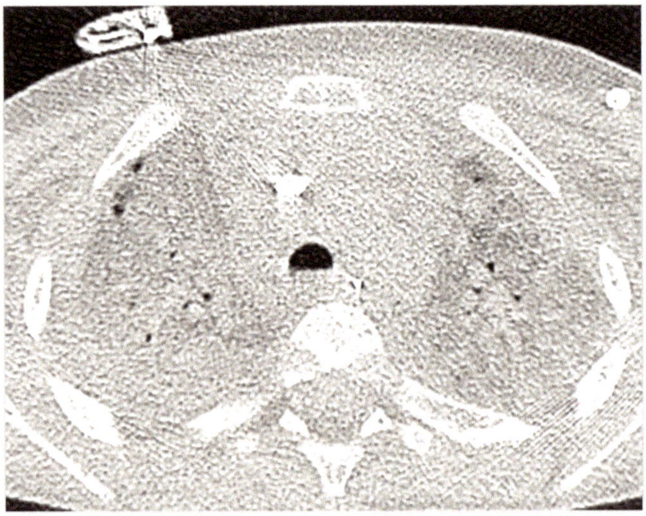

Fig. 6.25 Bleomycin-induced diffuse alveolar damage in a young child. CT image. Acute interstitial pneumonia necessitating mechanical ventilation. Bilateral diffuse, dense ground-glass opacities in both lungs.

The best-known types of pulmonary drug toxicity and their characteristic triggers are summarized in ▶ Table 6.8 (▶ Fig. 6.27). An excellent, regularly updated list of published pulmonary adverse drug effects can be consulted on the internet website www.pneumotox.com.

6.2.3 Parenchymal Lung Diseases due to Extrinsic Noxae

Several chemical and physical toxic substances can cause diffuse parenchymal lung diseases. Some common causes will be briefly discussed here.

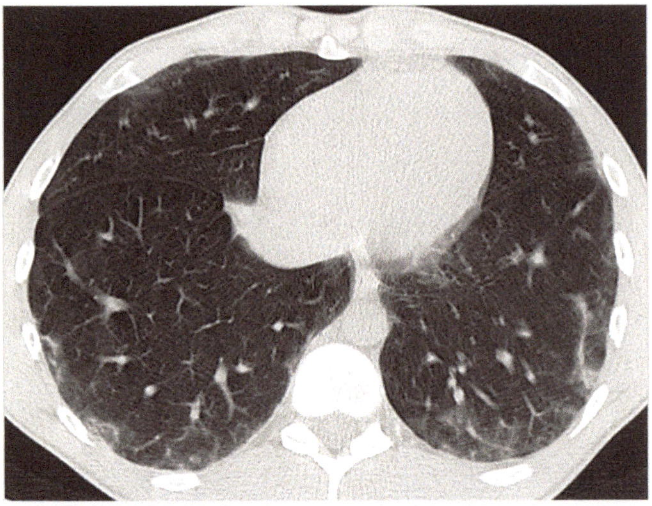

Fig. 6.26 Infliximab-induced organizing pneumonia. CT image. Bilateral subpleural consolidation and ground-glass opacities.

Table 6.8 Examples of pulmonary drug toxicity and typical triggers[91]

Lung disease	Typical trigger drugs
Diffuse alveolar damage	Bleomycin, busulfan, cyclophosphamide, gold salts
Nonspecific interstitial pneumonia	Amiodarone (see ▶ Fig. 6.27), methotrexate, chlorambuzil
Organizing pneumonia	Bleomycin, gold salts, methotrexate, amiodarone, Nitrofurantoin, penicillamine, sulfasalazine, cyclophosphamide
Eosinophilic pneumonia	Penicillamine, sulfasalazine, nitrofurantoin, nonsteroidal anti-inflammatories
Pulmonary hemorrhage	Anticoagulants, amphotericin B, cytarabine, penicillamine, cyclophosphamide

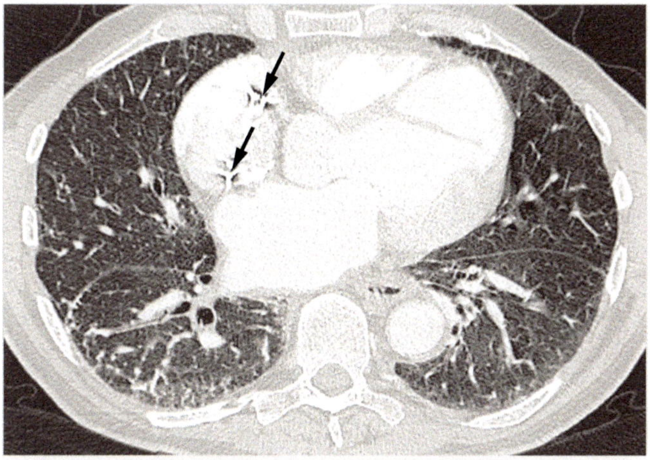

Fig. 6.27 Amiodarone-induced lung disease. CT image. Nonspecific interstitial pneumonia pattern with intralobular lines and ground-glass opacities. Besides, cardiomegaly; electrodes of implantable cardioverter defibrillator in the right atrium (*arrows*).

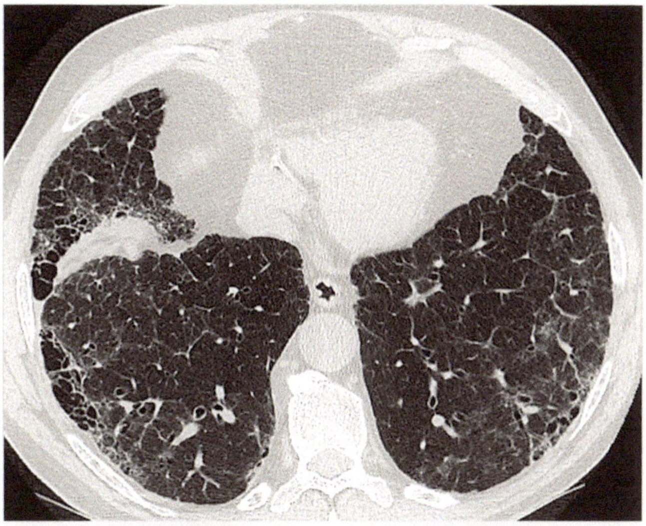

Fig. 6.28 Asbestosis. CT image. Lung fibrosis with basal and subpleural predominance.

Chemical Noxae

Lung damage due to inorganic dusts is often sustained in occupational settings, with asbestos dust and quartz dust being the principle causative agents. Asbestos dust leads to lung fibrosis in addition to pleural changes (▶Fig. 6.28), while quartz dust results in a granulomatous disease (▶Fig. 6.29) with a similar radiologic appearance to that of sarcoidosis. Myriad, mainly accidentally inhaled, substances can cause chemical irritation of the lung parenchyma (▶Fig. 6.30).

Allergic reactions play a pivotal role in the lung damage caused by organic substances. Hypersensitivity pneumonitis is caused by numerous organic substances and is implicated in a number of occupational diseases. Pulmonary drug toxicity could also be regarded as lung reaction to chemical noxae and should, therefore, be mentioned here.

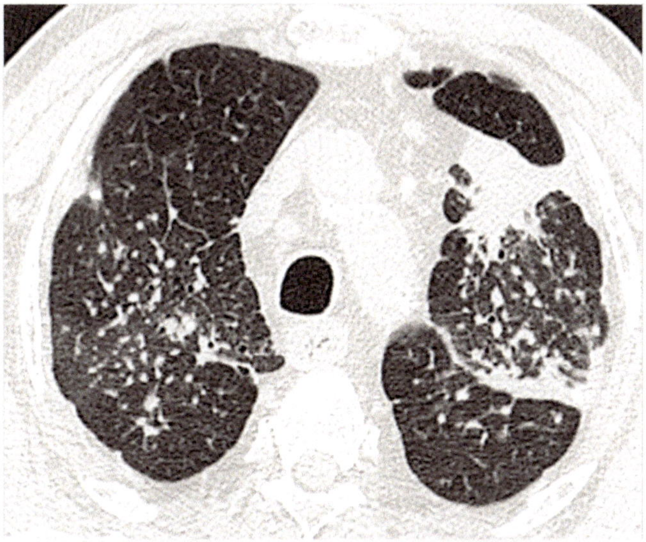

Fig. 6.29 Silicosis. CT image. Multiple small nodules with perilymphatic distribution pattern as well as consolidation in the left upper lobe (progressive massive fibrosis).

Physical Noxae

The most common physical noxae causing parenchymal lung damage are electromagnetic or particle radiation. This is of practical importance as an adverse effect of radiotherapy. As from a threshold dose of 20 Gy there is a risk of development of *radiation pneumonitis*, in more than 40 Gy this is highly probable.[96,97,98] Mostly, onset of this disease is seen 4 to 12 weeks after lung irradiation (▶Fig. 6.31). During the acute phase, ground-glass opacity and consolidation are identified in the irradiated lung tissue, with progression to *radiation fibrosis* over the course of several months (▶Fig. 6.32).

The radiologic findings may increase for as long as 2 years before a stable state is reached.[96] Radiation fibrosis is characterized by consolidation, loss of volume of the affected tissue, and traction bronchiectasis. As a result of modern radiotherapy procedures, irregular delineation of radiation pneumonitis may be encountered due to inhomogeneous distribution of the radiation dose in the lung tissue. Radiation pneumonitis manifests on histology similarly to organizing pneumonia and is mainly asymptomatic and confined to the irradiated lung areas. In certain cases, lung irradiation triggers organizing pneumonia, which is not confined to the irradiated lung and is usually symptomatic.[99]

6.3 Granulomatous Parenchymal Lung Diseases

6.3.1 Sarcoidosis

Sarcoidosis is a systemic disease of unknown origin and is histologically characterized by noncaseous, epithelioid cell granulomas.

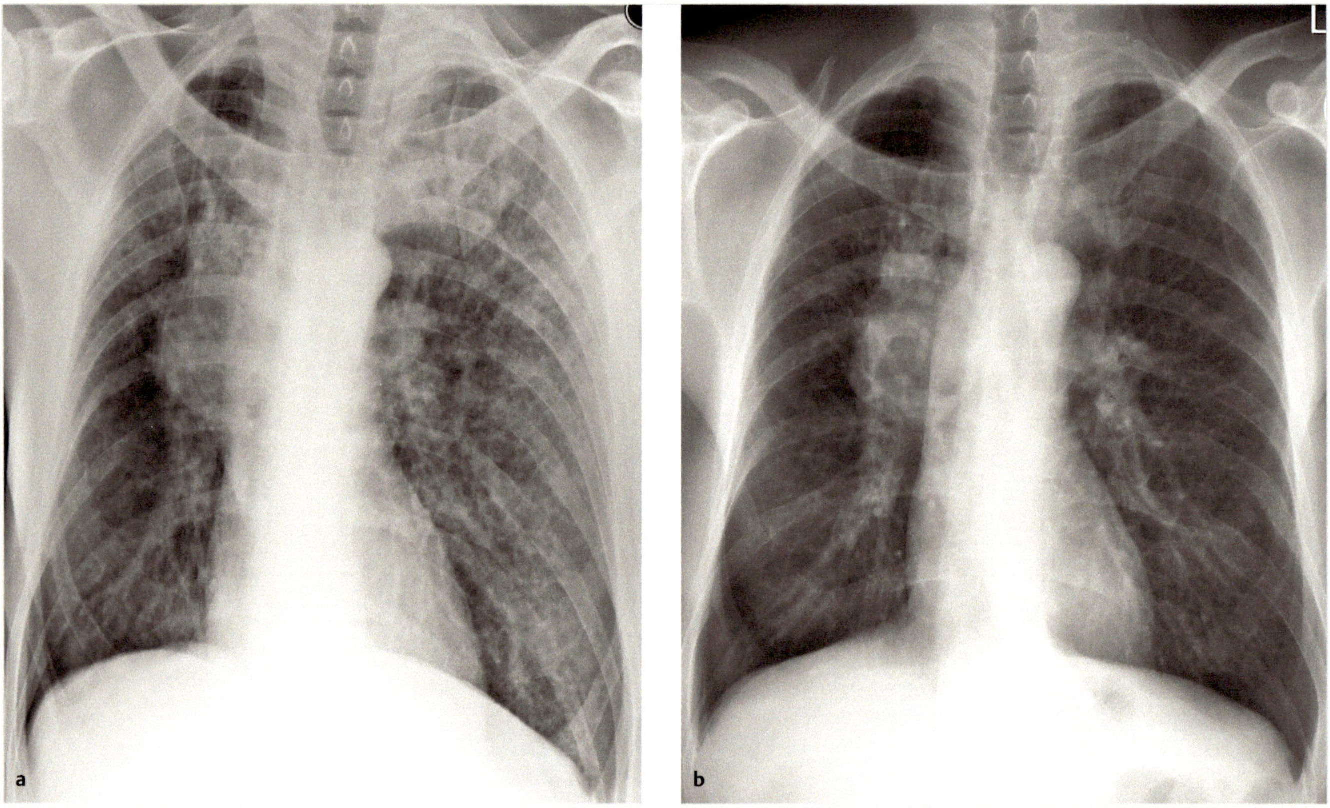

Fig. 6.30 Acute smoke gas intoxication. Radiographs. Besides, right central lung carcinoma. **(a)** On the first day of smoke gas inhalation, diffuse ground-glass opacity. **(b)** Normalization of findings 4 days later.

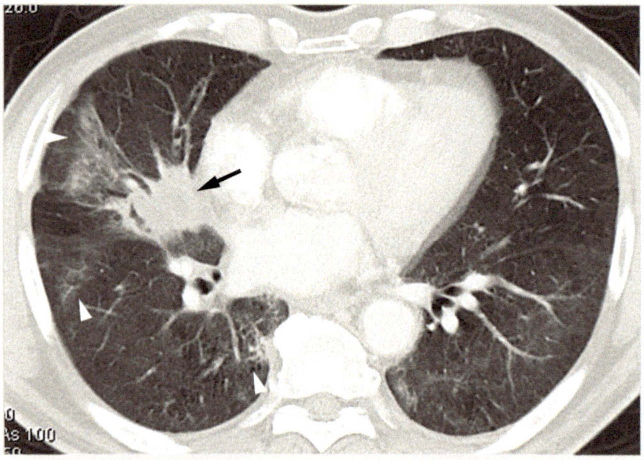

Fig. 6.31 Acute radiation pneumonitis. CT image. Central lung carcinoma in the middle lobe (*arrow*); ground-glass opacities in the middle and right lower lobe (*arrowheads*).

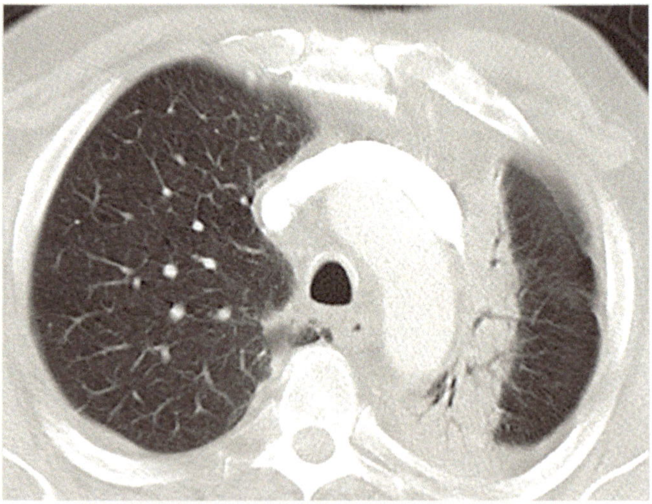

Fig. 6.32 Radiation fibrosis. CT image. Paramediastinal consolidation in the left lower lobe secondary to left upper lobe resection and adjuvant radiotherapy.

Sarcoidosis is thought to be linked to a genetic predisposition.[100] Myriad triggers are known such as infections caused by various microorganisms (e.g., *Mycobacterium tuberculosis*, other mycobacteria, *Rickettsia*, *Borrelia*, *Mycoplasma*, and different viruses), but also by organic and inorganic substances (aluminum, zirconium, mineral fibers, silicates, clay, talcum, pine pollen, and starch).[101,102,103,104,105] Sarcoidosis is also associated with other diseases, such as chronic inflammatory bowel diseases[18] and testicular carcinoma.[106]

Because of an undesired immune reaction, sarcoidosis results in formation of characteristic *granulomas*. On histology, the granulomas are seen to contain epithelioid histiocytes, occasionally multinucleated giant cells, activated T lymphocytes, monocytes, and fibroblasts. The epithelioid cells produce more than 40 enzymes, including angiotensin-converting enzyme. This is utilized for a laboratory test commonly used to access disease activity. In active disease, there is propagation of the activated T helper cells (CD4-positive cells), and elevated CD4/CD8 quotients can then be measured in the bronchoalveolar lavage.

Sarcoidosis affects, in particular, young and middle-aged adults. In around half of cases, it is diagnosed as an incidental finding. Of the affected patients, 21% have respiratory symptoms and 16% erythema nodosum, while eye symptoms (uveitis) and other forms of skin effervescences at 7 and 4%, respectively, are less common.[100] Occasionally, uncharacteristic general symptoms are observed (weakness, weight loss, fever, or joint ache). Acute courses with rapid onset of severe symptoms tend to have a better prognosis than the chronic form, which progresses to lung fibrosis in around 20% of cases.

> **Note**
>
> *Löfgren syndrome* with its characteristic triad of bihilar lymphadenopathy, erythema nodosum, and arthralgia constitutes a particularly acute disease course.[107]

Sarcoidosis mainly presents with bilateral hilar lymphadenopathy, pulmonary infiltrates, eye and skin lesions, and the less common involvement of other organs.[108] Over 90% of all patients exhibit sarcoid lesions of the lungs and intrathoracic lymph nodes.[109] Diagnosis necessitates evidence of noncaseous epithelioid cell granulomas with concomitant characteristic clinical and radiologic features. Other causes of granulomas must be ruled out.

The overall mortality rate is less than 5%.[103] The predominant cause of death is progressive lung fibrosis: less commonly, acute involvement of the heart and central nervous system.

Staging

Several radiologic staging systems of sarcoidosis were used in the past (▶Table 6.9). The current ATS/ERS/WASOG classification system, employed since 1999, is derived from some of the former staging systems, which can still be encountered in everyday practice and in some cases in the literature.

All systems use the presence of bihilar lymphadenopathy and lung involvement for staging. Some of the older systems, e.g., that of DeRemee (see ▶Table 6.9), do not recognize any terminal stage to mark the presence of lung fibrosis. Likewise, normal radiographic findings are not featured in all classification schemes. Currently, the staging system used is that of the American Thoracic Society, European Respiratory Society, and World Association of Sarcoidosis and Other Granulomatous Disorders. This system entails a synthesis of the earlier classification schemes and comprises five stages[113]:

- *Stage 0*: no radiologic signs of sarcoidosis.
- *Stage I*: bihilar and possibly paratracheal lymphadenopathy, no radiologic evidence of lung involvement (although often identifiable on biopsy).
- *Stage II*: bihilar lymphadenopathy and pulmonary opacities.
- *Stage III*: pulmonary opacities with no evidence of lymphadenopathy.
- *Stage IV*: advanced lung fibrosis with honeycombing, hilar distortion, bullae, cysts, and emphysema.

Staging is based on the disease appearance on a PA chest radiograph. CT may occasionally suggest another stage, for example, lung involvement identifiable only on CT. The CT findings should not alter the determination of the stage.[113]

Individual patients may not necessarily experience the disease stages in the order presented above. The main role of staging is to help estimate the prognosis, which is essentially determined by the stage at the time of diagnosis. Hence, remission at a more advanced disease stage is less likely (e.g., 65% in stage I and only 20% in stage III[108]).

Radiologic Findings

Lymphadenopathy

Bihilar lymphadenopathy which is characteristic of stages I and II can usually be easily detected on the radiograph (▶Fig. 6.33). But the presence of concomitant mediastinal lymphadenopathy may often not be identifiable on chest radiography. At CT, in one-third of cases only bilateral enlargement of the hilar, but not the mediastinal, lymph nodes is observed. Enlargement of the paratracheal or aortopulmonary lymph nodes alone is rare and involvement of only the posterior mediastinum is extremely rare.

When lymphadenopathy is seen in sarcoidosis, it almost always involves bilateral symmetric hilar lymph nodes, unlike its closest counterparts on differential diagnosis (e.g., lymphoma, tuberculosis, or metastases). Lymphadenopathy virtually always precedes involvement of the skin or eyes. If characteristic skin or eye findings are detected, the absence of bihilar lymphadenopathy rules out clinically suspected sarcoidosis.

In some cases, lymph node enlargement can persist indefinitely after resolution of sarcoidosis; hence, evidence of lymphadenopathy gives no insights into disease activity. Enlarged

Table 6.9 Various historic staging systems versus the currently recommended classification (Joint Statement of the American Thoracic Society, the European Respiratory Society, and the World Association of Sarcoidosis and Other Granulomatous Disorders from 1999)

Radiologic finding	Scadding 1961[110]	DeRemee 1983[111]	Chrétien 1983[112]	ATS 1999[113]
Normal findings		0		0
Bihilar lymphadenopathy	1	I	I	I
Lung involvement with bihilar lymphadenopathy	2	II	IIa	II
Lung involvement without bihilar lymphadenopathy	3	III	IIb	III
Lung fibrosis	4		III	IV

lymph nodes may calcify, occasionally assuming an egg shell-like appearance. In differential diagnosis this may also be suggestive of silicosis.

Pulmonary Opacities

In over three-quarters of cases, the most salient finding on the radiograph is a nodular pattern with apical predominance (▶Fig. 6.34). Numerous sharply marginated, small nodules with a perilymphatic distribution pattern are typically seen on CT (▶Fig. 6.35).

Less common is a random distribution pattern of the nodules in the lung parenchyma. Ground-glass opacity may be observed at times. But this does not reflect an alveolar inflammatory reaction but rather shows countless, minute granulomas in the lung parenchyma. They are too small to be visualized on CT due to its limited spatial resolution. Their presence results in diffusely increased density (▶Fig. 6.36). Occasionally, interlobular septal thickening is observed (▶Fig. 6.37) but this is neither the only nor the most dominant finding.

Confluence of individual granulomas to form larger cohesive consolidations is seen in 10 to 20% of cases. These may over time undergo fibrotic shrinkage: *progressive massive fibrosis* (PMF). On rare occasions, largish individual nodules or a central mass are identified as a solitary manifestation of pulmonary sarcoidosis.

In stage IV, the characteristic signs of fibrosis are observed with hilar elevation, distortion of the lobar fissures, and bundling of the pulmonary vascular structures as well as traction bronchiectasis. Besides, large fibrotic consolidations are common (progressive massive fibrosis). Emphysematous parenchymal lung destruction is also seen (▶Fig. 6.38).

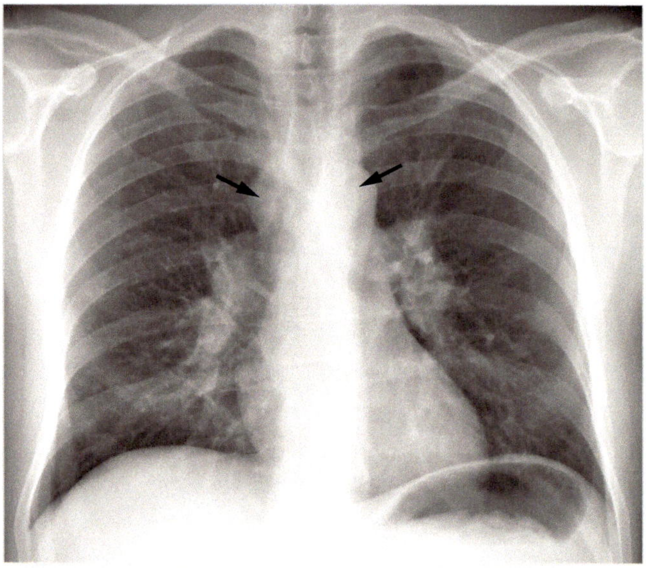

Fig. 6.33 Sarcoidosis I. Radiograph. Bihilar and mediastinal lymphadenopathy (*arrows*) as well as bilateral, enlarged, and polycyclic-bounded hila.

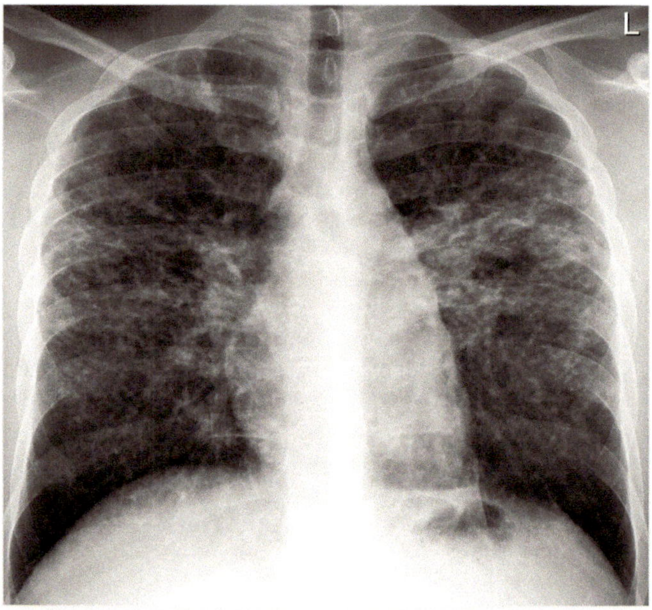

Fig. 6.34 Sarcoidosis II. Radiograph. Small nodular pattern with apical predominance, in addition bihilar and mediastinal lymphadenopathy.

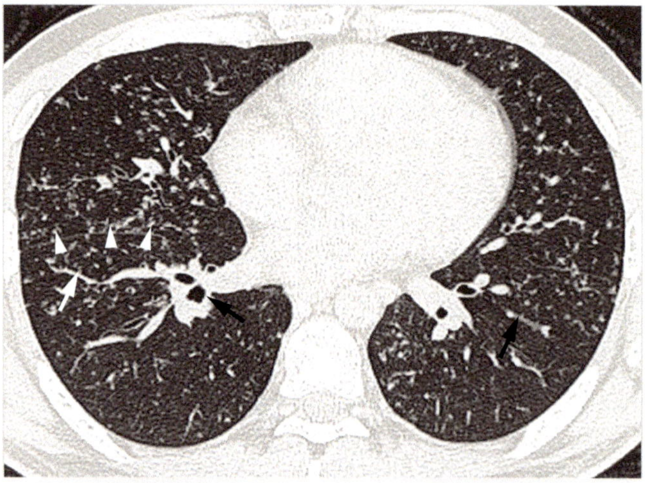

Fig. 6.35 Sarcoidosis II. CT image. Numerous sharply marginated micronodules with perilymphatic distribution pattern along the bronchovascular structures (*arrows*) and subpleural distribution along the lobar fissure (*arrowheads*).

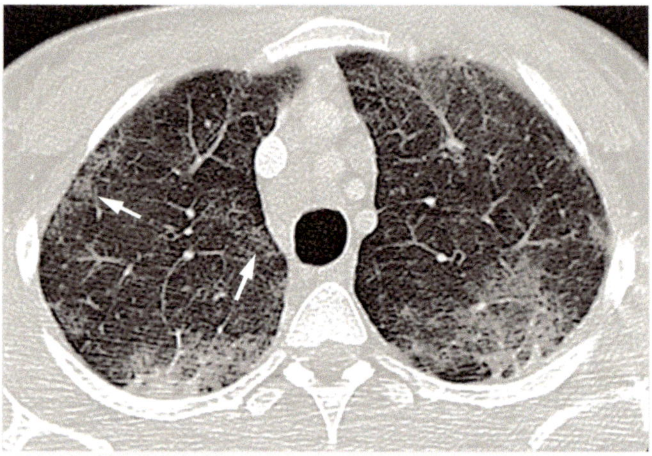

Fig. 6.36 Sarcoidosis II. CT image. Atypical image with predominantly ground-glass opacity and only a slight micronodular pattern (*arrows*).

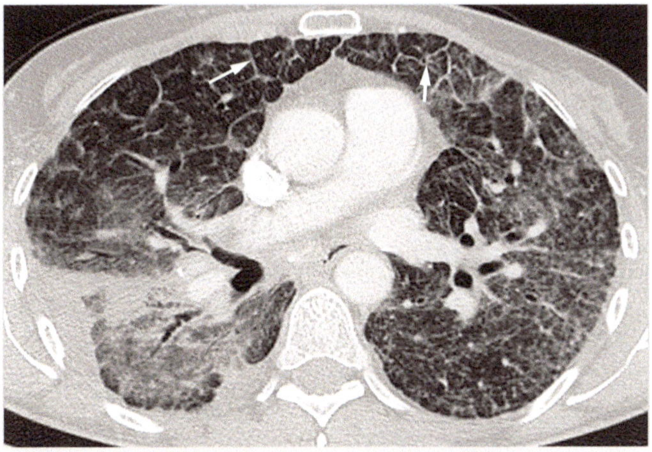

Fig. 6.37 Sarcoidosis IV. CT image. Interlobular septal thickening (*arrows*) as well as right perihilar progressive massive fibrosis.

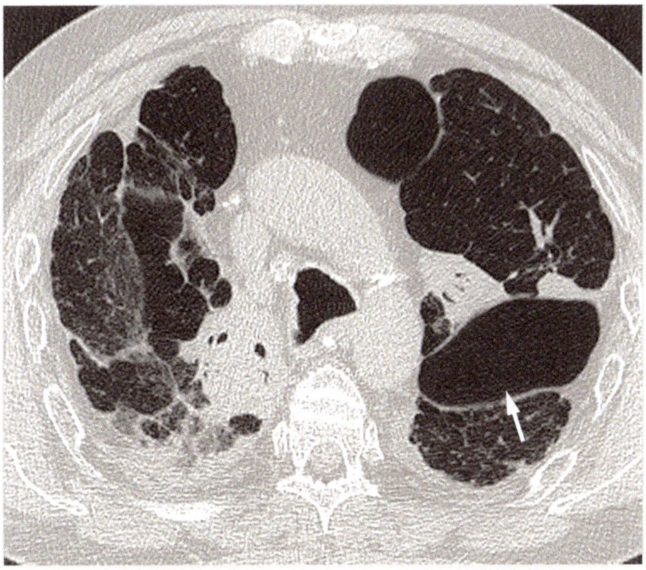

Fig. 6.38 Sarcoidosis IV. CT image. Emphysema-like image with large bullae (*arrow*).

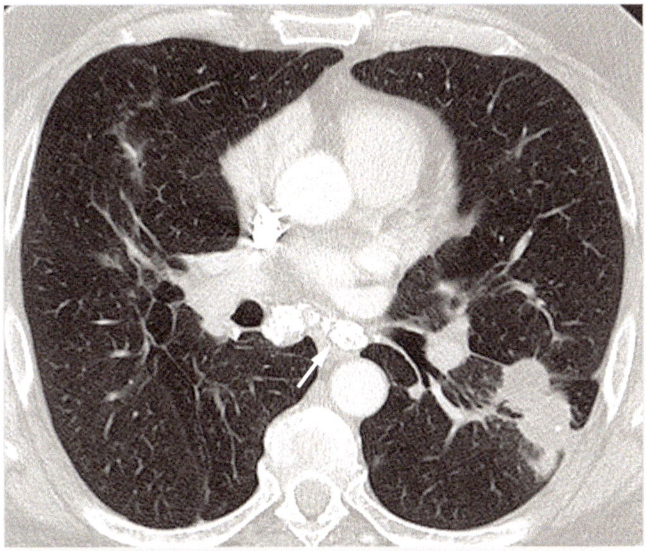

Fig. 6.39 Necrotizing sarcoid granulomatosis. CT image. Few nodules with bizarre shape. In addition, calcified mediastinal lymph nodes (*arrow*).

Differential Diagnosis

Lymphadenopathy and eggshell-like, calcified lymph nodes are also observed in *silicosis*, which exhibits very similar radiologic findings. A characteristic perilymphatic distribution pattern of sharply marginated, small nodules is visualized in both diseases. It is not possible in the individual case to distinguish the radiologic image of silicosis from that of sarcoidosis, especially since at an advanced stage the two diseases tend to result in progressive massive fibrosis. A criterion that may help overcome this differential diagnostic dilemma is that silicosis tends to affect the lung periphery, whereas sarcoidosis is initially seen in the central pulmonary region.

Other important conditions to be taken into account in differential diagnosis are *metastases of malignant tumors* and *malignant lymphomas*. These can cause enlargement of the mediastinal and hilar lymph nodes. Metastatic lung involvement, unlike sarcoidosis, typically exhibits a basal predominance as well as a random rather than a perilymphatic distribution pattern in the lung parenchyma. Carcinomatous lymphangitis is also associated with a perilymphatic distribution pattern of pulmonary nodules as well as smooth or irregular interlobular septal thickening. Unlike sarcoidosis, the most predominant finding is linear opacity, in particular interlobular septal thickening.

6.3.2 Other Granulomatous Parenchymal Lung Diseases

Other idiopathic, noninfectious types of granulomatous parenchymal lung diseases are rarely encountered.

Necrotizing sarcoid granulomatosis is a distinct disease entity. While the histologic image resembles that of sarcoidosis, it is thought to be independent of sarcoidosis due to the presence of necrosis within the granulomas as well as its different radiologic, serologic, and immunologic findings.[114] The clinical presentation is variable and determined by the extent of lung involvement. This ranges from an asymptomatic radiologic incidental finding to severe general symptoms such as fever, night sweats, weight loss, general weakness, chest pain, and cough.[115] Likewise, the eyes (uveitis), liver, and central nervous system may be affected.[116,117,118] Characteristic radiologic features include solitary or multiple pulmonary nodules as well as consolidation with upper lobe predominance (▶Fig. 6.39).[119] Unlike in sarcoidosis, concomitant lymphadenopathy is rare.[117,120,121] Diagnosis is based on histology, usually after examination of material taken from a pulmonary nodule during biopsy.

6.4 Other Types of Diffuse Parenchymal Lung Diseases

This heterogeneous group comprises relatively rare diseases characterized by cystic changes and includes pulmonary

Langerhans cell histiocytosis and lymphangioleiomyomatosis. Besides, various types of diffuse lung diseases that cannot be otherwise classified are assigned to this group, especially pulmonary alveolar proteinosis, vasculitis with pulmonary involvement, and diffuse types of eosinophilic pneumonia.[122]

6.4.1 Pulmonary Langerhans Cell Histiocytosis

The cause of pulmonary Langerhans cell histiocytosis (PLCH) is unknown. A pathogenetic finding is nodular proliferation of Langerhans cells. This disease presents in childhood as manifestation of syndromes with multiorgan involvement (▶Table 6.10) or as an autonomous disease. In the latter case, it mainly affects younger, heavy smokers. The mean age at the time of diagnosis is between 20 and 40 years.[123]

The most common pulmonary symptoms are cough, exertional dyspnea, and chest pain. Around one-quarter of the affected patients remain asymptomatic up to the time of diagnosis. In 20% of patients, spontaneous pneumothorax is the initial clinical feature.

On radiologic imaging, pulmonary Langerhans cell histiocytosis is characterized by multiple, mainly ill-defined nodules measuring up to 10 mm. They often exhibit areas of central colliquation leading to cavitation (▶Fig. 6.40) and finally form cysts (▶Fig. 6.41). The findings show apical predominance and spare the costophrenic angles. In certain cases, nodules regress after smoking cessation. Extremely rarely, pulmonary Langerhans cell histiocytosis presents as a solitary nodule or mass (▶Fig. 6.43).[124]

6.4.2 Lymphangioleiomyomatosis

Lymphangioleiomyomatosis or lymphangiomyomatosis (LAM) affects almost exclusively middle-aged women. It is characterized by multiple pulmonary cysts and is thought to be a low grade, destructive, metastatic, neoplastic disease.[125] Two types are known: a sporadic type and a type associated with tuberous sclerosis.[126] Histologic confirmation is not necessarily required for a definitive diagnosis. The diagnostic criteria are essentially based on radiologic imaging and, to an extent, on the clinical findings (▶Table 6.11). Often, lymphangioleiomyomatosis is first diagnosed after onset of spontaneous pneumothorax. Smoking can exacerbate existing lymphangioleiomyomatosis.

When lymphangioleiomyomatosis involves only mild cystic changes, the radiograph may be normal. Otherwise, a reticular pattern is seen. There may also be pneumothorax or a pleural effusion. CT findings are characteristic and exhibit multiple thin-walled cysts (▶Fig. 6.42a). Renal

Table 6.10 Forms of pulmonary Langerhans cell histiocytosis[100]

Disease onset	Designations	Characteristics
Childhood	Abt–Letterer–Siwe disease	Young children, fulminant multiorgan involvement (liver, spleen, lymph nodes, lung, bones)
	Hand–Schüller–Christian syndrome	Children, disseminated chronic disease; classic triad: osteolysis, exophthalmos, diabetes insipidus; in 30% of cases systemic organ involvement, including the lungs
	Eosinophilic granuloma (histiocytosis X)	Solitary or multiple nodules in bones (osteolysis) or lung
Adulthood	Pulmonary Langerhans cell histiocytosis	Smokers aged 20 to 40 years, in general only pulmonary involvement

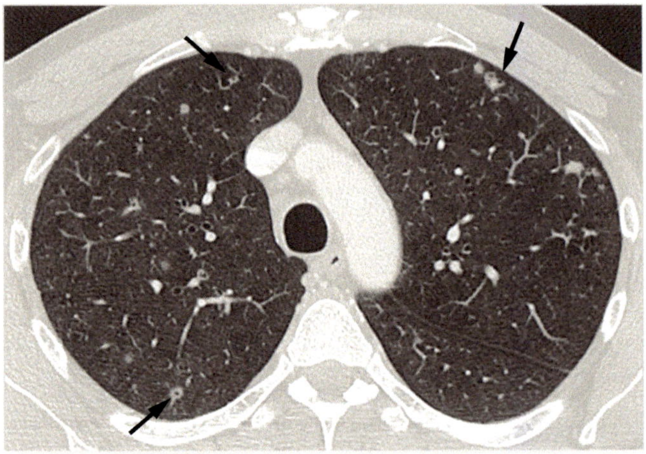

Fig. 6.40 **Pulmonary Langerhans cell histiocytosis.** CT image. Multiple bilateral, ill-defined nodules, some with cavitation (*arrows*).

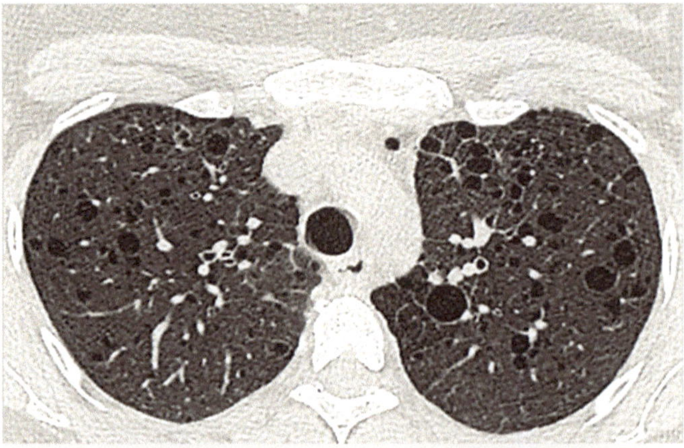

Fig. 6.41 **Pulmonary Langerhans cell histiocytosis.** CT image. Multiple bilateral, thin-walled cysts; no nodules present on this image.

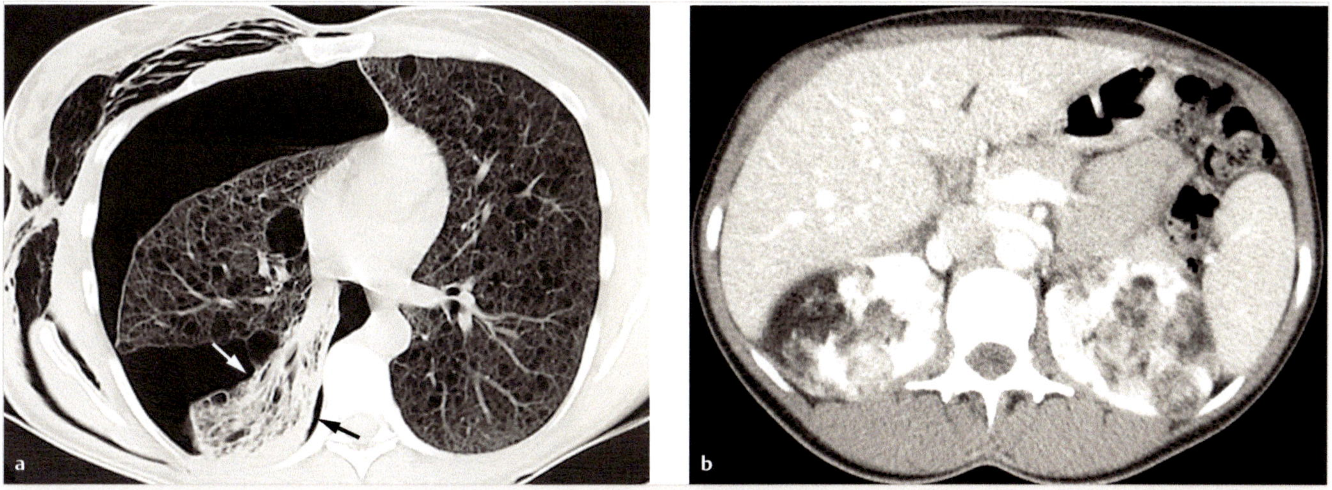

Fig. 6.42 **Lymphangioleiomyomatosis. (a)** On chest CT image multiple bilateral, thin-walled cysts. Large spontaneous pneumothorax on the right, with tension component: mediastinal displacement toward the left and chest wall emphysema due to positive pressure in the right hemithorax. Besides, extensive atelectasis of the right lower lobe (*arrows*). **(b)** On the abdominal CT image, angiomyolipomas in both kidneys: hypodense, fat-containing masses in both kidneys.

Table 6.11 Diagnostic criteria of lymphangioleiomyomatosis[127]

Diagnosis "lymphangioleiomyomatosis"	Chest CT[a]	Other findings
Definitive	Characteristic of lymphangioleiomyomatosis *or* Consistent with lymphangioleiomyomatosis	Lung biopsy findings consistent with lymphangioleiomyomatosis
	Characteristic of lymphangioleiomyomatosis	Renal angiomyolipoma *or* Chylous pleural effusion or ascites or Lymphangioleiomyoma and lymph node involvement in lymphangioleiomyomatose or Definitive or probable tuberous sclerosis complex[b]
Probable	Characteristic of lymphangioleiomyomatosis	Consistent clinical manifestations (pneumothorax or for lymphangioleiomyomatosis typical restrictive lung function)
	Consistent with lymphangioleiomyomatosis	Renal angiomyolipoma *or* chylous pleural effusion or ascites
Possible	Characteristic of lymphangioleiomyomatosis *or* Consistent with lymphangioleiomyomatosis	

[a]Chest CT characteristic of lymphangioleiomyomatosis: more than 10 thin-walled cysts, possibly centrilobular micronodules in patients with tuberous sclerosis, no other findings of interstitial lung disease. Chest CT consistent with lymphangioleiomyomatosis: 2–10 cysts
[b]Tuberous sclerosis complex is probable if at least one primary or secondary criterion has been met. A definition of the criteria can be consulted in European Respiratory Society.[128]

angiomyolipomas and retroperitoneal lymphangioleiomyomas are commonly identified on abdominal CT (▸Fig. 6.42b). Their presence helps to confirm diagnosis of lymphangioleiomyomatosis in association with characteristic findings on chest CT (see ▸Table 6.11).

6.4.3 Pulmonary Alveolar Proteinosis

Pulmonary alveolar proteinosis (PAP) is a rare disease of which three types are distinguished[129]:

- Most common, the adult *idiopathic* type.
- Occasionally, *secondary* to several underlying diseases or inhalation of toxic substances (inhalation of silicates, cement dust, aluminum dust, titanium dioxide, nitrogen dioxide, glass fibers, underlying malignant hematologic diseases; immunodeficiency, e.g., due to immunosuppressive or cytotoxic treatments, viral infections).
- Rarely, *congenital* in neonates.

PAP is caused by an imbalance between surfactant production and clearance, leading to accumulation of surfactant-like proteins in the alveoli.[130,131,132] Granulocyte-macrophage colony-stimulating factor regulates surfactant balance and the immune response.[129] An elevated granulocyte-macrophage colony-stimulating factor level in the peripheral blood and bronchoalveolar lavage serves as a diagnostic marker.

Pulmonary alveolar proteinosis presents clinically as progressive dyspnea persisting over months to years and dry or minimally productive cough. Less common manifestations are weight loss, low fever, exhaustion, chest pain, and hemoptysis.[133,134] The adult idiopathic type affects, in particular,

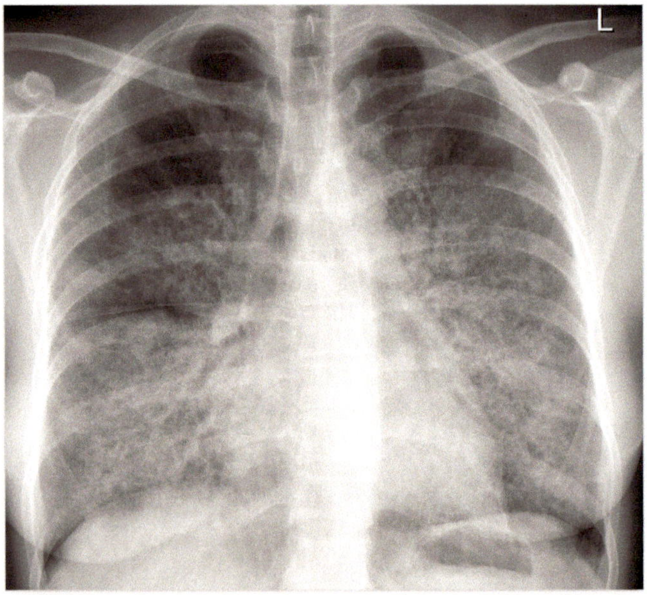

Fig. 6.43 Pulmonary alveolar proteinosis. Radiograph. Bilateral diffuse ground-glass opacity, with lung apices and costophrenic angles spared.

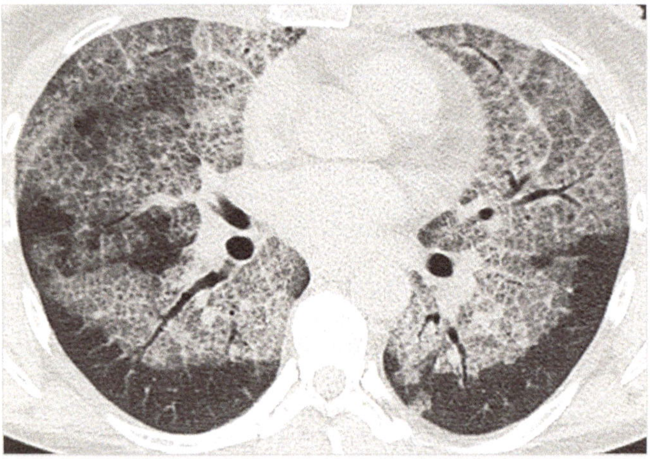

Fig. 6.44 Pulmonary alveolar proteinosis. CT image. Bilateral crazy-paving pattern with geographic outline.

middle-aged smokers. There is also impaired lung diffusion capacity and mild to moderate restrictive lung function.

Bilateral, symmetrical pulmonary opacities are observed in most cases on radiographs, with the lung apices and costophrenic angles remaining relatively unaffected (▶ Fig. 6.44); occasionally, asymmetrical opacities or extensive diffuse consolidation with no particular predominance can also be identified. The intensity of opacities ranges from ground-glass opacity to consolidation with air bronchograms. There is frequently a disparity between the pronounced changes evidenced on the radiograph and the rather mild symptoms that are apparent.[129]

The CT image is characteristic. The most salient findings are sharply marginated, bilateral ground-glass opacities, often with a geographic outline, exhibiting interlobular septal thickening as well as intralobular lines in these areas.[129] Because of its appearance, this image is known as *crazy-paving pattern* (▶ Fig. 6.45).

Note

Differential diagnosis of crazy-paving pattern[129,135]:

- Pulmonary alveolar proteinosis.
- Hydrostatic pulmonary edema in association with congestive heart failure.
- Pneumonia, in particular, *P. jirovecii* pneumonia.
- Alveolar hemorrhage.
- Lepidic growth of adenocarcinoma.
- Carcinomatous lymphangitis.
- Diffuse alveolar damage.
- Radiation pneumonitis.
- Drug-induced lung disease.
- Pulmonary veno-occlusive disease.
- Lipoid pneumonia.

The primary line of treatment for idiopathic pulmonary alveolar proteinosis is whole-lung lavage. Both lungs undergo lavage either synchronously or successively. Imaging shows immediate and widespread regression of pulmonary opacity after lavage. On average, this achieves symptom relief for more than 1 year, but usually repeat lavage is required.

6.4.4 Vasculitis and Other Autoimmune Diseases of the Lung

Chest involvement in idiopathic vasculitis of the large vessels, which presents on imaging studies as apparent vascular disease, is described in Chapter 14.3. This present chapter focuses on vasculitis of the small vessels, which can be identified in radiology only on the basis of the subsequent changes of the lung parenchyma.

Several forms of vasculitis with a highly variable incidence of lung involvement are known. Only those diseases with a high incidence of lung involvement are discussed here. All types of vasculitis that commonly affect the lung are accompanied by anti-neutrophil cytoplasmic antibodies (ANCA): granulomatous polyangiitis (Wegener granulomatosis), microscopic polyangiitis, and eosinophilic granulomatosis with polyangiitis (Churg–Strauss syndrome).

Granulomatous Polyangiitis (Wegener Granulomatosis)

Granulomatous polyangiitis (use of the alternate term, Wegener granulomatosis, is no longer recommended by some American medical societies[136]) is a systemic disease of unknown origin. In 90% of cases, it affects the lung and almost always the upper respiratory tract. Kidney involvement is also common.[137] Diagnosis requires that at least two of the following four criteria be met.

> **Note**
>
> Diagnostic criteria for granulomatous polyangiitis (Wegener granulomatosis), of which at least two must be met[138]:
> - Oral ulcers or nasal discharge.
> - Abnormal chest radiograph (nodules, cavities, or fixed infiltrates).
> - Microhematuria.
> - Granulomatous inflammation on biopsy.

Granulomatous polyangiitis affects the small and medium-sized vessels, presenting usually first in the respiratory tract and with a tendency to generalization. Pulmonary symptoms consist of cough, dyspnea, fever, and chest pain; hemoptysis may also be present.[139] The diagnostic marker in 90% of cases of active granulomatous polyangiitis is elevated levels of c-ANCA (cytoplasmic ANCA).[140,141] On rare occasions, eosinophilia is seen. Diagnosis is mainly based on biopsy.[142]

Imaging shows two main patterns of lung involvement[137]:

- In 70% of cases, pulmonary *nodules* or large masses measuring up to 10 cm are observed. Multiple masses are usually found, but the number of nodules tends to be fewer than 10, with multiple nodules seen only in exceptional cases. In the course of disease, the nodules can often "come and go," with regressive nodules frequently resulting in pulmonary scars. Many of these nodules are cavitating (▶ Fig. 6.46). They usually have ill-defined or spiculated margins. Occasionally, the nodules are surrounded by ground-glass opacity (halo sign), attesting to perifocal hemorrhage.
- Diffuse bilateral *ground-glass opacities* present secondary to pulmonary hemorrhage (▶ Fig. 6.47). The subpleural space often remains unaffected. Areas with intensive bleeding also contain consolidations caused by complete air displacement from the affected alveolar spaces.

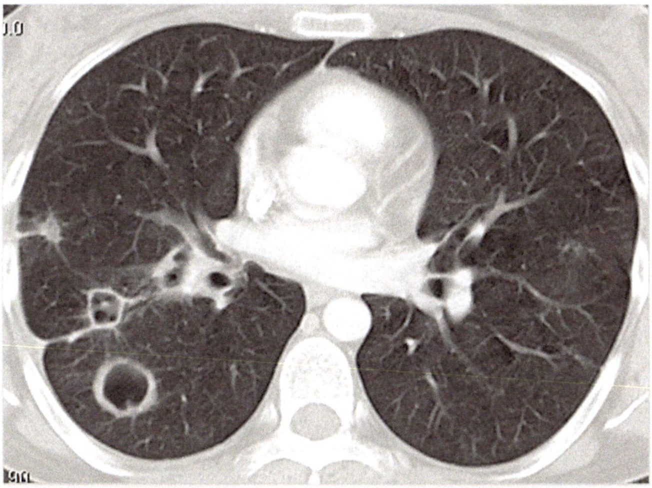

Fig. 6.45 **Granulomatous polyangiitis (Wegener granulomatosis).** CT image. Multiple nodules with some cavitation.

Besides, on CT wall thickening of the trachea and major bronchi as well as stenosis of the central airways may also be identified. A pleural effusion is not unusual.[137]

Eosinophilic Granulomatosis with Polyangiitis (Churg–Strauss Syndrome)

Eosinophilic granulomatosis with polyangiitis (former term: Churg–Strauss syndrome) is characterized by a triad of asthma, hypereosinophilia, and necrotizing vasculitis. Diagnosis requires that at least four of the six following criteria be met.[143]

> **Note**
>
> Diagnostic criteria for eosinophilic granulomatosis with polyangiitis (Churg–Strauss syndrome). Four criteria must be met[144]:
> - Asthma.
> - Peripheral blood eosinophilia with more than 10% eosinophils in the differential blood count.
> - Mononeuropathy (mononeuritis multiplex) or polyneuropathy.
> - Changing pulmonary opacities.
> - Abnormalities of the paranasal sinuses.
> - Evidence of extravascular eosinophilic leukocytes on biopsy.

Onset of asthma is seen later than in the normal population, generally as from age 40 years. Apart from the skin, the lung is the organ most commonly affected. Disease courses with fatal outcome are frequently caused by cardiac involvement with arteritis of the coronary arteries and myocarditis. The mortality rate is meanwhile lower than that of other forms of vasculitis.[145] Pulmonary hemorrhage and glomerulonephritis are less common. Laboratory tests often show elevated p-ANCA (perinuclear ANCA).

Eosinophilic granulomatosis with polyangiitis has three different clinical phases of variable progression and intensity[146]:

- *Phase 1*: prodromal phase with asthma and allergic rhinitis which can persist for several years.

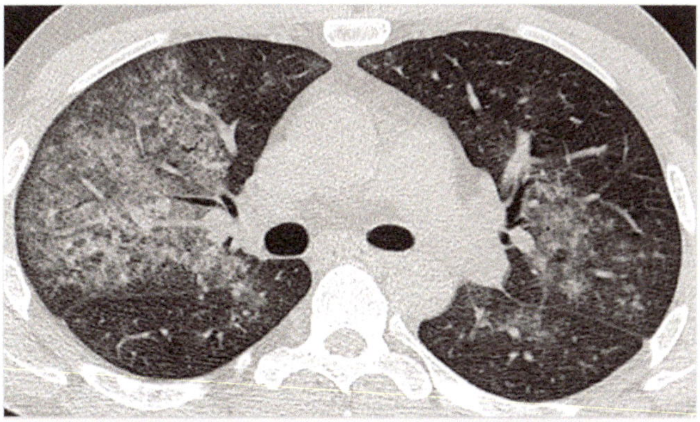

Fig. 6.46 **Granulomatous polyangiitis (Wegener granulomatosis).** CT image. Bilateral diffuse ground-glass opacities, not affecting the subpleural region, consistent with diffuse alveolar hemorrhage.

6

- *Phase 2*: phase with considerable blood eosinophilia and eosinophilic tissue infiltrates, which can manifest as eosinophilic pneumonia.
- *Phase 3*: life-threatening phase with vasculitis.

On histology, there is necrotizing vasculitis of the small vessels and eosinophilic infiltrates with necrotizing granulomas.

In phases 2 and 3, chest radiographs show bilateral, nonsegmental consolidation with no clear predominance. This image resembles that seen in Löffler syndrome, chronic eosinophilic pneumonia, or organizing pneumonia.[143,147] The most salient findings on CT are bilateral ground-glass opacity and consolidation with an almost symmetrical distribution pattern. These manifestations are often seen in the peripheral and, rarely, in the peribronchial regions or are patchily distributed (▶ Fig. 6.48).[146,147,148,149] Interlobular septal thickening can be identified on CT in half of cases.[147] Asthma, which is almost always present, additionally causes radiologic findings described in Chapter 7.1.

Microscopic Polyangiitis

Microscopic polyangiitis is a nongranulomatous, systemic necrotizing form of vasculitis affecting mainly the kidneys and less commonly the lungs. It is the leading cause of *pulmorenal syndrome* observed in association with glomerulonephritis and pulmonary hemorrhage. Clinical symptoms include dyspnea and hemoptysis, in addition to skin lesions, peripheral neuritis, and gastrointestinal bleeding. In laboratory tests, 70% of cases are p-ANCA positive. In general, p-ANCA demonstrates anti-myeloperoxidase (MPO) specificity, hence the name *MPO vasculitis*.[150]

Radiology often demonstrates more or less extensive bilateral ground-glass opacities as a correlate of diffuse pulmonary hemorrhage, a condition that is mainly caused by microscopic polyangiitis, in addition to granulomatous polyangiitis (Wegener granulomatosis).[143] Lung fibrosis is identified in around one-quarter of cases with lung involvement (▶ Fig. 6.49).[151]

Goodpasture Syndrome

Goodpasture syndrome is caused by a type IIa allergic reaction (see ▶ Table 7.1), with antibody formation against antigens of the basement membrane of the blood vessels, giving rise to glomerulonephritis and diffuse pulmonary hemorrhage. This rare disease predominantly affects younger men and is diagnosed on detection of anti-glomerular basement membranes antibodies in the peripheral blood.[152]

Radiology usually exhibits an image typical of diffuse alveolar hemorrhage: bilateral diffuse ground-glass opacities, with the subpleural region remaining relatively unaffected (▶ Fig. 6.50).[143]

6.5 Summary

Diffuse parenchymal lung diseases can be assigned to four large categories:

- Idiopathic interstitial pneumonias.
- Diffuse parenchymal lung diseases of known origin.
- Granulomatous parenchymal lung diseases.
- Other parenchymal lung diseases.

6.5.1 Idiopathic Interstitial Pneumonia

In terms of prognosis, idiopathic interstitial pneumonia constitutes a very heterogeneous group of diffuse parenchymal lung diseases. They are divided into common, rare, familial, and unclassifiable interstitial pneumonias, and often further broken down into chronic fibrosing, acute fibrosing, or subacute fibrosing as well as smoking-related interstitial pneumonias.

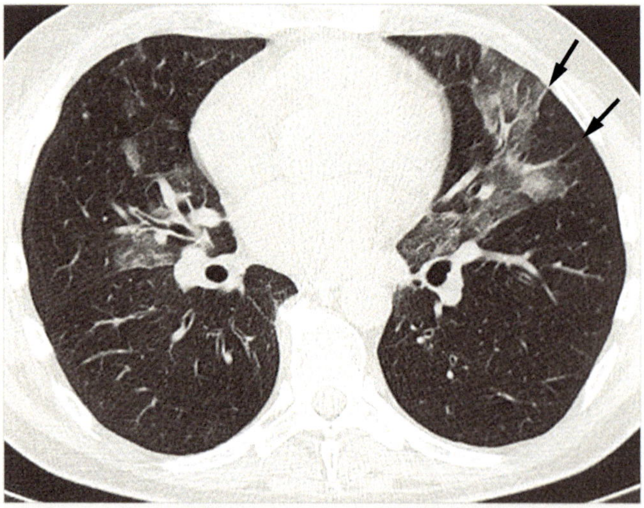

Fig. 6.47 Eosinophilic granulomatosis with polyangiitis (Churg–Strauss syndrome). CT image. Bilateral ground-glass opacities as well as interlobular septal thickening (*arrows*).

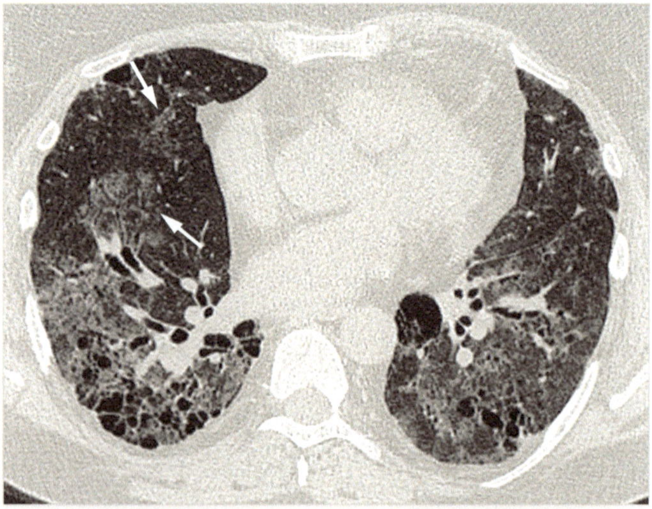

Fig. 6.48 Microscopic polyangiitis. CT image. The most salient findings are signs of lung fibrosis (traction bronchiectasis, honeycombing in the lower lobes, and intralobular lines). Additional ground-glass opacities are consistent with mild, diffuse pulmonary hemorrhage (*arrows*).

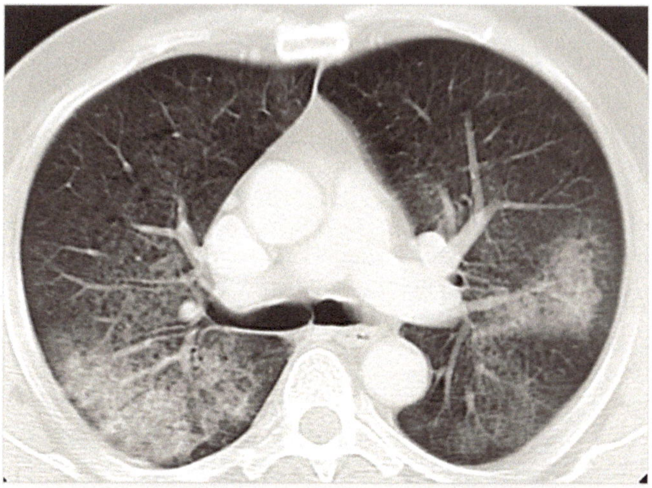

Fig. 6.49 **Goodpasture syndrome.** CT image. Diffuse alveolar hemorrhage with bilateral ground-glass opacities, sparing the subpleural region.

CT plays a key role in diagnosis of idiopathic interstitial pneumonia. Characteristic CT findings in *usual interstitial pneumonia* (UIP) include:

- Reticular opacities.
- Subpleural, basal predominance.
- Honeycombing.

The following findings are deemed inconsistent with usual interstitial pneumonia:

- Involvement of mainly the upper and middle zones or
- Peribronchovascular predominance or
- Predominantly, ground-glass opacities (more than reticular opacities) or
- Numerous micronodules (bilateral, with apical predominance) or
- Multiple cysts (outside areas with honeycombing) or
- Diffuse mosaic attenuation pattern, air trapping, or
- Segmental consolidation.

A diagnosis of usual interstitial pneumonia is confirmed in the presence of all UIP characteristic CT findings and in the absence of any inconsistent results. Lung biopsy is not needed. If only honeycombing is absent, usual interstitial pneumonia is possible but not definite (probable UIP pattern).

Some of the remaining types of idiopathic interstitial pneumonia exhibit typical radiologic manifestations but differential diagnosis is not as clear cut as for usual interstitial pneumonia. Surgical lung biopsy is therefore recommended for a definitive diagnosis in such cases. Radiologic findings:

- *Idiopathic nonspecific interstitial pneumonia* (NSIP): This frequently exhibits ground-glass opacities and intralobular lines but usually only mild or no honeycombing, which is a diagnostic criterion for differentiation versus usual interstitial pneumonia.
- *Cryptogenic organizing pneumonia* (COP): Typical manifestations are antibiotic-refractory, mainly bilateral, consolidations. However, only a solitary consolidation is observed in 10% of cases.
- *Acute interstitial pneumonia* (AIP): A severe acute disease with high mortality. Imaging shows bilateral ground-glass opacities and consolidation, similar to those of adult respiratory distress syndrome.
- *Smoking-related, idiopathic interstitial pneumonia:* They constitute a continuum of histologic findings of variable intensity. Whereas in respiratory bronchiolitis-interstitial lung disease (RB-ILD) the pathologic changes are confined to the small bronchioles, in desquamative interstitial pneumonia (DIP) the alveoli are also affected. RB-ILD is mainly characterized by small centrilobular nodules, and DIP by bilateral ground-glass opacity.

Thanks to a comprehensive classification system, it is possible to reach a diagnosis for around 90% of cases of idiopathic interstitial pneumonia. But that leaves at least 10% unclassifiable diseases.

6.5.2 Diffuse Parenchymal Lung Diseases of Known Origin

In *collagen vascular diseases*, lung involvement is common. NSIP pattern is the most frequent radiologic and pathologic finding. *Rheumatoid arthritis* is an exception in that it is predominantly associated with an UIP pattern. Less commonly, virtually all other interstitial pneumonias are seen with a variable incidence (see ▸Table 6.6). Many other manifestations are known, in particular diseases of the small airways and vascular involvement with pulmonary hypertension. Lung involvement frequently determines the prognosis.

For the detection of pulmonary complications of collagen vascular diseases, CT is vastly superior to chest radiography and is commonly used to exclude complications.[10] This may entail considerable radiation exposure for the, often young, patients; therefore, all technical means of reducing the radiation dose should be exploited.

Numerous chemical and physical noxae can cause diffuse or local lung damage. Clinically important is *pulmonary drug toxicity* resulting in drug-induced lung disease. Up-to-date information on the pulmonary adverse effects of almost 1,000 substances can be consulted on the website www.pneumotox.com. Occupational diffuse parenchymal lung diseases, especially those caused by inorganic and organic dusts, are discussed in Section 18.4.

Radiation pneumonitis, the most common manifestation of physical lung damage, presents as an adverse effect of radiotherapy. Pulmonary radiation doses above 20 Gy can trigger this, and doses above 40 Gy regularly do so.

6.5.3 Granulomatous Parenchymal Lung Diseases

Sarcoidosis, a systemic granulomatous disease of unknown origin, is often associated with bihilar and mediastinal lymphadenopathy as well as with lung involvement. Staging, which is of prognostic relevance (see ▸Table 6.9), is based on detection of pathologic changes on chest radiography. CT findings are not taken into account in staging. The classic pulmonary manifestation on radiography is a small nodular pattern with apical predominance. On CT, a small nodular pattern with perilymphatic distribution is typically observed. Common atypical findings are extensive ground-glass opacities and interlobular septal thickening. At advanced stages, confluence of individual granulomas to form larger consolidations may be seen (progressive massive fibrosis). Lung fibrosis is observed in the terminal stage.

Other granulomatous diseases, such as necrotizing sarcoid granulomatosis, are rare and must be included in the differential diagnosis of pulmonary nodules and masses. They do not exhibit any pathognomonic radiologic features.

6.5.4 Other Diffuse Parenchymal Lung Diseases

Two relatively rare parenchymal lung diseases are characterized by multiple pulmonary cysts: pulmonary Langerhans cell histiocytosis (PLCH) and lymphangioleiomyomatosis (LAM). Spontaneous pneumothorax is often the first manifestation of both diseases. The most important CT findings are summarized in ▶Table 6.12.

Pulmonary *Langerhans cell histiocytosis* occurs in younger smokers and is also seen in childhood in association with certain syndromes. Apart from cysts, there are mainly small, centrilobular nodules that can undergo cavitation and may form cysts. These findings exhibit apical predominance; the costophrenic angles are spared.

Lymphangioleiomyomatosis affects exclusively middle-aged women. Diagnosis is confirmed on detection of extrapulmonary findings, such as renal angiomyolipomas and lymphangioleiomyomas. Some cases present sporadically, while others are seen in settings of tuberous sclerosis complex.

Table 6.12 CT findings in pulmonary Langerhans cell histiocytosis and lymphangioleiomyomatosis

Pulmonary Langerhans cell histiocytosis	Lymphangioleiomyomatosis
• Thin-walled cysts • Centrilobular nodules, possibly cavitating • Apical predominance, sparing the costophrenic angles	• Thin-walled cysts • Renal angiomyolipomas (hypodense to fat-containing masses) • Retroperitoneal lymphangioleiomyomas (cystic or soft tissue-dense masses)

Assigned to the category of other diffuse parenchymal lung diseases are also other diseases such as pulmonary alveolar proteinosis and diffuse types of eosinophilic pneumonia.

Pulmonary alveolar proteinosis affects, in particular, middle-aged smokers. The underlying pathogenesis involves impaired surfactant clearance, leading to accumulation of surfactant-like proteins in the alveoli. The CT image is characteristic: bilateral ground-glass opacities with a geographic outline and an overlying reticular pattern. This combination is known as crazy-paving pattern.

Vasculitis is difficult to diagnose since both the symptoms and the radiologic findings are nonspecific and can be confused with infections, collagen vascular diseases and malignant diseases. The mere fact that vasculitis is included in differential diagnosis represents an important step toward a correct diagnosis and treatment. Clinical findings suggestive of vasculitis:

- Ulcerative or deforming lesions of the upper airways.
- Mononeuritis multiplex.
- Rapidly progressive glomerulonephritis.
- Diffuse alveolar hemorrhage.
- Multiple pulmonary nodules, especially cavitating nodules.

Various forms of vasculitis of the small vessels exhibit a different range of radiologic findings (▶Table 6.13):

- *Granulomatous polyangiitis (Wegener granulomatosis)*: Cavitating nodules as well as bilateral ground-glass opacities and consolidation are two typical patterns of findings. In general, an elevated c-ANCA titer is measured.
- *Eosinophilic granulomatosis with polyangiitis (Churg–Strauss syndrome)*: The combination of asthma, eosinophilia, and pulmonary opacities is suggestive of this disease. Unlike in eosinophilic pneumonia, extrapulmonary symptoms are often exhibited additionally (e.g., neuropathy). A raised p-ANCA titer can support the diagnosis.
- *Microscopic polyangiitis*: Lung fibrosis is observed in one-quarter of cases.
- *Goodpasture syndrome*: Rapidly progressive kidney failure in younger male patients is suggestive of this disorder in the presence of concomitant bilateral ground-glass opacities (diffuse pulmonary hemorrhage).

Onset of diffuse alveolar hemorrhage is typical of, but not specific to, vasculitis of the small vessels.

Table 6.13 Radiologic findings in vasculitis

Granulomatous polyangiitis (Wegener granulomatosis)	Eosinophilic granulomatosis with polyangiitis (Churg–Strauss syndrome)	Microscopic polyangiitis
• Nodules and masses, often cavitating • Diffuse bilateral ground-glass opacities • Less commonly: wall thickening or stenosis of the trachea and major bronchi • Pleural effusion	• Bilateral ground-glass opacities, often peripheral, less commonly peribronchial • Interlobular septal thickening • Signs of asthma	• Diffuse bilateral ground-glass opacities • Signs of lung fibrosis: intralobular lines, honeycombing, traction bronchiectasis

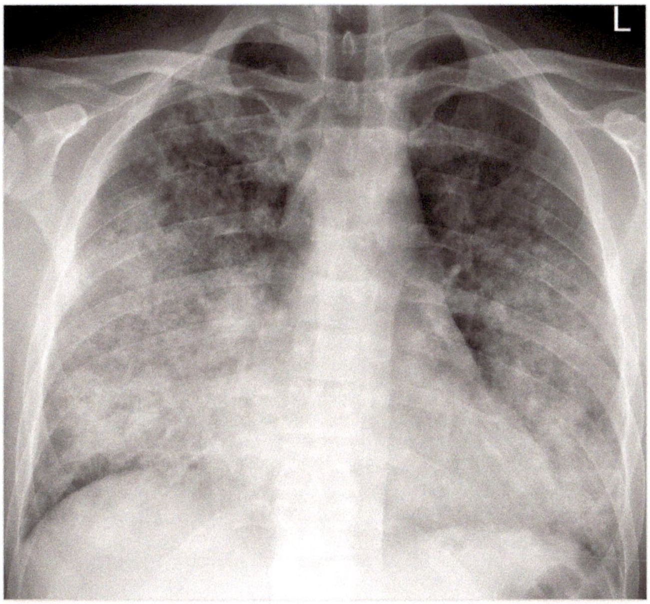

Fig. 6.50 Diffuse alveolar hemorrhage. Radiograph. Extensive bilateral ground-glass opacities.

> **Note**
>
> Differential diagnosis of diffuse alveolar hemorrhage[143,153,154]:
> - Granulomatous polyangiitis (Wegener granulomatosis)
> - Microscopic polyangiitis
> - Eosinophilic granulomatosis with polyangiitis (Churg–Strauss syndrome) (relatively rare)
> - Immune complex vasculitis:
> - Goodpasture syndrome.
> - Schönlein–Henoch purpura.
> - Cryoglobulinemic vasculitis.
> - Secondary vasculitis in autoimmune diseases:
> - Systemic lupus erythematosus.
> - Rheumatoid arthritis.
> - Anti-phospholipid syndrome.
> - Mixed connective tissue disease.
> - Polymyositis-dermatomyositis.
> - Impaired coagulation.
> - Stem cell transplantation.
> - Lung transplantation.
> - Mitral stenosis.
> - Pulmonary drug toxicity.
> - Inhalation trauma.

On radiology, diffuse alveolar hemorrhage manifests as bilateral, diffuse ground-glass opacities (▶Fig. 6.51), while on CT the subpleural region is often seen to be unaffected.

References

[1] American Thoracic Society. European Respiratory Society. International multidisciplinary consensus classification of the idiopathic interstitial pneumonias. Am J Respir Crit Care Med 2002;165(2):277–304

[2] Fishbein MC. Diagnosis: to biopsy or not to biopsy: assessing the role of surgical lung biopsy in the diagnosis of idiopathic pulmonary fibrosis. Chest 2005;128(5, Suppl 1):520S–525S

[3] Bensard DD, McIntyre RC Jr, Waring BJ, Simon JS. Comparison of video thoracoscopic lung biopsy to open lung biopsy in the diagnosis of interstitial lung disease. Chest 1993;103(3):765–770

[4] Kim TS, Han J, Chung MP, Chung MJ, Choi YS. Disseminated dendriform pulmonary ossification associated with usual interstitial pneumonia: incidence and thin-section CT-pathologic correlation. Eur Radiol 2005;15(8):1581–1585

[5] Webb WR, Müller NL, Naidich DP. High-Resolution CT of the Lung. 4th ed. Philadelphia, PA: Wolters Kluwer/Lippincott Williams & Wilkins; 2009

[6] Raghu G, Remy-Jardin M, Myers JL, et al; American Thoracic Society, European Respiratory Society, Japanese Respiratory Society, and Latin American Thoracic Society. Diagnosis of Idiopathic Pulmonary Fibrosis. An Official ATS/ERS/JRS/ALAT Clinical Practice Guideline. Am J Respir Crit Care Med 2018;198(5):e44–e68

[7] Lynch DA, Sverzellati N, Travis WD, et al. Diagnostic criteria for idiopathic pulmonary fibrosis: a Fleischner Society White Paper. Lancet Respir Med 2018;6(2):138–153

[8] Copley SJ, Wells AU, Sivakumaran P, et al. Asbestosis and idiopathic pulmonary fibrosis: comparison of thin-section CT features. Radiology 2003;229(3):731–736

[9] Travis WD, Matsui K, Moss J, Ferrans VJ. Idiopathic nonspecific interstitial pneumonia: prognostic significance of cellular and fibrosing patterns: survival comparison with usual interstitial pneumonia and desquamative interstitial pneumonia. Am J Surg Pathol 2000;24(1):19–33

[10] Antoniou KM, Margaritopoulos G, Economidou F, Siafakas NM. Pivotal clinical dilemmas in collagen vascular diseases associated with interstitial lung involvement. Eur Respir J 2009;33(4):882–896

[11] Kinder BW, Collard HR, Koth L, et al. Idiopathic nonspecific interstitial pneumonia: lung manifestation of undifferentiated connective tissue disease? Am J Respir Crit Care Med 2007;176(7):691–697

[12] Cottin V, Donsbeck AV, Revel D, Loire R, Cordier JF. Nonspecific interstitial pneumonia. Individualization of a clinicopathologic entity in a series of 12 patients. Am J Respir Crit Care Med 1998;158(4):1286–1293

[13] Daniil ZD, Gilchrist FC, Nicholson AG, et al. A histologic pattern of nonspecific interstitial pneumonia is associated with a better prognosis than usual interstitial pneumonia in patients with cryptogenic fibrosing alveolitis. Am J Respir Crit Care Med 1999;160(3):899–905

[14] Katzenstein AL, Fiorelli RF. Nonspecific interstitial pneumonia/fibrosis. Histologic features and clinical significance. Am J Surg Pathol 1994;18(2):136–147

[15] Kim TS, Lee KS, Chung MP, et al. Nonspecific interstitial pneumonia with fibrosis: high-resolution CT and pathologic findings. AJR Am J Roentgenol 1998;171(6):1645–1650

[16] Hartman TE, Swensen SJ, Hansell DM, et al. Nonspecific interstitial pneumonia: variable appearance at high-resolution chest CT. Radiology 2000;217(3):701–705

[17] MacDonald SL, Rubens MB, Hansell DM, et al. Nonspecific interstitial pneumonia and usual interstitial pneumonia: comparative appearances at and diagnostic accuracy of thin-section CT. Radiology 2001;221(3):600–605

[18] Black H, Mendoza M, Murin S. Thoracic manifestations of inflammatory bowel disease. Chest 2007;131(2):524–532

[19] Cordier JF, Loire R, Brune J. Idiopathic bronchiolitis obliterans organizing pneumonia. Definition of characteristic clinical profiles in a series of 16 patients. Chest 1989;96(5):999–1004

[20] Lee KS, Kullnig P, Hartman TE, Müller NL. Cryptogenic organizing pneumonia: CT findings in 43 patients. AJR Am J Roentgenol 1994;162(3):543–546

[21] Müller NL, Staples CA, Miller RR. Bronchiolitis obliterans organizing pneumonia: CT features in 14 patients. AJR Am J Roentgenol 1990;154(5):983–987

[22] Travis WD, Costabel U, Hansell DM, et al; ATS/ERS Committee on Idiopathic Interstitial Pneumonias. An official American Thoracic Society/European Respiratory Society statement: Update of the international multidisciplinary classification of the idiopathic interstitial pneumonias. Am J Respir Crit Care Med 2013;188(6):733–748

[23] Akira M, Yamamoto S, Sakatani M. Bronchiolitis obliterans organizing pneumonia manifesting as multiple large nodules or masses. AJR Am J Roentgenol 1998;170(2):291–295

[24] Katzenstein AL, Myers JL, Mazur MT. Acute interstitial pneumonia. A clinicopathologic, ultrastructural, and cell kinetic study. Am J Surg Pathol 1986;10(4):256–267

[25] Olson J, Colby TV, Elliott CG. Hamman-Rich syndrome revisited. Mayo Clin Proc 1990;65(12):1538–1548

[26] Tomashefski JF Jr. Pulmonary pathology of the adult respiratory distress syndrome. Clin Chest Med 1990;11(4):593–619

[27] Askin FB. Back to the future: the Hamman-Rich syndrome and acute interstitial pneumonia. Mayo Clin Proc 1990;65(12):1624–1626

[28] Bouros D, Nicholson AC, Polychronopoulos V, du Bois RM. Acute interstitial pneumonia. Eur Respir J 2000;15(2):412–418

[29] Vourlekis JS, Brown KK, Cool CD, et al. Acute interstitial pneumonitis. Case series and review of the literature. Medicine (Baltimore) 2000;79(6):369–378

[30] Primack SL, Hartman TE, Ikezoe J, Akira M, Sakatani M, Müller NL. Acute interstitial pneumonia: radiographic and CT findings in nine patients. Radiology 1993;188(3):817–820

[31] Johkoh T, Müller NL, Taniguchi H, et al. Acute interstitial pneumonia: thin-section CT findings in 36 patients. Radiology 1999;211(3):859–863

[32] Ichikado K, Johkoh T, Ikezoe J, et al. Acute interstitial pneumonia: high-resolution CT findings correlated with pathology. AJR Am J Roentgenol 1997;168(2):333–338

[33] Tomiyama N, Müller NL, Johkoh T, et al. Acute respiratory distress syndrome and acute interstitial pneumonia: comparison of thin-section CT findings. J Comput Assist Tomogr 2001;25(1):28–33

[34] Marten K. Interstitielle Lungenerkrankungen bei Rauchern. Fortschr Röntgenstr 2007;179:268–275

[35] Niewoehner DE, Kleinerman J, Rice DB. Pathologic changes in the peripheral airways of young cigarette smokers. N Engl J Med 1974;291(15):755–758

[36] Heyneman LE, Ward S, Lynch DA, Remy-Jardin M, Johkoh T, Müller NL. Respiratory bronchiolitis, respiratory bronchiolitis-associated interstitial lung disease, and desquamative interstitial pneumonia: different entities or part of the spectrum of the same disease process? AJR Am J Roentgenol 1999;173(6):1617–1622

[37] Gruden JF, Webb WR. CT findings in a proved case of respiratory bronchiolitis. AJR Am J Roentgenol 1993;161(1):44–46

[38] Turner-Warwick M. Connective tissue disorders and the lung. Aust N Z J Med 1986;16(2):257–262

[39] Moon J, du Bois RM, Colby TV, Hansell DM, Nicholson AG. Clinical significance of respiratory bronchiolitis on open lung biopsy and its relationship to smoking related interstitial lung disease. Thorax 1999;54(11):1009–1014

[40] Carrington CB, Gaensler EA, Coutu RE, FitzGerald MX, Gupta RG. Natural history and treated course of usual and desquamative interstitial pneumonia. N Engl J Med 1978;298(15):801–809

[41] Hartman TE, Primack SL, Kang EY, et al. Disease progression in usual interstitial pneumonia compared with desquamative interstitial pneumonia. Assessment with serial CT. Chest 1996;110(2):378–382

[42] Yousem SA, Colby TV, Gaensler EA. Respiratory bronchiolitis-associated interstitial lung disease and its relationship to desquamative interstitial pneumonia. Mayo Clin Proc 1989;64(11):1373–1380

[43] Gaensler EA, Goff AM, Prowse CM. Desquamative interstitial pneumonia. N Engl J Med 1966;274(3):113–128

[44] Liebow AA, Steer A, Billingsley JG. Desquamative interstitial pneumonia. Am J Med 1965;39:369–404

[45] Hartman TE, Primack SL, Swensen SJ, Hansell D, McGuinness G, Müller NL. Desquamative interstitial pneumonia: thin-section CT findings in 22 patients. Radiology 1993;187(3):787–790

[46] Ichikawa Y, Kinoshita M, Koga T, Oizumi K, Fujimoto K, Hayabuchi N. Lung cyst formation in lymphocytic interstitial pneumonia: CT features. J Comput Assist Tomogr 1994;18(5):745–748

[47] Reddy TL, Tominaga M, Hansell DM, et al. Pleuroparenchymal fibroelastosis: a spectrum of histopathological and imaging phenotypes. Eur Respir J 2012;40(2):377–385

[48] Antoniou KM, Margaritopoulos GA, Tomassetti S, Bonella F, Costabel U, Poletti V. Interstitial lung disease. Eur Respir Rev 2014;23(131):40–54

[49] Fischer A, Antoniou KM, Brown KK, et al; "ERS/ATS Task Force on Undifferentiated Forms of CTD-ILD". An official European Respiratory Society/American Thoracic Society research statement: interstitial pneumonia with autoimmune features. Eur Respir J 2015;46(4):976–987

[50] Kim EJ, Collard HR, King TE Jr. Rheumatoid arthritis-associated interstitial lung disease: the relevance of histopathologic and radiographic pattern. Chest 2009;136(5):1397–1405

[51] Tanaka N, Kim JS, Newell JD, et al. Rheumatoid arthritis-related lung diseases: CT findings. Radiology 2004;232(1):81–91

[52] Inui N, Enomoto N, Suda T, Kageyama Y, Watanabe H, Chida K. Anti-cyclic citrullinated peptide antibodies in lung diseases associated with rheumatoid arthritis. Clin Biochem 2008;41(13):1074–1077

[53] Lee HK, Kim DS, Yoo B, et al. Histopathologic pattern and clinical features of rheumatoid arthritis-associated interstitial lung disease. Chest 2005;127(6):2019–2027

[54] Tansey D, Wells AU, Colby TV, et al. Variations in histological patterns of interstitial pneumonia between connective tissue disorders and their relationship to prognosis. Histopathology 2004;44(6):585–596

[55] Yoshinouchi T, Ohtsuki Y, Fujita J, et al. Nonspecific interstitial pneumonia pattern as pulmonary involvement of rheumatoid arthritis. Rheumatol Int 2005;26(2):121–125

[56] Bouros D, Wells AU, Nicholson AG, et al. Histopathologic subsets of fibrosing alveolitis in patients with systemic sclerosis and their relationship to outcome. Am J Respir Crit Care Med 2002;165(12):1581–1586

[57] Fujita J, Yoshinouchi T, Ohtsuki Y, et al. Non-specific interstitial pneumonia as pulmonary involvement of systemic sclerosis. Ann Rheum Dis 2001;60(3):281–283

[58] Kim DS, Yoo B, Lee JS, et al. The major histopathologic pattern of pulmonary fibrosis in scleroderma is nonspecific interstitial pneumonia. Sarcoidosis Vasc Diffuse Lung Dis 2002;19(2):121–127

[59] Douglas WW, Tazelaar HD, Hartman TE, et al. Polymyositis-dermatomyositis-associated interstitial lung disease. Am J Respir Crit Care Med 2001;164(7):1182–1185

[60] Cottin V, Thivolet-Béjui F, Reynaud-Gaubert M, et al; Groupe d'Etudes et de Recherche sur les Maladies "Orphelines" Pulmonaires. Interstitial lung disease in amyopathic dermatomyositis, dermatomyositis and polymyositis. Eur Respir J 2003;22(2):245–250

[61] Won Huh J, Soon Kim D, Keun Lee C, et al. Two distinct clinical types of interstitial lung disease associated with polymyositis-dermatomyositis. Respir Med 2007;101(8):1761–1769

[62] Ito I, Nagai S, Kitaichi M, et al. Pulmonary manifestations of primary Sjogren's syndrome: a clinical, radiologic, and pathologic study. Am J Respir Crit Care Med 2005;171(6):632–638

[63] Parambil JG, Myers JL, Lindell RM, Matteson EL, Ryu JH. Interstitial lung disease in primary Sjögren syndrome. Chest 2006;130(5):1489–1495

[64] Lamblin C, Bergoin C, Saelens T, Wallaert B. Interstitial lung diseases in collagen vascular diseases. Eur Respir J Suppl 2001;32:69s–80s

[65] Nicholson AG, Colby TV, Wells AU. Histopathological approach to patterns of interstitial pneumonia in patient with connective tissue disorders. Sarcoidosis Vasc Diffuse Lung Dis 2002;19(1):10–17

[66] Biederer J, Schnabel A, Muhle C, Gross WL, Heller M, Reuter M. Correlation between HRCT findings, pulmonary function tests and bronchoalveolar lavage cytology in interstitial lung disease associated with rheumatoid arthritis. Eur Radiol 2004;14(2):272–280

[67] Altman RD, Medsger TA Jr, Bloch DA, Michel BA. Predictors of survival in systemic sclerosis (scleroderma). Arthritis Rheum 1991;34(4):403–413

[68] Cain HC, Noble PW, Matthay RA. Pulmonary manifestations of Sjögren's syndrome. Clin Chest Med 1998;19(4):687–699, viii

[69] Davidson BK, Kelly CA, Griffiths ID. Ten year follow up of pulmonary function in patients with primary Sjögren's syndrome. Ann Rheum Dis 2000;59(9):709–712

[70] Deheinzelin D, Capelozzi VL, Kairalla RA, Barbas Filho JV, Saldiva PH, de Carvalho CR. Interstitial lung disease in primary Sjögren's syndrome. Clinical-pathological evaluation and response to treatment. Am J Respir Crit Care Med 1996;154(3 Pt 1):794–799

[71] Kim EA, Lee KS, Johkoh T, et al. Interstitial lung diseases associated with collagen vascular diseases: radiologic and histopathologic findings. Radiographics 2002;22(Spec No):S151–S165

[72] Fathi M, Dastmalchi M, Rasmussen E, Lundberg IE, Tornling G. Interstitial lung disease, a common manifestation of newly diagnosed polymyositis and dermatomyositis. Ann Rheum Dis 2004;63(3):297–301

[73] Hirakata M, Nakamura K, Kaburaki J, et al. [Interstitial lung disease in patients with connective tissue diseases] Nihon Kyobu Shikkan Gakkai Zasshi 1995;33(Suppl):268–276

[74] Marie I, Hachulla E, Chérin P, et al. Interstitial lung disease in polymyositis and dermatomyositis. Arthritis Rheum 2002;47(6):614–622

[75] Marie I, Hatron PY, Hachulla E, Wallaert B, Michon-Pasturel U, Devulder B. Pulmonary involvement in polymyositis and in dermatomyositis. J Rheumatol 1998;25(7):1336–1343

[76] Akira M, Hara H, Sakatani M. Interstitial lung disease in association with polymyositis-dermatomyositis: long-term follow-up CT evaluation in seven patients. Radiology 1999;210(2):333–338

[77] Mino M, Noma S, Taguchi Y, Tomii K, Kohri Y, Oida K. Pulmonary involvement in polymyositis and dermatomyositis: sequential evaluation with CT. AJR Am J Roentgenol 1997;169(1):83–87

[78] Bankier AA, Kiener HP, Wiesmayr MN, et al. Discrete lung involvement in systemic lupus erythematosus: CT assessment. Radiology 1995;196(3):835–840

[79] Fenlon HM, Doran M, Sant SM, Breatnach E. High-resolution chest CT in systemic lupus erythematosus. AJR Am J Roentgenol 1996;166(2):301–307

[80] Devaraj A, Wells AU, Hansell DM. Computed tomographic imaging in connective tissue diseases. Semin Respir Crit Care Med 2007;28(4):389–397

[81] Asherson RA, Cervera R, Piette JC, et al. Catastrophic antiphospholipid syndrome. Clinical and laboratory features of 50 patients. Medicine (Baltimore) 1998;77(3):195–207

[82] Hoffbrand BI, Beck ER. „" Unexplained" dyspnea and shrinking lungs in systemic lupus erythematosus. BMJ 1965;1(5445):1273–1277

[83] Jeanmenne T, Singh NK, Pick M. Shrinking lung syndrome. BMJ Case Rep 2009;2009:bcr08.2008.0825

[84] Tavoni A, Vitali C, Cirigliano G, Frigelli S, Stampacchia G, Bombardieri S. Shrinking lung in primary Sjögren's syndrome. Arthritis Rheum 1999;42(10):2249–2250

[85] Ahmed S, Herrick A, O'Driscoll BR. Shrinking lung syndrome in patients without systemic lupus erythematosus: comment on the concise communication by Tavoni et al. Arthritis Rheum 2001;44(1):243–245

[86] Hardy K, Herry I, Attali V, Cadranel J, Similowski T. Bilateral phrenic paralysis in a patient with systemic lupus erythematosus. Chest 2001;119(4):1274–1277

[87] Hemmati I, Blocka K. Shrinking lung syndrome masked by pleuropericarditis: a case report and review of the literature. Clin Rheumatol 2012;31(12):1741–1744

[88] Murin S, Wiedemann HP, Matthay RA. Pulmonary manifestations of systemic lupus erythematosus. Clin Chest Med 1998;19(4):641–665, viii

[89] Sharp GC, Irvin WS, Tan EM, Gould RG, Holman HR. Mixed connective tissue disease--an apparently distinct rheumatic disease syndrome associated with a specific antibody to an extractable nuclear antigen (ENA). Am J Med 1972;52(2):148–159

[90] Kozuka T, Johkoh T, Honda O, et al. Pulmonary involvement in mixed connective tissue disease: high-resolution CT findings in 41 patients. J Thorac Imaging 2001;16(2):94–98

[91] Rossi SE, Erasmus JJ, McAdams HP, Sporn TA, Goodman PC. Pulmonary drug toxicity: radiologic and pathologic manifestations. Radiographics 2000;20(5):1245–1259

[92] Carson CW, Cannon GW, Egger MJ, Ward JR, Clegg DO. Pulmonary disease during the treatment of rheumatoid arthritis with low dose pulse methotrexate. Semin Arthritis Rheum 1987;16(3):186–195

[93] Hacking JC, Flower CD. Causes and investigation of increasing dyspnoea in rheumatoid arthritis. Ann Rheum Dis 1995;54(1):17–19

[94] Kremer JM, Alarcón GS, Weinblatt ME, et al. Clinical, laboratory, radiographic, and histopathologic features of methotrexate-associated lung injury in patients with rheumatoid arthritis: a multicenter study with literature review. Arthritis Rheum 1997;40(10):1829–1837

[95] Padley SP, Adler B, Hansell DM, Müller NL. High-resolution computed tomography of drug-induced lung disease. Clin Radiol 1992;46(4):232–236

[96] Choi YW, Munden RF, Erasmus JJ, et al. Effects of radiation therapy on the lung: radiologic appearances and differential diagnosis. Radiographics 2004;24(4):985–997, discussion 998

[97] Libshitz HI, Southard ME. Complications of radiation therapy: the thorax. Semin Roentgenol 1974;9(1):41–49

[98] Movsas B, Raffin TA, Epstein AH, Link CJ Jr. Pulmonary radiation injury. Chest 1997;111(4):1061–1076

[99] Oie Y, Saito Y, Kato M, et al. Relationship between radiation pneumonitis and organizing pneumonia after radiotherapy for breast cancer. Radiat Oncol 2013;8:56

[100] Du Bois RM, Richeldi L. Interstitial Lung Diseases. Sheffield: European Respiratory Society; 2009

[101] Baughman RP, Lower EE, du Bois RM. Sarcoidosis. Lancet 2003;361(9363):1111–1118

[102] Drent M, Bomans PH, Van Suylen RJ, Lamers RJ, Bast A, Wouters EF. Association of man-made mineral fibre exposure and sarcoidlike granulomas. Respir Med 2000;94(8):815–820

[103] Hunninghake GW, Costabel U, Ando M, et al. ATS/ERS/WASOG statement on sarcoidosis. American Thoracic Society/European Respiratory Society/World Association of Sarcoidosis and other Granulomatous Disorders. Sarcoidosis Vasc Diffuse Lung Dis 1999;16(2):149–173

[104] McGrath DS, Goh N, Foley PJ, du Bois RM. Sarcoidosis: genes and microbes--soil or seed? Sarcoidosis Vasc Diffuse Lung Dis 2001;18(2):149–164

[105] Nilsson K, Påhlson C, Lukinius A, Eriksson L, Nilsson L, Lindquist O. Presence of Rickettsia helvetica in granulomatous tissue from patients with sarcoidosis. J Infect Dis 2002;185(8):1128–1138

[106] Leatham EW, Eeles R, Sheppard M, et al. The association of germ cell tumours of the testis with sarcoid-like processes. Clin Oncol (R Coll Radiol) 1992;4(2):89–95

[107] Löfgren SH, Lundberg G. Erythema Nodosum. Studies on Etiology and Pathogenesis in 185 Adult Cases. Stockholm: Kungl. Boktryckeriet, P. A. Norstedt; 1946

[108] James DG, Turiaf J, Hosoda Y, et al. Description of sarcoidosis: Report of the Subcommittee on Classification and Definition. Ann N Y Acad Sci 1976;278:742

[109] Morgenthau AS, Iannuzzi MC. Recent advances in sarcoidosis. Chest 2011;139(1):174–182

[110] Scadding JG. Prognosis of intrathoracic sarcoidosis in England. A review of 136 cases after five years' observation. BMJ 1961;2(5261):1165–1172

[111] DeRemee RA. The roentgenographic staging of sarcoidosis. Historic and contemporary perspectives. Chest 1983;83(1):128–133

[112] Chrétien J, Marsac J, Saltiel JC, eds. Ninth International Conference on Sarcoidosis and Other Granulomatous Disorders. Paris: Pergamon Press; 1983

[113] American Thoracic Society. Statement on sarcoidosis. Joint Statement of the American Thoracic Society (ATS), the European Respiratory Society (ERS) and the World Association of Sarcoidosis and Other Granulomatous Disorders (WASOG) adopted by the ATS Board of Directors and by the ERS Executive Committee, February 1999. Am J Respir Crit Care Med 1999;160(2):736–755

[114] Costabel U. Seltene Lungenkrankheiten. Grosshansdorf: Inter-Pneu-Verlag; 2002

[115] Claussen M, Kirsten D, Amthor M, Magnussen H. Epitheloidzellige Granulomatose mit beidseitigen grossflächigen Lungenverschattungen. Med Klin (Munich) 1996;91(4):199–204

[116] Baur X, Büchele W, Gokel M, Hacker H, Remberger K, Sunder-Plassmann L. 25jähriger Mann mit multiplen Lungenrundherden. Internist (Berl) 1987;28(2):128–133

[117] Koss MN, Hochholzer L, Feigin DS, Garancis JC, Ward PA. Necrotizing sarcoid-like granulomatosis: clinical, pathologic, and immunopathologic findings. Hum Pathol 1980;11(5, Suppl):510–519

[118] Rosen Y, Moon S, Huang CT, Gourin A, Lyons HA. Granulomatous pulmonary angiitis in sarcoidosis. Arch Pathol Lab Med 1977;101(4):170–174

[119] Niimi H, Hartman TE, Müller NL. Necrotizing sarcoid granulomatosis: computed tomography and pathologic findings. J Comput Assist Tomogr 1995;19(6):920–923

[120] Chittock DR, Joseph MG, Paterson NA, McFadden RG. Necrotizing sarcoid granulomatosis with pleural involvement. Clinical and radiographic features. Chest 1994;106(3):672–676

[121] Churg A. Pulmonary angiitis and granulomatosis revisited. Hum Pathol 1983;14(10):868–883

[122] Wells AU. Managing diagnostic procedures in idiopathic pulmonary fibrosis. Eur Respir Rev 2013;22(128):158–162

[123] Abbott GF, Rosado-de-Christenson ML, Franks TJ, Frazier AA, Galvin JR. From the archives of the AFIP: pulmonary Langerhans cell histiocytosis. Radiographics 2004;24(3):821–841

[124] Khoor A, Myers JL, Tazelaar HD, Swensen SJ. Pulmonary Langerhans cell histiocytosis presenting as a solitary nodule. Mayo Clin Proc 2001;76(2):209–211

[125] McCormack FX, Travis WD, Colby TV, Henske EP, Moss J. Lymphangioleiomyomatosis: calling it what it is: a low-grade, destructive, metastasizing neoplasm. Am J Respir Crit Care Med 2012;186(12):1210–1212

[126] Xu KF, Lo BH. Lymphangioleiomyomatosis: differential diagnosis and optimal management. Ther Clin Risk Manag 2014;10:691–700

[127] Johnson SR, Cordier JF, Lazor R, et al; Review Panel of the ERS LAM Task Force. European Respiratory Society guidelines for the diagnosis and management of lymphangioleiomyomatosis. Eur Respir J 2010;35(1):14–26

[128] European Respiratory Society. ERS LAM Task force diagnostic criteria and recommended assessments for patients with tuberous sclerosis complex (TSC), Appendix 2. Available at: http://www.erj.ersjournals.com/content/suppl/2010/06/01/35.1.14.DC1/ERS_LAM_guidelines_appendix_2.doc

[129] Frazier AA, Franks TJ, Cooke EO, Mohammed TL, Pugatch RD, Galvin JR. From the archives of the AFIP: pulmonary alveolar proteinosis. Radiographics 2008;28(3):883–899, quiz 915

[130] Doerschuk CM. Pulmonary alveolar proteinosis--is host defense awry? N Engl J Med 2007;356(6):547–549

[131] Katzenstein AA. Katzenstein and Askin's Surgical Pathology of Non-Neoplastic Lung Disease. 4th ed. Edinburgh: Elsevier Saunders; 2006

[132] Uchida K, Beck DC, Yamamoto T, et al. GM-CSF autoantibodies and neutrophil dysfunction in pulmonary alveolar proteinosis. N Engl J Med 2007;356(6):567–579

[133] Ioachimescu OC, Kavuru MS. Pulmonary alveolar proteinosis. Chron Respir Dis 2006;3(3):149–159

[134] Presneill JJ, Nakata K, Inoue Y, Seymour JF. Pulmonary alveolar proteinosis. Clin Chest Med 2004;25(3):593–613, viii

[135] Hansell DM, Bankier AA, MacMahon H, McLoud TC, Müller NL, Remy J. Fleischner Society: glossary of terms for thoracic imaging. Radiology 2008;246(3):697–722

[136] Falk RJ, Gross WL, Guillevin L, et al. Granulomatosis with polyangiitis (Wegener's): an alternative name for Wegener's granulomatosis. J Am Soc Nephrol 2011;22(4):587–588

[137] Martinez F, Chung JH, Digumarthy SR, et al. Common and uncommon manifestations of Wegener granulomatosis at chest CT: radiologic-pathologic correlation. Radiographics 2012;32(1):51–69

[138] Leavitt RY, Fauci AS, Bloch DA, et al. The American College of Rheumatology 1990 criteria for the classification of Wegener's granulomatosis. Arthritis Rheum 1990;33(8):1101–1107

[139] Olivencia-Simmons I. Wegener's granulomatosis: symptoms, diagnosis, and treatment. J Am Acad Nurse Pract 2007;19(6):315–320

[140] Pretorius ES, Stone JH, Hellman DB, Fishman EK. Wegener's Granulomatosis: CT evolution of pulmonary parenchymal findings in treated disease. Crit Rev Computed Tomogr 2004;45(1):67–85

[141] Uehara A, Sato T, Iwashiro A, Yokota S. PR3-ANCA in Wegener's granulomatosis prime human mononuclear cells for enhanced activation via TLRs and NOD1/2. Diagn Pathol 2009;4:23

[142] Seo P, Stone JH. The antineutrophil cytoplasmic antibody-associated vasculitides. Am J Med 2004;117(1):39–50

[143] Castañer E, Alguersuari A, Gallardo X, et al. When to suspect pulmonary vasculitis: radiologic and clinical clues. Radiographics 2010;30(1):33–53

[144] Masi AT, Hunder GG, Lie JT, et al. The American College of Rheumatology 1990 criteria for the classification of Churg-Strauss syndrome (allergic granulomatosis and angiitis). Arthritis Rheum 1990;33(8): 1094–1100

[145] Solans R, Bosch JA, Pérez-Bocanegra C, et al. Churg-Strauss syndrome: outcome and long-term follow-up of 32 patients. Rheumatology (Oxford) 2001;40(7):763–771

[146] Kim YK, Lee KS, Chung MP, et al. Pulmonary involvement in Churg-Strauss syndrome: an analysis of CT, clinical, and pathologic findings. Eur Radiol 2007;17(12):3157–3165

[147] Worthy SA, Müller NL, Hansell DM, Flower CD. Churg-Strauss syndrome: the spectrum of pulmonary CT findings in 17 patients. AJR Am J Roentgenol 1998;170(2):297–300

[148] Choi YH, Im JG, Han BK, Kim JH, Lee KY, Myoung NH. Thoracic manifestation of Churg-Strauss syndrome: radiologic and clinical findings. Chest 2000;117(1):117–124

[149] Silva CIS, Müller NL, Fujimoto K, Johkoh T, Ajzen SA, Churg A. Churg-Strauss syndrome: high resolution CT and pathologic findings. J Thorac Imaging 2005;20(2):74–80

[150] Schnabel A, Gross WL. Pulmonale Vaskulitis. Lungenbeteiligung bei systemischen Gefässentzündungen. Pneumologie 2000;54(6): 232–242

[151] Tzelepis GE, Kokosi M, Tzioufas A, et al. Prevalence and outcome of pulmonary fibrosis in microscopic polyangiitis. Eur Respir J 2010;36(1):116–121

[152] Salama AD, Levy JB, Lightstone L, Pusey CD. Goodpasture's disease. Lancet 2001;358(9285):917–920

[153] Brown KK. Pulmonary vasculitis. Proc Am Thorac Soc 2006;3(1):48–57

[154] Marten K, Schnyder P, Schirg E, Prokop M, Rummeny EJ, Engelke C. Pattern-based differential diagnosis in pulmonary vasculitis using volumetric CT. AJR Am J Roentgenol 2005;184(3):720–733

Chapter 7

Immunologic Diseases of the Lung

7 Immunologic Diseases of the Lung

II

Immunologic diseases of the lung may present in the bronchial system, lung parenchyma, and the pulmonary vessels. The classification system used in this book with breakdown into allergic, eosinophilic, and vascular pulmonary diseases is—just like other attempts to categorize these—arbitrary and inevitably results in overlapping. For example, allergic bronchopulmonary aspergillosis can be assigned to both the allergic and eosinophilic pulmonary disease groups. These overlaps will be pointed out in the introductory text to the respective sections.

7.1 Allergic Pulmonary Diseases

Allergic reactions essentially involve four different immune mechanisms. These are summarized in ▶Table 7.1. These different types of allergic reaction account for varying degrees for the diseases presented here.

7.1.1 Asthma

Asthma is characterized by major changes in intrapulmonary respiratory tract resistance within a very short period of time. This is caused by reversible bronchoconstriction, increased mucus secretion, and edema of the bronchial mucosa, giving rise to reversible hyperinflation of the airspaces. In two-thirds of asthma patients, this involves allergic bronchial asthma. The bronchial changes described above are caused by an allergic type I reaction. The remaining third of patients have nonallergic, intrinsic asthma.

The main clinical manifestations are cough and attack-like shortness of breath, in particular, at night and in the morning, wheezing, and transparent, viscous sputum. With regard to lung function, asthma is associated with increased lung volume and higher functional residual volume. Concomitant reduced vital capacity attests to the presence of peripheral obstruction and resultant air trapping. Severe complications are very rare. Pneumothorax or mediastinal emphysema is seen especially in children. Increased endobronchial mucus viscosity may cause hyperinflation due to an endobronchial valve mechanism. The resultant clinical picture is similar to that of tension pneumothorax.

The use of chest radiography is controversial in different guidelines.[1,2] The following conditions may constitute an indication for chest radiography:

- Patients to be admitted to the hospital because of asthma.
- Suspected pneumonia or pneumothorax.
- Before mechanical ventilation.
- In cases of poor response to treatment.
- If methotrexate treatment is intended.

In around one-quarter of patients, treatment-relevant findings are identified on imaging. At times, CT may be indicated for severe asthma to exclude differential diagnoses, in particular, to rule out malformations, dysplasia, tumors, bronchiolitis, bronchiectasis, pulmonary embolisms, and various types of diffuse parenchymal lung diseases.[1,3]

The radiologic findings in asthma are summarized in ▶Table 7.2; also see ▶Fig. 7.1 and ▶Fig. 7.2.

7.1.2 Allergic Bronchopulmonary Aspergillosis

In industrialized countries, allergic bronchopulmonary aspergillosis is the most common eosinophilic lung disease. It predominantly affects long-term asthma patients and patients with cystic fibrosis. *Aspergillus* antigens, usually belonging to *Aspergillus fumigatus*, trigger types I and III allergic reactions in the bronchial mucosa.[4] Type I reaction causes a bronchial spasm, as seen in asthma, as well as blood eosinophilia. Type III reaction causes damage to the bronchial wall tissues, giving rise over time to bronchiectasis.

In general, diagnosis is clinically suspected and is confirmed with radiology and serology.[5] Diagnostic criteria are presented in ▶Table 7.3; rarely all criteria are met at the same time.

Table 7.1 Types of allergic reactions and associated allergic pulmonary diseases

Allergy type	Description	Pulmonary diseases
Type I	Classic immediate-type allergy: • Immunoglobulin-E-mediated: – Mast cell activation – Histamine release • Reaction in seconds to minutes	• Allergic bronchopulmonary aspergillosis • Asthma
Type II	Cytotoxicity: antibody production → opsonization of autologous structures (antibody marking)	
• Type IIa	Destruction by immune system	Goodpasture syndrome
• Type IIb	Activation	
Type III	Formation of immune complexes: antibodies against soluble antigens: • Multivalent complex formation • Deposition in capillaries or complement activation	• Hypersensitivity pneumonitis • Allergic bronchopulmonary aspergillosis
Type IV	Delayed-type: T cell activation by soluble antigens → macrophage activation	Hypersensitivity pneumonitis

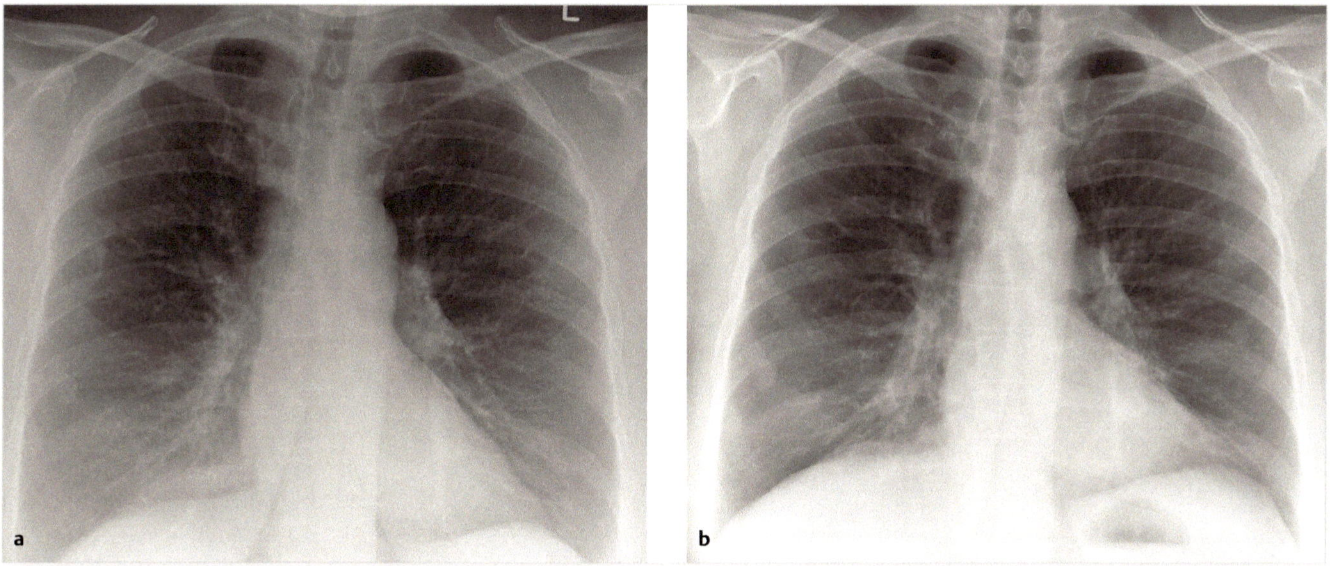

Fig. 7.1 **Lung hyperinflation in asthma.** Radiographs. **(a)** On clinical deterioration, bilateral, low-riding diaphragm as a sign of hyperinflation. **(b)** The findings revert to normal on clinical improvement.

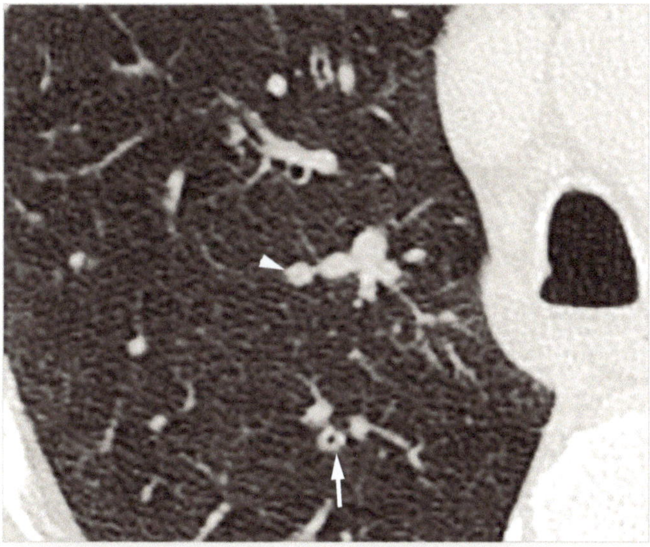

Fig. 7.2 **Bronchial wall thickening (*arrow*) and mucoid impaction (*arrowhead*) in asthma.** CT image.

Table 7.2 Radiologic findings in asthma

Diagnostic imaging	Findings
Radiograph (▸Fig. 7.1)	• Signs of hyperinflation: – Low-riding diaphragm – Diaphragmatic flattening – Expansion of the intercostal spaces • Thickening of the subsegmental bronchial walls • Prominent hila (vascular, lymphadenopathy)
CT (▸Fig. 7.2)	• Bronchial wall thickening • Linear opacities • Reduced lung density • Mucoid impaction • Small centrilobular opacities • Cylindrical bronchiectasis • Rarely, consolidation

Allergic bronchopulmonary aspergillosis progresses in five clinical stages[7]:

- *Stage 1*: Acute stage (initial manifestation with cough, fever, transient pulmonary infiltrates, and bronchial obstruction).
- *Stage 2*: Remission of clinical and immunologic parameters.
- *Stage 3*: Exacerbation.
- *Stage 4*: Corticosteroid dependence.
- *Stage 5*: Fibrosis.

Radiologic changes may be absent in early stages. Findings include transient pulmonary infiltrates and evidence of mucoid impaction: tubular (toothpaste sign), branching consolidation (gloved finger sign), in particular, in the apical and central lung regions, and occasionally areas of lobular or segmental atelectasis.[4,8] In advanced stages, central bronchiectasis and

Table 7.3 Diagnostic criteria for allergic bronchopulmonary aspergillosis[4,6]

Diagnostic examination	Diagnostic criteria
Clinical examination	• Asthma • Immediate skin reaction to *Aspergillus* antigens
Serology	• Blood eosinophilia • Precipitation antibodies against *Aspergillus* antigens • Elevated serum immunoglobulin E levels (correlates with disease activity)
Imaging	• Pulmonary infiltrates • Central bronchiectasis

lung fibrosis are observed as well. Radiologic findings (▶Table 7.4) can be distinguished as transient (▶Fig. 7.3) and chronic manifestations (▶Fig. 7.4).

7.1.3 Hypersensitivity Pneumonitis

More than 200 inhalative allergens are known to trigger allergic reactions in the lung. ▶Table 7.5 gives a brief overview of these, often occupational, diseases. Pulmonary hypersensitivity involves types III (formation of immune complexes) and IV (T cell-mediated, delayed-type) allergic reactions.[9]

Clinical onset of hypersensitivity pneumonitis involves acute, flu-like symptoms, cough, and shortness of breath around 4 to 12 hours after contact with the allergen. Pathologic manifestations include neutrophilic and lymphocytic alveolitis as well as alveolar damage. Alveolitis may resolve or progress to lung fibrosis.

Three stages of hypersensitivity pneumonitis may be observed; they can merge or be coexisting in an individual patient. These are determined by the duration and extent of allergen exposure as well as by the immune response:

- *Acute hypersensitivity pneumonitis*: Flu-like symptoms develop within a few hours after exposure to the allergen. If there is no further exposure to the allergen, the symptoms resolve within a few days. This stage is rarely seen on radiologic images since there is generally no indication for radiographic examination. If a radiograph has been obtained, it may show bilateral, more or less extensive, consolidation and small, rounded opacities(▶Fig. 7.5).[11]
- *Subacute hypersensitivity pneumonitis*: The acute phase of the disease resolves within a few days. Then, or in the intervals between several acute flares, a discrete nodular pattern is seen on the radiograph (▶Fig. 7.6). The CT findings are virtually pathognomonic: multiple centrilobular ground-glass nodules and diffuse ground-glass opacity or mosaic

Table 7.4 Radiologic findings in allergic bronchopulmonary aspergillosis

Transient findings	Chronic findings
• Consolidation (often recurrence at same location) • Mucoid impaction (toothpaste or gloved finger sign) • Atelectasis • Pleural effusion	• Central bronchiectasis • Fibrosis • Bronchoceles • Mycetoma (in particular in the middle fields)

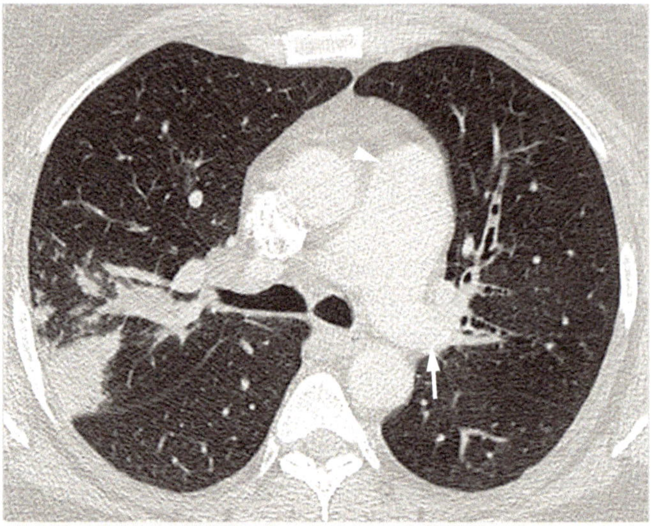

Fig. 7.3 Allergic bronchopulmonary aspergillosis. CT image. Transient findings with consolidation in right upper lobe (*arrowheads*); mucoid impaction in the left upper lobe (*arrow*).

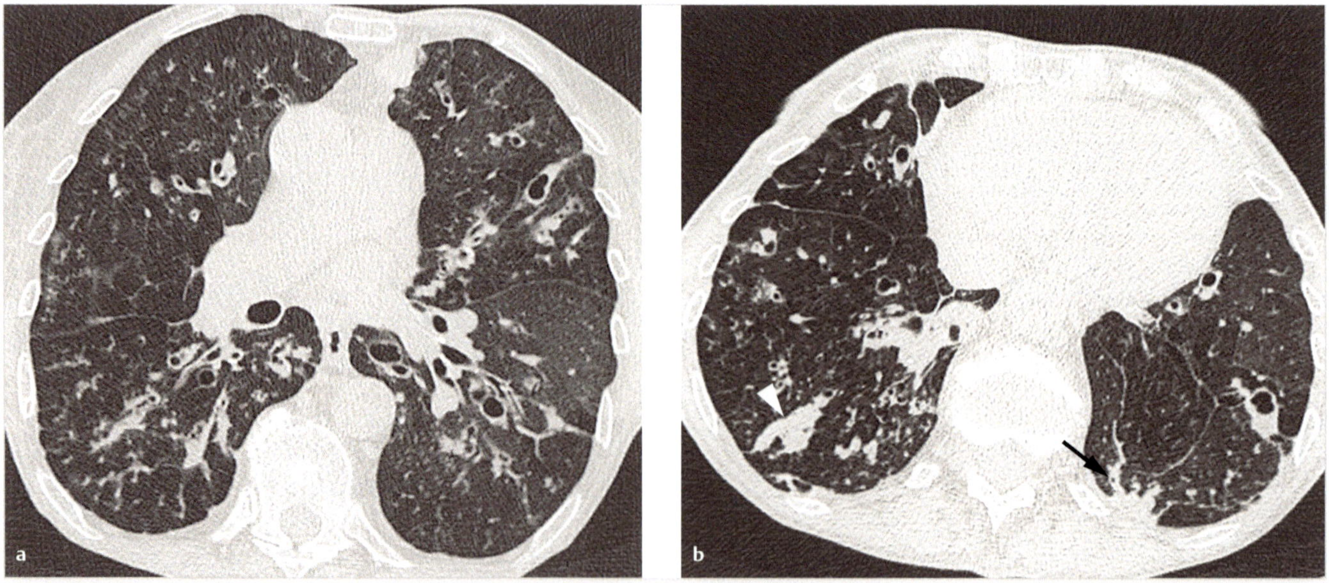

Fig. 7.4 Allergic bronchopulmonary aspergillosis. CT images. Chronic findings. **(a)** Multiple areas of central bronchiectasis. **(b)** Besides, fibrosis (*arrow*) and → (*arrowhead*).

pattern (▶Fig. 7.7). Occasionally, small cysts are observed as well. The findings can completely resolve in the absence of exposure to the allergen.

- *Chronic hypersensitivity pneumonitis*: Long-lasting hypersensitivity pneumonitis can cause development of lung fibrosis (▶Fig. 7.8). If contact with the allergen persists, subacute and acute disease manifestations can coincide.

Table 7.5 Hypersensitivity pneumonitis listed in ICD-10 under Code J67[10]

Disease entity	Examples
Farmer lung	• Haymaker lung • Harvester lung • Moldy hay disease
Bird fancier lung	• Pigeon fancier lung • Budgerigar fancier lung
Suberosis	• Corkworker lung • Corkhandler lung
Bagassosis	
Maltworker lung	
Mushroom-worker lung	
Maple-bark-stripper lung	
Air-conditioner and humidifier lung	
Hypersensitivity pneumonitis due to other organic dusts	• Fishmeal-worker lung • Cheese-washer lung • Coffee-worker lung • Furrier lung • Sequoiosis

While the latter entities are reversible, lung fibrosis secondary to chronic hypersensitivity pneumonitis is irreversible. This is characterized by restriction on pulmonary function tests. In radiologic findings, variable amounts of pulmonary fibrosis (honeycombing, intralobular lines, traction bronchiectasis) and ground-glass opacity are seen (▶Table 7.6). Unlike other forms of pulmonary fibrosis, chronic hypersensitivity pneumonitis is not associated with basal predominance. Likewise, there is little involvement of the costophrenic angles, whereas these are the main location affected by other forms of fibrosis (see Chapter 6). Imaging criteria for differential diagnosis are summarized in ▶Table 7.7.

7.2 Eosinophilic Lung Diseases

Eosinophilic lung diseases are characterized by pulmonary infiltrates and an increase in circulating or tissue eosinophils. The clinical spectrum of disease comprises acute and chronic forms. At least one of the diagnostic criteria listed below must be met for diagnosis of eosinophilic lung disease[4,14]:

- Pulmonary infiltrates and peripheral eosinophilia.
- Tissue eosinophilia in transbronchial or open lung biopsy.
- Elevated eosinophil count in bronchoalveolar lavage.

This chapter covers acute eosinophilic pneumonia (AEP) and chronic eosinophilic pneumonia (CEP) as well as idiopathic hypereosinophilia syndrome. Other diseases associated with eosinophilia are discussed elsewhere:

- *Allergic bronchopulmonary aspergillosis*: This was already introduced in the section on allergic pulmonary diseases.

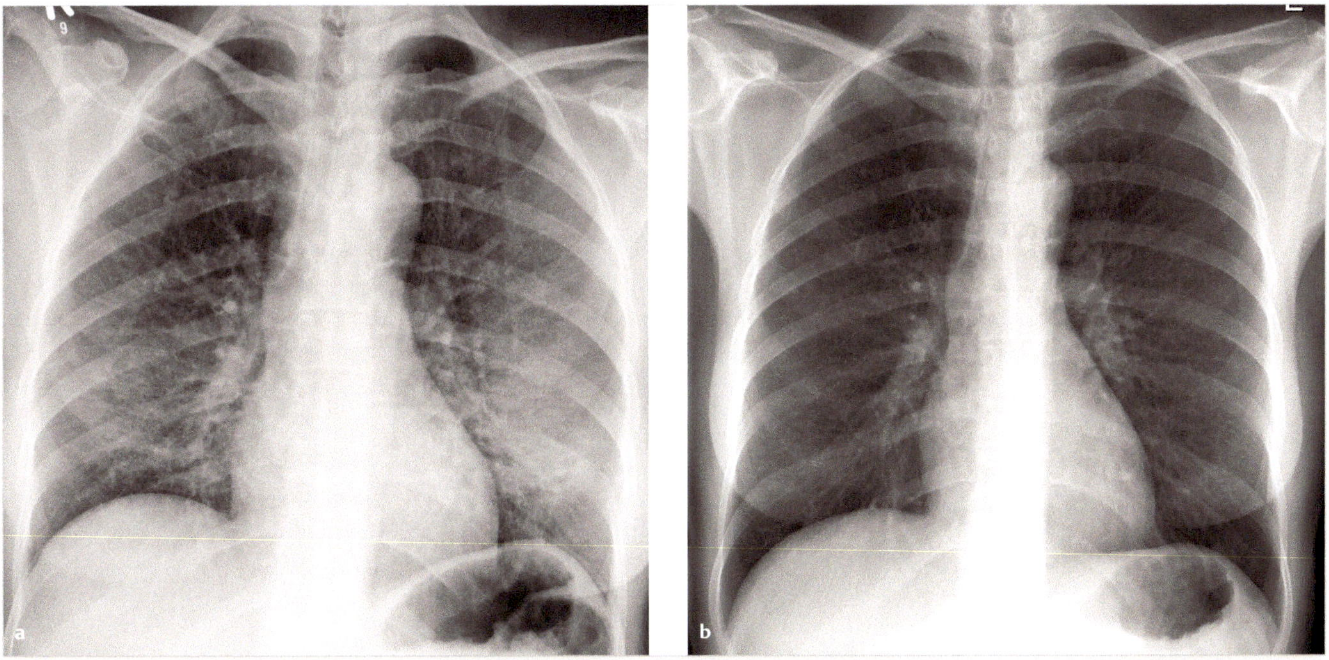

Fig. 7.5 Acute hypersensitivity pneumonitis. Radiographs. **(a)** Bilateral consolidation in the middle and lower fields. **(b)** Two weeks later, consolidations have completely resolved.

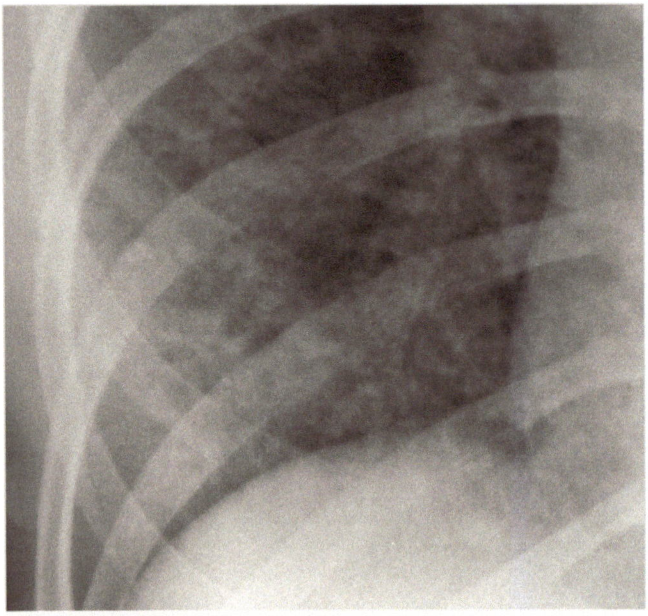

Fig. 7.6 Subacute hypersensitivity pneumonitis. Magnified section of radiograph. Subtle nodular pattern and diffuse ground-glass opacities.

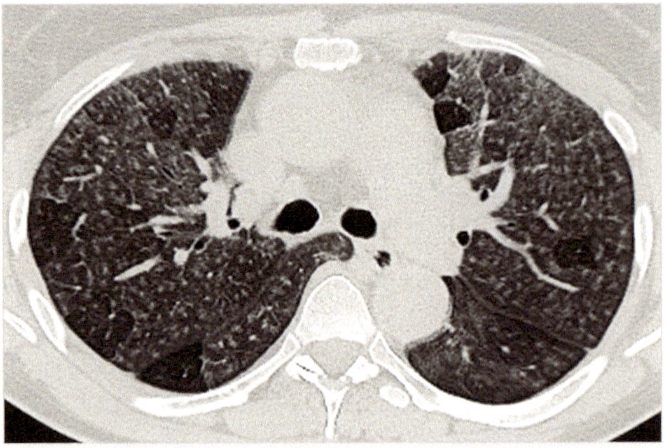

Fig. 7.7 Subacute hypersensitivity pneumonitis. CT image. Mosaic pattern and multiple centrilobular ground-glass nodules.

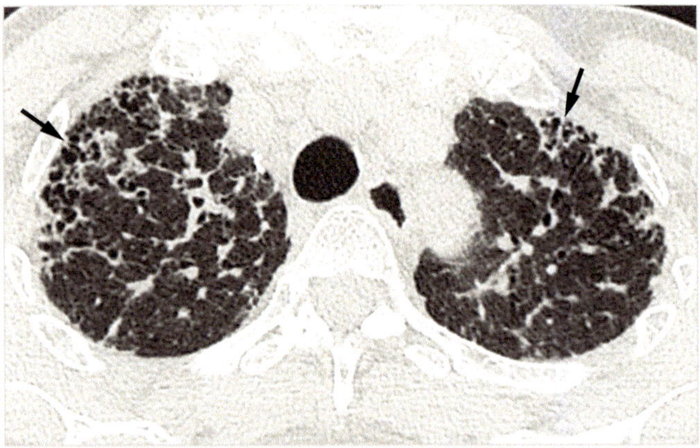

Fig. 7.8 Chronic hypersensitivity pneumonitis. CT image. Subpleural honeycombing (*arrows*) in both upper lobes, intralobular lines, and few thickened interlobular septa. These findings are not confined to the periphery and are without basal predominance.

- *Eosinophilic granulomatosis with polyangiitis or Churg–Strauss syndrome*: This will be discussed in the section on vasculitis.
- *Pulmonary drug toxicity*: This can also present as eosinophilia.
- *Pulmonary parasitosis*: Rare diseases in developed countries can also cause pulmonary eosinophilia either due to direct parasite invasion or secondary to an allergic reaction. Serology is generally used to detect the implicated parasite as the radiologic findings are usually nonspecific. A compact overview of the predominantly tropical and subtropical pulmonary parasitoses can be consulted in the publication by Jeong and coauthors.[4]

Table 7.6 Radiologic findings in hypersensitivity pneumonitis. The different forms may overlap

Forms of hypersensitivity pneumonitis	Radiologic findings
Acute hypersensitivity pneumonitis	• Bilateral diffuse consolidation • Small rounded opacities
Subacute hypersensitivity pneumonitis	• Mosaic pattern or diffuse ground-glass opacities • Centrilobular ground-glass nodules (airspace nodules) • Occasional cysts
Chronic hypersensitivity pneumonitis	• Signs of fibrosis: – Intralobular lines – Honeycombing – Traction bronchiectasis – Interlobular septal thickening • Ground-glass opacities • Random distribution of findings • No basal or peripheral predominance

7.2.1 Simple Pulmonary Eosinophilia (Loeffler Syndrome)

Simple pulmonary eosinophilia (SPE), or Loeffler syndrome, is a benign form of AEP. It gives rise to no, or only mild, symptoms in the lung and spontaneously regresses within a month but peripheral blood eosinophilia persists. The cause of this disease is largely unknown but in certain cases parasite infection, allergic bronchopulmonary aspergillosis, or pulmonary drug toxicity may be involved.[4,15]

The most salient radiologic findings observed in SPE are transient and migratory nonsegmental areas of consolidation. These are often located peripherally and poorly marginated, with apical predominance (▶Fig. 7.9). CT often demonstrates additional ground-glass opacities. Nodules surrounded by ground-glass opacities is a different radiological manifestation of SPE (▶Fig. 7.10).[4,14,16–18]

7.2.2 Acute Eosinophilic Pneumonia

AEP presents as an acute feverish illness that lasts for a few days. It is accompanied by hypoxemia and radiographic evidence of pulmonary opacities. Its cause is unknown. Eosinophil count is raised over 25% in bronchoalveolar lavage samples. Initially, peripheral blood eosinophilia is usually absent but may develop in the ensuing course. The disease promptly responds to corticosteroids and, unlike CEP (see below), tends not to recur on discontinuation of treatment.[4,19,20] It may be difficult to diagnose incipient AEP on radiologic imaging and clinical examination. Differential diagnosis is broad and includes atypical bacterial or viral pneumonia, acute interstitial pneumonia, hydrostatic pulmonary edema, and adult respiratory distress syndrome.[4,21]

On radiographs, a bilateral reticular pattern is typically seen, often accompanied by ground-glass opacity, less commonly by consolidation or poorly marginated nodules (▶ Fig. 7.11). Pleural effusion is often present. On CT scans, bilateral randomly distributed ground-glass opacities are observed; interlobular septal thickening is often seen as well (▶ Fig. 7.12).[4,21,22]

Table 7.7 Differentiation between chronic hypersensitivity pneumonitis and idiopathic pulmonary fibrosis: incidence of CT findings[12,13]

CT finding	Chronic hypersensitivity pneumonitis	Idiopathic pulmonary fibrosis
Honeycombing	+	+ + +
Traction bronchiectasis	+ +	+ + +
Basal predominance	+/-	+ + +
Peripheral predominance	+	+ + +

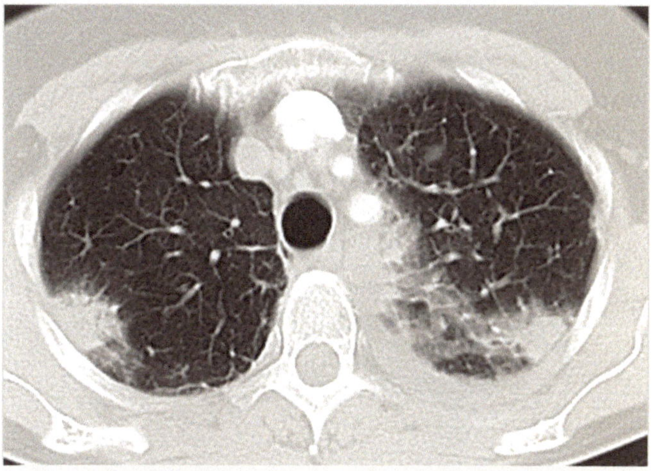

Fig. 7.9 Simple pulmonary eosinophilia (Loeffler syndrome). CT image. Bilateral peripheral, poorly marginated consolidations, also ground-glass opacities in left upper lobe.

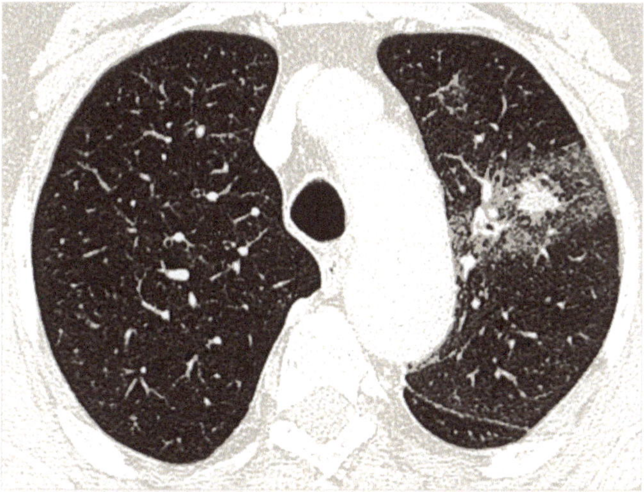

Fig. 7.10 Simple pulmonary eosinophilia (Loeffler syndrome). CT image. Nodule surrounded by ground-glass opacity in left upper lobe.

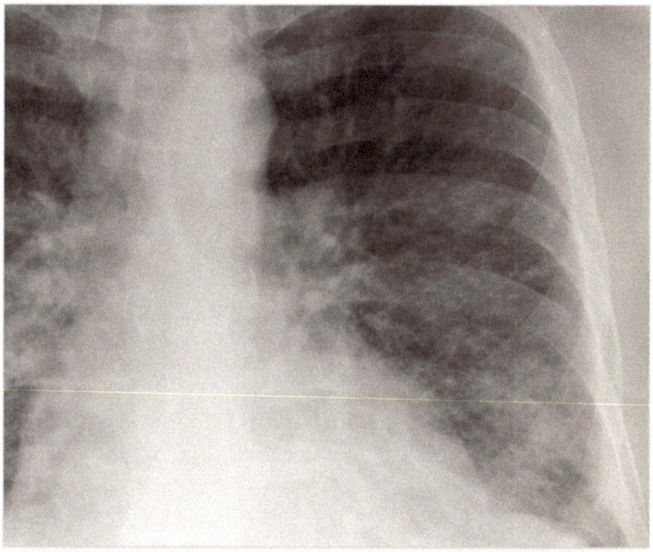

Fig. 7.11 Acute eosinophilic pneumonia. Magnified section of radiograph. Diffuse reticular pattern and overlying ground-glass opacity.

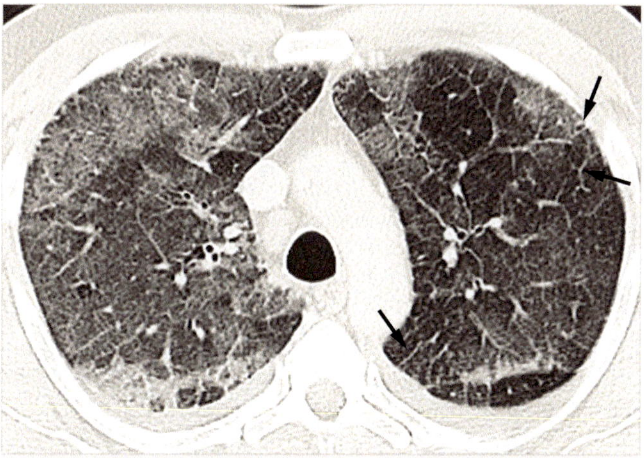

Fig. 7.12 Acute eosinophilic pneumonia. CT image. Patchy bilateral ground-glass opacities; besides, few thickened interlobular septa (*arrows*).

7.2.3 Chronic Eosinophilic Pneumonia

CEP is of insidious onset with fever, night sweats, cough, loss of appetite, and weight loss. Around half of patients have preexisting asthma.[23] Several months may elapse before CEP is diagnosed. Peripheral blood eosinophilia is usually mild to moderate, occasionally severe. Elevated serum immunoglobulin E levels are seen in two-thirds of cases. Massive eosinophilia in bronchoalveolar lavage is a salient finding that often suggests the diagnosis.[24,25]

Radiographs typically exhibit bilateral peripheral consolidation in the upper lobes (▶Fig. 7.13). However, these are seen in fewer than half of cases.[26] CT shows nonsegmental, bilateral peripheral consolidation (▶Fig. 7.14), less commonly also ground-glass opacity, nodules, and intralobular lines (see ▶Table 7.8). Occasionally, a pleural effusion is observed.[4]

7.2.4 Bronchocentric Granulomatosis

On histology, bronchocentric granulomatosis (BG) is seen to cause necrotizing granulomatous inflammation of the bronchial and bronchiolar epithelium with chronic inflammation of the surrounding lung parenchyma. Some patients with BG have asthma and peripheral blood eosinophilia. That clinical picture may be associated with allergic bronchopulmonary aspergillosis.

Radiologic findings of BG include cavitating nodules, masses, or consolidations (▶Fig. 7.15). Most findings are unilateral and, ultimately, nonspecific. The diagnosis is rarely suspected on radiologic images and BG is usually diagnosed with tissue sampling.[4,27–29]

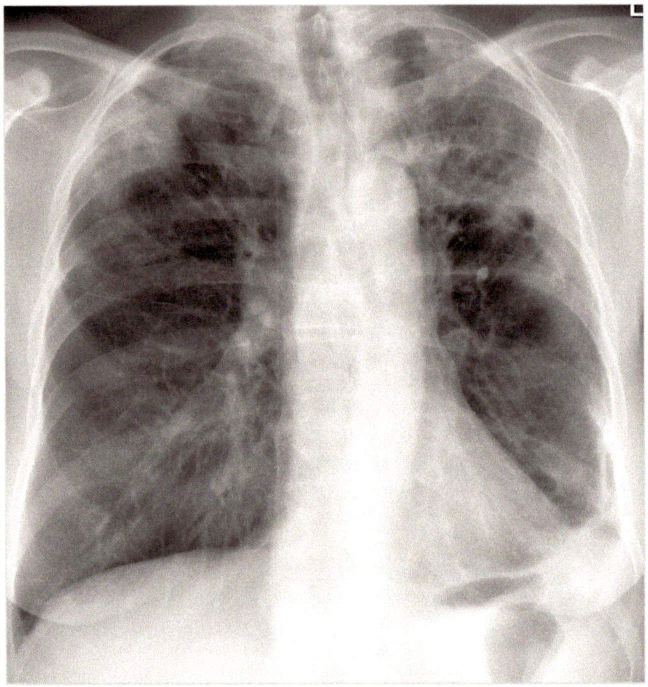

Fig. 7.13 Chronic eosinophilic pneumonia. Radiograph. Bilateral, apical peripheral consolidation.

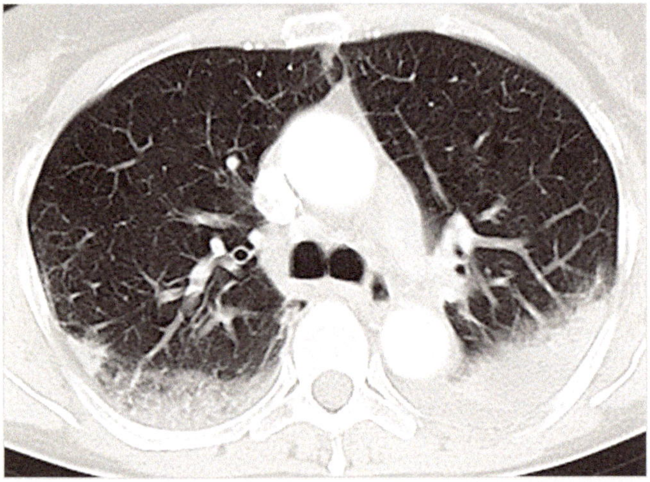

Fig. 7.14 Chronic eosinophilic pneumonia. CT image. Bilateral peripheral consolidation.

Table 7.8 Radiologic findings in eosinophilic pneumonia

Diagnostic imaging	Simple pulmonary eosinophilia (Loeffler syndrome)	Acute eosinophilic pneumonia	Chronic eosinophilic pneumonia
Radiography	• Peripheral consolidation, unilateral or bilateral, apical predominance • Nodules, surrounded by ground-glass opacities	• Reticular pattern • Ground-glass opacities • Less commonly consolidation and poorly marginated nodules	• Bilateral peripheral consolidation
CT		• Patchy areas of ground-glass opacity • Interlobular septal thickening	• Nonsegmental bilateral consolidation • Apical predominance • Less commonly: ground-glass opacities, nodules, intralobular lines

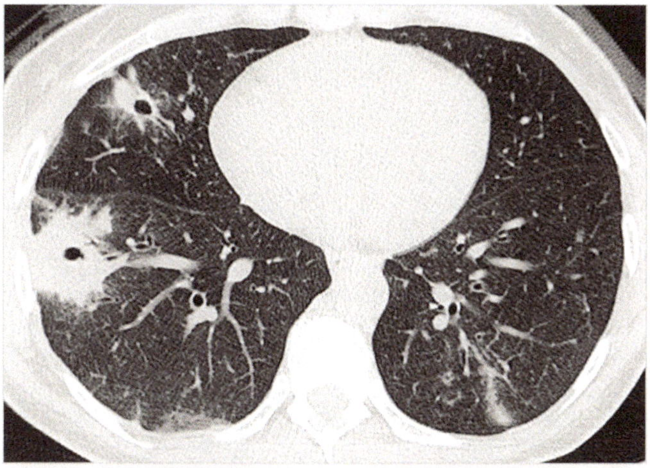

Fig. 7.15 Bronchocentric granulomatosis. CT image. Bilateral nodules and consolidation with central cavitation.

7.2.5 Idiopathic Hypereosinophilic Syndrome

The cause of idiopathic hypereosinophilic syndrome (IHS) is unknown. In addition to peripheral blood eosinophilia (eosinophil count of more than 1,500/mm^3 over at least 6 months), there is also tissue infiltration by eosinophils, causing tissue damage.[4,30,31] IHS predominantly affects men aged 30 to 40 years[32] and has a predilection for the heart and central nervous system; lung involvement is seen in 40% of patients.[4] Massively elevated eosinophil counts are identified in bronchoalveolar lavage. The main histologic findings are infiltration of the affected organs by eosinophils, architectural destruction, and necrosis.[30]

The radiologic findings are often nonspecific and consist of focal or diffuse, nonsegmental opacities, often obscured by hydrostatic pulmonary edema. The latter is caused by congestive heart failure as a sequela of the underlying disease. CT shows bilateral nodules with or without surrounding ground-glass opacity as well as focal or diffuse ground-glass opacities (▶Fig. 7.16).[4]

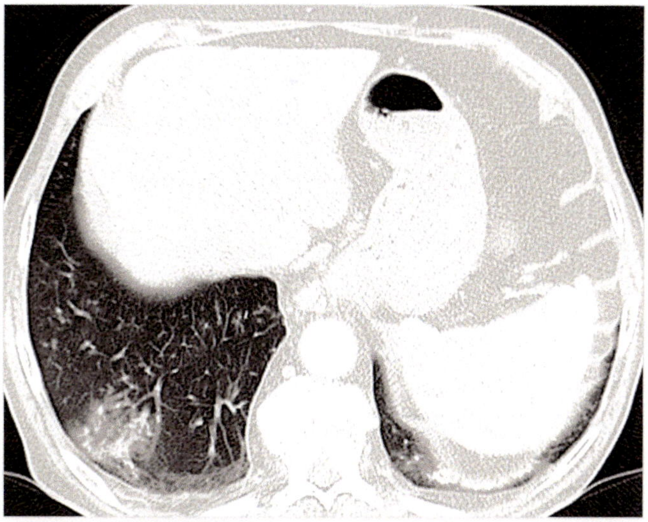

Fig. 7.16 Idiopathic hypereosinophilic syndrome. CT image. Bizarre nodule in the right lower lobe surrounded by ground-glass opacity.

7.3 Summary

Allergic pulmonary diseases include asthma, allergic bronchopulmonary aspergillosis, and hypersensitivity pneumonitis:

- *Asthma*: Radiology plays only a limited role in diagnosis of asthma and is generally restricted to patients whose clinical condition calls for hospitalization or even mechanical ventilation. Imaging is used, in particular, for differential diagnosis and to exclude complications.
- *Allergic bronchopulmonary aspergillosis*: This is the most common eosinophilic lung disease and is seen mainly in long-term asthma patients. It is diagnosed by evidence of antibodies to *Aspergillus* antigens. Imaging demonstrates bilateral infiltrates, mucoid impaction, atelectasis, and central bronchiectasis.
- *Hypersensitivity pneumonitis*: Subacute hypersensitivity pneumonitis exhibits highly characteristic findings on CT with diffuse or bilateral ground-glass opacity or mosaic pattern and centrilobular nodules, and occasionally also small cysts. It may become chronic, giving rise to lung fibrosis. Unlike other forms of pulmonary fibrosis, it is associated with apical predominance.

Eosinophilic pneumonia is characterized by infiltration of the lung parenchyma by eosinophilic leukocytes, radiographically presenting as migratory pulmonary infiltrates. In SPE (Loeffler syndrome) and CEP, blood eosinophilia suggests the diagnosis. SPE presents as AEP with a short course and few symptoms, whereas chronic pneumonia has an insidious course persisting over several months. A summary of the main radiologic findings is given in ▶Table 7.8.

References

[1] Chung KF, Wenzel SE, Brozek JL, et al. International ERS/ATS guidelines on definition, evaluation and treatment of severe asthma. Eur Respir J 2014;43(2):343–373

[2] American College of Radiology. ACR appropriateness criteria - acute respiratory illness in immunocompetent patients. Available at: https://acsearch.acr.org/docs/69446/Narrative/. Accessed November 9, 2017

[3] Lommatzsch M, Virchow JC. Severe asthma: definition, diagnosis and treatment. Dtsch Arztebl Int 2014;111(50):847–855

[4] Jeong YJ, Kim KI, Seo IJ, et al. Eosinophilic lung diseases: a clinical, radiologic, and pathologic overview. Radiographics 2007;27(3):617–637, discussion 637–639

[5] Rosenberg M, Patterson R, Mintzer R, Cooper BJ, Roberts M, Harris KE. Clinical and immunologic criteria for the diagnosis of allergic bronchopulmonary aspergillosis. Ann Intern Med 1977;86(4):405–414

[6] Ricketti AJ, Greenberger PA, Patterson R. Serum IgE as an important aid in management of allergic bronchopulmonary aspergillosis. J Allergy Clin Immunol 1984;74(1):68–71

[7] Patterson R, Greenberger PA, Radin RC, Roberts M. Allergic bronchopulmonary aspergillosis: staging as an aid to management. Ann Intern Med 1982;96(3):286–291

[8] Franquet T, Müller NL, Giménez A, Guembe P, de La Torre J, Bagué S. Spectrum of pulmonary aspergillosis: histologic, clinical, and radiologic findings. Radiographics 2001;21(4):825–837

[9] Ando M, Suga M, Kohrogi H. A new look at hypersensitivity pneumonitis. Curr Opin Pulm Med 1999;5(5):299–304

[10] American Medical Association. ICD-10-CM, 2018 - The Complete Official Codebook. Chicago, IL: American Medical Association; 2017

[11] Silver SF, Müller NL, Miller RR, Lefcoe MS. Hypersensitivity pneumonitis: evaluation with CT. Radiology 1989;173(2):441–445

[12] Adler BD, Padley SP, Müller NL, Remy-Jardin M, Remy J. Chronic hypersensitivity pneumonitis: high-resolution CT and radiographic features in 16 patients. Radiology 1992;185(1):91–95

[13] Grenier P, Chevret S, Beigelman C, Brauner MW, Chastang C, Valeyre D. Chronic diffuse infiltrative lung disease: determination of the diagnostic value of clinical data, chest radiography, and CT and Bayesian analysis. Radiology 1994;191(2):383–390

[14] Allen JN, Davis WB. Eosinophilic lung diseases. Am J Respir Crit Care Med 1994;150(5 Pt 1):1423–1438

[15] Ford RM. Transient pulmonary eosinophilia and asthma. A review of 20 cases occurring in 5,702 asthma sufferers. Am Rev Respir Dis 1966;93(5):797–803

[16] Bain GA, Flower CD. Pulmonary eosinophilia. Eur J Radiol 1996;23(1):3–8

[17] Johkoh T, Müller NL, Akira M, et al. Eosinophilic lung diseases: diagnostic accuracy of thin-section CT in 111 patients. Radiology 2000;216(3):773–780

[18] Kim Y, Lee KS, Choi DC, Primack SL, Im JG. The spectrum of eosinophilic lung disease: radiologic findings. J Comput Assist Tomogr 1997;21(6):920–930

[19] Ogawa H, Fujimura M, Matsuda T, Nakamura H, Kumabashiri I, Kitagawa S. Transient wheeze. Eosinophilic bronchobronchiolitis in acute eosinophilic pneumonia. Chest 1993;104(2):493–496

[20] Philit F, Etienne-Mastroïanni B, Parrot A, Guérin C, Robert D, Cordier JF. Idiopathic acute eosinophilic pneumonia: a study of 22 patients. Am J Respir Crit Care Med 2002;166(9):1235–1239

[21] Cheon JE, Lee KS, Jung GS, Chung MH, Cho YD. Acute eosinophilic pneumonia: radiographic and CT findings in six patients. AJR Am J Roentgenol 1996;167(5):1195–1199

[22] King MA, Pope-Harman AL, Allen JN, Christoforidis GA, Christoforidis AJ. Acute eosinophilic pneumonia: radiologic and clinical features. Radiology 1997;203(3):715–719

[23] Fox B, Seed WA. Chronic eosinophilic pneumonia. Thorax 1980; 35(8):570–580

[24] Dejaegher P, Demedts M. Bronchoalveolar lavage in eosinophilic pneumonia before and during corticosteroid therapy. Am Rev Respir Dis 1984;129(4):631–632

[25] Naughton M, Fahy J, FitzGerald MX. Chronic eosinophilic pneumonia. A long-term follow-up of 12 patients. Chest 1993;103(1): 162–165

[26] Jederlinic PJ, Sicilian L, Gaensler EA. Chronic eosinophilic pneumonia. A report of 19 cases and a review of the literature. Medicine (Baltimore) 1988;67(3):154–162

[27] Katzenstein AL, Liebow AA, Friedman PJ. Bronchocentric granulomatosis, mucoid impaction, and hypersensitivity reactions to fungi. Am Rev Respir Dis 1975;111(4):497–537

[28] Liebow AA. The J. Burns Amberson lecture--pulmonary angiitis and granulomatosis. Am Rev Respir Dis 1973;108(1):1–18

[29] Robinson RG, Wehunt WD, Tsou E, Koss MN, Hochholzer L. Bronchocentric granulomatosis: roentgenographic manifestations. Am Rev Respir Dis 1982;125(6):751–756

[30] Chusid MJ, Dale DC, West BC, Wolff SM. The hypereosinophilic syndrome: analysis of fourteen cases with review of the literature. Medicine (Baltimore) 1975;54(1):1–27

[31] Winn RE, Kollef MH, Meyer JI. Pulmonary involvement in the hypereosinophilic syndrome. Chest 1994;105(3):656–660

[32] Spry CJ, Davies J, Tai PC, Olsen EG, Oakley CM, Goodwin JF. Clinical features of fifteen patients with the hypereosinophilic syndrome. Q J Med 1983;52(205):1–22

Chapter 8

Chronic Obstructive Pulmonary Disease

8 Chronic Obstructive Pulmonary Disease

Chronic obstructive pulmonary disease (COPD) is a chronic illness with progressive obstruction of the airways which cannot be completely reversed with medication based on bronchodilators or corticosteroids. It consists of chronic bronchitis or pulmonary emphysema.[1]

COPD is one of the leading causes of death worldwide. Smoking is by far the main risk factor for COPD, followed by environmental influences such as air pollution and the adverse effects of organic or inorganic dust, often in occupational settings. In rare cases, a genetic defect causes α1-antitrypsin deficiency, leading to development of pulmonary emphysema.

The main symptoms of COPD are as follows:

- *Chronic cough*: This occurs, in particular, in the morning and generally persists over months or years.
- *Expectoration*: There is less sputum production in pulmonary emphysema than in chronic bronchitis or bronchiectasis. If hemoptysis occurs, differential diagnosis must be carried out to exclude, for example, lung carcinoma or mycobacteriosis.
- *Dyspnea*: At the outset, only exertional dyspnea is present. This deteriorates in the course of disease, leading to progressive immobility.

COPD is considered a systemic disease. In addition to immobility-related muscle loss, the increased breathing effort needed leads to higher energy consumption. This places greater demands on the cardiovascular system. Besides, low blood oxygen saturation levels lead to chronic myocardial ischemia. The ensuing vicious circle increases the patient's debility, in turn leading to greater immobility.

Based on the spirometry lung function test, COPD is classified into different stages (▶Table 8.1).

Three manifest forms of COPD, which may also overlap, are distinguished: pulmonary emphysema, chronic bronchitis, and bronchiectasis.

8.1 Pulmonary Emphysema

Pulmonary emphysema is a condition involving irreversible expansion of the terminal air spaces with destruction of the alveolar walls, leading to rarefaction of the pulmonary capillary bed. The ensuing rise in pulmonary circulation resistance can cause pulmonary hypertension.

Computed tomography (CT) is able to visualize the underlying pathomorphologic changes in greater detail than are radiographs. Likewise, classification of the different types of pulmonary emphysema as presented in the next section is based on CT morphology.

8.1.1 Emphysema on Computed Tomography

In general, destruction of the lung parenchyma with simultaneous expansion of the terminal air spaces results in lower density of the affected lung tissue on CT. While this is obvious in most cases of inhomogeneous emphysema, it may at times be difficult to identify in diffuse emphysema.

Emphysema is best visualized in a narrow lung window (e.g., width 700 HU, center -700 HU; ▶Fig. 8.1). Emphysematous portions of the lung can be displayed in a dual window with a window width of 1. The voxels whose density is above the center of the CT window appear white, and the remaining voxels are black. The center of the CT window is selected such that emphysematous lung tissue appears black and normal lung tissue white (▶Fig. 8.2). For thin slices (1–2 mm), a value of -950 HU is generally used[3]; for thick slices, a value of -910 HU is more suitable.[4] Minimum intensity projections have proved particularly useful for detection of subtle centrilobular emphysema (see Table 1.3).

Three main types of pulmonary emphysema are distinguished depending on their distribution within the lobule:

- *Centrilobular* emphysema: This is a type of emphysema mainly caused by smoking which starts in the central portions of the acini and goes on to affect the entire lobule. Centrilobular emphysema is associated with apical predominance. On CT, rounded areas of low density with a diameter of around 1 cm can be seen. The lobular structures are preserved (▶Fig. 8.3).

The severity is graded as:

- Trace if less than 0.5%.
- Mild if 0.5 to 5%.
- Moderate if more than 5%.

Table 8.1 Stages of chronic obstructive pulmonary disease according to the Global Initiative for Chronic Obstructive Lung Disease based on lung function parameters[2]

Stage	FEV1/FVC	FEV1
I	<0.7	≥80% predicted
II	<0.7	50–80% predicted
III	< 0.7	30–50% predicted
IV	< 0.7	<30% predicted *or*
		<50% predicted and chronic respiratory failure

Abbreviations: FEV1, 1-second capacity, forced expiratory volume in 1 second; FVC, forced vital capacity.

CT of the lung show visual centrilobular emphysema.[1] But as the disease progresses it becomes increasingly more difficult to identify centrilobular emphysema as such on CT. This process is characterized by two newly defined subtypes of severe centrilobular emphysema[1]:

- Confluent centrilobular emphysema: The centrilobular distribution of emphysema is no longer clearly visualized on CT. In most cases, the hypodense areas have no visible boundary (▶ Fig. 8.4). Normal lung tissue can be identified between hypodense areas of the lung. Architectural distortion has not occurred yet.
- Advanced destructive emphysema: This is the most advanced stage of centrilobular emphysema with homogeneously reduced density of the lung parenchyma. There is clear evidence of architectural distortion and vascular rarefaction. On radiologic imaging, this condition may be indistinguishable from panlobular emphysema (▶ Fig. 8.5).

• *Panlobular emphysema*: Panlobular emphysema leads to diffuse destruction of the lung parenchyma; the lobular structures are no longer visible. This type of emphysema is caused by a genetically mediated α1-antitrypsin deficiency. It is typically associated with basal and anterior predominance and can even be seen in young patients with this genetic predisposition (▶ Fig. 8.6). Disease progression can be halted with continuous substitution therapy.

• *Paraseptal emphysema*: Destruction of the lung parenchyma begins in the subpleural space or along the interlobular septa (▶ Fig. 8.7), in particular in the apical regions. Paraseptal emphysema often causes spontaneous pneumothorax. It is graded as mild if the juxtapleural lucencies do not exceed 1-cm diameter, and as substantial in case of larger lesions.[1] This type of emphysema is associated with a leptosomatic habitus which, because of the resultant effect of gravity on the lungs, is thought to give rise to particularly negative pleural pressure in the apical lung regions. This in turn increases the mechanical stress on the subpleural lung parenchyma, causing paraseptal emphysema in the apical lung regions.[5–7] Often, mixed types of paraseptal emphysema are seen in association with the two aforementioned types. Minimal paraseptal emphysematous abnormalities are a common incidental finding even in young nonsmokers. Therefore, it is reasonable to ignore up to five small (≤1 cm) subpleural emphysematous areal at the lung apices.[1,8,9]

Bullous emphysema is a pulmonary emphysema subtype that is frequently observed in association with paraseptal emphysema.[6] The term *bulla* is used to denote sharply marginated, air-containing cavities measuring more than 1 cm and enclosed in a thin wall (▶ Fig. 8.8). Occasionally, bullae are also seen in the absence of recognizable emphysema. In young patients, spontaneous pneumothorax is often caused by bullae predominantly located in the apical lung regions and the apical lower lobes. The rare *vanishing lung syndrome* has been described in young males who develop often asymmetric giant bullous emphysema occupying at least one-third of a hemithorax. It is sometimes associated with centrilobular emphysema or bronchiectasis; smoking, cannabis abuse, and α1-antitrypsin deficiency are known predisposing factors.[10,11]

A special type of focal emphysema (so-called *paracicatricial emphysema*) is seen adjacent to areas of scarring, usually and mainly caused by sarcoidosis, silicosis, or tuberculosis.[12]

Quantification of pulmonary emphysema is advisable for clarification of issues such as treatment planning prior to endobronchial valve implantation or before lung volume reduction surgery as well as for drug trials. Several methodical approaches are available[6]:

• For threshold value techniques analysis software is used to calculate the proportion of voxels of the total lung volume

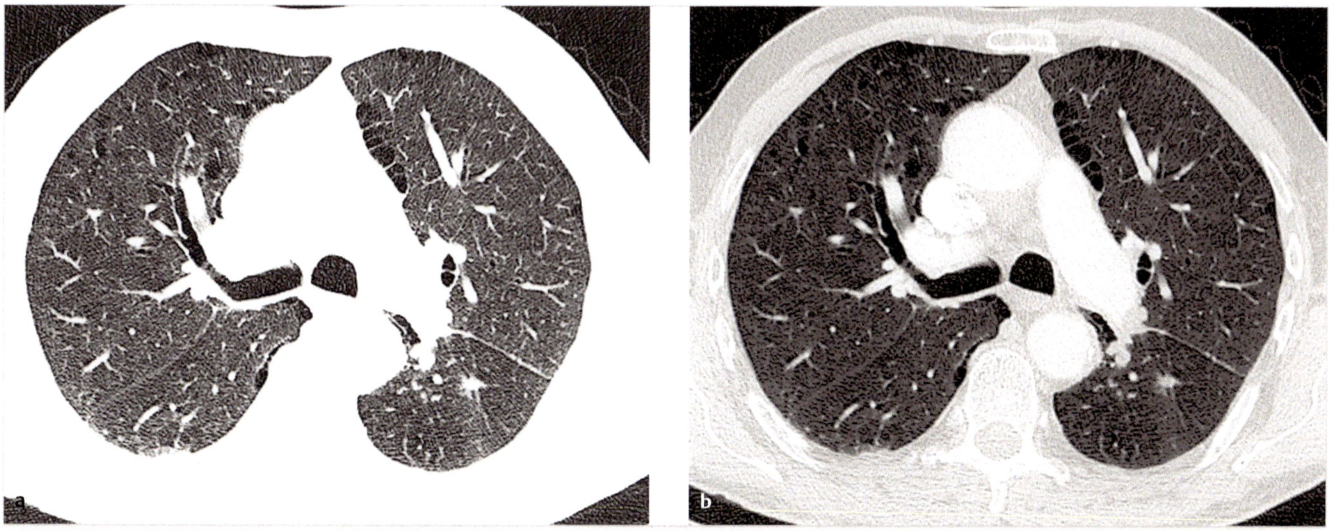

Fig. 8.1 Subtle centrilobular and paraseptal emphysema. CT images. **(a)** In a narrow lung window (700/-700 HU). **(b)** In a standard window (1,700/-500 HU).

8

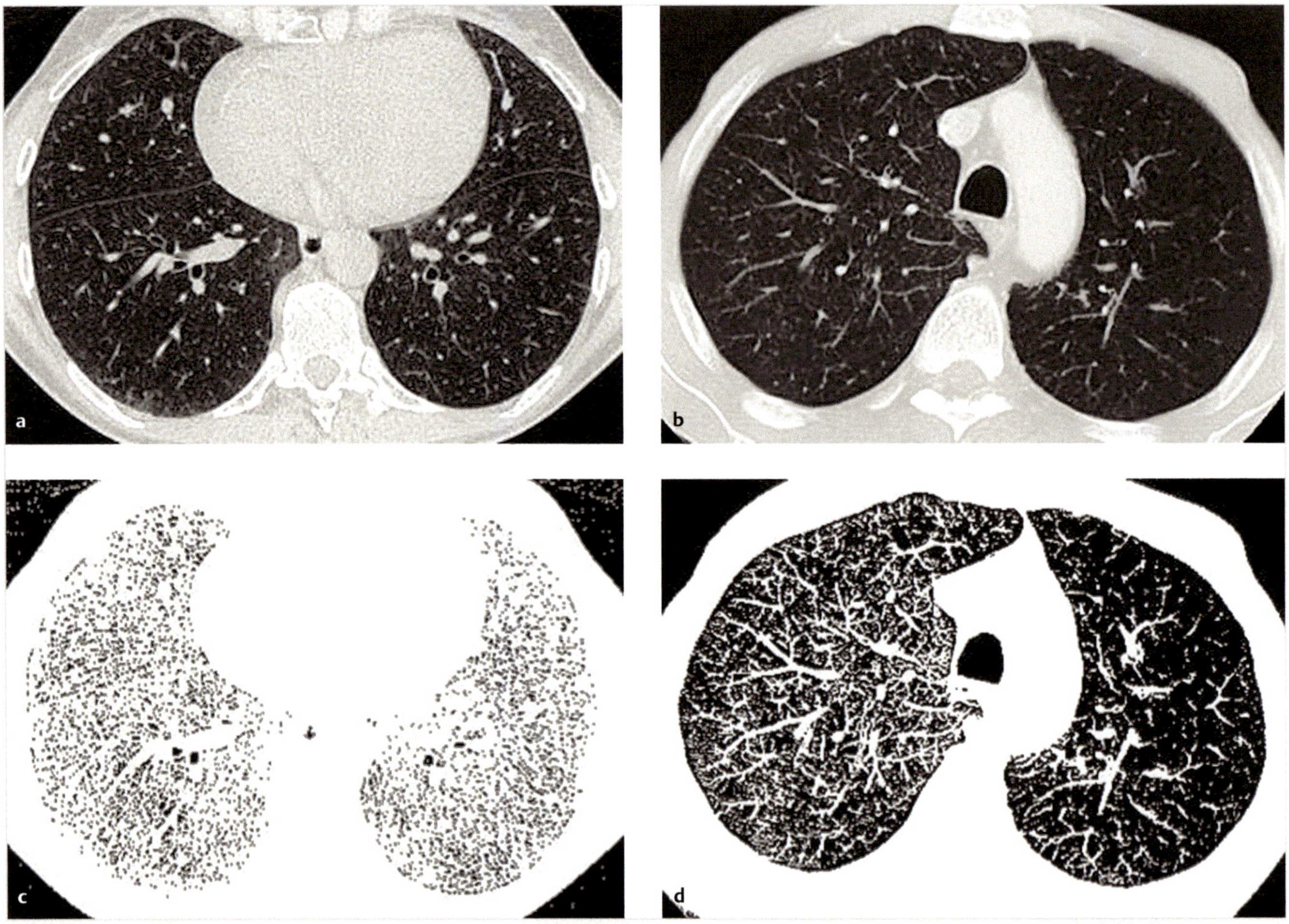

Fig. 8.2 **Severe centrilobular emphysema.** CT images, window 1/-950 HU. **(a)** Normal findings in lung window. **(b)** Pulmonary emphysema in lung window. **(c)** Image **a** in dual window. **(d)** Image **b** in dual window.

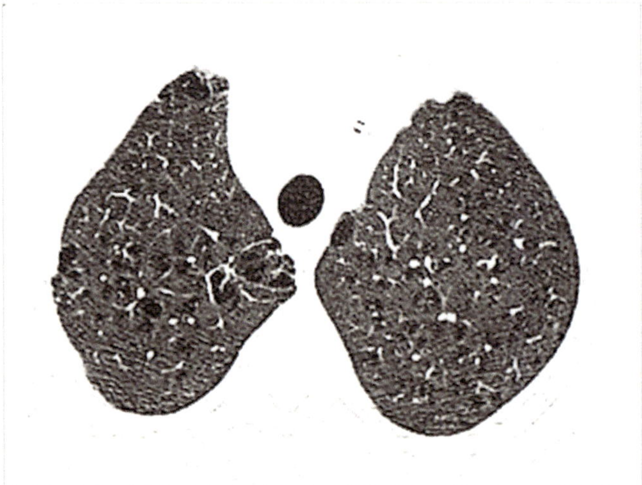

Fig. 8.3 **Centrilobular emphysema.** CT image. Incipient centrilobular emphysema with rounded areas of low density.

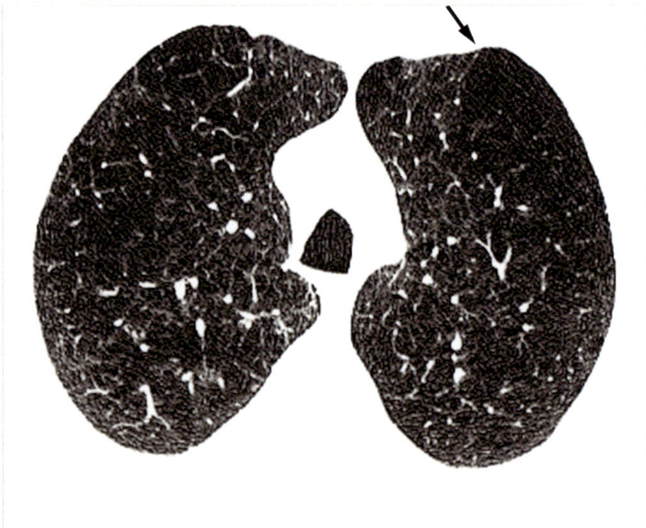

Fig. 8.4 **Confluent centrilobular emphysema.** CT image. Largish confluent hypodense areas in the left upper lobe (*arrows*).

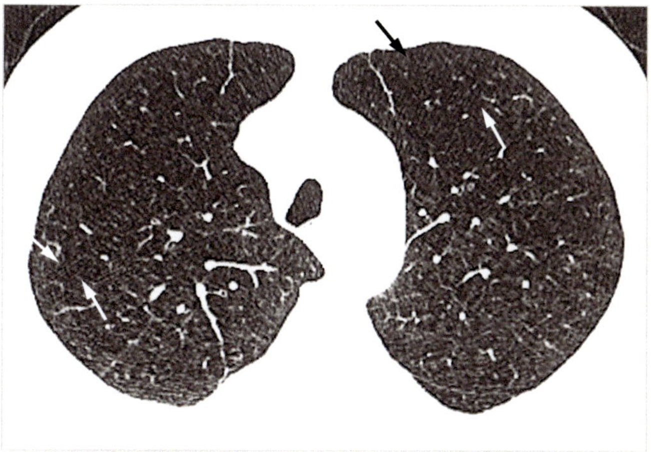

Fig. 8.5 **Advanced destructive emphysema.** CT image. Diffuse reduction in the density of the lung parenchyma and destruction of the lobular structure (*arrows*).

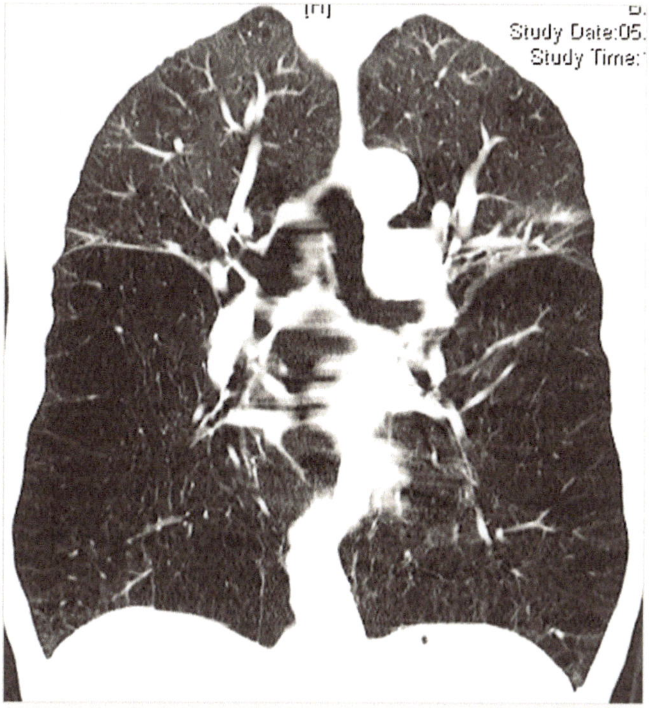

Fig. 8.6 **α1-antitrypsin deficiency emphysema**. CT image, coronal reformatting. Panlobular emphysema with basal predominance.

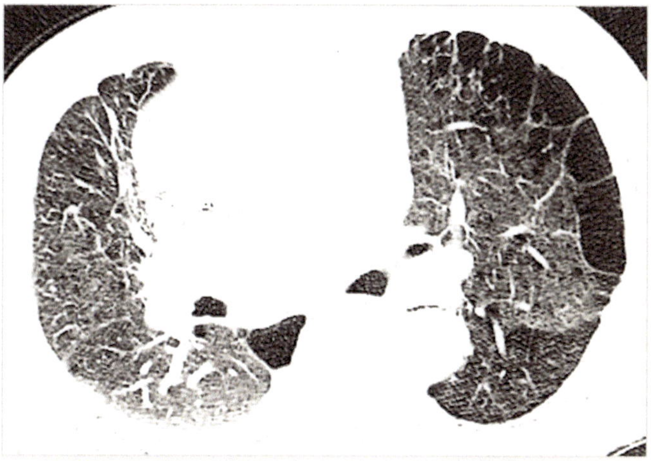

Fig. 8.7 **Paraseptal emphysema.** CT image. In addition, mild centrilobular emphysema.

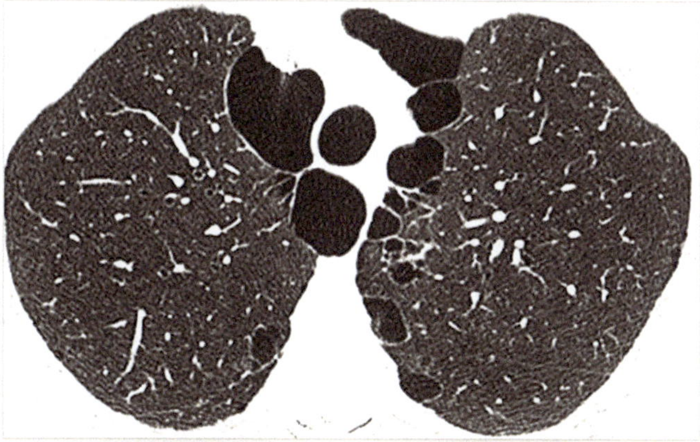

Fig. 8.8 **Bullous emphysema.** CT image. Bilateral emphysematous bullae.

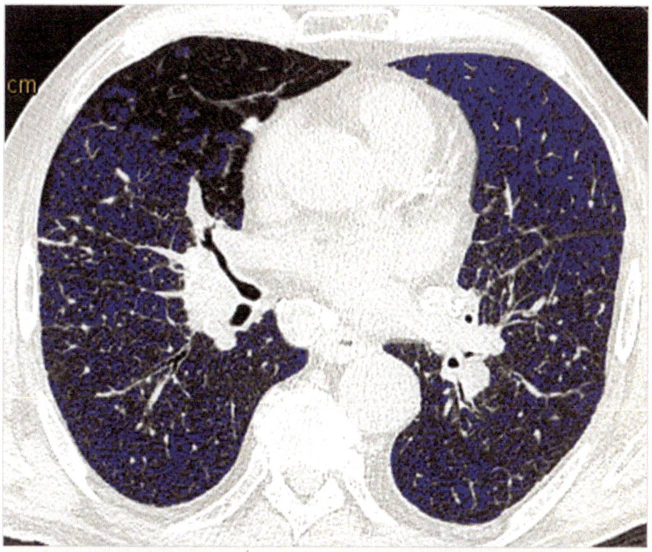

Fig. 8.9 **Emphysema.** CT image, software-based emphysema quantification. Voxels with CT density below -950 HU are shown in blue on the image.

with a density below a certain threshold value (usually -950 HU) (▶Fig. 8.9). Here, it is assumed that the voxels below the threshold value represent the emphysematous lung areas.

- Techniques based on the lung density histogram show the frequency distribution of CT density. Various parameters can be defined, mainly the mean lung density, the emphysema index, and the 5th percentile of lung density, which decreases in line with increasing emphysema.[6,13]
- The total CT density of the lung parenchyma is a summary parameter of existing pulmonary emphysema that, like histogram analysis, does not give any insight into the spatial distribution of emphysema.
- New approaches are based on texture analysis of CT images and provide quantitative assessment of different types of emphysema and their regional distribution.[14]

8.1.2 Emphysema on Chest Radiography

Bullae are the only sign of emphysema directly visible on chest radiography (▶Fig. 8.10).[6] Emphysema can be indirectly identified on the radiograph on the basis of hyperinflation of the lung parenchyma and changes in the pulmonary vascular architecture (▶Table 8.2 and ▶Fig. 8.11, ▶Fig. 8.12, and ▶Fig. 8.13). The vascular changes have a sensitivity of around 40%, while signs of lung hyperinflation have only low specificity.[6] In symptomatic patients, the combination of hyperinflation and vascular changes has a good positive predictive value for the presence of pulmonary emphysema. However, that does not apply for asymptomatic patients.[15]

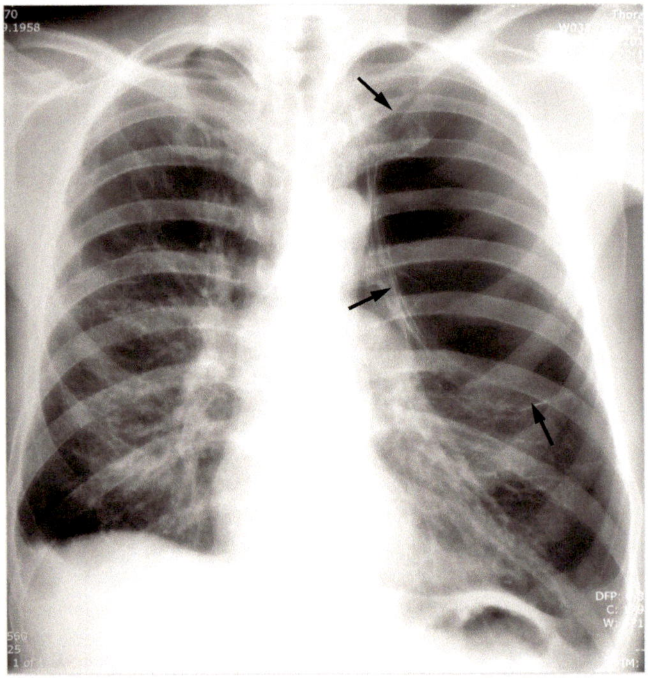

Fig. 8.10 Bullous emphysema. Radiograph. Large emphysematous bulla in the left upper lobe (*arrows*).

Besides, the sequelae of pulmonary emphysema or treatment side effects are also often seen on the radiograph:

- In longstanding disease, apart from the radiologic emphysema signs, the sequelae of long-term corticosteroid treatment, especially an osteoporotic thoracic spine, possibly with vertebral fractures, can be observed.

Table 8.2 Direct and important indirect signs of emphysema on radiographs[6]

Direct signs	Indirect signs
Bullae	• Vascular changes: – Rarefaction of vasculature – Reduced caliber of pulmonary vessels with tapering toward the periphery • Hyperinflation of the lung parenchyma: – Diaphragmatic flattening – Widened retrosternal space – Chest deformity: Barrel- or bell-shaped chest

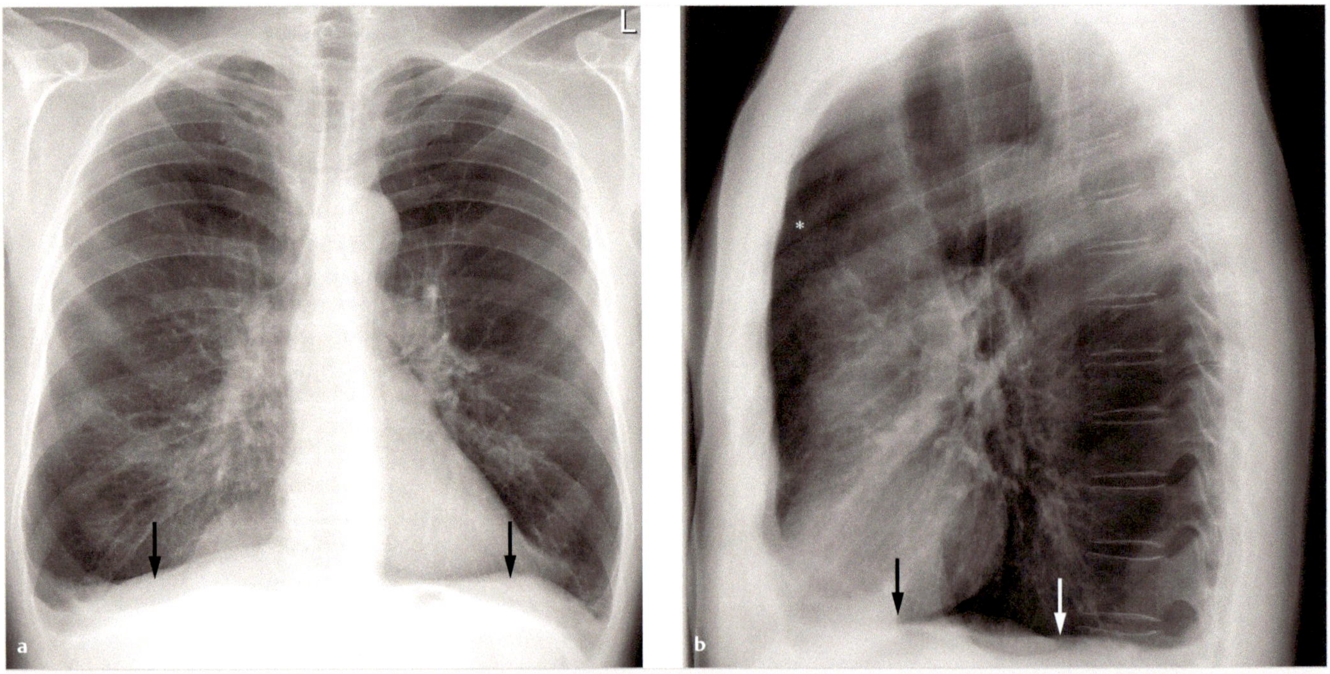

Fig. 8.11 Emphysema. Radiographs. Low-riding, flattened diaphragm, bilateral **(a, b)** (*arrows*), widened retrosternal space **(b)** (*asterisk*), and rarefaction of pulmonary vasculature. **(a)** Posteroanterior view. **(b)** Lateral view.

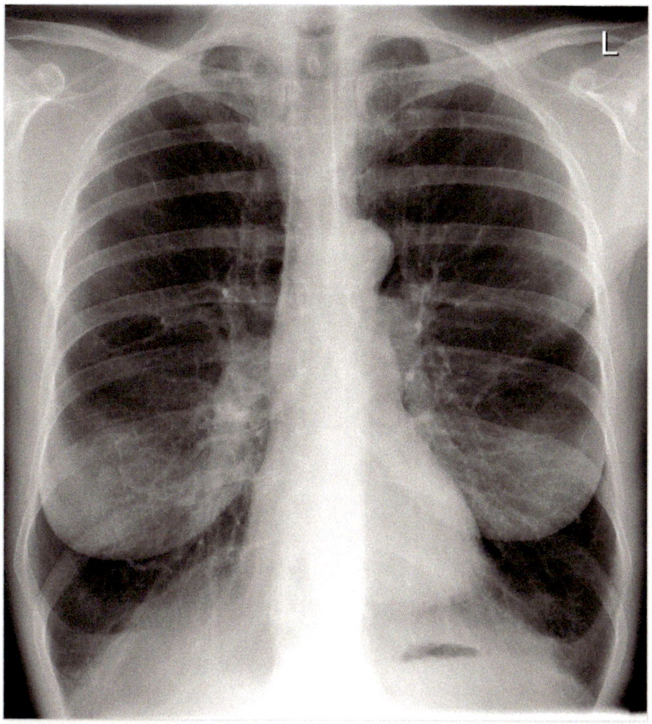

Fig. 8.12 **Emphysema.** Radiograph. Barrel-shaped chest deformity.

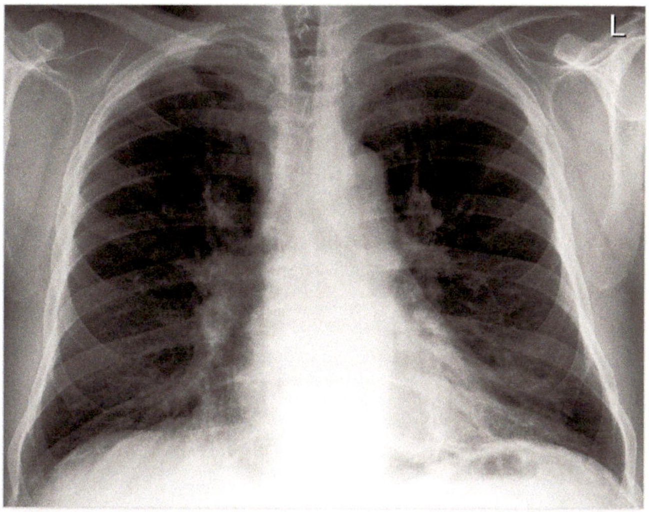

Fig. 8.13 **Emphysema.** Radiograph. Bell-shaped chest deformity.

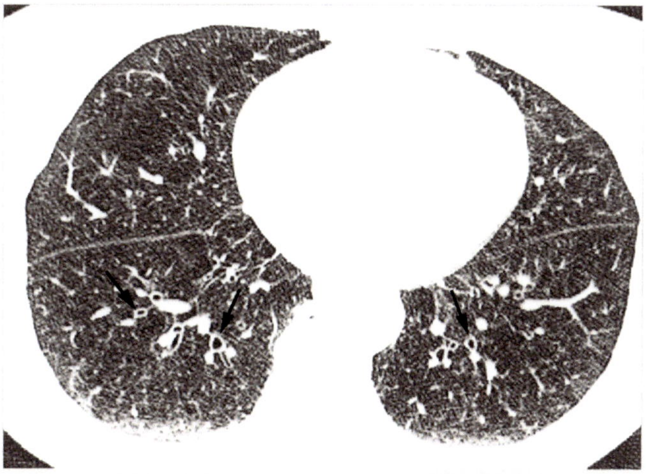

Fig. 8.14 **Chronic bronchitis.** CT image. Bronchi in both lower lobes (*arrows*) of normal caliber but with thickened walls.

- The development of pulmonary hypertension is accompanied by corresponding signs on radiography, such as an enlarged pulmonary trunk or dilated central pulmonary arteries with a change in arterial caliber toward the periphery.

8.2 Chronic Bronchitis

The main symptoms of chronic bronchitis are chronic cough and expectoration, with the latter more copious than in the case of pulmonary emphysema. The majority of patients do not develop obstructive pulmonary function disorder; this condition is known as simple chronic bronchitis.

Note

Based on the definition of the World Health Organization, chronic bronchitis is present if symptoms with expectoration have persisted for 2 years, manifesting at least over 3 months per year.[16] All other causes of chronic cough and expectoration should be excluded.[17]

Bronchial wall thickening is a characteristic radiologic finding of chronic bronchitis. In less than half of the cases, this may be identified on radiographs, in particular, in orthogonally viewed bronchi.[18] These changes are much more apparent on CT (▶ Fig. 8.14); bronchial wall thickening can also be quantified on CT using appropriate software. Wall thickness and the resultant luminal constriction vary in the course of disease. Wall irregularities can be identified on thin CT slices.[19]

Acute exacerbation of COPD cannot be reliably distinguished from pneumonia based on its clinical manifestations. In the presence of a corresponding clinical picture, chest radiography for patients requiring hospital admission is required to exclude community-acquired pneumonia.[20]

In addition to differentiating pneumonia from acute exacerbation of COPD, imaging can exclude other causes of chronic cough and expectoration, such as malignant tumors or bronchiectasis. However, imaging is not useful for diagnosis of chronic bronchitis itself.

Small airway disease is a common feature of COPD and can be seen in combination with any form of emphysema, but also as predominant feature of COPD in the absence of emphysema. CT directly visualizes inflammatory small airway disease as small peripheral centrilobular micronodular opacities. Obstructive small airway disease can be identified by air trapping, especially on expiratory CT scans.[1]

II

8.3 Bronchiectasis

Bronchiectasis is a condition characterized by irreversible dilation of the bronchial lumens with bronchial wall thickening.[21,22] Common causes include[23,24]:

- Viral childhood infection.
- Allergic bronchopulmonary aspergillosis.
- Cystic fibrosis.
- Bronchiolitis obliterans.
- Lung fibrosis (traction bronchiectasis).

It mainly involves chronic or resolved inflammation.

Traction bronchiectasis is a special type of *bronchiectasis* in which dilation of the bronchial lumen is caused by traction of the bronchial wall rather than by chronic inflammatory processes of the bronchial wall itself. This results from lung fibrosis causing contracture of the peribronchial connective tissue.

Note

N!

Following pneumonia, bronchial dilation can at times persist for several months before regressing. These changes should not be misinterpreted as bronchiectasis since the latter is not reversible.

Three types of bronchiectasis are distinguished depending on the extent of bronchial wall deformity[23]:

- *Cylindrical bronchiectasis* (▶ Fig. 8.15): Lack of tapering of the bronchial lumen toward the periphery or smooth dilation of the bronchial lumen.
- *Varicose bronchiectasis* (▶ Fig. 8.16): Irregular dilation of the bronchial lumen.
- *Cystic bronchiectasis* (▶ Fig. 8.17): Dilation of the bronchial lumen by over 1 cm, giving rise to cyst-like structures (very large, rather ovoid [saccular] cysts are occasionally called *sacciform bronchiectasis*).

This differentiation system describes the pathologic or radiologic aspect and gives insights into the intensity of the pathologic process but is of no direct relevance for treatment.

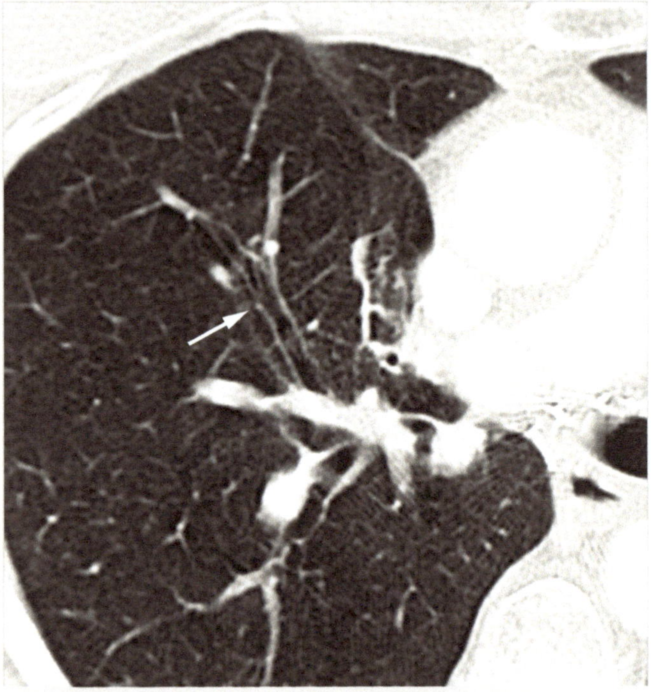

Fig. 8.15 Cylindrical bronchiectasis in the middle lobe (*arrow*). CT image.

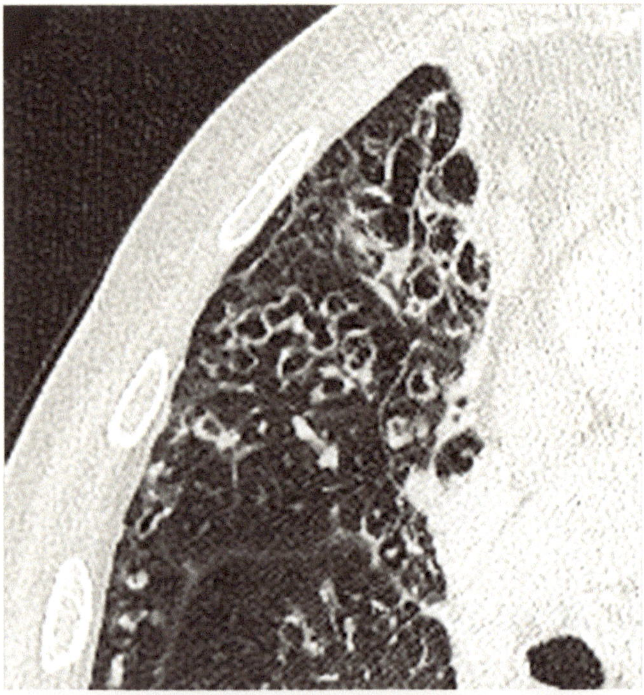

Fig. 8.16 Varicose bronchiectasis in the middle lobe. CT image.

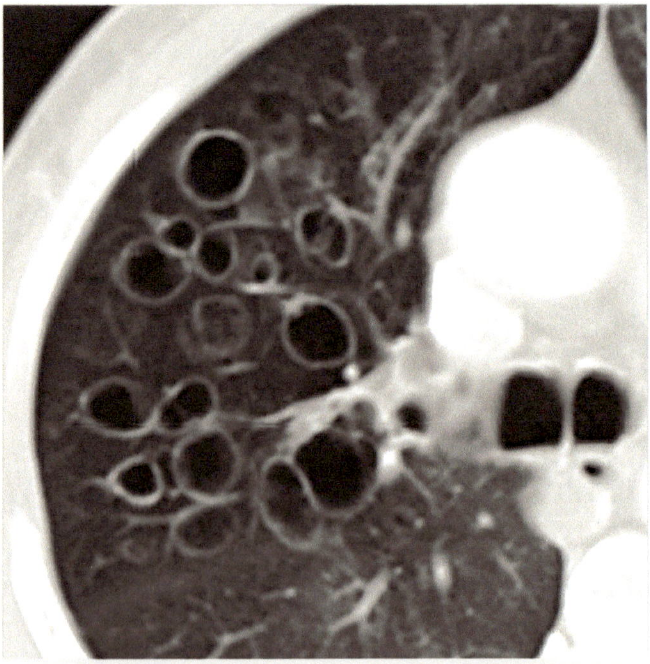

Fig. 8.17 Cystic bronchiectasis in the right upper lobe. CT image.

On chest radiography, the thickened and atypically widely spaced bronchial walls of tangentially imaged bronchi manifest as a *tram-track sign*. The thick, parallel lines correspond to a longitudinal image of the dilated bronchus with wall thickening (▶Fig. 8.18). Areas of extensive, in particular cystic or orthogonally projected, bronchiectasis are seen on the radiograph as ring-shaped opacity similar to cavitating nodules (▶Fig. 8.19).

On CT, bronchial dilation and bronchial wall thickening are directly recognizable. A characteristic finding is the *signet ring sign*: when bronchiectasis is seen in cross-section, the dilated bronchus appears as the ring and the accompanying pulmonary artery of normal caliber as its smaller signet (▶Fig. 8.20). False-positive results may be caused by a pulmonary artery of reduced caliber (e.g., in the presence of regional oligemia secondary to chronic pulmonary embolism), while false-negative findings may result from dilated pulmonary arteries.[23] Discrete cylindrical bronchiectasis can be detected only through subtle image analysis confirming the lack of peripheral tapering of the bronchial lumen. Often, concomitant inflammation of the small airways (tree-in-bud pattern) and of the adjacent parenchyma (peribronchial opacity; ▶Fig. 8.21) is seen on CT. Occasionally, dilated bronchial arteries may manifest in severe bronchiectatic disease (▶Fig. 8.22) and frequently cause hemoptysis.

Bronchiectasis exhibits the characteristic findings of certain genetically mediated syndromes:

- *Cystic fibrosis or mucoviscidosis* (▶Fig. 8.23): This is the most common genetic disease with a prevalence of around 1:2,000 live births. Due to a genetic defect, highly viscous mucus is produced, resulting in reduced bronchial clearance in the lungs. The disease first manifests in childhood. Frequent concomitant findings include mucoid impaction, atelectasis, and inflammatory consolidation. Pulmonary emphysema and bullae may present as secondary findings.
- *Primary ciliary dyskinesia or Kartagener syndrome* (▶Fig. 8.24): This is a rare disease characterized by a combination of situs inversus and bronchiectasis; it is caused by genetically mediated ciliary dyskinesia of the bronchial mucosa, with reduced clearance.

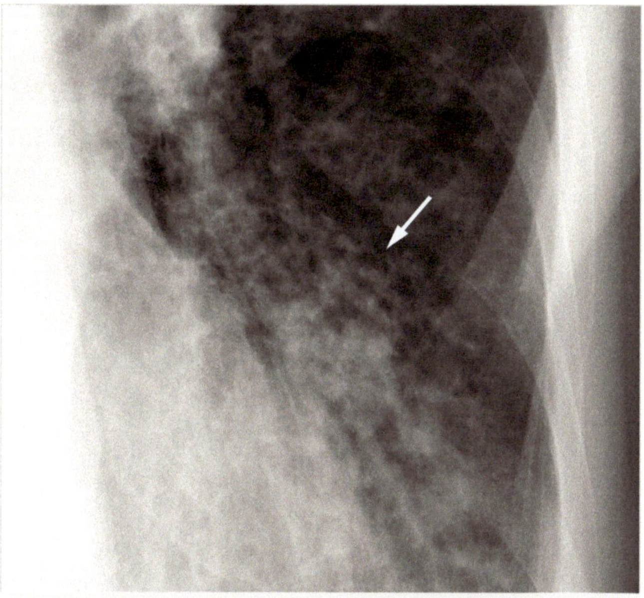

Fig. 8.18 Bronchiectasis. Magnified section of radiograph. Tram-track sign due to thickened bronchial walls and dilated bronchial lumen in cylindrical bronchiectasis (*arrow*).

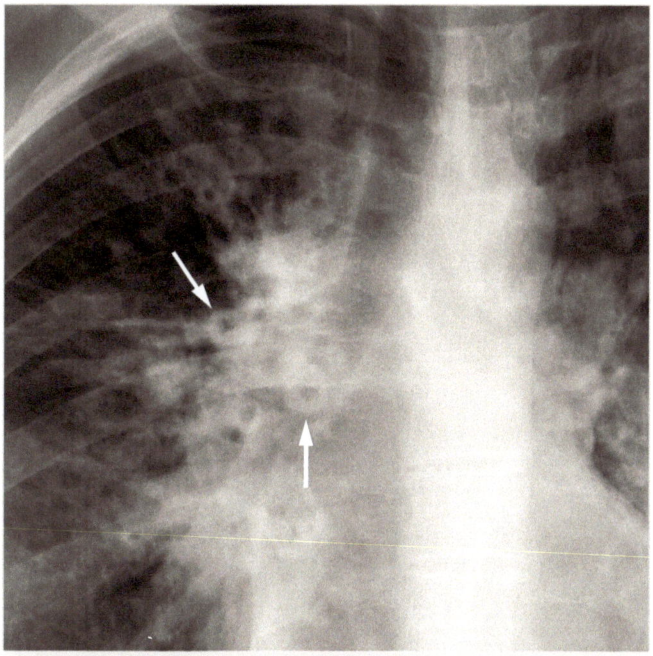

Fig. 8.19 Bronchiectasis. Magnified section of radiograph. Rounded structures with central brightening correspond to orthograde image of bronchiectasis (*arrows*).

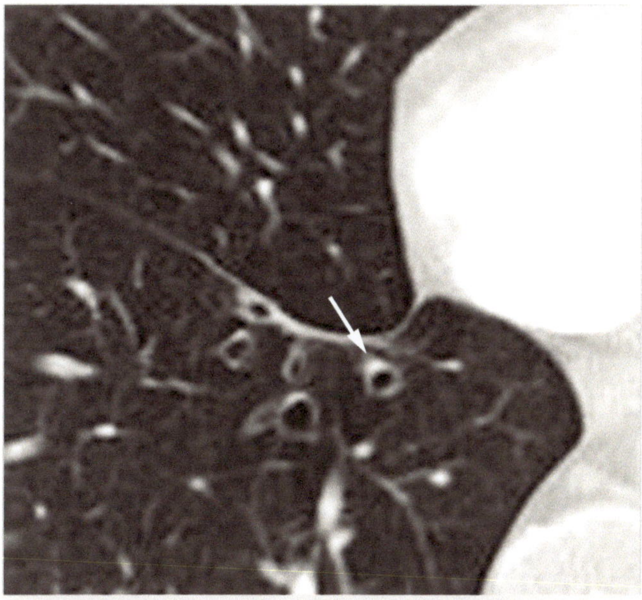

Fig. 8.20 Bronchiectasis. CT image. Signet ring sign with dilated bronchus and accompanying pulmonary artery of normal caliber (*arrow*).

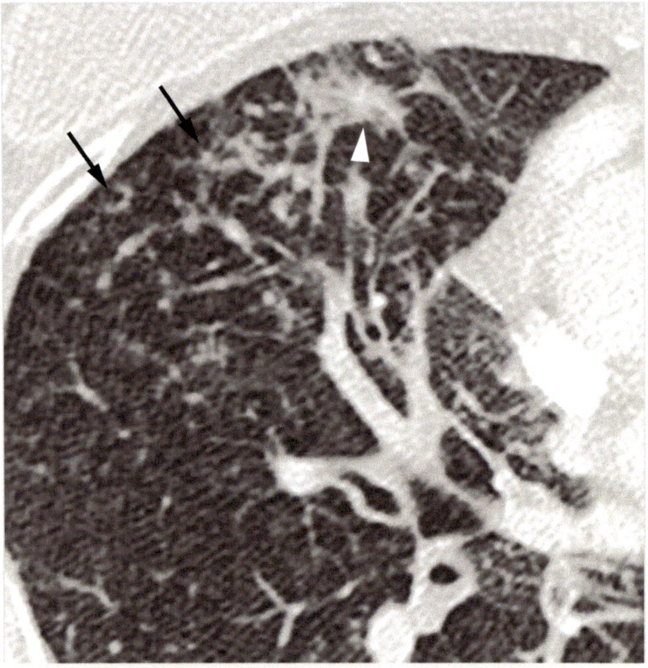

Fig. 8.21 **Bronchiectasis and concomitant inflammation of the lung parenchyma.** CT image. Same patient as in ▶Fig. 8.15 at another time point. Tree-in-bud pattern (*arrows*) and ground-glass opacity (*arrowhead*) in the middle lobe as a sign of acute inflammation of the small airways and lung parenchyma.

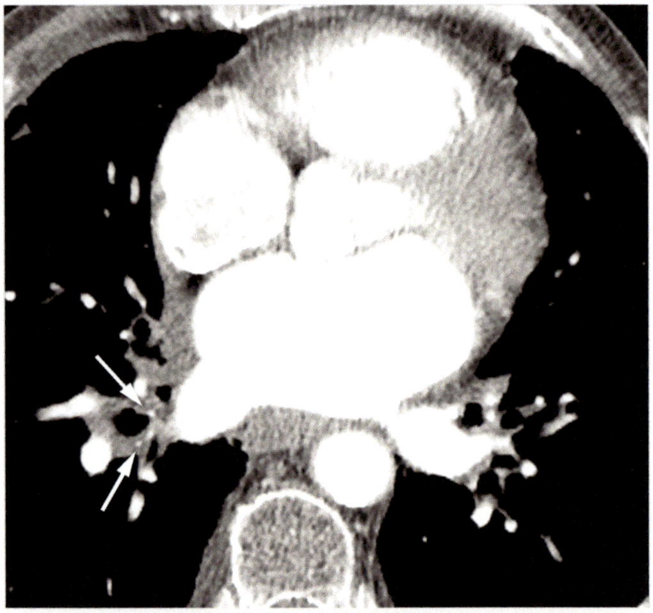

Fig. 8.22 **Bronchiectasis.** CT image. Dilated right hilar bronchial arteries (*arrows*).

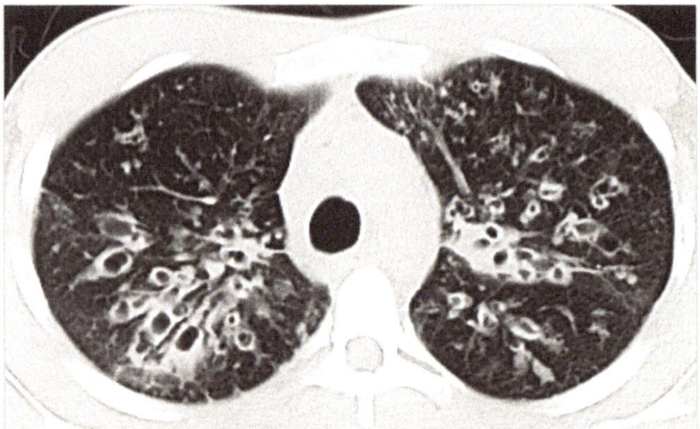

Fig. 8.23 **Cystic fibrosis.** CT image. Extensive varicose bronchiectasis, bilateral.

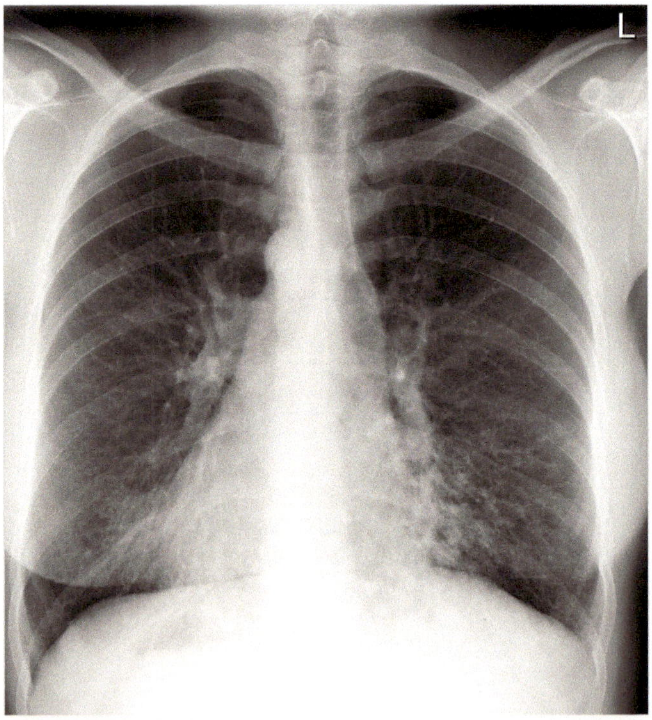

Fig. 8.24 **Primary ciliary dyskinesia.** Radiograph. Situs inversus, bronchiectasis, and pneumonia-induced consolidation.

8.4 Summary

COPD is a widespread disease. Smoking is the main risk factor for COPD, followed by environmental influences, such as air pollution. It comprises three disease entities: emphysema, chronic bronchitis, and bronchiectasis, which in the individual case may account to varying degrees for the clinical picture. The characteristic symptoms of COPD are chronic cough, expectoration, and dyspnea.

In *emphysema*, the pathologic changes occurring in the lobule are differentiated into three general types in accordance with their distribution pattern:

- *Centrilobular emphysema*: This is mainly caused by smoking.
- *Panlobular emphysema*: This tends to be associated with basal and anterior predominance and is caused by a genetically mediated α1-antitrypsin deficiency.
- *Paraseptal emphysema*: This presents in combination with the two aforementioned types or on its own.

Table 8.3 Radiologic findings in bronchiectasis

Diagnostic imaging	Findings
Radiography	• Tram-track sign • Ring-shaped opacity • Reticular pattern
CT	• Signet ring sign • Dilation of the bronchial lumen • Bronchial wall thickening • Lack of tapering of the bronchial lumen toward the periphery • Cystic structures • Concomitant inflammatory processes: – Ground-glass opacity – Consolidation – Tree-in-bud pattern

In particular, paraseptal emphysema tends to give rise to the formation of large, air-containing cystic structures (bullae) and, in turn, to bullous emphysema. In the early stages, emphysema is hard to detect on radiographs. Bullae are the only direct sign of emphysema. Lung hyperinflation and vascular rarefaction constitute indirect signs of emphysema. The emphysema types described above can be directly visualized on CT. Early types of emphysema are best visualized in a narrow lung window. Several methods are used for quantification of emphysema. These are based on analysis of lung density using special software.

Chronic bronchitis is defined as persistent cough and expectoration over 2 successive years, manifesting at least over 3 months per year. Clinical diagnosis is made after exclusion of other causes of the manifested symptoms. Imaging is used, on the one hand, to exclude other causes of cough and expectoration and, on the other hand, for differential diagnosis between pneumonia and acute exacerbation of COPD. Bronchial wall thickening serves as a radiologic correlate of chronic bronchitis with variable constriction of the bronchial lumen.

Irreversible dilation of the bronchial lumen, mainly accompanied by thickening of the walls of the affected bronchus, is termed *bronchiectasis*. Bronchiectatic areas are predilection sites for recurrent pulmonary infections. These are mainly caused by viral childhood infection, allergic bronchopulmonary aspergillosis, cystic fibrosis, and bronchiolitis obliterans. Depending on the extent of changes, three types are distinguished: cylindrical, varicose, and cystic bronchiectasis. A summary of the radiologic findings in bronchiectasis is given in ▶Table 8.3.

References

[1] Lynch DA, Austin JHM, Hogg JC, et al. CT-definable subtypes of chronic obstructive pulmonary disease: a statement of the Fleischner Society. Radiology 2015;277(1):192–205

[2] Rabe KF, Hurd S, Anzueto A, et al; Global Initiative for Chronic Obstructive Lung Disease. Global strategy for the diagnosis, management, and prevention of chronic obstructive pulmonary disease: GOLD executive summary. Am J Respir Crit Care Med 2007;176(6):532–555

[3] Gevenois PA, Koob MC, Jacobovitz D, De Vuyst P, Yernault JC, Struyven J. Whole lung sections for computed tomographic-pathologic correlations. Modified Gough-Wentworth technique. Invest Radiol 1993;28(3):242–246

[4] Müller NL, Staples CA, Miller RR, Abboud RT. "Density mask". An objective method to quantitate emphysema using computed tomography. Chest 1988;94(4):782–787

[5] Churg A, Wright JL. Proteases and emphysema. Curr Opin Pulm Med 2005;11(2):153–159

[6] Litmanovich D, Boiselle PM, Bankier AA. CT of pulmonary emphysema--current status, challenges, and future directions. Eur Radiol 2009;19(3):537–551

[7] Wright JL, Churg A. Advances in the pathology of COPD. Histopathology 2006;49(1):1–9

[8] Barr RG, Berkowitz EA, Bigazzi F, et al; COPDGene CT Workshop Group. A combined pulmonary-radiology workshop for visual evaluation of COPD: study design, chest CT findings and concordance with quantitative evaluation. COPD 2012;9(2):151–159

[9] Mets OM, van Hulst RA, Jacobs C, van Ginneken B, de Jong PA. Normal range of emphysema and air trapping on CT in young men. AJR Am J Roentgenol 2012;199(2):336–340

[10] Stern EJ, Webb WR, Weinacker A, Müller NL. Idiopathic giant bullous emphysema (vanishing lung syndrome): imaging findings in nine patients. AJR Am J Roentgenol 1994;162(2):279–282

[11] Davies P, Bradley C. Vanishing lung syndrome: giant bullous emphysema. Lancet 2017;390(10112):2583

[12] Jeong YJ, Lee KS, Chung MP, Han J, Johkoh T, Ichikado K. Chronic hypersensitivity pneumonitis and pulmonary sarcoidosis: differentiation from usual interstitial pneumonia using high-resolution computed tomography. Semin Ultrasound CT MR 2014;35(1):47–58

[13] Ley-Zaporozhan J, Ley S, Kauczor HU. Morphological and functional imaging in COPD with CT and MRI: present and future. Eur Radiol 2008;18(3):510–521

[14] Yang J, Angelini ED, Smith BM, et al. Explaining radiological emphysema subtypes with unsupervised texture prototypes: MESA COPD study. Paper presented at: Medical Computer Vision and Bayesian and Graphical Models for Biomedical Imaging: MICCAI 2016 International Workshops, MCV and BAMBI. Athens, Greece, October 21, 2016, Revised selected papers. MCV (Workshop) (2016 Athens, Greece) 2017:69–80

[15] Sutinen S, Christoforidis AJ, Klugh GA, Pratt PC. Roentgenologic criteria for the recognition of nonsymptomatic pulmonary emphysema. Correlation between roentgenologic findings and pulmonary pathology. Am Rev Respir Dis 1965;91:69–76

[16] World Health Organization. Chronic cor pulmonale. Report of an expert committee. World Health Organ Tech Rep Ser 1961;213:35

[17] Hartman TE, Tazelaar HD, Swensen SJ, Müller NL. Cigarette smoking: CT and pathologic findings of associated pulmonary diseases. Radiographics 1997;17(2):377–390

[18] DiMango EA, Lubetsky H, Austin JHM. Assessment of bronchial wall thickening on posteroanterior chest radiographs in acute asthma. J Asthma 2002;39(3):255–261

[19] Zompatori M, Sverzellati N, Gentile T, Spaggiari L, Laporta T, Fecci L. Imaging of the patient with chronic bronchitis: an overview of old and new signs. Radiol Med (Torino) 2006;111(5):634–639

[20] Wedzicha JA, Miravitlles M, Hurst JR, et al. Management of COPD exacerbations: a European Respiratory Society/American Thoracic Society guideline. Eur Respir J 2017;49(3):1600791

[21] Grenier P, Maurice F, Musset D, Menu Y, Nahum H. Bronchiectasis: assessment by thin-section CT. Radiology 1986;161(1):95–99

[22] Naidich DP, McCauley DI, Khouri NF, Stitik FP, Siegelman SS. Computed tomography of bronchiectasis. J Comput Assist Tomogr 1982;6(3):437–444

[23] Hartman TE, Primack SL, Lee KS, Swensen SJ, Müller NL. CT of bronchial and bronchiolar diseases. Radiographics 1994;14(5):991–1003

[24] Teel GS, Engeler CE, Tashijian JH, duCret RP. Imaging of small airways disease. Radiographics 1996;16(1):27–41

Chapter 9

Tumors of the Lung

9 Tumors of the Lung

9.1 Hamartoma

Hamartomas (synonyms: chondroid hamartoma, chondromatous hamartoma, chondrohamartoma, hamartochondroma, chondroma) are the most common type of benign lung tumor and account for 8% of all lung neoplasms. As a malformation tumor, the hamartoma may contain fatty tissue, cartilage, epithelial tissue, and connective tissue. They are more common than leiomyomatous hamartomas.[1] Two-thirds of hamartomas are asymptomatic incidental findings identified on radiographs in middle-aged patients, with men affected around two to three times more often than women. Only in around one-third of cases do hamartomas exhibit symptoms caused by bronchial obstruction, with chronic cough, hemoptysis, and fever.[2]

Hamartomas usually occur in the lung parenchyma, and less commonly in the endobronchial region (3–20% of cases).[2] They generally manifest as peripheral, smoothly marginated, occasionally polycyclic, nodules usually measuring 1 to 2.5 cm, with a maximum diameter of 4 cm. Endobronchial hamartomas can cause inflammatory changes and atelectasis, which can lead to an atypical radiological appearance. Hamartomas containing larger amounts of chondromatous tissue typically exhibit "popcorn-like" chondroid matrix calcifications (▶Fig. 9.1); on computed tomography (CT), these are seen in 50% of the larger nodules.[3] On rare occasions, diffuse calcifications are identified.[4] Around half of hamartomas are found on CT to contain fat with a density of between –40 and –120 HU (▶Fig. 9.2); this is considered a reliable predictor of nodule benignity.[1] Identification of fat in a smoothly marginated nodule is considered virtually pathognomonic for a hamartoma. Other fat-containing nodules are seen very rarely in the lung, in particular benign pulmonary lipomas and lipoid pneumonia.

Around half of hamartomas exhibit an identifiable growth and are usually slow growing with around 3-mm-diameter increase per year.[2] Fast-growing hamartomas are observed on rare occasions and may have doubling times of less than 1 year. Often, lesion growth is an indication for surgical resection of the nodule because of a suspected malignant tumor.

A biopsy is not needed if characteristic findings have been identified on CT: smoothly marginated nodule, fat-equivalent CT density, or popcorn-like calcifications as well as no or only slow growth. Otherwise, biopsy or resection is needed, in particular in the absence of characteristic CT results or on identification of fast growth suggestive of malignancy.

Treatment is based, as far as possible, on parenchymal-sparing resection of the hamartoma. However, resection is needed only for symptomatic patients or for patients with a suspected malignant growth when biopsy cannot be performed or was inconclusive.[2]

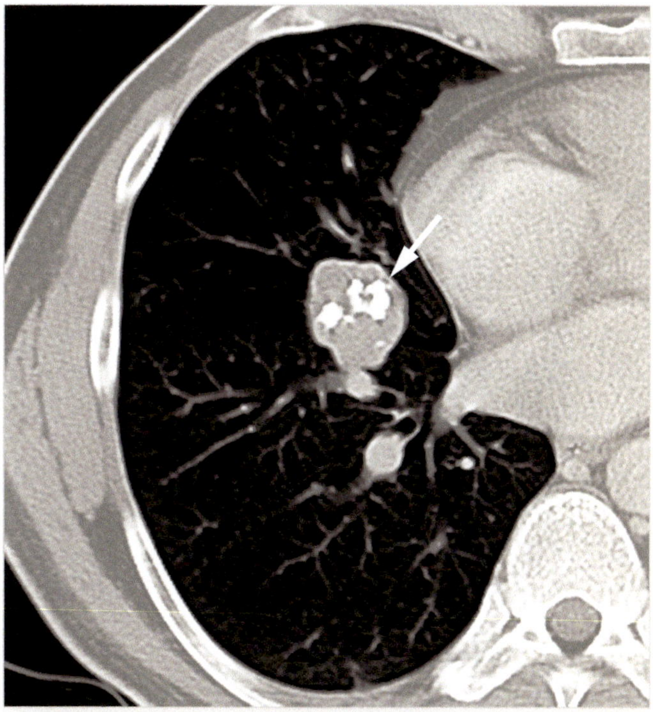

Fig. 9.1 Hamartoma. CT image. Typical popcorn-like calcifications (*arrow*).

9.2 Atypical Adenomatous Hyperplasia

Atypical adenomatous hyperplasia (AAH) is a preinvasive precursor lesion of adenocarcinoma of the lung. It entails

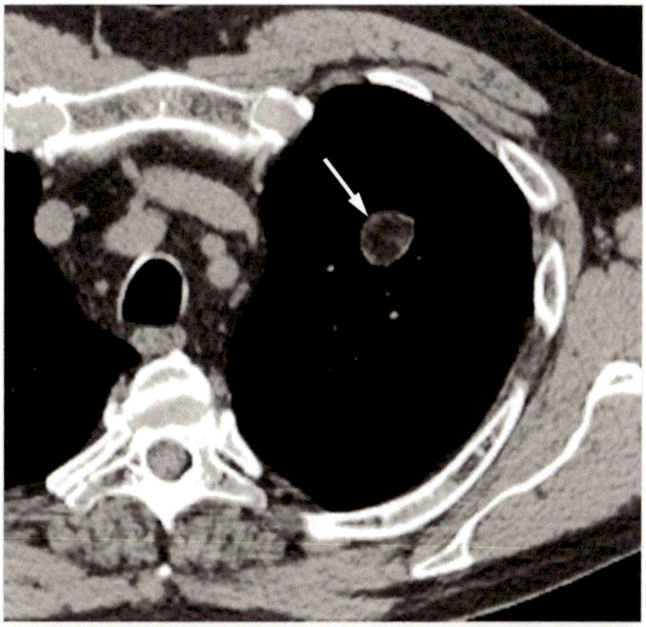

Fig. 9.2 Hamartoma. CT image. Hypodense components with fat-equivalent density (*arrow*).

9

II

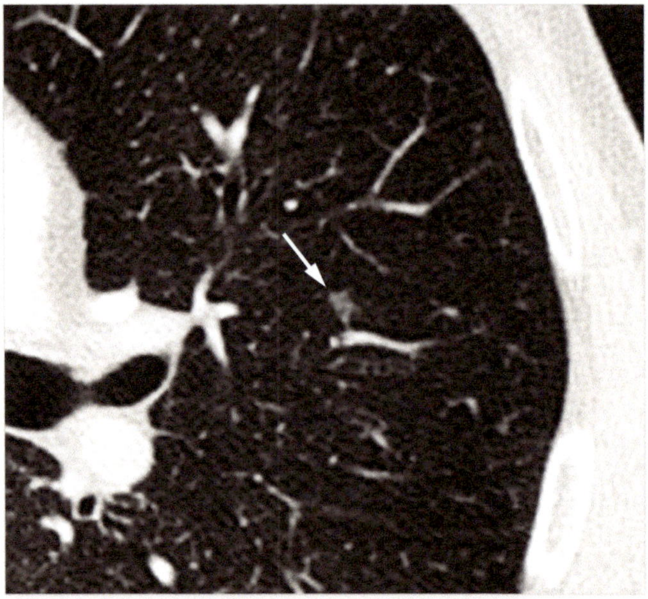

Fig. 9.3 Atypical adenomatous hyperplasia. CT image. Small ground-glass nodule (*arrow*).

discrete proliferation of type II pneumocytes or Clara cells along the alveolar walls and occasionally also the respiratory bronchioles. The transition from AAH to adenocarcinoma in situ (AIS) is not well definable. Often, foci of AAH are found in proximity to adenocarcinomas and only discovered by chance during pathological evaluation of the resected specimens.

AAH cannot be identified on chest radiography since it causes too little change in the density of the lung parenchyma. On CT, it manifests, if at all visible, as a small ground-glass nodule with very low density (▶Fig. 9.3). Its diameter is usually less than 5 mm but there are also reports of AAH nodules of more than 1 cm.[5,6,7] The majority of the small AAH nodules detected in surgical resected specimens cannot be located even retrospectively on CT.[7] AAH nodules may not change in size over several years, or they grow only very slowly.[8] AAH nodules manifesting on CT as ground-glass nodules have only a very low probability of progressing to adenocarcinoma.[5]

AAH should be included in differential diagnosis of focal ground-glass nodules. The main reason for long-term monitoring of such lesions is that they could potentially progress to adenocarcinoma. Monitoring is required beyond the 2-year period that is sufficient for solid nodules because of the very slow development of signs of malignant growth in ground-glass nodules; hence, a follow-up of 5 years is recommended.[9]

9.3 Lung Cancer

Lung cancer is the leading cause of malignancy-related deaths worldwide. Several predisposing factors are known: cigarette smoking is responsible for 80% of lung cancers. Around 9 to 15% of lung cancers are attributable to occupational exposure to noxae.[10] The most compelling evidence is the link between asbestos dust exposure and lung cancer; additional smoking exponentially increases the risk for lung cancer. Other physical and chemical noxae include:

- Radon and other radioactive isotopes.
- Quartz dust.
- Chromium.
- Nickel as well as nickel compounds.
- Beryllium.
- Arsenic.
- Cadmium.
- Wolfram- and cobalt-containing dusts.
- Polycyclic aromatic hydrocarbons.
- Dichlorodimethyl ether.
- Diesel engine exhaust emissions.

A genetic predisposition is thought to be implicated especially in younger patients.

Lung cancer has a male predominance, with 2.5 times more men than women affected in developed countries. However, that gender difference has decreased in recent years, no doubt due to changing smoking habits among women. Lung cancer is predominantly diagnosed in persons aged over 60 years and only very rarely before age 40 years.

There are no early clinical symptoms. When lung cancer becomes clinically apparent, it often has already undergone lymphogenous or hematogenous spread. Hence, the diagnosis is often only made at advanced tumor stages. That explains the poor prognosis for lung cancer: the overall 5-year survival rate is below 18%.[11] The prognosis is essentially better for early stage cancers, with a 5-year survival rate of 92% for stage IA1.[12] The close relation between the disease stage and prognosis in combination with the lack of early symptoms suggests a potential benefit of lung cancer screening in populations at risk.

9.3.1 Classification

Based on their histology, lung cancers are classified into two main groups with considerably different prognoses and requiring different treatment approaches: small cell and nonsmall cell lung cancers. Around 80% of lung cancers are nonsmall cell lung cancers and 20% are small cell lung cancers.

Nonsmall Cell Lung Cancer

The World Health Organization Classification of Lung Tumors of 2004 recognizes five types of nonsmall cell lung cancers[10]:

- Adenocarcinoma.
- Squamous cell carcinoma.
- Large cell carcinoma.
- Adenosquamous carcinoma (mixed form composed of squamous cell carcinoma and adenocarcinoma).
- Sarcomatoid carcinoma.

The former bronchioloalveolar carcinoma comprised a group of very heterogeneous carcinomas with highly variable prognoses. Today, those carcinomas previously known as bronchioloalveolar carcinoma are classified as various types of adenocarcinomas (see following sections). This facilitates their assignment to treatment regimens and improves prognosis assessment.[13]

Adenocarcinoma

Adenocarcinoma is the most common type of nonsmall cell lung cancer and occurs predominantly in the lung periphery. It also increasingly occurs in nonsmokers and younger patients without the typical risk factors, especially in women.

In the vast majority of cases, these are invasive adenocarcinomas. However, in recent years noninvasive or minimally invasive types of adenocarcinoma have drawn attention, in particular due to results from lung cancer screening trials. For that reason, a current *histologic classification of adenocarcinomas* is now presented below. One aspect of relevance for radiologists is the relationship between the CT morphology and histology of adenocarcinomas.[14]

Because of the new insights into the biologic behavior of incidentally detected small adenocarcinomas, it was necessary to revise the previous concepts used for classification of adenocarcinomas, in particular with regard to treatment and prognosis. Hence, in 2011 a new system for classification of lung adenocarcinoma, jointly compiled by the International Association for the Study of Lung Cancer, American Thoracic Society, and European Respiratory Society, was published.[8] As for other tumor entities, importance is now ascribed to tumor invasiveness and noninvasiveness. In an invasive carcinoma, the tumor breaches the basement membrane. Growth along the alveolar walls with wallpaper-like lining of the alveoli and preservation of aeration of the affected alveoli is termed "lepidic growth." Recognition of a lepidic growth pattern does not exclude tumor invasiveness. Different types of adenocarcinoma are distinguished in accordance with tumor size and invasiveness (▶Fig. 9.4):

- *Preinvasive lesions*: The term adenocarcinoma in situ refers to a cancer without an invasive component; it corresponds to one of the former types of bronchoalveolar carcinoma. The size of adenocarcinomas in situ is usually less than 2 cm, and as per their definition never more than 3 cm; they have no invasive component and are slow growing. Strictly speaking, AAH is also classified as a preinvasive lesion which is, however, a precursor lesion rather than an adenocarcinoma.
- *Minimally invasive adenocarcinoma* (MIA): These tumors measuring up to 3 cm exhibit a lepidic growth pattern and have an invasive component of less than 5 mm.
- *Invasive adenocarcinoma*: These adenocarcinomas exhibit a solid or lepidic growth pattern with an invasive component of over 5 mm in size. The rare tumors with a predominantly lepidic growth pattern are called *lepidic predominant adenocarcinomas* (LPAs) and have a better prognosis than other invasive adenocarcinomas. By contrast, adenocarcinomas classified as solid or micropapillary on histology have a particularly unfavorable prognosis.[13] Invasive adenocarcinomas account for the vast majority of adenocarcinomas of the lung seen in clinical routine practice.

The various growth patterns have different imaging manifestations. In principle, a lepidic growth pattern can often be identified on imaging as an area of ground-glass density. A solid growth pattern manifests on CT either as a consolidation or as a ground-glass nodule of increasing density.[5] That a nodule exhibits purely ground-glass density does not rule out an invasive carcinoma.[14]

Different growth patterns (see ▶Fig. 9.4) produce different imaging findings:

- *Solid nodule, often with spiculated margins* (▶Fig. 9.5): Course spicules of more than 2 mm are correlated with a higher probability of lymphogenous metastasis and vascular invasion as well as with a poorer prognosis.[5,16] Open bronchi

9

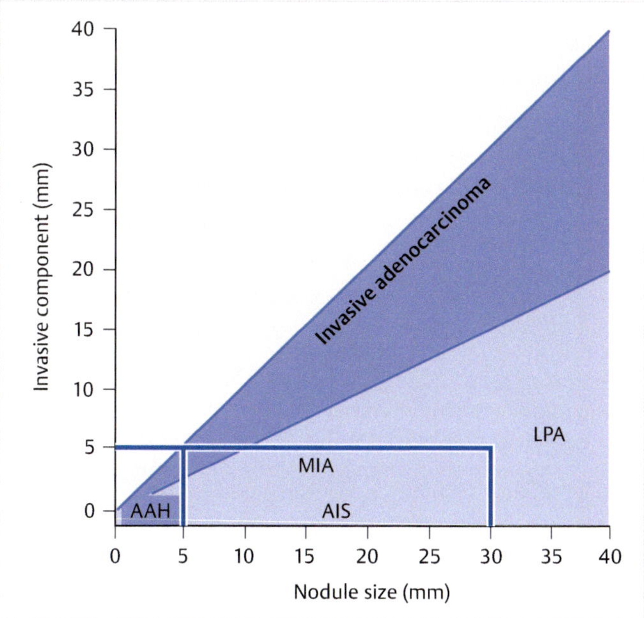

Fig. 9.4 Classification of adenocarcinomas based on invasiveness and size. AAH, atypical adenomatous hyperplasia; AIS, adenocarcinoma in situ; LPA, lepidic predominant adenocarcinoma; MIA, minimally invasive adenocarcinoma.

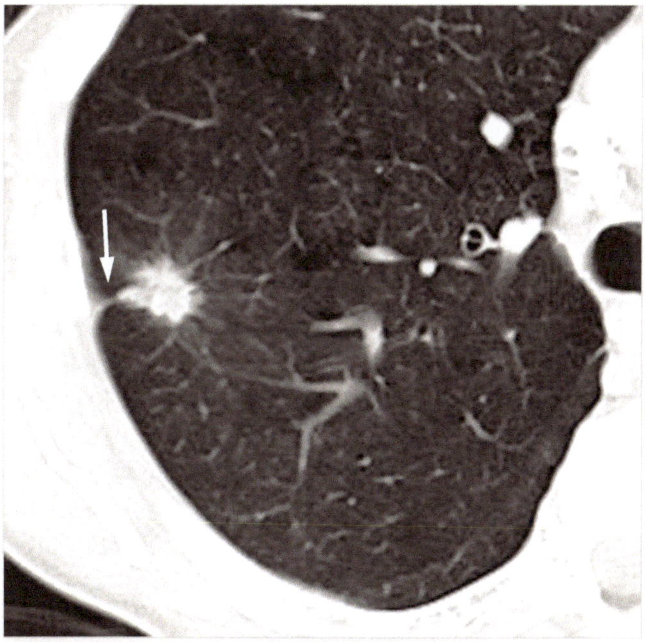

Fig. 9.5 Pulmonary nodule. CT image. Small cell lung cancer. Coarse spicules, "corona radiata" as sign of malignancy. Distal subsegmental atelectasis, "pleural finger" (*arrow*).

within the nodule—positive air bronchogram (▶ Fig. 9.6)—can be identified especially in adenocarcinomas[16,17,18,19] and should serve as a criterion for differential diagnosis versus benign tumor of the lung.[20,21]

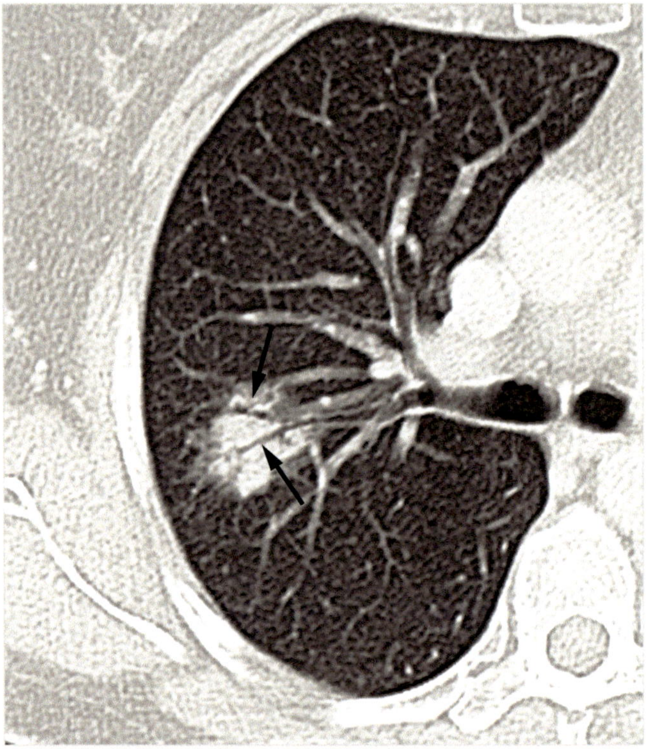

Fig. 9.6 Adenocarcinoma. CT image. Positive air bronchogram (*arrows*).

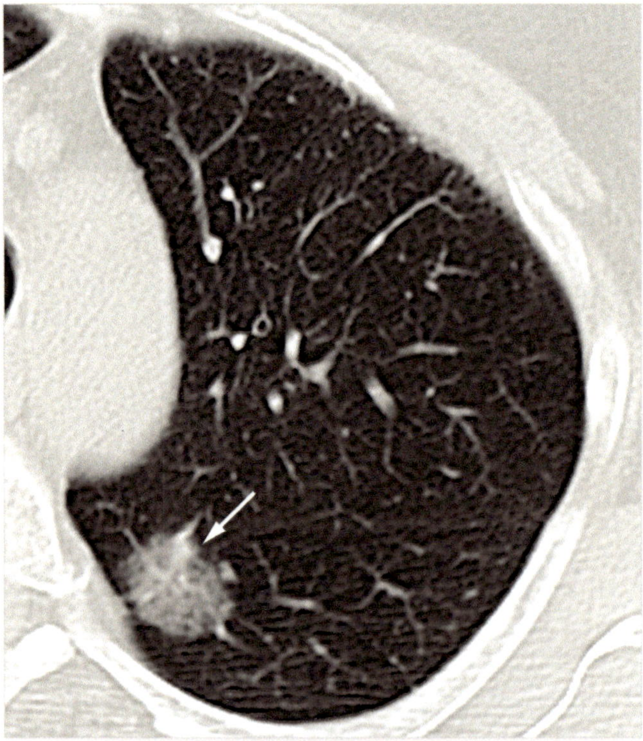

Fig. 9.8 Part-solid nodule. CT image. Adenocarcinoma with small solid component (*arrow*) inside a larger ground-glass nodule.

- *Ground-glass nodule* (▶ Fig. 9.7): A focal lesion with ground-glass density. It often represents an adenocarcinoma with a lepidic growth pattern, a growth pattern involving wallpaper-like, tumor-cell lining of the airspaces, which continue to be aerated.
- *Part-solid nodule* (▶ Fig. 9.8): A focal lesion with a solid and a ground-glass component; the latter is usually caused by a lepidic growth pattern (▶ Fig. 9.9). This CT morphology is particularly seen in adenocarcinomas containing a mixture of solid and lepidic growth patterns (often MIA with a diameter up to 3 cm, or larger LPA).

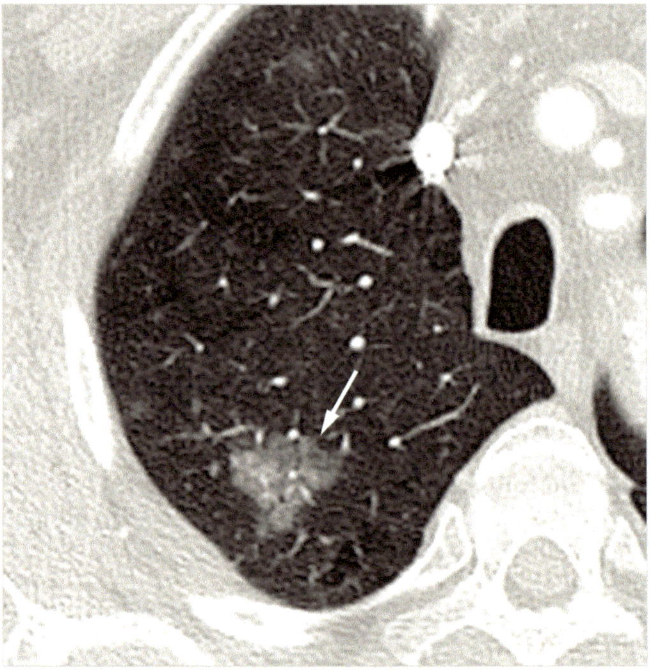

Fig. 9.7 Ground-glass nodule. CT image. Adenocarcinoma with lepidic growth pattern (*arrow*).

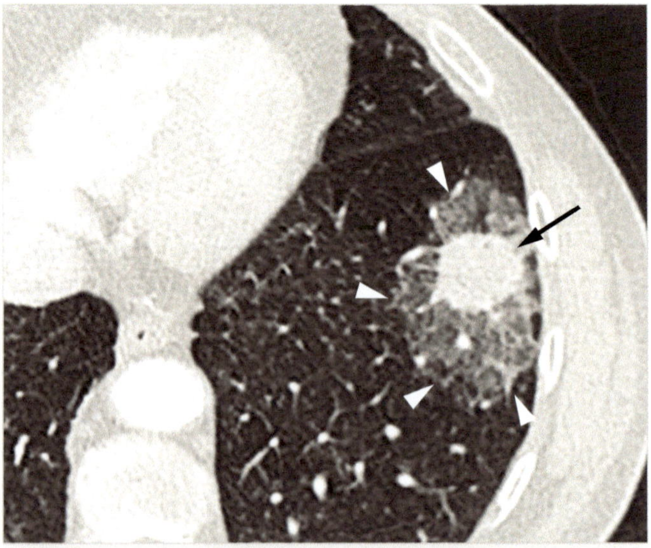

Fig. 9.9 Lepidic predominant adenocarcinoma. CT image. Solid central tumor component (*arrow*) surrounded by extensive ground-glass opacities (*arrowheads*).

- *Lobar opacities* (▶ Fig. 9.10): Consolidations and ground-glass opacities within a lobe, or in a number of lung lobes in the case of multifocal opacities, are interpreted as a characteristic manifestation of pneumonic-type lung adenocarcinoma.[22] The increase in the density of the implicated lung parenchyma is due to tumor growth as well as the mucinous component which results in the areas of consolidation exhibiting lower density than that of muscle on CT.[8] The pulmonary vessels traversing the tumor mass can be identified on CT as a CT angiogram sign after intravenous contrast administration.[23,24,25,26]

Synchronous multifocal adenocarcinomas are not uncommon; in 8 to 22% of resected pulmonary adenocarcinomas, additional lesions of the sequence AAH → AIS → invasive adenocarcinoma were identified histologically.[27,28] Ground-glass nodule metastases are very rare; hence, such multiple adenocarcinomas tend to be viewed as synchronous primary tumors rather than lung metastases.[8,29]

Squamous Cell Carcinoma

In the past, squamous cell carcinoma was the most common type of nonsmall cell lung cancer, but today it is less common than adenocarcinoma, probably as a result of changing smoking habits. Squamous cell carcinomas are frequently located in the hilar region. They may undergo central liquefaction and then present as thick-walled cavity. Mediastinal invasion is common due to their central predominance. Some of these tumors can be quite easily surgically dissected from their surrounding structures, such as blood vessels or bronchi. Therefore, not every vascular contact of squamous cell carcinoma on staging imaging should be interpreted as vascular invasion.

Squamous cell carcinomas located at the lung periphery manifest as solid or cavitary nodules, usually with spicules. Unlike adenocarcinoma, squamous cell carcinoma does not present as subsolid nodule since it does not exhibit a lepidic growth pattern.

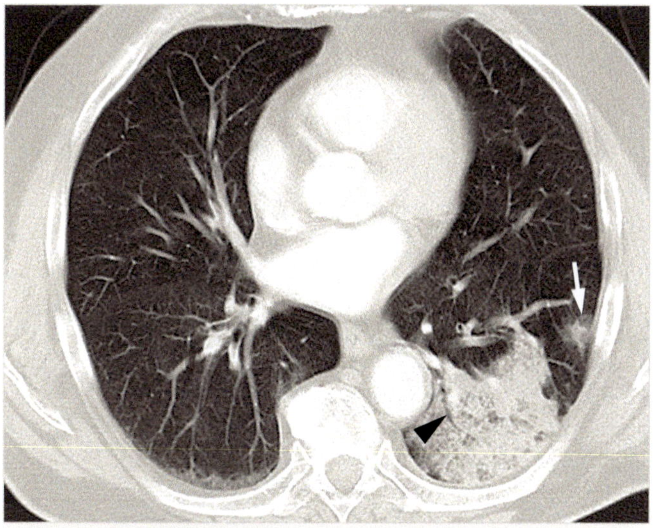

Fig. 9.10 Pneumonic-type adenocarcinoma. CT image. Consolidations and ground-glass opacities in the left lower lobe, multifocal (*arrow*). Positive air bronchogram within the tumor (*arrowhead*).

Squamous cell carcinomas can grow very quickly. The fastest growing lung cancer reported in the literature was a squamous cell carcinoma with a tumor doubling time of only 7.5 days.[30] However, the tumor doubling time is usually between 1 month and 2 years, as for other lung cancer entities.[31,32,33]

Other Nonsmall Cell Lung Cancers

A common feature of the adenosquamous, large cell, and sarcomatoid carcinomas is their peripheral predominance and nodular or mass-like appearance.

On histology, *adenosquamous carcinoma* is seen to contain features of both adenocarcinoma and squamous cell carcinoma. It cannot be distinguished on imaging from these two tumor entities.

The term *large cell lung carcinoma* is a collective term for undifferentiated, nonsmall cell lung cancers of different histologic etiology. Often, these are cancers that have undergone such profound dedifferentiation that their adeno- or squamous cell carcinoma heritage can no longer be identified on light microscopy. Neuroendocrine large cell carcinoma belongs to the group of neuroendocrine tumors, like typical and atypical carcinoids as well as small cell lung cancer.[34] With respect to their differentiation at histopathology, they are classified as being between the carcinoids and small cell lung cancer.[35,36] On imaging, large cell neuroendocrine carcinomas are generally seen as peripheral nodules or masses. Less commonly, they are found in central lung regions where they cause atelectasis or mucus retention.[37] Peripheral large cell carcinomas usually have a smoothly marginated and lobulated, occasionally spiculated, appearance. Necrosis is very common and calcification is not uncommon.[38]

Sarcomatoid carcinomas are rare, predominantly peripheral, lung tumors with aggressive growth, which are relatively large at the time of diagnosis. These tumors often have extensive areas of central necrosis and tend to invade the pleura and chest wall.

Small Cell Lung Cancer

Small cell lung cancer accounts for around 20% of all lung cancers.[34] Due to tumor biology, treatment and prognosis greatly differ from nonsmall cell lung cancer described above. Since it is often associated with ectopic hormone production, it frequently causes paraneoplastic syndromes, in particular Cushing syndrome or Schwartz–Bartter syndrome (syndrome of inappropriate secretion of antidiuretic hormone).[39,40,41]

Because of its fast growth, small cell lung cancer usually better responds to chemo- and radiotherapy than nonsmall cell lung cancer. The remission rate is around 90%, and complete remission is not uncommon.[42] But, unfortunately, early recurrences after initially successful treatment are very common. In the absence of distant metastases and when disease is limited to one hemithorax (limited disease), long-term remission is observed in 20 to 25% of cases, which can be regarded as a cure. By contrast, more advanced tumor stages (extensive disease) continue to be incurable, but with palliative treatment, life expectancy can be prolonged.[42]

	Nodule	Peripheral mass	Cavity	Infiltrate	Pleural thickening	Central mass	Atelectasis	Pleural effusion
Localization	Peripheral					Central		Central or peripheral
Schematic diagram	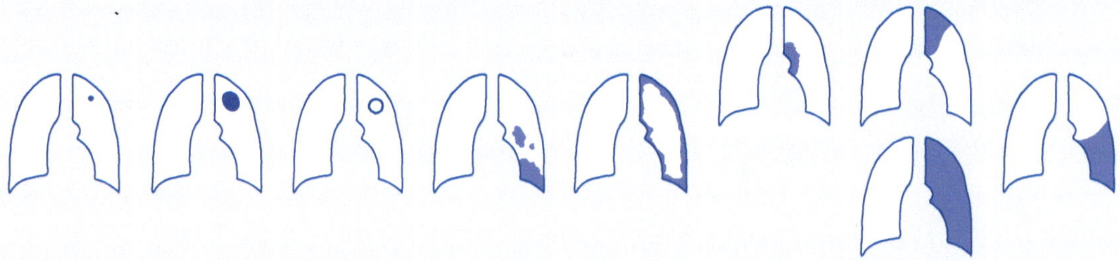							
Adenocarcinoma	++	++	(+)	+	(+)	(+)	(+)	++
Squamous cell carcinoma	+	+	+	–	–	++	++	+
Large-cell carcinoma	+	++	–	–	–	+	(+)	+
Small-cell carcinoma	(+)	(+)	–	–	–	+++	+	+

Fig. 9.11 **Radiologic appearance of peripheral and central lung cancers.** Incidence of occurrence in different histologic types.

One-fifth of all small cell lung cancers contain components of nonsmall cell lung cancer, usually of squamous cell carcinomas.[43]

Around 90% of small cell lung cancers are found in the central lung region and have their origin in the mucosa of the mainstem bronchus or lobar bronchi.[21] Early extensive lymphogenous and hematogenous metastasis is typical. Less commonly, small cell lung cancer manifests as a peripheral nodule, typically with large hilar and mediastinal lymph node metastases by the time of diagnosis.[44]

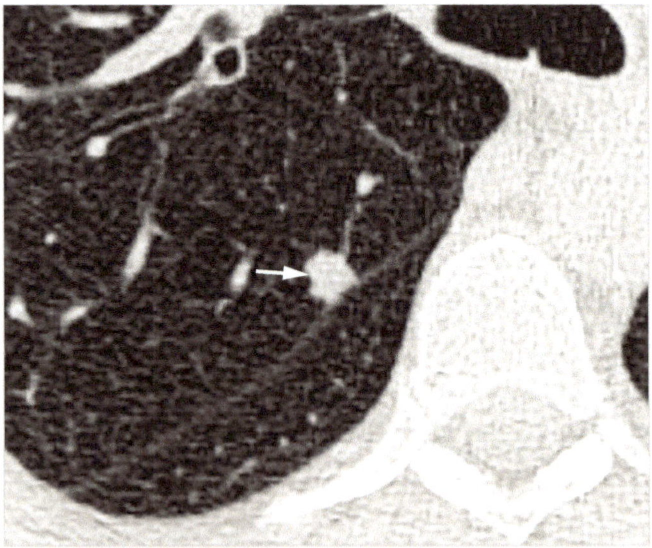

Fig. 9.12 **Lobulated nodule.** CT image. Adenocarcinoma (*arrow*).

9.3.2 Imaging Findings

The imaging findings of lung carcinoma are determined by its location and biologic features. Half of all lung cancers are found at the periphery. These can be directly seen on radiographs once they have reached a certain size, whereas central lung carcinomas can often only be identified through indirect signs. The typical radiologic findings are presented in ▸Fig. 9.11.

Peripheral Lung Cancer

The *pulmonary nodule*, defined as a rounded or irregular opacity of either solid or subsolid (part-solid or ground-glass) density, is a common presentation of small peripheral lung cancer.[45,46] At times, the nodule has a lobulated appearance (▸Fig. 9.12) because of its histologic heterogeneity with variable growth rates.[21] Its ill-defined or spiculated margins are known as *corona radiata* (see ▸Fig. 9.5) and may be caused by tumor invasion into the surrounding lung, a desmoplastic reaction of the body to the tumor, or interstitial edema.[21,47,48,49] That explains the difficulties in delineating the tumor margins and determining its exact size on radiological imaging. Often, additional findings are identified. A pleural finger (see ▸Fig. 9.5) is a subsegmental atelectasis caused by the tumor and seen on CT as linear opacity extending from the nodule toward the pleura. Rigler sign (umbilical retraction sign) is the term used to denote retraction of the tumor contour at the entry point of vessels into the tumor.[50] For differential diagnosis of pulmonary nodules, please see Section 21.1. Small nodule-like lung cancers are frequently overlooked on radiographs and only diagnosed on CT. That is particularly true for ground-glass nodules or part-solid nodules. These are often incidental findings and, as small tumors, are usually asymptomatic.

A *mass* is a focal lesion larger than 3 cm, which is a typical appearance of larger peripheral lung cancers. The image characteristics of such lung cancers do not differ from those described in the above sections. The larger the mass, the more likely it is to impair aeration of more distal lung regions. Occasionally, adenocarcinomas contain larger ground-glass components, too.

The term *cavity* (or cavern) is used to denote the large air-filled hollows seen at the center of pulmonary nodules or masses. On chest radiography, they manifest as ring shadows (▶Fig. 9.13). Cavities are formed by areas of central necrosis that connect with and drain into the bronchial system. Squamous cell carcinomas tend to develop thick-walled cavities.[51,52] Less commonly, adenocarcinomas also have cavities which tend to be more thin-walled than those seen in squamous cell carcinomas. Cavities are uncommon in small cell lung cancer.

Adenocarcinomas, in particular of pneumonic type, may manifest as *consolidation*, as seen in pneumonia (see ▶Fig. 9.10). In advanced tumor stages, multiple, or even bilateral, consolidations may occasionally be seen. Often, ground-glass components may be identified on CT at the periphery of the nodules. These must be distinguished from inflammatory opacities, such as poststenotic pneumonia seen in central lung cancers.

Diffuse pleural invasion is a rare manifestation of adenocarcinomas, with direct tumor spread along the pleura (▶Fig. 9.14). This causes usually irregular *pleural thickening*, as seen in pleural mesothelioma or pleural dissemination from other tumors.[21,43] Concomitant pleural effusion may be seen but that is not necessarily the case.

Occasionally, extensive scars are seen on histology around lung cancers, which gave rise to the concept of a *scar carcinoma* developing in a pre-existing scar. But it is also thought that the scar may have been formed as a result of a strong desmoplastic tissue reaction to the cancer. The existence of scar carcinomas is therefore disputed.[21,40,44,53,54,55]

Central Lung Carcinoma

Most small cell lung cancers and squamous cell carcinomas have their origin in the central bronchial system. The latter tends to exhibit an endobronchial growth pattern and may cause atelectasis of distal peripheral lung areas. By contrast, the former tends to cause extrinsic compression of the bronchial system. Because of the *central tumor localization*, early invasion of the mediastinum, great blood vessels, and nerves often occurs. The phrenic nerve adjacent to the hilum is occasionally invaded by central lung carcinomas. This can be diagnosed already on a radiograph from the high-riding diaphragm. It is often difficult to distinguish between central lung cancer and their mediastinal lymph node metastases. Hence, staging problems may arise when trying to differentiate between mediastinal invasion by the primary tumor (T4) and mediastinal lymph node metastases (N2). Apart from atelectasis, bronchial and vascular stenosis has other effects: incomplete bronchial obstruction is conducive to onset of poststenotic pneumonia and, less commonly, a valve mechanism causes hyperinflation of the distal lung. Higher-grade stenosis of the central pulmonary arteries resulting from the tumor can lead to hypoperfusion of the affected lung. CT is able to directly visualize pulmonary artery stenosis; occasionally, even radiographs may demonstrate a reduced caliber of the affected pulmonary arteries and rarefaction of the pulmonary vascular bed.

Endobronchial growth of central lung carcinomas causes hypoventilation of the lung parenchyma distal to the tumor.

9

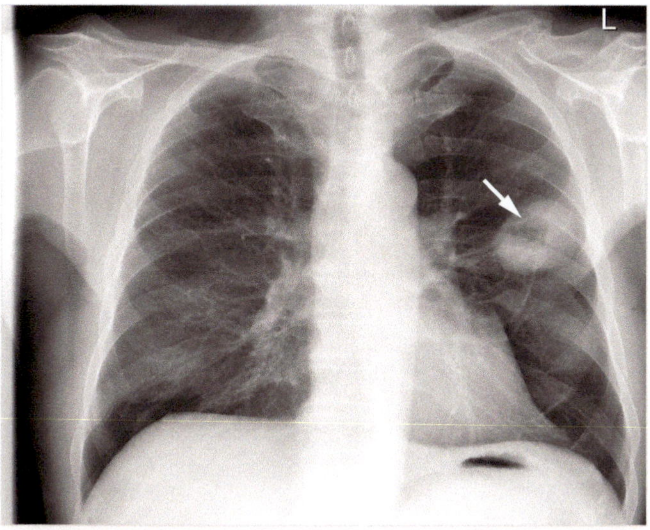

Fig. 9.13 Cavity. Radiograph. Squamous cell carcinoma in the left upper lobe with thick-walled cavity (*arrow*).

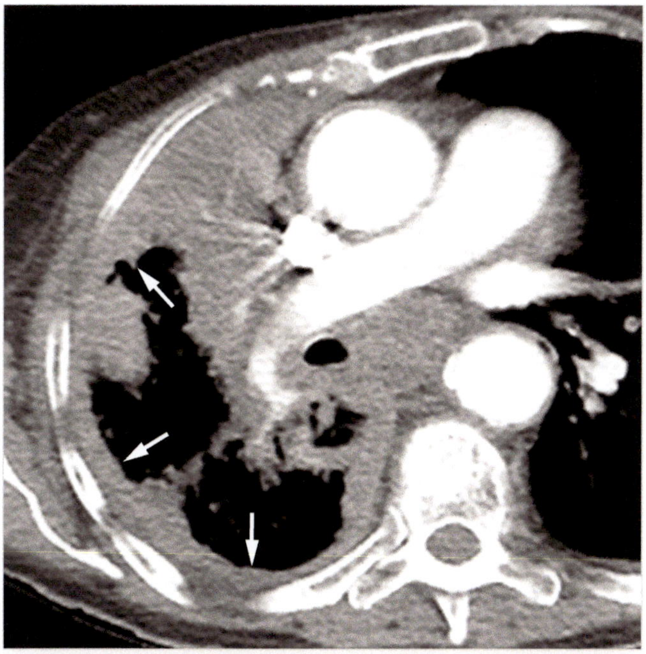

Fig. 9.14 Adenocarcinoma with diffuse subpleural tumor growth (*arrows*). CT image.

A tumor in the mainstem bronchus gives rise to *atelectasis* of the entire lung, while central tumors of the lobar bronchi cause atelectasis of an individual lung lobe. On radiographs often only the atelectasis but not the tumor can be identified. A central right upper lobe tumor may be visible within the atelectasis on the radiograph if it projects from the outer contour of the atelectatic lobe (▶ Fig. 9.15). This manifestation is known as the "Golden-S sign," first described by Ross Golden.[56,57] Left-sided upper lobe atelectasis is also suggestive of a tumor even if no evidence of a tumor can be found on chest radiography. Even on CT, differentiation of a tumor from atelectasis can be challenging. Positron emission tomography (PET)-CT, which is often indicated, improves tumor within the atelectasis.

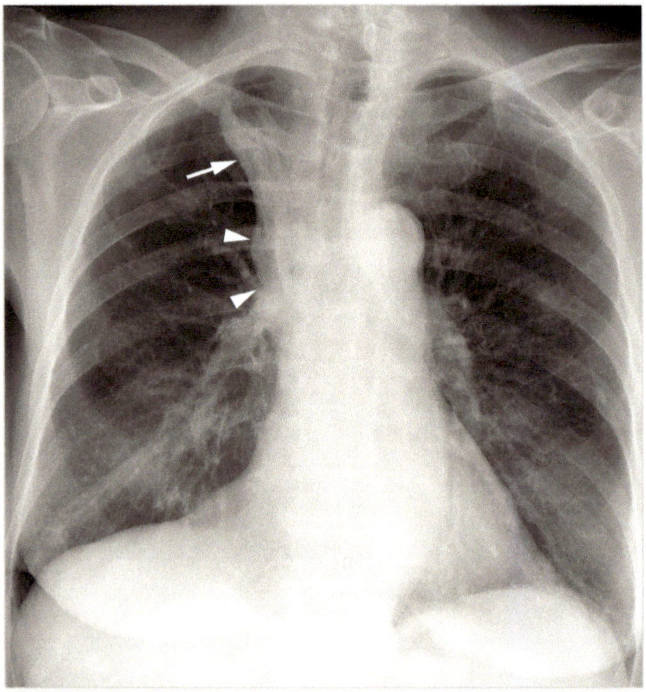

Fig. 9.15 Central lung cancer in the right upper lobe. Radiograph. Right upper lobe atelectasis (*arrow*) and ensuing right high-riding diaphragm. The central tumor projects laterally from the atelectasis: Golden-S sign (*arrowheads*).

Other Tumor Manifestations

A *pleural effusion* presents in association with all the tumor manifestations described above and is an indication of the presence of pleural dissemination. But it can also be caused by atelectasis and is not malignant in such a case. The presence of pleural effusion at the time of staging should therefore not automatically be interpreted as pleural dissemination (M1a). Pleural nodules of soft-tissue density are likewise indicative of malignant pleural disease.

A *Pancoast tumor* is a tumor that grows cranially from the apex of lung and invades the soft tissues of the superior thoracic aperture (▶ Fig. 9.16). It is also known as a *superior sulcus tumor*. Its first symptom is often treatment-refractory shoulder and arm pain on the affected side. This is followed by neurologic deficits secondary to tumor invasion of the brachial plexus.

Lymph node metastases present on imaging as enlarged lymph nodes or as lymph nodes with a hypodense center. On radiographs, they can be identified as hilar enlargement, a mediastinal mass, or diffuse expansion of the upper mediastinum (▶ Fig. 9.17). Small cell lung cancer is typically associated with extensive mediastinal lymphadenopathy. Upper venous congestion is caused by extrinsic vascular compression, tumor-related thrombosis, or, less commonly, direct vascular invasion if the superior vena cava or the brachiocephalic veins are affected.

9.3.3 Staging

Diagnostic imaging plays an important role in noninvasive staging of lung cancer. Invasive staging is dominated by bronchoscopic and surgical techniques, especially in determining the tumor extent in the bronchial system and in lymph node staging. The purpose of these staging examinations is to determine the extension of the primary tumor and

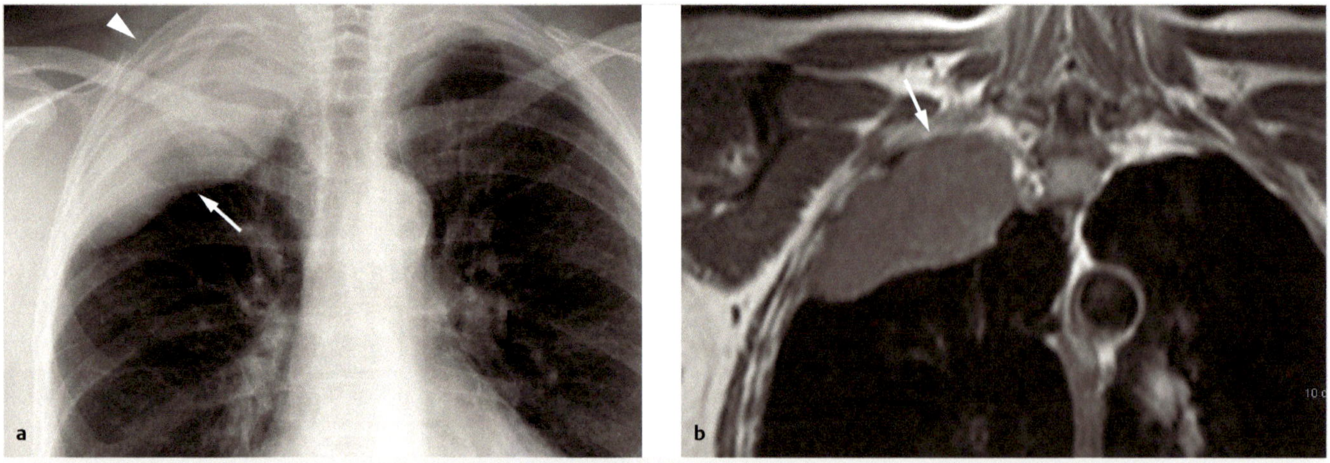

Fig. 9.16 Pancoast tumor. Lung cancer in the right upper lobe growing cranially into the soft tissues of the superior thoracic aperture. **(a)** Radiograph. Right apical tumor (*arrow*) and tumor-related opacity in the soft tissues of the upper thoracic inlet (*arrowhead*). **(b)** Coronal T1-weighted MRI image without intravenous contrast. Tumor invasion of the fatty tissues of the upper thoracic inlet (*arrow*).

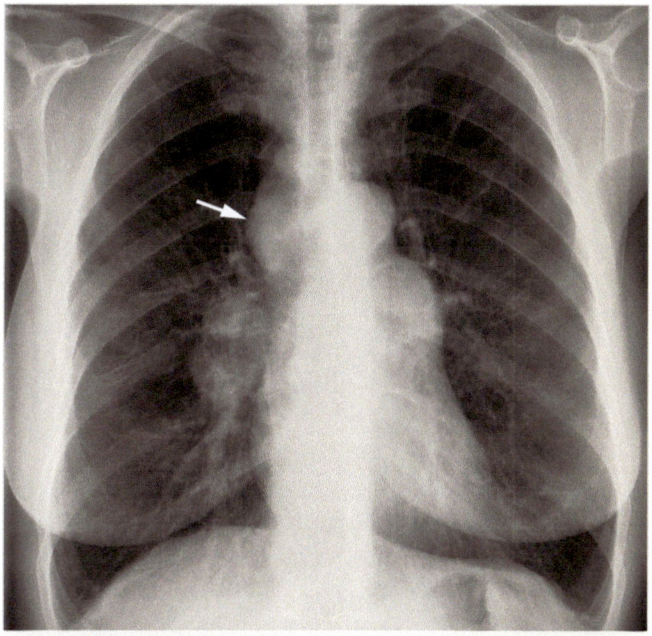

Fig. 9.17 Mediastinal lymph node metastasis (*arrow*) of a right central adenocarcinoma. Radiograph.

its relationship to neighboring structures, and the presence and extent of lymph node metastasis as well as of distant metastasis.

The TNM classification system devised by the International Union for Cancer Control (*Union Internationale Contre le Cancer* [UICC]) is used for tumor staging. The current 8th version was published in 2016.[58] TNM staging is described in detail in ▸Table 9.1. From the TNM tumor formula, a tumor stage (▸Table 9.2) is calculated to determine the appropriate stage-related treatment. This also permits insights into the prognosis.

Note

In the past, a simplified staging system was used for small cell lung cancer: classification into very limited disease, limited disease, and extensive disease. That classification system was deemed obsolete with the advent of differentiated treatment approaches; complete staging of small cell lung cancer is also needed based on the TNM tumor formula.

▸Table 9.3 lists imaging procedures recommended for complete lung cancer staging; significant differences exist between European and U.S. guidelines, particularly in terms of staging for distant metastases.[59,60] Additional examination techniques may be needed for clinically suspicious findings or for clarification of any hitherto unclear imaging results.

Local Tumor Extension (T Descriptor)

The T descriptor (see ▸Table 9.1) gives information on the tumor size and on invasion of surrounding structures. For example, categories T1 and T2 are used to describe a tumor confined to the lung and measuring up to 5 cm. The advanced categories T3 and T4 are used to describe a tumor measuring more than 5 cm, which extends beyond the lung borders or is associated with separate tumor nodules(s) in the affected lung.

Categories T1 and T2 are further subdivided in accordance with the *tumor size (diameter)* in greatest dimension. This reflects the prognosis which is largely determined by the tumor size: for nonmetastatic, nonsmall cell lung carcinomas (T1a) measuring up to 1 cm, the 5-year survival rate is 92%, while for those measuring 4 to 5 cm (T2b) it is only 60%.[12]

Invasion of the pleura can often only be suspected from the imaging results and only reliably diagnosed from the resected specimen.[61,62] The more longitudinal the tumor contact with the pleura appears on CT, the greater the probability of pleural invasion. Distal atelectasis (pleural finger) can mimic tumor contact with the visceral pleura.

Tumors affecting the *mainstem bronchus* are evaluated in terms of their involvement of the carina as T2 (no invasion) or T4 (in the case of invasion of the carina or trachea). In such settings, diagnostic imaging is less reliable than bronchoscopy since it is hardly able to visualize superficial invasion of the mucosa.

It is difficult to distinguish between invasion of large mediastinal vessels and mere *vascular contact* with radiologic imaging. The greater the contact surface area and the greater the proportion of vessel with tumor contact, the more probable is vascular invasion. In general, a contact surface area of at least 3 cm or tumor contact of more than one-third of the vessel circumference is viewed as a criterion of potential invasion. Squamous cell carcinomas can, however, often be detached intraoperatively from the blood vessels even if CT had suggested tumor invasion. Magnetic resonance imaging (MRI) with dynamic sequences may be helpful: visible tumor mobility versus the vascular wall makes invasion unlikely. Conversely, subtle changes in the signal intensity of the vascular wall are suggestive of tumor invasion.

For assessment of the *extrapulmonary extension* of Pancoast tumors, MRI of the upper thoracic inlet is recommended in addition to the usual staging examinations.[59,60] MRI is superior to CT in visualizing invasion of the relevant structures, such as the brachial plexus (▸Fig. 9.18).[63,64]

Satellite nodules associated with separate nodule(s) in the same lobe as the primary tumor are classified as T3, while tumor nodules in different (ipsilateral) lobes than that of the primary tumor are classified as T4. Contralateral pulmonary tumor manifestations are classified as distant metastasis (M1a; see below). That said, small, usually benign pulmonary nodules occur extremely frequently independently of lung carcinoma.[62] In the vast majority of cases, pulmonary nodules of less than 10 mm are not tumorous satellite nodules but incidental benign nodules.[65] By contrast, nodules measuring more than 10 mm should be viewed as satellite nodules because of their high probability of malignancy or as synchronous second primary lung cancer, depending on their imaging and pathologic findings.[66]

Table 9.1 Clinical TNM staging based on 8th edition of UICC[58]

Descriptors	Definitions
T descriptor (primary tumor)	
Tx	Cytologic evidence of tumor but no correlate on imaging or bronchoscopy
T0	No evidence of primary tumor
Tis	Carcinoma in situ
T1	Tumor 3 cm in greatest dimension surrounded by lung or visceral pleura, without invasion of the bronchi more proximal than the lobar bronchus
T1a(mi)	Minimally invasive adenocarcinoma
T1a	Tumor ≤1 cm in greatest dimension
T1b	Tumor >1 cm but ≤2 cm in greatest dimension
T1c	Tumor >2 cm but ≤3 cm in greatest dimension
T2	Tumor >3 cm but ≤5 cm in greatest dimension
	With invasion of the visceral pleura or
	With invasion of the mainstem bronchus regardless of distance from the carina or
	Atelectasis or obstructive inflammation that extents to the hilar region, involving part or all of the lung
T2a	Tumor >3 cm but ≤4 cm in greatest dimension
T2b	Tumor >4 cm but ≤5 cm in greatest dimension
T3	Tumor >5 cm but ≤7 cm in greatest dimension or With separate tumor nodule(s) in the same lung lobe or With invasion of the: • Chest wall (including parietal pleura und superior sulcus tumors) • Phrenic nerve • Parietal pericardium
T4	Tumor >7 cm in greatest dimension or
	With separate tumor nodule(s) in different ipsilateral lung lobes or
	With invasion of the: • Diaphragm • Mediastinum • Heart • Great vessels • Trachea or carina • Recurrent laryngeal nerve • Esophagus • Vertebral body
N descriptor (regional lymph node metastasis)	
Nx	Regional lymph nodes cannot be assessed
N0	No regional lymph node metastasis
N1	Metastasis in ipsilateral peribronchial or
	Ipsilateral hilar lymph node(s) or
	Intrapulmonary lymph node(s) (including involvement by direct extension)
N2	Metastasis in ipsilateral mediastinal or
	Subcarinal carinal lymph node(s)
N3	Metastasis in contralateral mediastinal or
	Contralateral hilar or
	Ipsi- or contralateral scalene or supraclavicular lymph node(s)
M descriptor (distant metastasis)	
M0	No distant metastasis
M1	Distant metastasis present

(*Continue*)

Table 9.1 (*Continue*) Clinical TNM staging based on 8th edition of UICC[108]

Descriptors	Definitions
• M1a	Intrathoracic metastasis • Separate tumor nodule(s) in contralateral lobe or • Pleural or pericardial tumor nodule(s) or • Malignant pleural effusion or • Malignant pericardial effusion
• M1b	Single extrathoracic metastasis
• M1c	Multiple extrathoracic metastases in one or more organs

Table 9.2 TNM tumor formula and resultant tumor stage based on 8th edition of UICC, and 5-year survival rates[12,58]

Stage	T descriptor	N descriptor	M descriptor	5-year survival
Occult carcinoma	Tx	N0	M0	
Stage 0	Tis	N0	M0	
Stage IA1	T1a(mi) T1a	N0	M0	92%
Stage IA2	T1b	N0	M0	83%
Stage IA3	T1c	N0	M0	77%
Stage IB	T2a	N0	M0	68%
Stage IIA	T2b	N0	M0	60%
Stage IIB	T1a-c T2a-b T3	N1 N1 N0	M0 M0 M0	53%
Stage IIIA	T1a-c T2a-b T3 T4	N2 N2 N1 N0–1	M0 M0 M0 M0	36%
Stage IIIB	T1a-c T2a-b T3 T4	N3 N3 N2 N2	M0 M0 M0 M0	26%
Stage IIIC	T3–4	N2	M0	13%
Stage IVA	Any T	Any N	M1a-b	10%
Stage IVB	Any T	Any N	M1c	0%

Table 9.3 Radiologic imaging for lung cancer staging; recommendations vary significantly among guidelines[59,60]

Modality	Recommended for	Remarks	Alternative
Chest CT	All stages	With IV contrast	Unenhanced if IV contrast contraindicated
Upper abdominal CT	All stages	With IV contrast	Ultrasound if IV contrast contraindicated
Brain MRI	Stages IIB-IV	With IV contrast	If contraindicated, alternatively brain CT with IV contrast
PET-CT	Stages IB–IIIB, optional stage IA	If treatment with curative intent planned	If contraindicated, alternatively skeletal scintigraphy or whole-body MRI
Chest MRI	Recommended for sulcus superior tumors	With IV contrast	Unenhanced if IV contrast contraindicated

Abbreviations: CT, computed tomography; IV, intravenous; MRI, magnetic resonance imaging.

II

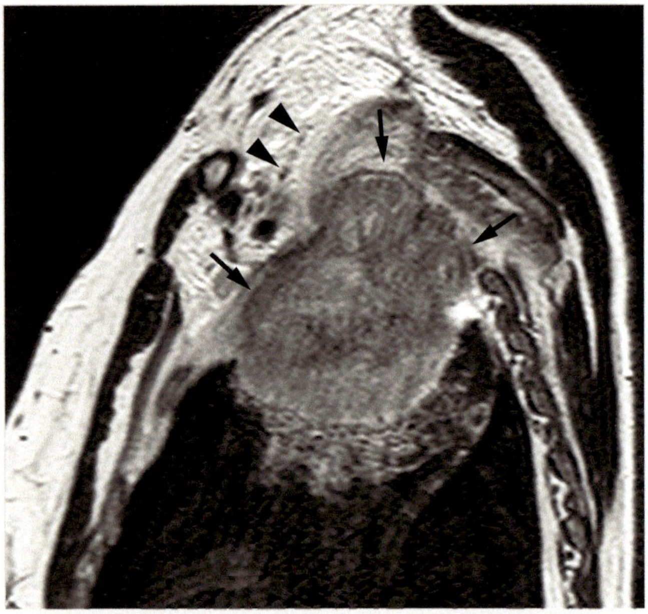

Fig. 9.18 Pancoast tumor. Sagittal T1-weighted MRI image without intravenous contrast. Lung cancer growing cranially from the apex of lung into the superior thoracic aperture (*arrows*). The structures of the brachial plexus can be well recognized as areas of low signal intensity (*arrowheads*) and have not been invaded by the tumor.

Regional Lymph Node Metastasis (N Descriptor)

The N descriptor defines the extent of lymph node metastases: N1 describes ipsilateral hilar or intrapulmonary metastases, N2 only ipsilateral mediastinal or subcarinal metastases, and N3 more extensive involvement of the lymph nodes, in particular of the contralateral mediastinal or hilar lymph nodes. A special aspect here is that subcarinal metastases in lymph node station 7 (see ▶Table 2.2) are always classified as N2 regardless of their location. Involvement of the supraclavicular or scalene lymph nodes is also defined as N3 if there is ipsilateral metastasis, whereas more distant lymph nodes (cervical or abdominal) have no implications for the N category as they are then assigned to the distant metastases M category (M1b or M1c).

On *CT imaging*, enlarged lymph nodes are interpreted as suspected metastases. In general, 10 mm is considered the upper limit for the short axis of mediastinal lymph nodes,[67] even if the maximum size of normal lymph nodes is between 7 and 11 mm depending on the lymph node station.[68]

> **Note**
>
> The long axis of a lymph node is not relevant for suspicion of lymph node metastasis.

Using these criteria, sensitivity of lymph node staging with CT is less than 60% and specificity is around 80%.[69] False-negative results may be obtained for micrometastases in normal-sized lymph nodes and false-positive results in the case of enlarged lymph nodes secondary to an inflammation.

On *PET-CT*, lymph nodes with a standard uptake value of at least 2.5 are classified as suspected metastases regardless of their size. PET-CT is superior to CT in visualizing lymph node metastasis, and in studies was found to have a sensitivity of around 70 to 90% and a specificity of around 90%.[10,69,70,71,72,73] For the diagnosis, the uptake of the primary tumor on FDG-PET should also be considered. For example, caution is advised in cases of a primary tumor with intense FDG uptake but only slightly increased FDG uptake by the enlarged lymph nodes: these should not automatically be interpreted as lymph node metastases.

No imaging modality, including PET-CT, is able to reliably diagnose mediastinal lymph node metastases. Therefore, if suspicious mediastinal lymph nodes are identified on CT or PET, tissue sampling should be performed (usually using a bronchoscopic or surgical technique) before reaching any treatment decision.[59,60] This helps avoid overstaging resulting from imaging findings due to inflammatory mediastinal lymphadenopathy, and at the same time can rule out contralateral lymph node metastasis (N3) not detected with imaging.

Distant Metastasis (M Descriptor)

For almost half of newly diagnosed lung carcinomas, distant metastases are identified at the time of diagnosis, usually in the lung, liver, adrenal glands, brain, and bones.[62] The metastatic sites are identified with staging examinations. Since metastases confined to the thorax have a better prognosis than more distant metastasis, the M category is subdivided into:

- *M1a*: Metastasis confined to the chest, i.e., contralateral pulmonary or pleural (malignant pleural effusion or pleural masses) as well as malignant pericardial effusion.
- *M1b*: Single extrathoracic metastasis thus enabling an oligometastatic treatment concept.
- *M1c:* Multiple extrathoracic metastases.

Additional imaging procedures may be required for differential diagnosis between metastases and incidental findings, in particular in the following situations:

- *Liver lesions*: This is particularly true in the case of a solitary lesion identified in the first examination. Differential diagnosis should include benign liver lesions, predominantly hemangiomas, which are common incidental findings. If reliable differentiation cannot be made with lesion morphology at staging CT, ultrasound or MRI may help obviate the need for biopsy if typical benign features are present.
- *Adrenal gland mass*: The commonly encountered benign adenomas are the most important differential diagnosis of metastasis. Often, supplementary unenhanced CT scans, dynamic contrast CT, or MRI with chemical shift imaging is able to make that distinction noninvasively.
- *Contralateral pulmonary nodules*: Please see T descriptor category details. In general, nodules of less than 10 mm in size are probably benign, while larger ones tend to be malignant. If treatment is based on that distinction, tissue sampling of a contralateral nodule is necessary.

PET-CT is used primarily for detection of distant metastases at atypical sites. For the more advanced tumor stages, there is a greater probability of still detecting unexpected distant metastases on PET-CT after the staging CT of the chest and upper abdomen (7.5% in stage I, 24% in stage III).[74]

> **Note**
>
> Any suspect metastatic nodules identified on imaging should be verified through histology in the absence of unequivocal clinical or imaging findings. Incorrect exclusion of patients from curative intention-to-treat regimens must definitely be avoided.

9.3.4 Treatment Concepts

The treatment concepts for nonsmall cell and small cell lung cancers differ greatly. In addition to the tumor stage (see above), the patient's age and comorbidities must be taken into account.[10]

Nonsmall Cell Lung Cancer

In general, cure can be the treatment intention up to stage IIIA. For contralateral lymph node metastases (stage IIIB) or distant metastases (stage IV), a cure is usually no longer possible; hence, palliative treatment is the remaining option.

In *stages I and II* if functional and technical operability is assured, the treatment of choice is lobectomy with systematic ipsilateral, mediastinal lymphadenectomy. More radical surgery may be necessary depending on the local findings, such as supplementary bronchoangioplastic procedures or pneumonectomy. In cases of inoperability, radiotherapy with curative intent may be delivered alternatively. Adjuvant chemotherapy has also proved beneficial in stage II, and in individual cases in stage IB, too. Adjuvant radiotherapy may be considered in individual cases, e.g., if there is chest wall invasion.

Stage III (IIIA and certain constellations in stage IIIB: T4N0–1) require, depending on tumor extension and regional lymph node involvement, a tailored multimodal treatment concept consisting of surgery, chemotherapy, and/or radiotherapy.

In *more advanced tumor stages* (other IIIB and IV), chemotherapy alone is administered provided that this is compatible with the patient's general condition. In certain oligometastatic settings, a curative intention to treat can still be considered in stage IV with resection of any distant metastasis and of the primary tumor.

Small Cell Lung Cancer

The mainstay treatment for small cell lung cancer is chemotherapy; in the absence of distant metastasis and if the tumor extension is amenable to radiotherapy, this can be used in combination with radiotherapy of the primary tumor. In early tumor stages (T1–2, N0–1), surgery constitutes an additional treatment option. This is done in combination with neoadjuvant or adjuvant chemotherapy. Because of the risk of occult brain metastasis, prophylactic whole-brain irradiation is recommended.

9.3.5 Early Detection and Lung Cancer Screening

Lung cancer rarely causes early symptoms and is thus generally diagnosed only at an already advanced stage. The prognosis is largely determined by the tumor stage (see ▶Table 9.2). Early stage tumors, in particular of nonsmall cell lung cancers, have a relatively good prognosis but are usually only discovered by chance. Against that background, the introduction of early detection programs for asymptomatic individuals at risk has been contemplated.

Screening based on *chest radiography* has not proved useful. While several large studies carried out in the 1970s and 1980s identified numerous asymptomatic lung cancers, it did not reduce lung cancer mortality.[75,76,77,78] This is thought to be mainly due to the low sensitivity of chest radiographs for detection of small lung cancers.

Conversely, *CT* has much higher sensitivity for detection of small lung cancers. Lung cancers exhibit high contrast versus the air-containing lung and can usually be identified even in the presence of increased image noise. This means that the radiation dose can be considerably reduced compared with normal chest CT scans. Studies have been performed since the early 1990s to investigate the suitability of this low-dose CT for lung cancer screening.[79,80,81,82,83,84,85,86] In 2010, a U.S. study with more than 53,000 subjects demonstrated a 20% reduction of lung cancer mortality. Participants were 55- to 74-year-old smokers with at least 30 pack years (number of cigarette packs per day multiplied by the number of years smoked).[87,88] The results of similar, albeit smaller, European studies are still pending; smaller published studies did not support the National Lung Screening Trial (NLST) findings.[89,90,91,92,93,94]

In the light of NLST data, multiple medical societies recommended early detection programs for individuals at risk.[91,95] The development or the existence and utilization of such programs vary greatly among different countries. In general, a trend toward the setup of such programs can be currently observed.

9.4 Carcinoid

Carcinoids are relatively rare malignant neuroendocrine tumors and account for less than 2% of lung tumors.[34] They are diagnosed in persons with a mean age of less than 50 years. On average, such patients are thus younger than lung cancer patients.[96] On histology, a distinction is made between typical carcinoids of low malignancy and atypical carcinoids of moderate malignancy and with a greater tendency to metastatic spread.[36] Typical carcinoid tumors are usually located centrally, and atypical carcinoids at the periphery.[97,98] Typical and atypical carcinoids cannot be reliably differentiated on imaging. Metastases occur in around 15% of patients, and like in lung cancer, particularly in the liver, bones, adrenal glands, and brain.[34,99]

A carcinoid is usually a smoothly marginated tumor that presents as a central mass with polycyclic margins (▶Fig. 9.19) or as

II

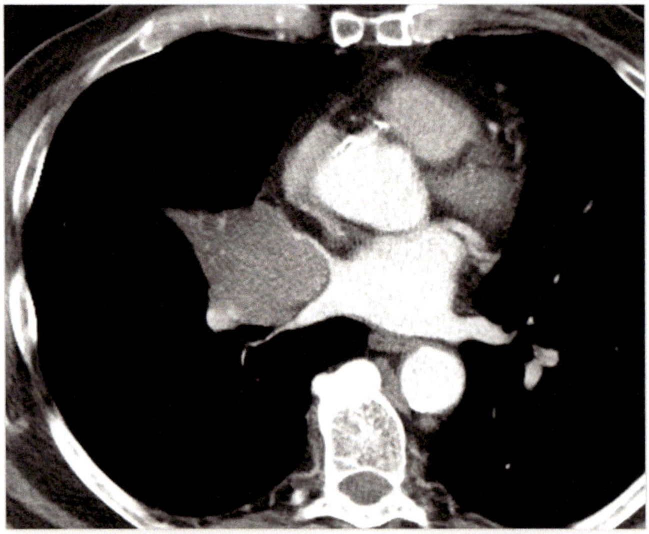

Fig. 9.19 Central atypical carcinoid. CT image. Relatively smoothly marginated mass with homogeneous contrast enhancement.

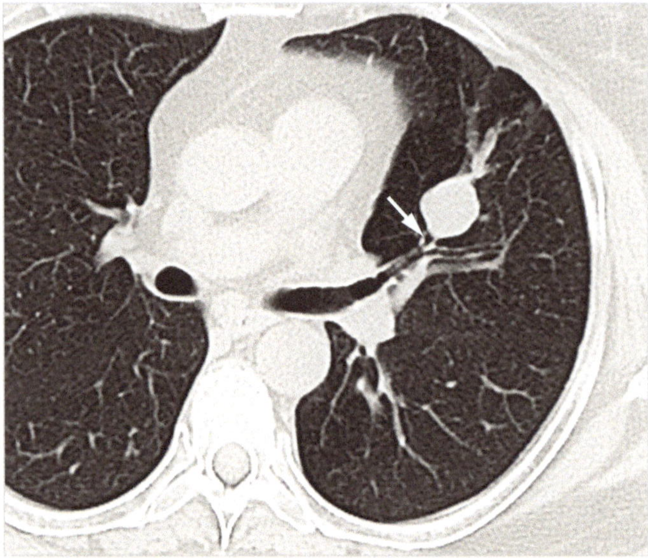

Fig. 9.20 Peripheral carcinoid. CT image. Smoothly marginated oval nodule originating from the inferior lingula segmental bronchus (*arrow*).

an oval peripheral nodule that grows with its long axis along the supply bronchus (▶Fig. 9.20). Often, carcinoids have a close spatial relationship to the bronchi; in such cases, an endoluminal component can be identified on CT. Occasionally, they present as purely intraluminal nodules (▶Fig. 9.21). The tumor-related bronchial obstruction characteristic of carcinoids may cause atelectasis, postobstructive pneumonia, or mucoid impaction peripheral to the tumor. Because of widespread vascularization, intense and mainly homogeneous contrast enhancement is observed on CT (see ▶Fig. 9.19). This makes it easier to delineate the tumor from distal atelectasis or postobstructive pneumonia.[34]

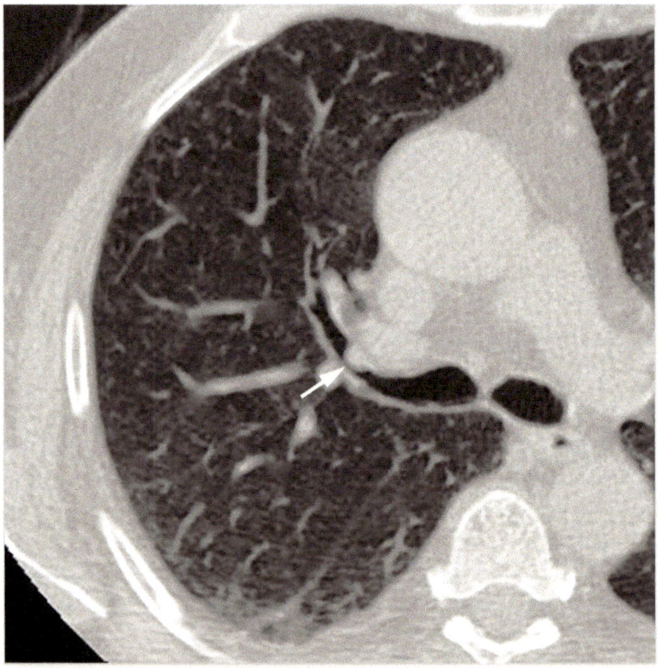

Fig. 9.21 Endobronchial central carcinoid in the right upper lobe bronchus (*arrow*). CT image.

Note

Typical imaging characteristics of carcinoids[34]:

- Smoothly marginated, often lobulated, central mass (see ▶Fig. 9.19) or oval peripheral nodule (see ▶Fig. 9.20).
- Occasionally, small, centrally located, endobronchial tumor (see ▶Fig. 9.21).
- Strong contrast enhancement on CT.
- Occasionally, calcifications visible on CT.
- Atelectasis, postobstructive pneumonia, or mucoid impaction in bronchi distal to tumor.

Locoregional hilar and mediastinal lymph node metastases are found, in particular, in association with atypical carcinoids.[100] Lymphadenopathy can be caused by lymph node metastasis as well as by an inflammatory reaction secondarily to recurrent postobstructive pneumonia.[101]

Nuclear medicine techniques are used to assess tumor extension, and also for differential diagnosis of lymphadenopathy. However, in the case of carcinoids the intense tracer uptake characteristic of malignancy is often absent on FDG-PET. But, on the other hand, thanks to an abundance of somatostatin receptors these tumors can generally be well visualized on scintigraphy when using specific tracers, e.g., octreotide scintigraphy.[102,103]

Carcinoid staging is performed in a similar manner to lung cancer; see also ▶Table 9.1.

9.5 Rare Malignant Tumors of the Lung

Adenoid cystic carcinomas of the lung typically present on CT as relatively smoothly marginated, solid nodules of low density. In most cases, no contrast enhancement can be identified (▶Fig. 9.22); likewise, FDG-PET often produces false-negative results for this tumor entity. Furthermore, the tumor usually exhibits a very slow growth pattern. Unlike other lung cancers, it predominantly affects younger patients. All these factors hamper the diagnosis of a malignant tumor.

Pulmonary *Kaposi sarcomas* tend to occur multifocally. On radiography and CT, they present as multiple nodules, usually with conspicuous spicules (▶Fig. 9.23). Kaposi sarcomas are found almost exclusively in AIDS patients.

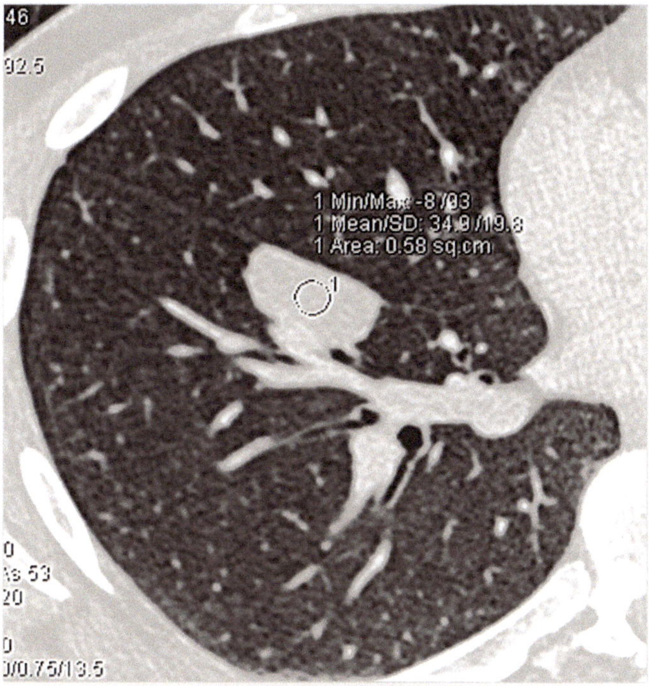

Fig. 9.22 Adenoid cystic carcinoma of the lung. CT image. Smoothly marginated nodule of relatively low density in a 30-year-old nonsmoker.

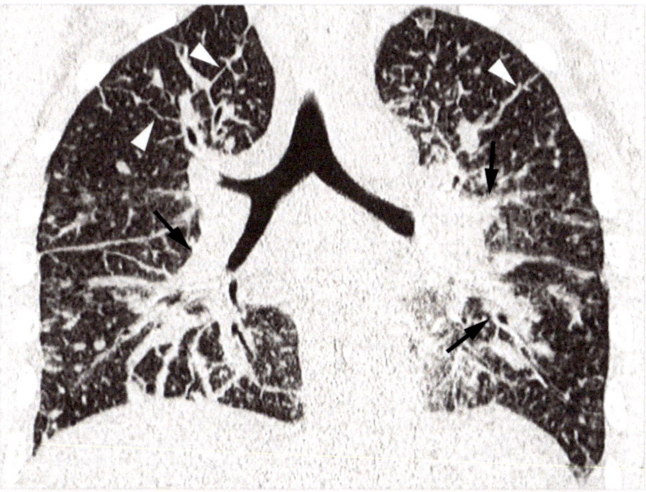

Fig. 9.24 Anaplastic lymphoma. Coronal CT image. Mediastinal and bilateral hilar lymphadenopathy with continuous extension of the lymphoma into the lung tissue (*arrows*). Interlobular septal thickening (*arrowheads*) with impaired lymph drainage secondary to hilar and mediastinal lymphoma.

9.6 Pulmonary Lymphoma

Primary pulmonary lymphomas are much less common than pulmonary manifestations of primary extrapulmonary lymphomas. Their appearance and spread patterns are very variable[104,105]:

- Direct extension from the affected hilar lymph nodes to the lung tissue (▶Fig. 9.24).
- Solitary or multiple pulmonary nodules or masses, usually with ill-defined margins (▶Fig. 9.25) and, in particular in Hodgkin lymphomas, with open intralesional bronchi.
- Solitary, predominantly peripheral consolidation, often with open intralesional bronchi (▶Fig. 9.26).

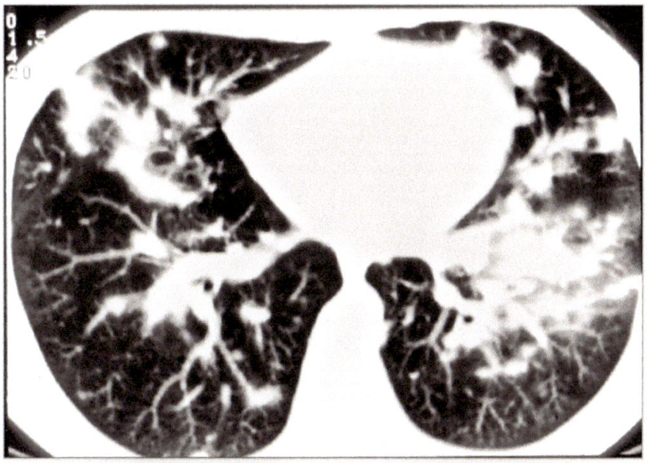

Fig. 9.23 Multiple Kaposi sarcomas. CT image. Bizarre nodules and masses in both lungs. (The image is provided courtesy of S. Diederich, Düsseldorf.)

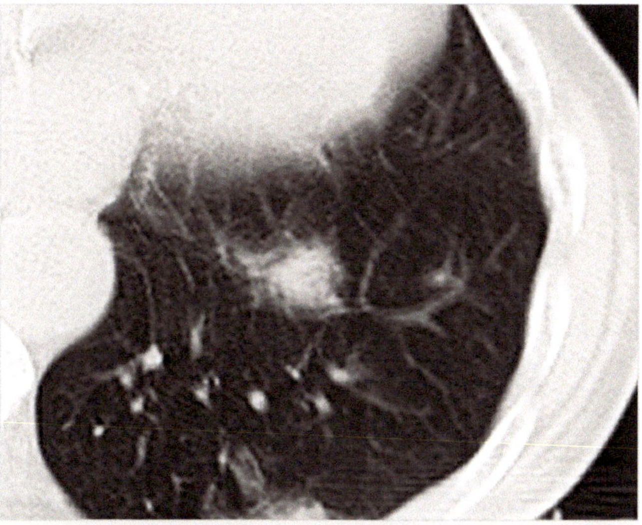

Fig. 9.25 Non-Hodgkin lymphoma. CT image. Multiple ill-defined nodules in the left lower lobe.

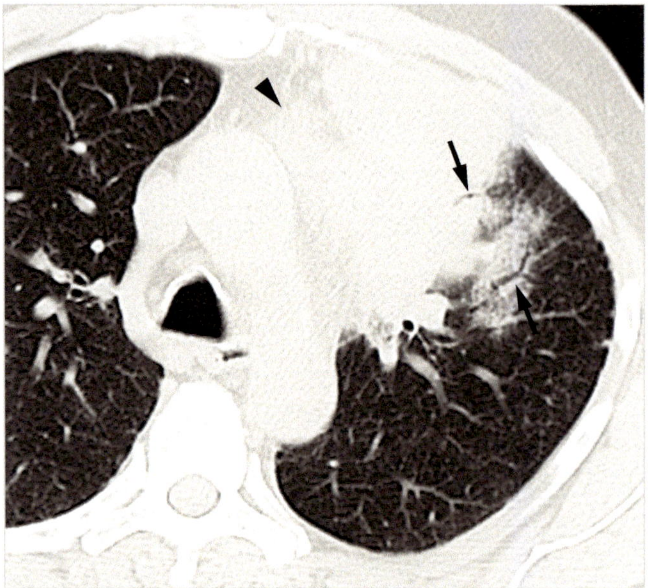

Fig. 9.26 Hodgkin disease. CT image. Mass in the left upper lobe with open intralesional bronchi (*arrows*); besides, mediastinal lymphadenopathy (*arrowhead*).

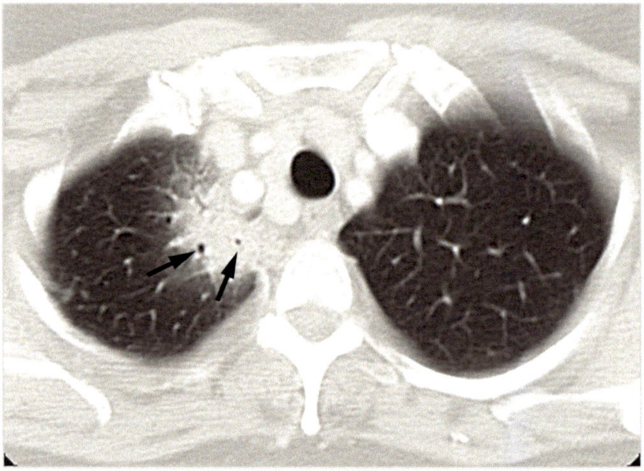

Fig. 9.28 BALToma. CT image. Solid mass in the right upper lobe, in which open bronchi can be identified (*arrows*).

- Diffuse lymphoma invasion, in particular as irregular ground-glass opacities (▶ Fig. 9.27).

The *BALToma* is a special type of lymphoma that originates from the bronchus-associated lymphatic tissue (BALT). In general, it presents as a solitary pulmonary mass (▶ Fig. 9.28).

There are no imaging findings pathognomonic for pulmonary lymphoma. If patients are known to have an extrapulmonary lymphoma, differential diagnosis of pulmonary findings is very broad and comprises, in particular, the following clinical disease entities:

- Pulmonary lymphoma.
- Pneumonia, also opportunistic pneumonia especially in patients who had undergone chemotherapy.

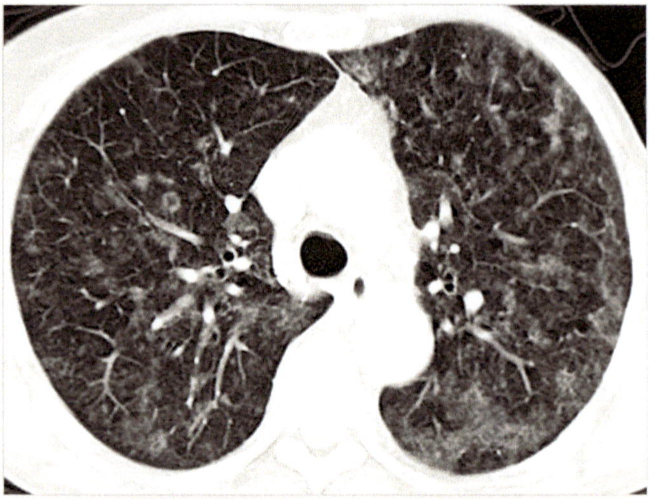

Fig. 9.27 Primary pulmonary non-Hodgkin lymphoma. CT image. Diffuse bilateral ill-defined ground-glass nodules, no mediastinal lymphadenopathy.

- Drug toxicity.
- Radiation pneumonitis secondary to radiotherapy.

Lymphoma staging calls for a comprehensive diagnostic work-up. This will entail at least CT imaging of the chest and abdomen, including the pelvis, as well as abdominal ultrasound since especially liver manifestations are not adequately visible on CT images.

9.7 Lung Metastases

Lung metastases are commonly observed systemic manifestations of the most diverse malignant tumors and are almost always the result of hematogenous spread to the lungs. On imaging, two types are distinguished: predominantly nodular metastasis and lymphangitic carcinomatosis, occurring occasionally in association with certain tumor entities.

9.7.1 Nodular Metastasis

Lung metastases are very often included in differential diagnosis of solitary or multiple nodules. By virtue of its capillary network, the lung is an organ predestined for hematogenous metastasis once a malignant tumor has embarked on hematogenous dissemination in the venous circulation. Even widespread pulmonary metastasis can remain clinically asymptomatic over a long period of time. This may be followed by onset of cough, poststenotic pneumonia, chest pain, and dyspnea.

For small lung metastases, radiographs do not have adequate sensitivity. Larger pulmonary metastases present as nodules or masses. Multiple metastases exhibit a patchy nodular pattern with basal predominance (▶ Fig. 9.29).

On CT, lung metastases generally manifest as solitary or multiple nodules of soft-tissue density. These may have well-defined or spiculated margins. Since lung metastases result from hematogenous spread, they do not have any preference for individual lobular structures and thus exhibit a random distribution. Typically, the nodules are of variable size (▶Fig. 9.30), and at times also have central cavities. Extremely rarely, the nodules exhibit ground-glass density; these are usually metastases with a lepidic growth pattern from a pulmonary adenocarcinoma. Calcified lung metastases are characteristic of an osteosarcoma and are very rarely seen in other primary tumors (▶Fig. 9.31).

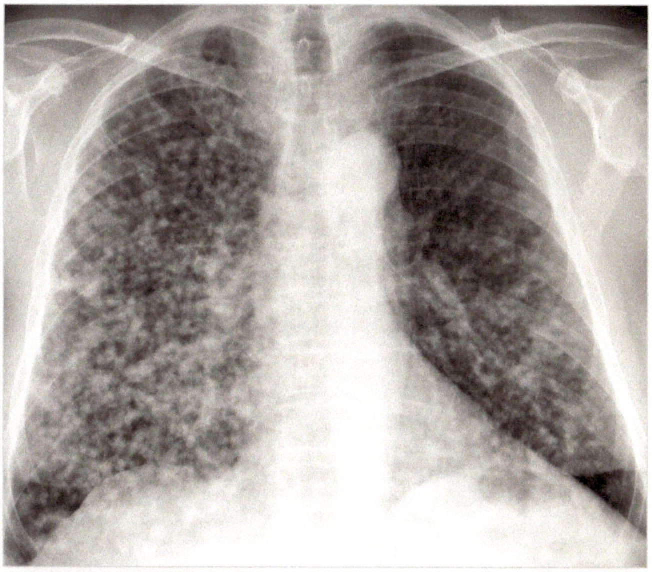

Fig. 9.29 Multiple lung metastases. Radiograph. Nodular pattern with basal predominance.

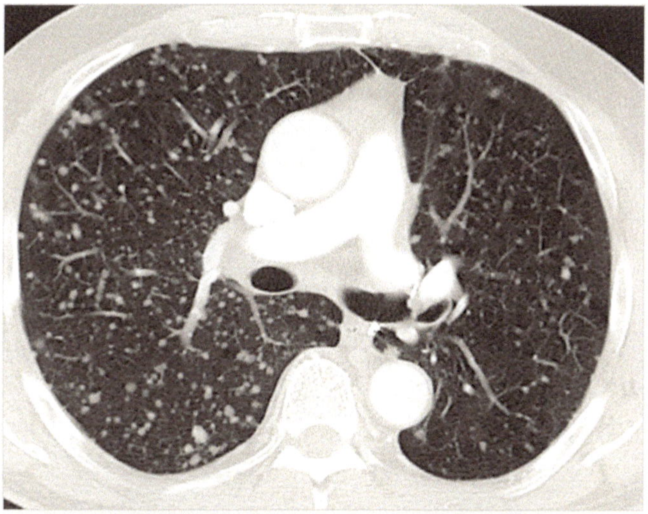

Fig. 9.30 Nodular metastases. CT image. Multiple well-defined nodules of variable size with random distribution.

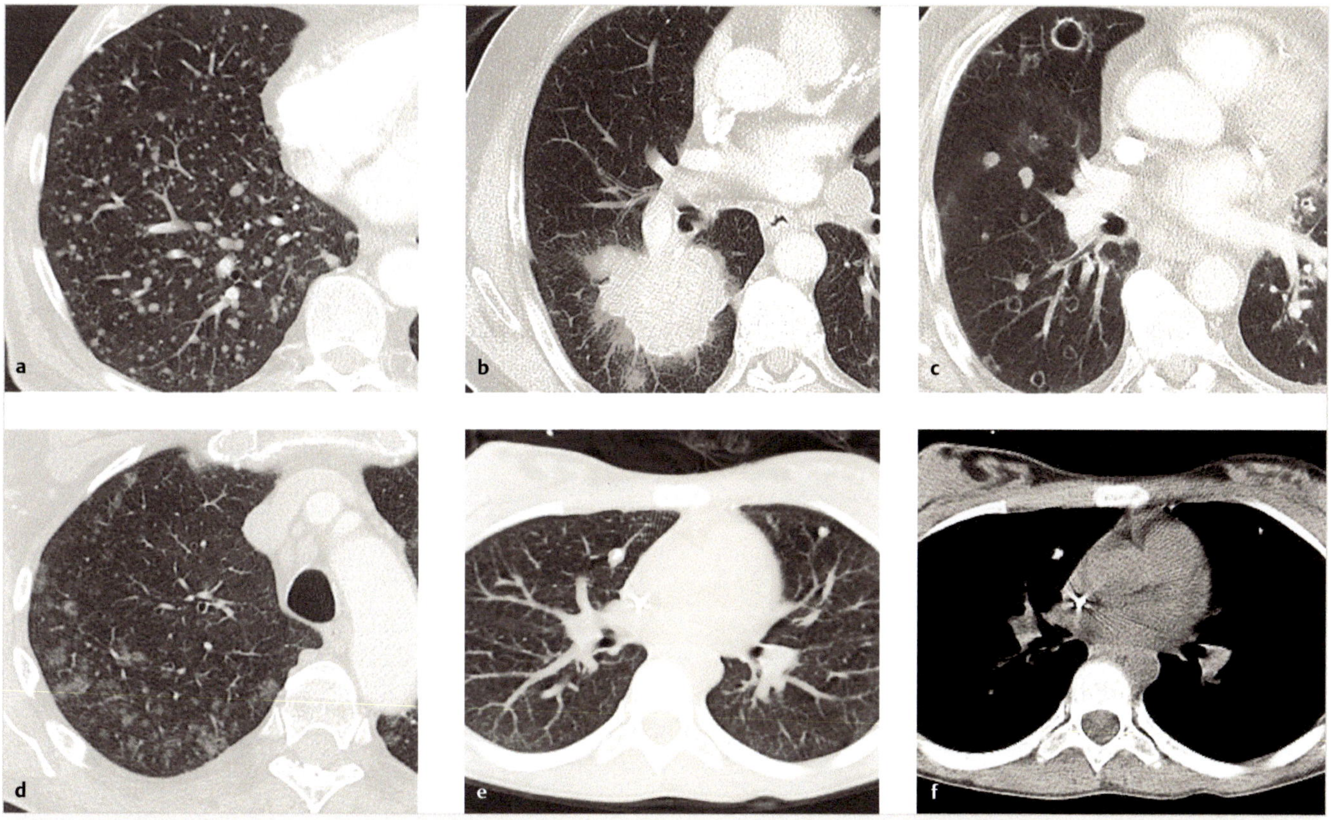

Fig. 9.31 Nodular metastases. Examples of different CT morphologies. **(a)** Well-defined nodules. **(b)** Spiculated mass. **(c)** Cavitary nodules. **(d)** Ground-glass nodules. **(e)** Calcified nodules in the lung window. **(f)** Calcified nodules in the soft tissue window (same image as **e**).

Note

CT findings in nodular metastases:

- Solitary or multiple nodules.
- Basal predominance.
- Random distribution in the lobular structures.
- Nodules of variable size.
- Smooth or spiculated margins.
- Usually of soft-tissue density, rarely cavitating, extremely rarely ground-glass nodules, certain tumor entities with calcification (especially osteosarcomas).

Occasionally, necrotic disintegration of subpleural metastases causes spontaneous pneumothorax, as seen in particular in sarcoma metastasis.[106]

Differential diagnosis of nodules in different clinical settings is discussed in detail in Section 21.2, with special focus on when lung metastases are likely and under which circumstances they should be considered unlikely.

9.7.2 Lymphangitic Carcinomatosis

Lymphangitic carcinomatosis is a characteristic type of metastasis seen in certain carcinomas, especially primary tumors of the breast, lung, stomach, pancreas, prostate gland, cervix, and thyroid gland as well as in patients with CUP syndrome (cancer of unknown primary).[107] In most cases, the tumor cells have spread hematogenously to the lung and go on to invade the lymphatic system and interstitium. Less commonly, the tumor cells spread per continuitatem from metastatic hilar or mediastinal lymph nodes.[108] Tumor growth unfolds along the lymphatic system of the axial interstitium as well as in the interlobular fissures, accompanied by edema responsible for the characteristic imaging findings.

Lymphangitic carcinomatosis typically presents clinically as dyspnea, which may precede the changes identified on imaging.

The most predominant finding on radiographs is a reticular pattern and interlobular septal thickening. Hilar or mediastinal lymphadenopathy and a pleural effusion may also be observed. However, these findings are nonspecific; moreover, half of patients diagnosed with lymphangitic carcinomatosis have a normal radiograph.[109,110]

The characteristic findings on CT are tumor extension along the lymphatic system and in the interstitium as well as edema caused by impaired lymphatic drainage of the lung following tumor-related obstruction of the lymph vessels (▸Fig. 9.32). Occasionally, tumor cell thrombi can be identified in the lymphatic system as nodular interlobular septal thickening, known as the *beaded septum sign*. In addition, because of longstanding edema or of a desmoplastic reaction to the tumor in the interstitium, interstitial fibrosis may give rise to the pathologic changes seen on CT imaging. The typical imaging findings are presented in ▸Table. 9.4 These findings may also be seen coincidently with multiple randomly distributed nodules consistent with concomitant nodular metastases (▸Fig. 9.33).

Table 9.4 Imaging findings in lymphangitic carcinomatosis[107]

Imaging modality	Findings
Radiography	• Reticular pattern • Interlobular septal thickening • Lymphadenopathy (hilar or mediastinal) • Pleural effusion
CT	• Thickening of the peribronchovascular connective tissue, smooth or nodular • Interlobular septal thickening, smooth or nodular (beaded septum sign) • Thickening of lung fissures, smooth or nodular • Diffuse, patchy or unilateral distribution • Lymphadenopathy (hilar or mediastinal) • Pleural effusion

Abbreviation: CT, computed tomography.

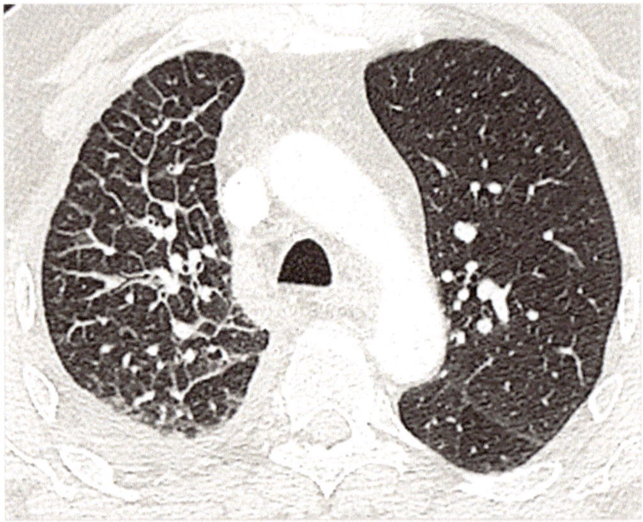

Fig. 9.32 Lymphangitic carcinomatosis. CT image. Smooth interlobular septal thickening in the right upper lobe and right pleural effusion.

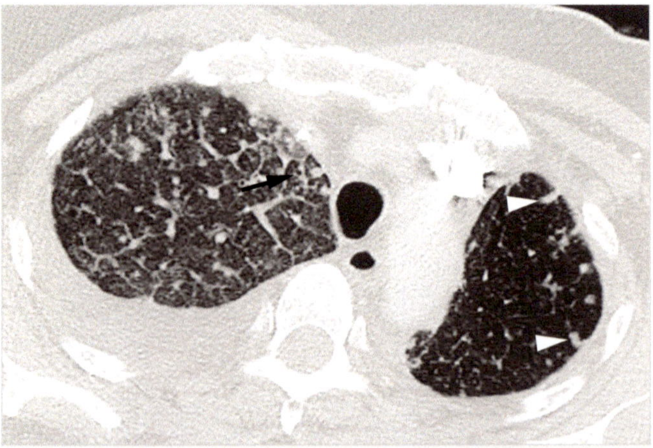

Fig. 9.33 Lymphangitic carcinomatosis. CT image. Nodular interlobular septal thickening beaded septum sign (*arrow*). Besides, multiple nodular metastases (*arrowheads*) as well as right pleural effusion.

The most important disorder to be considered for differential diagnosis is hydrostatic pulmonary edema, especially of cardiac or renal origin, which may cause similar findings on CT, with smooth interstitial thickening. Unilateral presentation of such findings is suggestive of lymphangitic carcinomatosis and makes pulmonary edema of a different origin unlikely. For differential diagnosis, please refer to Chapter 24.

9.8 Inflammatory Pseudotumor

Inflammatory pseudotumors are quasi-neoplastic masses that can occur in any organ, especially in the lung and the orbita.[111] Clinically and on imaging, they manifest as malignant tumors[112] with locally aggressive growth; occasionally, multifocal pseudotumors are seen. In histologic terms, they consist of inflammatory cells and myofibroblastic spindle cells, but there is widespread variability. The myriad names used in the literature reflect the heterogeneity of this disease entity.

> **Note**
>
> Synonymous designations for inflammatory pseudotumors[111]:
> - Plasma cell granuloma.
> - Inflammatory myofibroblastic tumor.
> - Histiocytoma.
> - Xanthoma.
> - Fibroxanthoma.
> - Xanthogranuloma.
> - Xanthomatous pseudotumor.
> - Plasma cell/histiocytoma complex.
> - Solitary mast cell granuloma.

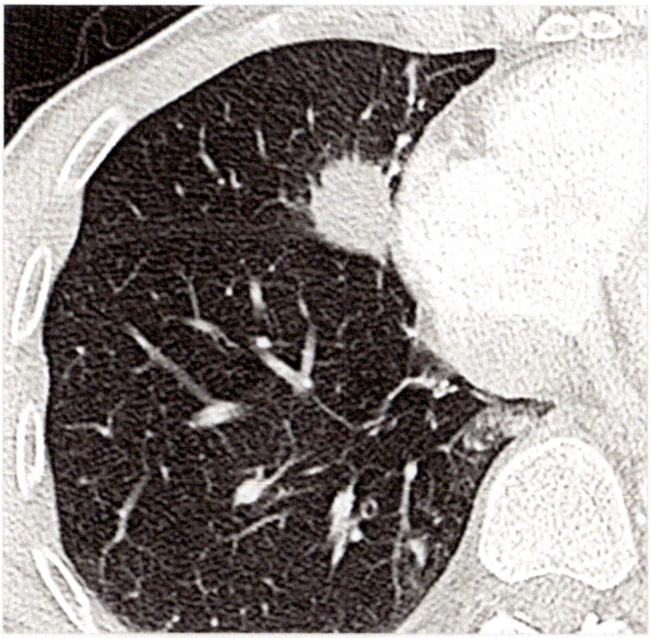

Fig. 9.34 Inflammatory pseudotumor. CT image. Spiculated nodule in the middle lobe.

In the majority of cases, these are thought to be low-grade fibrosarcomas; there are also reports of postinfectious and posttraumatic genesis as well as of autoimmune mechanisms.[111]

Inflammatory pseudotumors are the most common pulmonary masses identified in childhood but also occur in adults. They are usually accompanied by cough, fever, dyspnea, and hemoptysis; some patients are asymptomatic. The most typical imaging findings involve a solitary, peripheral, smoothly marginated, lobulated nodule or a mass with lower lobe predominance (▶Fig. 9.34). Calcifications may be observed, especially in children.[113]

9.9 Summary

Lung cancer accounts for the highest mortality rate from malignant tumors, and is mainly caused by cigarette smoking. Occupational exposure to organic or inorganic noxae causes lung cancer much less often; asbestos exposure is the best-known form of exposure. Pulmonary adenocarcinoma is increasingly found in younger nonsmokers, too; this is attributed to a genetic predisposition. Two histologic types requiring essentially different treatment concepts are described: small cell and nonsmall cell lung cancer. The latter accounts for 80% of lung carcinomas and is subclassified into adenocarcinomas, squamous cell carcinomas, and large cell carcinomas as well as a number of rarer types. Staging (see ▶Table 9.1 and ▶Table 9.2) and hence therapeutic decision-making are largely based on the imaging results. CT of the chest and upper abdomen as well as brain MRI (CT as a substitute for MRI if the latter is contraindicated) is recommended. If a potentially curative intention to treat can be considered, a PET-CT scan is needed additionally to rule out distant metastasis (see ▶Table 9.3). Often, extrapulmonary metastases are found in the adrenal glands, liver, bones, and brain. In early stages (stage I and II) of nonsmall cell lung cancer, treatment with curative intent is offered. The treatment of choice is surgical resection of at least the affected lung lobe, including the locoregional lymph nodes, or radiotherapy for inoperable cases. Locally advanced tumor stages (stage IIIA and certain stages IIIB) require a combination of chemotherapy, radiotherapy, and/or surgery; treatment with curative intent is still usually administered in stage IIIA. Palliative treatment is indicated if there are distant metastases or contralateral mediastinal lymph node metastases (stage IIIB–IV). Chemotherapy on its own is beneficial if this is compatible with the patient's general state. In principle, the first-line treatment for small cell lung cancer is chemotherapy. In the absence of distant metastasis, irradiation of the primary tumor may be possible in addition. Lobectomy plays a certain role for local tumor stages (T1/2 N0/1 M0) but is not a substitute for chemotherapy. Prophylactic whole-brain irradiation should also be performed in every stage.

Carcinoids are associated with a very variable course of disease and have the potential to undergo metastasis. They are relatively rare lesions, often found in the endobronchial region, are rounded and smoothly marginated. In most cases, they exhibit strong contrast enhancement on CT.

Primary pulmonary *lymphomas* are a rare entity. Much more common is secondary lung involvement following invasion per

9

continuitatem, originating from mediastinal lymphomas, or systemic spread. Thoracic and abdominal diagnostic work-up with CT and ultrasound is always needed.

II

Rare malignant tumors of the lung also include *adenoid cystic carcinoma*, which is usually a smoothly marginated nodule with slow growth, as well as *Kaposi sarcoma*, which is found almost exclusively in AIDS patients and typically manifests as multifocal spiculated nodules.

Hamartomas are common. These benign malformation tumors are usually asymptomatic nodules identified as incidental findings and are often slow growing. A smoothly marginated solitary pulmonary nodule with popcorn-like calcifications or evidence of fat on CT is considered virtually pathognomonic for a hamartoma. In the absence of pathognomonic CT findings or if the nodule exhibits growth suggestive of malignancy, biopsy is needed. Resection is indicated only if there are symptoms.

Systemic tumor spread often results in *lung metastases*. Two types are distinguished:

- *Nodular metastases*: Depending on the primary tumor, these are usually nodules or masses of soft-tissue density, less commonly cavitating nodules or extremely rarely ground-glass nodules. They constitute a common differential diagnosis of solitary or multiple pulmonary nodules.
- *Lymphangitic carcinomatosis*: Following mainly hematogenous dissemination to the lung (less commonly spread per continuitatem), the tumor spreads in the interstitium and along the lymph vessels. The most predominant imaging finding is smooth or nodular thickening of the axial connective tissue and interlobular fissures. For differential diagnosis, please see Chapter 24.

Inflammatory pseudotumors of the lung are common in childhood, but relatively less rare in adults. They are of heterogeneous histology and have a broad pathogenetic spectrum, ranging from postinfectious etiology to malignant tumor; in many cases, they are thought to be low-grade fibrosarcomas. Imaging usually demonstrates a smoothly marginated, solitary peripheral nodule or mass.

References

[1] Gaerte SC, Meyer CA, Winer-Muram HT, Tarver RD, Conces DJ Jr. Fat-containing lesions of the chest. Radiographics 2002;22(Spec No): S61–S78

[2] Hansen CP, Holtveg H, Francis D, Rasch L, Bertelsen S. Pulmonary hamartoma. J Thorac Cardiovasc Surg 1992;104(3):674–678

[3] Erasmus JJ, Connolly JE, McAdams HP, Roggli VL. Solitary pulmonary nodules: Part I. Morphologic evaluation for differentiation of benign and malignant lesions. Radiographics 2000;20(1):43–58

[4] Siegelman SS, Khouri NF, Scott WW Jr, et al. Pulmonary hamartoma: CT findings. Radiology 1986;160(2):313–317

[5] Godoy MCB, Naidich DP. Subsolid pulmonary nodules and the spectrum of peripheral adenocarcinomas of the lung: recommended interim guidelines for assessment and management. Radiology 2009;253(3):606–622

[6] Ishikawa H, Koizumi N, Morita T, et al. Ultrasmall pulmonary opacities on multidetector-row high-resolution computed tomography: a prospective radiologic-pathologic examination. J Comput Assist Tomogr 2005;29(5):621–625

[7] Koga T, Hashimoto S, Sugio K, et al. Lung adenocarcinoma with bronchioloalveolar carcinoma component is frequently associated with foci of high-grade atypical adenomatous hyperplasia. Am J Clin Pathol 2002;117(3):464–470

[8] Travis WD, Brambilla E, Noguchi M, et al. International association for the study of lung cancer/american thoracic society/european respiratory society international multidisciplinary classification of lung adenocarcinoma. J Thorac Oncol 2011;6(2):244–285

[9] MacMahon H, Naidich DP, Goo JM, et al. Guidelines for management of incidental pulmonary nodules detected on CT images: from the Fleischner Society 2017. Radiology 2017;284(1):228–243

[10] Goeckenjan G, Sitter H, Thomas M, et al; German Respiratory Society. German Cancer Society. Prevention, diagnosis, therapy, and follow-up of lung cancer. Interdisciplinary guideline of the German Respiratory Society and the German Cancer Society--abridged version [in German] Pneumologie 2011;65(8):e51–e75

[11] Osarogiagbon RU, Smeltzer MP, Faris N, Rami-Porta R, Goldstraw P, Asamura H. Comment on the Proposals for the Revision of the N Descriptors in the Forthcoming Eighth Edition of the TNM Classification for Lung Cancer. J Thorac Oncol 2016;11(10):1612–1614

[12] Kay FU, Kandathil A, Batra K, Saboo SS, Abbara S, Rajiah P. Revisions to the Tumor, Node, Metastasis staging of lung cancer (8th edition): Rationale, radiologic findings and clinical implications. World J Radiol 2017;9(6):269–279

[13] Brambilla E. The histologic reclassification of adenocarcinoma of the lung: implications for diagnosis and therapy. Am Soc Clin Oncol 2011;1092-9118/10/1-10. ASCO 2011 Annual Meeting, Educational Books

[14] Travis WD, Asamura H, Bankier AA, et al. The IASLC Lung Cancer Staging Project: Proposals for Coding T Categories for Subsolid Nodules and Assessment of Tumor Size in Part-Solid Tumors in the Forthcoming Eighth Edition of the TNM Classification of Lung Cancer. J Thorac Oncol 2016;11(8):1204–1223

[15] Aoki T, Tomoda Y, Watanabe H, et al. Peripheral lung adenocarcinoma: correlation of thin-section CT findings with histologic prognostic factors and survival. Radiology 2001;220(3):803–809

[16] Yoshino I, Nakanishi R, Kodate M, et al. Pleural retraction and intra-tumoral air-bronchogram as prognostic factors for stage I pulmonary adenocarcinoma following complete resection. Int Surg 2000;85(2):105–112

[17] Nakazono T, Sakao Y, Yamaguchi K, Imai S, Kumazoe H, Kudo S. Subtypes of peripheral adenocarcinoma of the lung: differentiation by thin-section CT. Eur Radiol 2005;15(8):1563–1568

[18] Takashima S, Maruyama Y, Hasegawa M, Saito A, Haniuda M, Kadoya M. High-resolution CT features: prognostic significance in peripheral lung adenocarcinoma with bronchioloalveolar carcinoma components. Respiration 2003;70(1):36–42

[19] Yabuuchi H, Murayama S, Murakami J, et al. High-resolution CT characteristics of poorly differentiated adenocarcinoma of the peripheral lung: comparison with well differentiated adenocarcinoma. Radiat Med 2000;18(6):343–347

[20] Kuriyama K, Tateishi R, Doi O, et al. Prevalence of air bronchograms in small peripheral carcinomas of the lung on thin-section CT: comparison with benign tumors. AJR Am J Roentgenol 1991;156(5):921–924

[21] Rosado-de-Christenson ML, Templeton PA, Moran CA. Bronchogenic carcinoma: radiologic-pathologic correlation. Radiographics 1994;14(2):429–446, quiz 447–448

[22] Detterbeck FC, Marom EM, Arenberg DA, et al. The IASLC Lung Cancer Staging Project: Background Data and Proposals for the Application of TNM Staging Rules to Lung Cancer Presenting as Multiple Nodules with Ground Glass or Lepidic Features or a Pneumonic Type of Involvement in the Forthcoming Eighth Edition of the TNM Classification. J Thorac Oncol 2016;11(5):666–680

[23] Gaeta M, Vinci S, Minutoli F, et al. CT and MRI findings of mucin-containing tumors and pseudotumors of the thorax: pictorial review. Eur Radiol 2002;12(1):181–189

[24] Im JG, Han MC, Yu EJ, et al. Lobar bronchioloalveolar carcinoma: "angiogram sign" on CT scans. Radiology 1990;176(3):749–753

[25] Lee HY, Lee KS, Han J, et al. Mucinous versus nonmucinous solitary pulmonary nodular bronchioloalveolar carcinoma: CT and FDG PET findings and pathologic comparisons. Lung Cancer 2009;65(2):170–175

[26] Miyake H, Matsumoto A, Terada A, Yoshida S, Takaki H, Mori H. Mucin-producing tumor of the lung: CT findings. J Thorac Imaging 1995;10(2):96–98

[27] Nakata M, Sawada S, Yamashita M, et al. Surgical treatments for multiple primary adenocarcinoma of the lung. Ann Thorac Surg 2004;78(4):1194–1199

[28] Zwirewich CV, Miller RR, Müller NL. Multicentric adenocarcinoma of the lung: CT-pathologic correlation. Radiology 1990;176(1):185–190

[29] Park CM, Goo JM, Kim TJ, et al. Pulmonary nodular ground-glass opacities in patients with extrapulmonary cancers: what is their clinical significance and how can we determine whether they are malignant or benign lesions? Chest 2008;133(6):1402–1409
[30] Shyu CL, Lee YC, Perng RP. Fast-growing squamous cell lung cancer. Lung Cancer 2002;36(2):199–202
[31] Aoki T, Nakata H, Watanabe H, et al. Evolution of peripheral lung adenocarcinomas: CT findings correlated with histology and tumor doubling time. AJR Am J Roentgenol 2000;174(3):763–768
[32] Hasegawa M, Sone S, Takashima S, et al. Growth rate of small lung cancers detected on mass CT screening. Br J Radiol 2000;73(876):1252–1259
[33] Winer-Muram HT, Jennings SG, Tarver RD, et al. Volumetric growth rate of stage I lung cancer prior to treatment: serial CT scanning. Radiology 2002;223(3):798–805
[34] Chong S, Lee KS, Chung MJ, Han J, Kwon OJ, Kim TS. Neuroendocrine tumors of the lung: clinical, pathologic, and imaging findings. Radiographics 2006;26(1):41–57, discussion 57–58
[35] Jiang SX, Kameya T, Shoji M, Dobashi Y, Shinada J, Yoshimura H. Large cell neuroendocrine carcinoma of the lung: a histologic and immunohistochemical study of 22 cases. Am J Surg Pathol 1998;22(5):526–537
[36] Travis WD, Linnoila RI, Tsokos MG, et al. Neuroendocrine tumors of the lung with proposed criteria for large-cell neuroendocrine carcinoma. An ultrastructural, immunohistochemical, and flow cytometric study of 35 cases. Am J Surg Pathol 1991;15(6):529–553
[37] Jung KJ, Lee KS, Han J, et al. Large cell neuroendocrine carcinoma of the lung: clinical, CT, and pathologic findings in 11 patients. J Thorac Imaging 2001;16(3):156–162
[38] Takamochi K, Yokose T, Yoshida J, et al. Calcification in large cell neuroendocrine carcinoma of the lung. Jpn J Clin Oncol 2003;33(1):10–13
[39] Boyars MC. Clinical manifestations of carcinoma of the lung. J Thorac Imaging 1991;7(1):21–28
[40] Haque AK. Pathology of carcinoma of lung: an update on current concepts. J Thorac Imaging 1991;7(1):9–20
[41] Müller NL, Miller RR. Neuroendocrine carcinomas of the lung. Semin Roentgenol 1990;25(1):96–104
[42] Kalemkerian GP. Staging and imaging of small cell lung cancer. Cancer Imaging 2012;11:253–258
[43] Yesner R. Histopathology of lung cancer. Semin Ultrasound CT MR 1988;9(1):4–26
[44] Pietra GG. The pathology of carcinoma of the lung. Semin Roentgenol 1990;25(1):25–33
[45] Austin JH, Müller NL, Friedman PJ, et al. Glossary of terms for CT of the lungs: recommendations of the Nomenclature Committee of the Fleischner Society. Radiology 1996;200(2):327–331
[46] Hansell DM, Bankier AA, MacMahon H, McLoud TC, Müller NL, Remy J. Fleischner Society: glossary of terms for thoracic imaging. Radiology 2008;246(3):697–722
[47] Heitzman ER, Markarian B, Raasch BN, Carsky EW, Lane EJ, Berlow ME. Pathways of tumor spread through the lung: radiologic correlations with anatomy and pathology. Radiology 1982;144(1):3–14
[48] Sobin LH, Gospodarowicz MK, Wittekind C. TNM Classification of Malignant Tumours. 7th ed. Hoboken, NJ: Wiley-Blackwell; 2010
[49] Theros EG. 1976 Caldwell Lecture: varying manifestation of peripheral pulmonary neoplasms: a radiologic-pathologic correlative study. AJR Am J Roentgenol 1977;128(6):893–914
[50] Rigler LG. An overview of cancer of the lung. Semin Roentgenol 1977;12(3):161–164
[51] Matthews MJ. Morphology of lung cancer. Semin Oncol 1974;1(3): 175–182
[52] Samet JM, Nero AV Jr. Indoor radon and lung cancer. N Engl J Med 1989;320(9):591–594
[53] Bakris GL, Mulopulos GP, Korchik R, Ezdinli EZ, Ro J, Yoon BH. Pulmonary scar carcinoma. A clinicopathologic analysis. Cancer 1983;52(3): 493–497
[54] Madri JA, Carter D. Scar cancers of the lung: origin and significance. Hum Pathol 1984;15(7):625–631
[55] Yesner R, Carter D. Pathology of carcinoma of the lung. Changing patterns. Clin Chest Med 1982;3(2):257–289
[56] Golden R. The effect of bronchostenosis upon the roentgen ray shadow in carcinoma of the bronchus. AJR Am J Roentgenol 1925;13:21–30
[57] Gupta P. The Golden S sign. Radiology 2004;233(3):790–791
[58] Goldstraw P, Chansky K, Crowley J, et al; International Association for the Study of Lung Cancer Staging and Prognostic Factors Committee, Advisory Boards, and Participating Institutions. International Association for the Study of Lung Cancer Staging and Prognostic Factors Committee Advisory Boards and Participating Institutions. The IASLC Lung Cancer Staging Project: Proposals for Revision of the TNM Stage Groupings in the Forthcoming (Eighth) Edition of the TNM Classification for Lung Cancer. J Thorac Oncol 2016;11(1):39–51
[59] Silvestri GA, Gonzalez AV, Jantz MA, et al. Methods for staging non-small cell lung cancer: Diagnosis and management of lung cancer, 3rd ed: American College of Chest Physicians evidence-based clinical practice guidelines. Chest 2013;143(5 Suppl):e211S–e250S
[60] Stamatis G. Staging of lung cancer: the role of noninvasive, minimally invasive and invasive techniques. Eur Respir J 2015;46(2):521–531
[61] Glazer HS, Duncan-Meyer J, Aronberg DJ, Moran JF, Levitt RG, Sagel SS. Pleural and chest wall invasion in bronchogenic carcinoma: CT evaluation. Radiology 1985;157(1):191–194
[62] UyBico SJ, Wu CC, Suh RD, Le NH, Brown K, Krishnam MS. Lung cancer staging essentials: the new TNM staging system and potential imaging pitfalls. Radiographics 2010;30(5):1163–1181
[63] Komaki R, Putnam JB Jr, Walsh G, Lee JS, Cox JD. The management of superior sulcus tumors. Semin Surg Oncol 2000;18(2):152–164
[64] MacDonald SLS, Hansell DM. Staging of non-small cell lung cancer: imaging of intrathoracic disease. Eur J Radiol 2003;45(1):18–30
[65] Kim YH, Lee KS, Primack SL, et al. Small pulmonary nodules on CT accompanying surgically resectable lung cancer: likelihood of malignancy. J Thorac Imaging 2002;17(1):40–46
[66] Detterbeck FC, Franklin WA, Nicholson AG, et al. The IASLC Lung Cancer Staging Project: Background Data and Proposed Criteria to Distinguish Separate Primary Lung Cancers from Metastatic Foci in Patients with Two Lung Tumors in the Forthcoming Eighth Edition of the TNM Classification for Lung Cancer. J Thorac Oncol 2016;11(5):651–665
[67] Armstrong P. Imaging of Diseases of the Chest. 2nd ed. St. Louis, MO: Mosby; 1995
[68] Glazer GM, Gross BH, Quint LE, Francis IR, Bookstein FL, Orringer MB. Normal mediastinal lymph nodes: number and size according to American Thoracic Society mapping. AJR Am J Roentgenol 1985;144(2):261–265
[69] Hellwig D, Baum RP, Kirsch C. FDG-PET, PET/CT and conventional nuclear medicine procedures in the evaluation of lung cancer: a systematic review. Nucl Med (Stuttg) 2009;48(2):59–69, quiz N8–N9
[70] Birim O, Kappetein AP, Stijnen T, Bogers AJ. Meta-analysis of positron emission tomographic and computed tomographic imaging in detecting mediastinal lymph node metastases in nonsmall cell lung cancer. Ann Thorac Surg 2005;79(1):375–382
[71] Gould MK, Kuschner WG, Rydzak CE, et al. Test performance of positron emission tomography and computed tomography for mediastinal staging in patients with non-small-cell lung cancer: a meta-analysis. Ann Intern Med 2003;139(11):879–892
[72] Silvestri GA, Gould MK, Margolis ML, et al. Noninvasive staging of non-small cell lung cancer: ACCP evidenced-based clinical practice guidelines (2nd edition). Chest 2007;132(3 Suppl):178S–201S
[73] Toloza EM, Harpole L, McCrory DC. Noninvasive staging of non-small cell lung cancer: a review of the current evidence. Chest 2003;123 (1, Suppl):137S–146S
[74] MacManus MP, Hicks RJ, Matthews JP, et al. High rate of detection of unsuspected distant metastases by pet in apparent stage III non-small-cell lung cancer: implications for radical radiation therapy. Int J Radiat Oncol Biol Phys 2001;50(2):287–293
[75] Fontana RS, Sanderson DR, Taylor WF, et al. Early lung cancer detection: results of the initial (prevalence) radiologic and cytologic screening in the Mayo Clinic study. Am Rev Respir Dis 1984;130(4):561–565
[76] Frost JK, Ball WC Jr, Levin ML, et al. Early lung cancer detection: results of the initial (prevalence) radiologic and cytologic screening in the Johns Hopkins study. Am Rev Respir Dis 1984;130(4):549–554
[77] Kubík A, Polák J. Lung cancer detection. Results of a randomized prospective study in Czechoslovakia. Cancer 1986;57(12):2427–2437
[78] Melamed MR, Flehinger BJ, Zaman MB, Heelan RT, Perchick WA, Martini N. Screening for early lung cancer. Results of the Memorial Sloan-Kettering study in New York. Chest 1984;86(1):44–53
[79] Diederich S, Wormanns D, Semik M, et al. Screening for early lung cancer with low-dose spiral CT: prevalence in 817 asymptomatic smokers. Radiology 2002;222(3):773–781
[80] Henschke CI, McCauley DI, Yankelevitz DF, et al. Early Lung Cancer Action Project: overall design and findings from baseline screening. Lancet 1999;354(9173):99–105
[81] Kaneko M, Eguchi K, Ohmatsu H, et al. Peripheral lung cancer: screening and detection with low-dose spiral CT versus radiography. Radiology 1996;201(3):798–802
[82] Nawa T, Nakagawa T, Kusano S, Kawasaki Y, Sugawara Y, Nakata H. Lung cancer screening using low-dose spiral CT: results of baseline and 1-year follow-up studies. Chest 2002;122(1):15–20

[83] Pastorino U, Bellomi M, Landoni C, et al. Early lung-cancer detection with spiral CT and positron emission tomography in heavy smokers: 2-year results. Lancet 2003;362(9384):593–597
[84] Sone S, Takashima S, Li F, et al. Mass screening for lung cancer with mobile spiral computed tomography scanner. Lancet 1998;351(9111):1242–1245
[85] Swensen SJ, Jett JR, Sloan JA, et al. Screening for lung cancer with low-dose spiral computed tomography. Am J Respir Crit Care Med 2002;165(4):508–513
[86] Tiitola M, Kivisaari L, Huuskonen MS, et al. Computed tomography screening for lung cancer in asbestos-exposed workers. Lung Cancer 2002;35(1):17–22
[87] Aberle DR, Adams AM, Berg CD, et al; National Lung Screening Trial Research Team. Reduced lung-cancer mortality with low-dose computed tomographic screening. N Engl J Med 2011;365(5):395–409
[88] Kramer BS, Berg CD, Aberle DR, Prorok PC. Lung cancer screening with low-dose helical CT: results from the National Lung Screening Trial (NLST). J Med Screen 2011;18(3):109–111
[89] Baldwin DR, Duffy SW, Wald NJ, Page R, Hansell DM, Field JK. UK Lung Screen (UKLS) nodule management protocol: modelling of a single screen randomised controlled trial of low-dose CT screening for lung cancer. Thorax 2011;66(4):308–313
[90] Becker N, Motsch E, Gross M-L, et al. Randomized study on early detection of lung cancer with MSCT in Germany: study design and results of the first screening round. J Cancer Res Clin Oncol 2012;138(9):1475–1486
[91] Kauczor H-U, Bonomo L, Gaga M, et al; European Society of Radiology (ESR). European Respiratory Society (ERS). ESR/ERS white paper on lung cancer screening. Eur Respir J 2015;46(1):28–39
[92] Pastorino U, Rossi M, Rosato V, et al. Annual or biennial CT screening versus observation in heavy smokers: 5-year results of the MILD trial. Eur J Cancer Prev 2012;21(3):308–315
[93] Saghir Z, Dirksen A, Ashraf H, et al. CT screening for lung cancer brings forward early disease. The randomised Danish Lung Cancer Screening Trial: status after five annual screening rounds with low-dose CT. Thorax 2012;67(4):296–301
[94] van Iersel CA, de Koning HJ, Draisma G, et al. Risk-based selection from the general population in a screening trial: selection criteria, recruitment and power for the Dutch-Belgian randomised lung cancer multi-slice CT screening trial (NELSON). Int J Cancer 2007;120(4): 868–874
[95] Wender R, Fontham ETH, Barrera E Jr, et al. American Cancer Society lung cancer screening guidelines. CA Cancer J Clin 2013;63(2):107–117
[96] Schreurs AJ, Westermann CJ, van den Bosch JM, Vanderschueren RG, Brutel de la Rivière A, Knaepen PJ. A twenty-five-year follow-up of ninety-three resected typical carcinoid tumors of the lung. J Thorac Cardiovasc Surg 1992;104(5):1470–1475
[97] Bosman FT, de la Riviere AB, Giard RW, Verhofstad AA, Cramer-Knijnenburg G. Amine and peptide hormone production by lung carcinoid: a clinicopathological and immunocytochemical study. J Clin Pathol 1984;37(8):931–936
[98] Grote TH, Macon WR, Davis B, Greco FA, Johnson DH. Atypical carcinoid of the lung. A distinct clinicopathologic entity. Chest 1988;93(2):370–375
[99] Rosado de Christenson ML, Abbott GF, Kirejczyk WM, Galvin JR, Travis WD. Thoracic carcinoids: radiologic-pathologic correlation. Radiographics 1999;19(3):707–736
[100] Gould PM, Bonner JA, Sawyer TE, Deschamps C, Lange CM, Li H. Bronchial carcinoid tumors: importance of prognostic factors that influence patterns of recurrence and overall survival. Radiology 1998;208(1):181–185
[101] Jeung MY, Gasser B, Gangi A, et al. Bronchial carcinoid tumors of the thorax: spectrum of radiologic findings. Radiographics 2002;22(2): 351–365
[102] Jadvar H, Segall GM. False-negative fluorine-18-FDG PET in metastatic carcinoid. J Nucl Med 1997;38(9):1382–1383
[103] Virgolini I, Patri P, Novotny C, et al. Comparative somatostatin receptor scintigraphy using in-111-DOTA-lanreotide and in-111-DOTA-Tyr3-octreotide versus F-18-FDG-PET for evaluation of somatostatin receptor-mediated radionuclide therapy. Ann Oncol 2001;12(Suppl 2):S41–S45
[104] Diederich S, Link TM, Zühlsdorf H, Steinmeyer E, Wormanns D, Heindel W. Pulmonary manifestations of Hodgkin's disease: radiographic and CT findings. Eur Radiol 2001;11(11):2295–2305
[105] Lee HJ, Im JG, Goo JM, et al. Peripheral T-cell lymphoma: spectrum of imaging findings with clinical and pathologic features. Radiographics 2003;23(1):7–26, discussion 26–28
[106] Seo JB, Im JG, Goo JM, Chung MJ, Kim MY. Atypical pulmonary metastases: spectrum of radiologic findings. Radiographics 2001;21(2):403–417
[107] Webb WR, Müller NL, Naidich DP. High-Resolution CT of the Lung. 4th ed. Philadelphia, PA: Wolters Kluwer/Lippincott Williams & Wilkins; 2009
[108] Davis SD. CT evaluation for pulmonary metastases in patients with extrathoracic malignancy. Radiology 1991;180(1):1–12
[109] Goldsmith HS, Bailey HD, Callahan EL, Beattie EJ Jr. Pulmonary lymphangitic metastases from breast carcinoma. Arch Surg 1967;94(4):483–488
[110] Sadoff L, Grossman J, Weiner H. Lymphangitic pulmonary metastases secondary to breast cancer with normal chest x-rays and abnormal perfusion lung scans. Oncology 1975;31(3–4):164–171
[111] Narla LD, Newman B, Spottswood SS, Narla S, Kolli R. Inflammatory pseudotumor. Radiographics 2003;23(3):719–729
[112] Umiker WO, Iverson L. Postinflammatory tumors of the lung; report of four cases simulating xanthoma, fibroma, or plasma cell tumor. J Thorac Surg 1954;28(1):55–63
[113] Agrons GA, Rosado-de-Christenson ML, Kirejczyk WM, Conran RM, Stocker JT. Pulmonary inflammatory pseudotumor: radiologic features. Radiology 1998;206(2):511–518

Chapter 10

Airway Diseases

10 Airway Diseases

10.1 Diseases of the Trachea and Mainstem Bronchi

10.1.1 Tracheal Stenosis and Stenosis of the Mainstem Bronchi

Benign tracheal stenosis usually occurs secondary to endotracheal tube cuff pressure alteration, typically in the middle trachea. The cuff pressure causes ischemic necrosis of the mucosa and subsequent fibrosis.[1,2] This results in short stenosis of the tracheal lumen. In addition, several other causes of stenosis of the trachea or central bronchi are known.

Note

Causes of tracheal stenosis[2]:

- Intubation.
- Penetrating or blunt trauma.
- Postinfectious, especially in tuberculosis.
- Anastomotic stenosis following lung transplant.
- Crohn disease.
- Sarcoidosis.
- Granulomatous polyangiitis or Wegner granulomatosis.
- Amyloidosis.
- Tracheobronchopathia osteochondroplastica.
- Perichondritis.

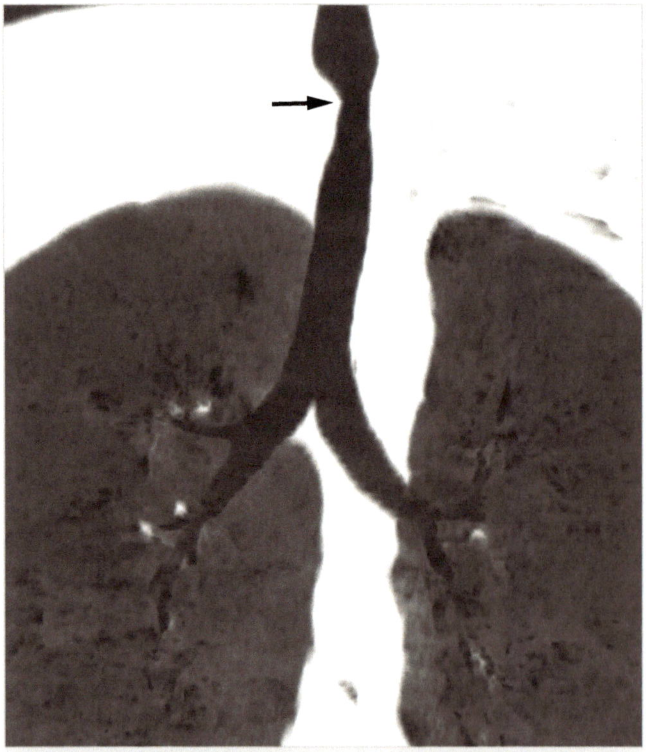

Fig. 10.1 Benign tracheal stenosis (*arrow*) secondary to mechanical ventilation. CT image, coronal MinIP.

Occasionally, tracheal stenosis can be identified on radiography. Computed tomography (CT) is able to reliably visualize stenosis even if, at times, this is not apparent on axial slices. Therefore, comparison of the tracheal lumen with adjacent and more distant slices is needed. Stenosis can be visualized more clearly on sagittal and paracoronal MPR (multiplanar reconstructions) or MinIP (minimum intensity projections) (▶Fig. 10.1),[3] with the latter angled along the course of the trachea. Typically, the area of stenosis has a symmetrical, hourglass shape measuring up to 2 cm in length.

10.1.2 Tracheal Diverticula

Tracheal diverticula (paratracheal air cysts) are rare and usually asymptomatic incidental findings identified on CT scans.[4] At times, chronic cough or recurrent infections, hemoptysis, stridor, or dyspnea may be observed. Occasionally, intubation difficulties lead to the diagnosis.[5]

Air accumulation in the superior thoracic aperture can sometimes be seen on radiography but CT is needed to reach the diagnosis (▶Fig. 10.2). A well-defined air accumulation is usually located right dorsal to the tracheal at the level of the superior thoracic aperture; an air-filled channel between the extraluminal air and the trachea can be identified.[5]

For differential diagnosis, other air-containing structures of the superior thoracic aperture must be taken into account, especially Zenker diverticulum of the esophagus, pharyngoceles, laryngoceles, apical lung hernias, bullae, and pneumomediastinum.[4,5] An important differential criterion is detection of a communication between the trachea and diverticulum on CT.

10.1.3 Tracheal Rupture

Traumatic tracheal rupture is rare but may occur secondary to chest trauma or iatrogenic tracheal injury during intubation. It usually affects the posterior tracheal wall, the softer membranous part.

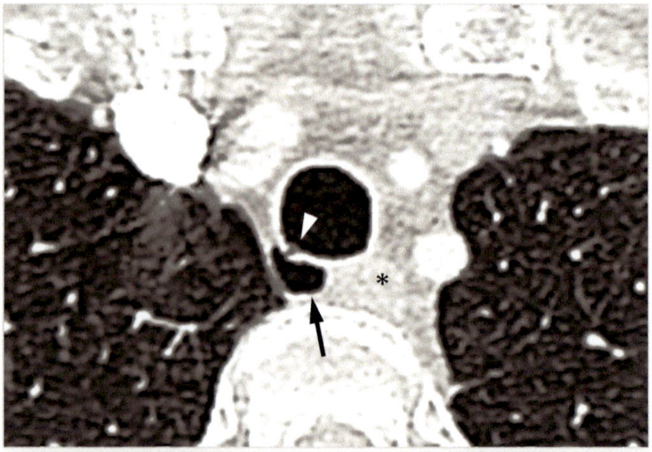

Fig. 10.2 Tracheal diverticulum. CT image. Retrotracheal, smoothly marginated air accumulation (*arrow*) right lateral to the esophagus (*asterisk*) with visible communication with the trachea (*arrowhead*).

Tracheal rupture cannot be directly identified on radiography; indirect signs include mediastinal and cervical soft-tissue emphysema. CT is usually able to directly demonstrate the defect in the tracheal wall (▶Fig. 10.3). Furthermore, abnormal distension of a tracheal tube cuff is an indirect sign of tracheal rupture.[6]

10.1.4 Foreign Body Aspiration

Foreign body aspiration occurs predominantly in children younger than 6 years of age who are capable of aspirating the most diverse objects. In adults, foreign bodies are generally aspirated accidentally while ingesting food, usually chicken or fish bones, less commonly dentures.[7] Predisposing factors include pathologic changes to the gastrointestinal tract, in particular esophageal stenosis, advanced age, mental retardation, or psychiatric disorders.

Note

Foreign bodies are often found in the right lower lobe. Since the right mainstem bronchus has a steeper course than the left, most foreign bodies pass to the right side and, due to gravity, are dislodged more distal into the right lower lobe bronchus.

Larger, metallic objects are visible on radiography but other foreign bodies, including chicken or fish bones, almost never.[7] CT is indicated if aspiration is suspected and no foreign bodies are radiographically seen. CT has very high sensitivity for detection of foreign bodies but does not have absolute specificity since, for example, endobronchial tumors can also mimic a foreign body (see ▶Fig. 10.5).

In almost half of cases, additional findings are identified on radiography, most commonly atelectasis, less often hyperinflation of parts of the lung due to a valve mechanism caused by the foreign body, or poststenotic pneumonia.[8] Around 20% of all cases of foreign body aspiration have a normal radiograph. On CT, inflammatory changes to the bronchial wall manifest as wall thickening or luminal constriction, in particular in the case of a longstanding foreign body. Furthermore, in addition to inflammation, mucoceles or bronchiectasis is also often observed over time distal to the foreign body (▶Fig. 10.4).

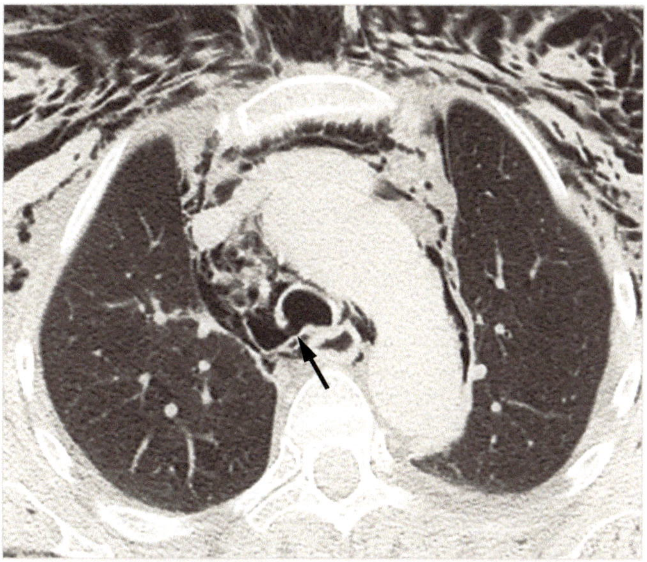

Fig. 10.3 **Tracheal rupture.** CT image. Gaping defect in the posterior tracheal wall (*arrow*) with massive mediastinal and soft-tissue emphysema.

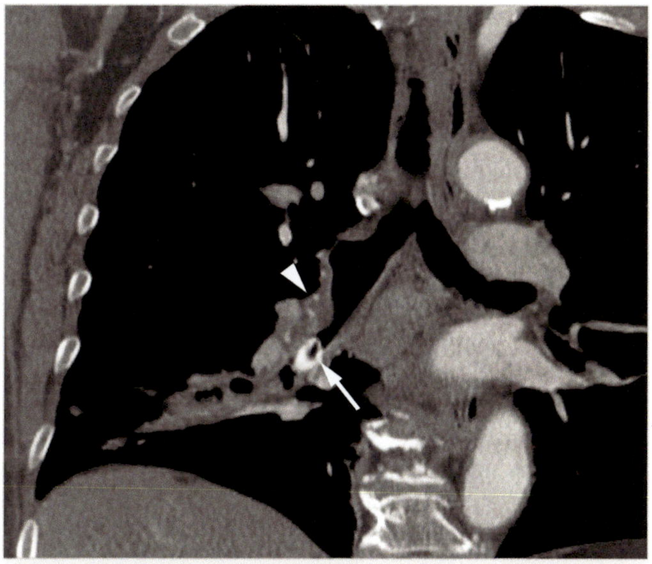

Fig. 10.4 **Aspirated chicken bone in the right lower lobe bronchus (*arrow*).** CT, coronal image. Granulation tissue in the intermediate bronchus (*arrowhead*) and impaired aeration of the distal bronchus as well as bronchiectasis.

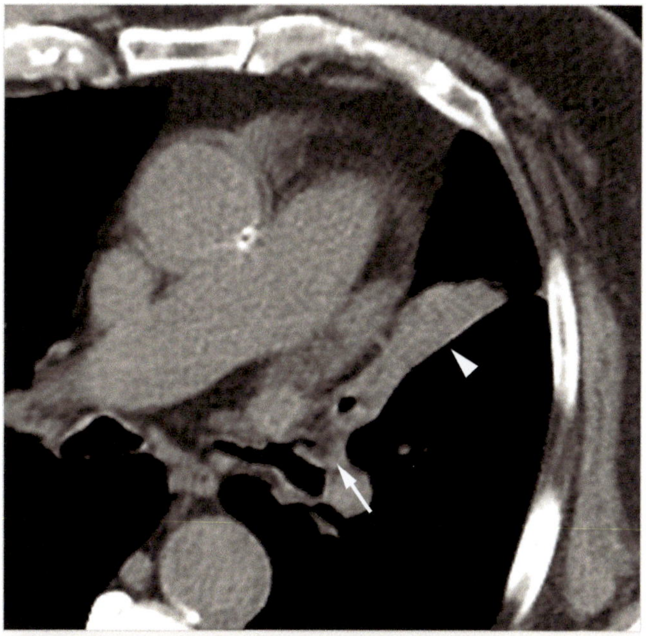

Fig. 10.5 **Bronchial lipoma.** CT image. Small, endobronchial mass of fat density (*arrow*) with distal atelectasis (*arrowhead*).

II

10.1.5 Benign Tumors

Benign tumors of the trachea and the mainstem bronchi are much less common than malignant tumors. These are smoothly marginated, rounded tumors that are rarely more than 2 cm in size. Clinically, these generally manifest as stridor. The predominant findings on histology are papillomas, adenomas of the submucosal mucous glands, hamartomas, and lipomas.[1]

On CT these tumors present as polycyclic endoluminal masses that do not extend beyond the borders of the specific organ. Hamartomas, too, may also be seen to contain fat on CT, like pulmonary hamartomas.[1] Likewise, lipomas characteristically exhibit fat-equivalent density on CT. Some endobronchial tumors cause atelectasis (▶Fig. 10.5).

10.1.6 Malignant Tumors

Malignant tumors of the trachea account for less than 1% of all thoracic tumors.[9] The most common tumors are squamous cell carcinomas (▶Fig. 10.6), followed by adenoid cystic carcinomas (▶Fig. 10.7); less common are mucoepidermoid tumors and carcinoids.[1] Clinically, only nonspecific early symptoms, such as dyspnea, stridor, hemoptysis, or dysphagia, are seen.

On radiographs, these tumors are rarely detected prospectively, although they can usually be identified retrospectively as constriction of the tracheal lumen.[1] CT is able to visualize both the endobronchial tumor component and the tumor extension. The tumor is seen as a more or less circular area of enhanced thickening surrounding the tracheal or mainstem bronchial wall, with, in some cases, a pronounced endoluminal exophytic component (see ▶Fig. 10.6).

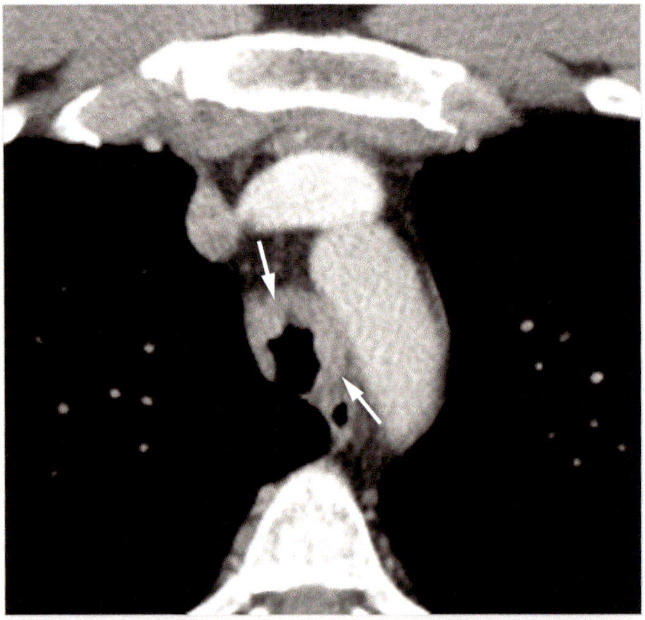

Fig. 10.6 Squamous cell carcinoma of the trachea (*arrows*). CT image.

10.1.7 Inflammatory and Other Systemic Diseases

Infections of the upper airways by human papillomaviruses cause *papillomatosis*. This disease usually affects children and is less common in adults. The usually multiple papillomas are classified as nonneoplastic lesions.[2] Occasionally, they may even be seen on radiographs, and on CT they regularly manifest as endoluminal nodules in the trachea (▶Fig. 10.8).

Perichondritis (relapsing polychondritis) belongs to the collagen vascular diseases, in which recurrent inflammatory processes successively destroy the tracheal and bronchial cartilage clasps, leading to constriction of the airways. On CT, diffuse wall thickening and narrowing of the tracheal lumen can be identified. The destruction of cartilage clasps may also be visible on CT in cases with calcified cartilage.[1]

Deposition of fibrillar proteins in various organs and tissues causes *amyloidosis*. In the tracheobronchial system, these proteins usually form diffuse deposits in the submucosa or, less commonly, a solitary mass. The mucosal surfaces generally remain intact. Calcification and ossification may be present. CT demonstrates subtle wall thickening and sometimes calcifications causing narrowing of the bronchial lumen (▶Fig. 10.9).

Osteochondral proliferations of unknown origin found in the anterior and lateral walls of the trachea and mainstem bronchi are known as *tracheobronchopathia osteochondroplastica*. The posterior walls are not affected since they do not contain cartilage. Thickened tracheal and bronchial cartilage clasps as well as, often multiple, exophytic nodules can be identified in the bronchial lumen on CT (▶Fig. 10.10); these findings are pathognomonic for this disease.[1,10,11,12]

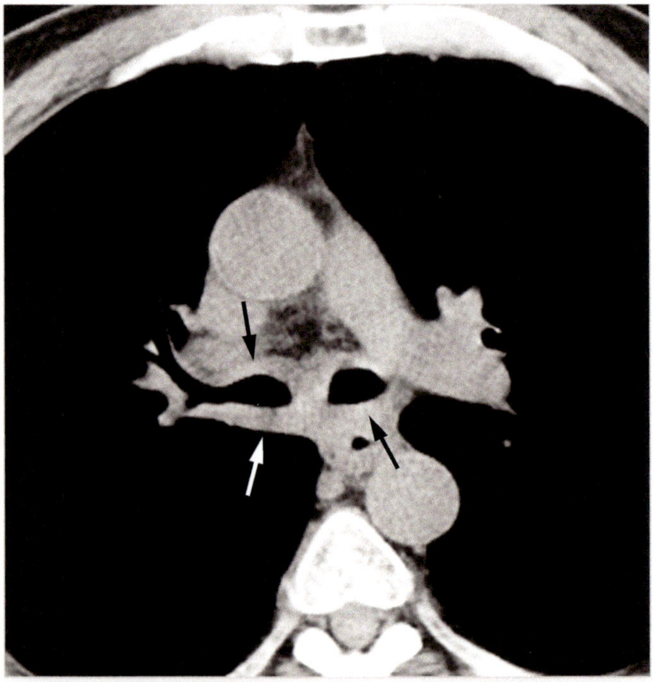

Fig. 10.7 Adenoid cystic carcinoma in both mainstem bronchi (*arrows*) and the trachea (not shown). CT image.

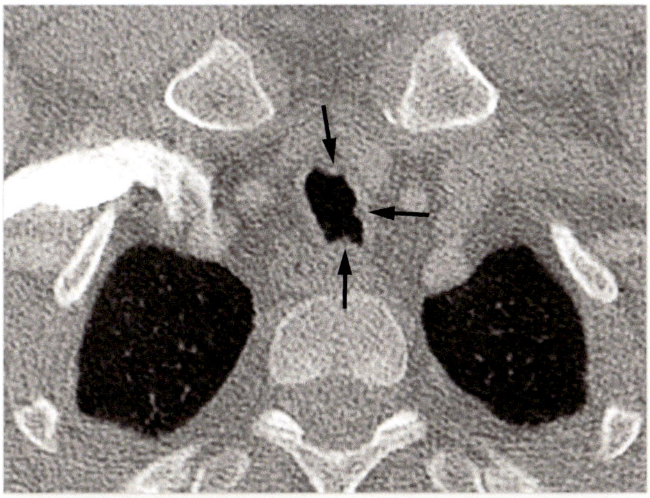

Fig. 10.8 **Tracheal papillomatosis (*arrows*).** CT image.

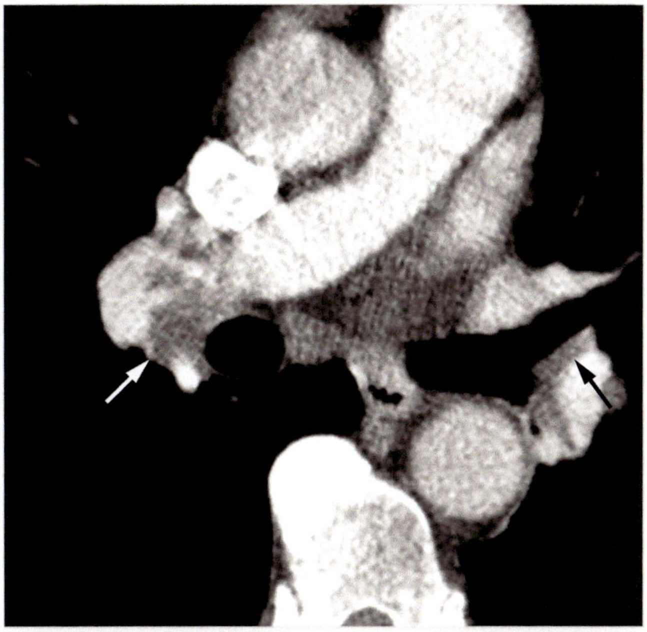

Fig. 10.9 **Amyloidosis.** CT image. Peribronchial masses of soft-tissue density (*arrows*).

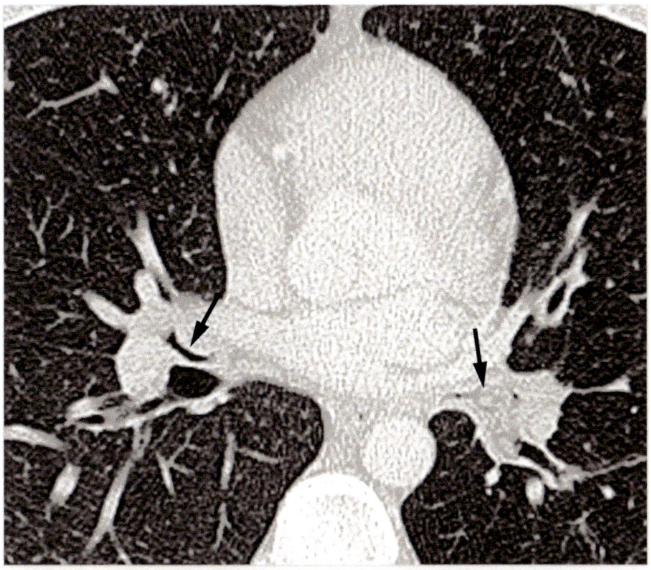

Fig. 10.10 **Tracheobronchopathia osteochondroplastica.** CT image. Endoluminal nodular proliferations in the bronchi of left lower lobe and middle lobe (*arrows*).

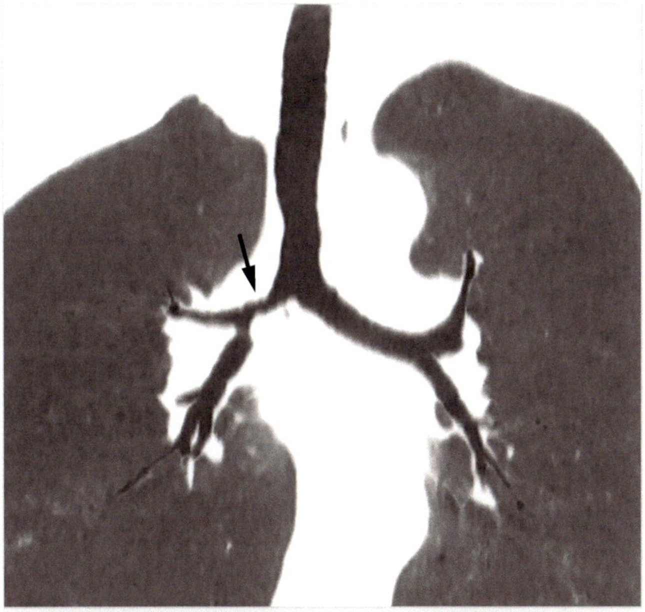

Fig. 10.11 **Granulomatosis with polyangiitis (Wegener granulomatosis).** CT, coronal MinIP. Irregular stenosis of the right mainstem bronchus (*arrow*).

Several systemic diseases also affect the tracheobronchial system. Sarcoidosis can, in particular, cause extrinsic compression of the bronchi because of mediastinal or hilar lymph node enlargement. There may also be granulomatous mucosal lesions of the trachea and mainstem bronchi but these rarely cause stenosis of any relevance. Tracheal involvement is an unusual late manifestation in granulomatous polyangiitis or Wegner granulomatosis. On CT, bronchial stenosis due to wall thickening can be identified (▶Fig. 10.11), which is secondary to granulomatous inflammation of the mucosa and submucosa as well as vasculitis.[1,13,14] Tracheobronchitis associated with *ulcerative colitis* is seen on CT as thickening of the bronchial walls, possibly with concomitant bronchiectasis.[1,15]

10.1.8 Saber Sheath Trachea

The term "saber sheath trachea" is used to describe narrowing of the coronal diameter of the trachea to less than half of the sagittal diameter (▶Fig. 10.12). This is typically associated with chronic obstructive pulmonary disease and is almost exclusively seen in males. Often, calcification of the cartilage clasps can be detected on CT.[1]

II

10.1.9 Tracheomalacia and Bronchomalacia

The term tracheo- and bronchomalacia is used to describe the flaccidity, and hence the reduced mechanical strength, of the tracheal and bronchial walls. This results in increased mobility and collapse susceptibility of the tracheobronchial system. A rare primary form is seen in children with congenital impairment of cartilage formation.[16] Secondary tracheo- and bronchomalacia results from intubation, chronic obstruction, trauma, or polychondritis (▶Fig. 10.13).[1] The pressure exerted by an enlarged thyroid gland can also cause tracheomalacia. The potential cause can be inferred on identification of goiter on radiography and narrowing of the tracheal lumen in a posteroanterior image cranial to the superior thoracic aperture.

The width of the tracheal or bronchial lumen varies according to the central airway pressure. The radiologic diagnostic criterion for this disease is identification of a difference of at least 50% in width of the tracheal lumen between the inspiratory and expiratory tracheal images.[1]

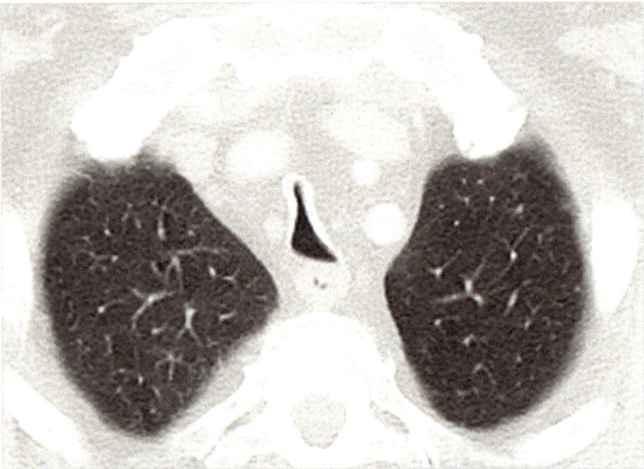

Fig. 10.12 **Saber sheath trachea.** CT image.

10.2 Small Airway Diseases

The distal bronchi with an internal diameter of less than 2 mm are known as the *small airways*. Normal bronchi of this size are not visible on CT. Pathologic changes to these bronchi can be identified on imaging from direct and indirect signs:

- *Direct imaging signs* (▶Fig. 10.14): These are due to inflammatory thickening of the bronchial wall and bronchiectasis as well as surrounding or endoluminal exudates. On CT, these findings correlate with centrilobular nodules and a tree-in-bud pattern.[17,18]
- *Indirect imaging signs* (▶Fig. 10.15): These stem from obliteration of the bronchial lumen and ensuing hyperinflation of the portions of the lung distal to the obstruction. The resulting mosaic-like reduced density of lung parenchyma due to air trapping reflects the patchy distribution of the pathologic changes (mosaic attenuation pattern).[17,19]

Classification of small airway diseases was formerly based, in general, on the histopathology findings and was inconsistent[18,20,21] since there was not always a direct correlation between the histopathological results and the clinical and imaging findings.[19] The present system used for classification of bronchial diseases also takes account of the clinical context and is illustrated in ▶Table 10.1. Some of these diseases are discussed in detail in the chapters on diffuse parenchymal lung diseases and immunologic diseases of the lung.

CT is the mainstay for *diagnosis* of these diseases, obviating the need for invasive procedures, i.e., biopsy, in the majority of cases. The diagnostic work-up includes a medical

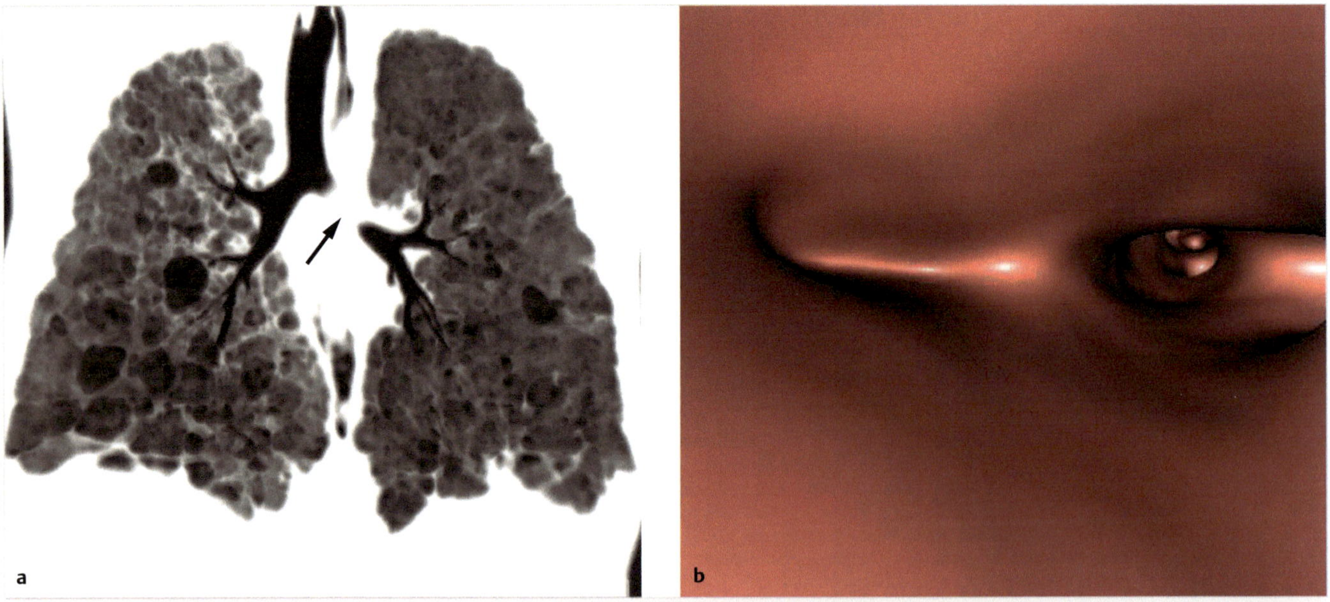

Fig. 10.13 **Bronchomalacia in newborn.** CT images. The pressure exerted by the adjacent gastric probe (not on the image) is causing high-grade stenosis of the left mainstem bronchus. **(a)** Coronal MinIP with stenosis of the left mainstem bronchus (*arrow*). Furthermore, lung fibrosis secondary to long-term ventilation. **(b)** Virtual bronchoscopy with extrinsic compression of the left mainstem bronchus.

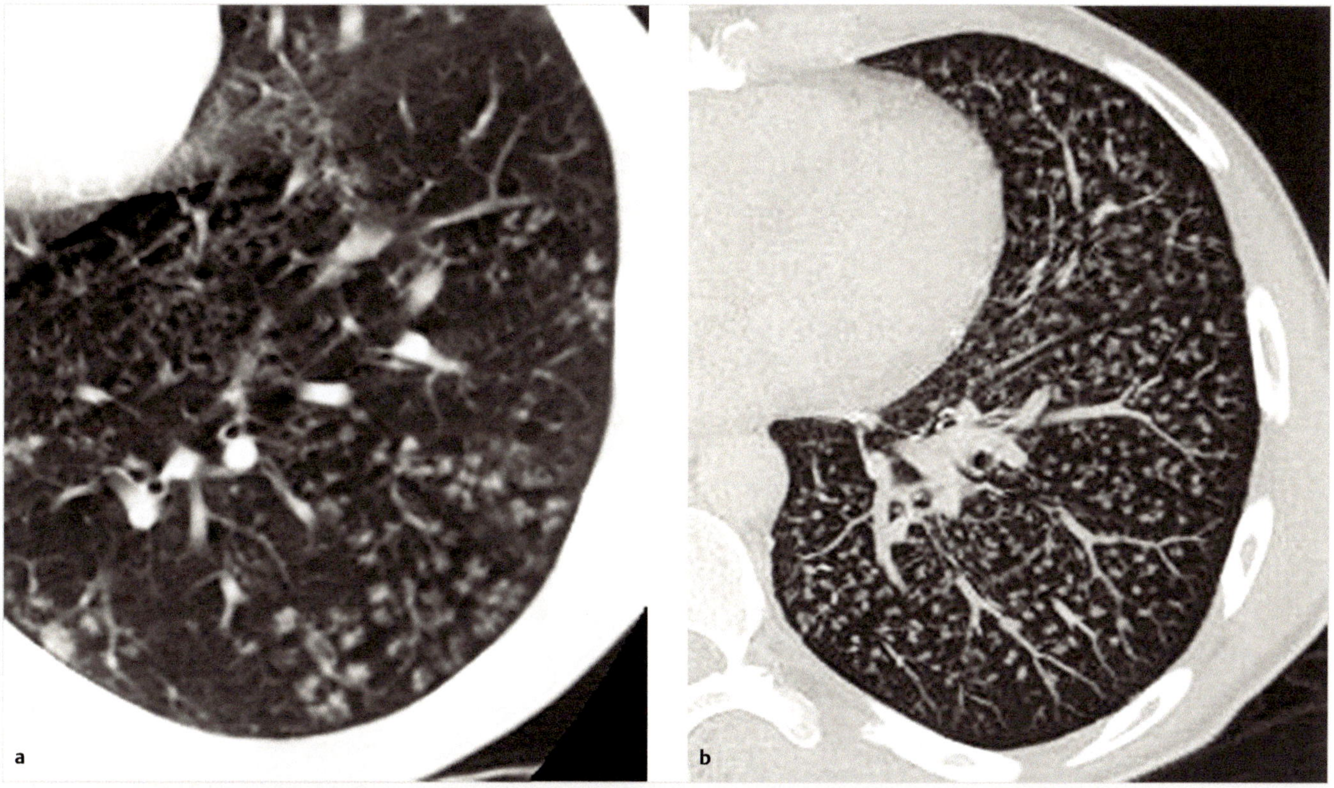

Fig. 10.14 **Direct signs of bronchiolitis.** CT images. **(a)** Centrilobular nodules. **(b)** Tree-in-bud pattern.

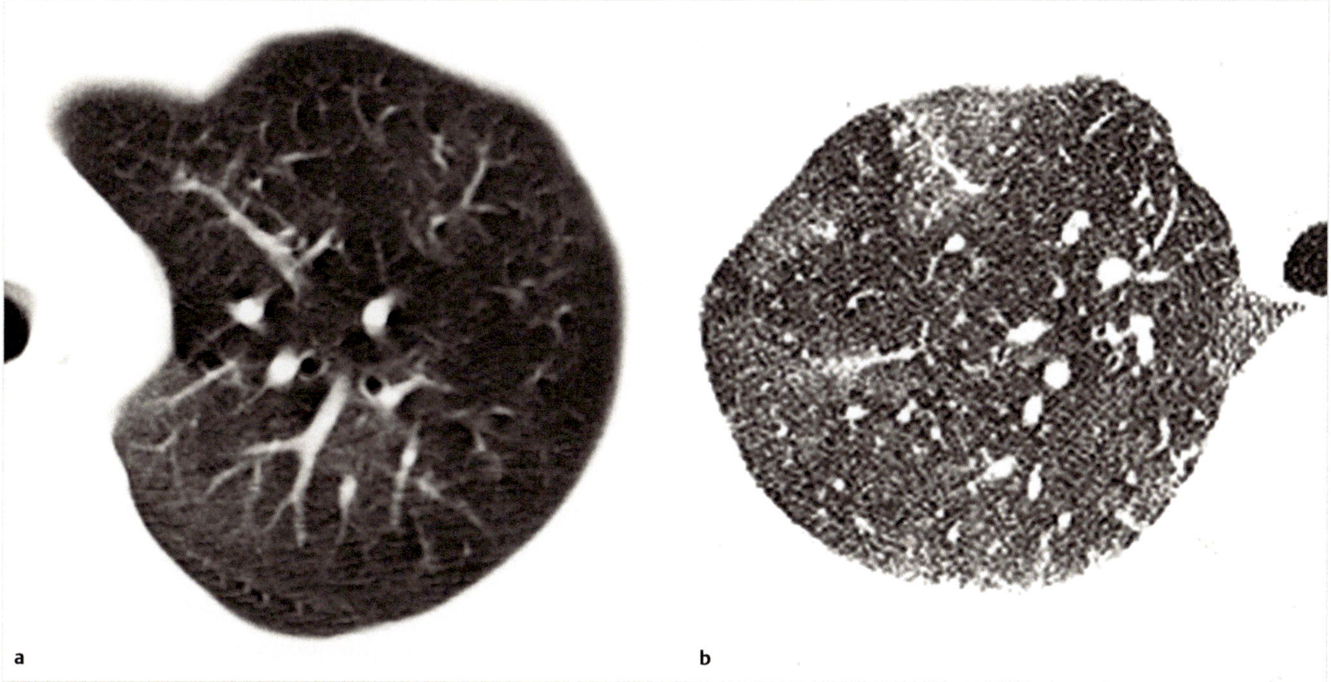

Fig. 10.15 **Indirect signs of bronchiolitis.** CT images. **(a)** Diffusely decreased lung parenchymal density. **(b)** Mosaic attenuation pattern.

history (infection, inhalation exposure, drug toxicity, organ transplant), physical examination, lung function test (airway obstruction), and chest radiography (hyperinflation). CT is indicated if small airway disease is suspected. CT differential diagnosis is presented in ▶Fig. 10.16.[17] Biopsy may be omitted in cases with typical clinical and imaging findings; if the findings are inconclusive, biopsy is necessary to establish a definitive diagnosis. Open surgery lung biopsy is superior to bronchoscopic biopsy since it yields a larger tissue specimen.

Table 10.1 Classification of small airway diseases[22]

Groups	Diseases
Primary bronchiolar diseases	• Constrictive bronchiolitis (obliterative bronchiolitis and bronchiolitis obliterans) • Acute bronchiolitis • Diffuse panbronchiolitis • Respiratory bronchiolitis • Mineral dust airway disease • Follicular bronchiolitis • Other primary bronchiolar disorders (e.g., diffuse aspiration bronchiolitis and lymphocytic bronchiolitis)
Diffuse parenchymal lung diseases with prominent bronchiolar involvement	• Hypersensitivity pneumonitis • Respiratory bronchiolitis with diffuse parenchymal lung disease • Other diffuse parenchymal lung diseases, e.g., Langerhans cell histiocytosis, sarcoidosis
Bronchiolar involvement in diseases also involving large airways	• Chronic obstructive pulmonary disease • Bronchiectasis, including cystic fibrosis • Asthma

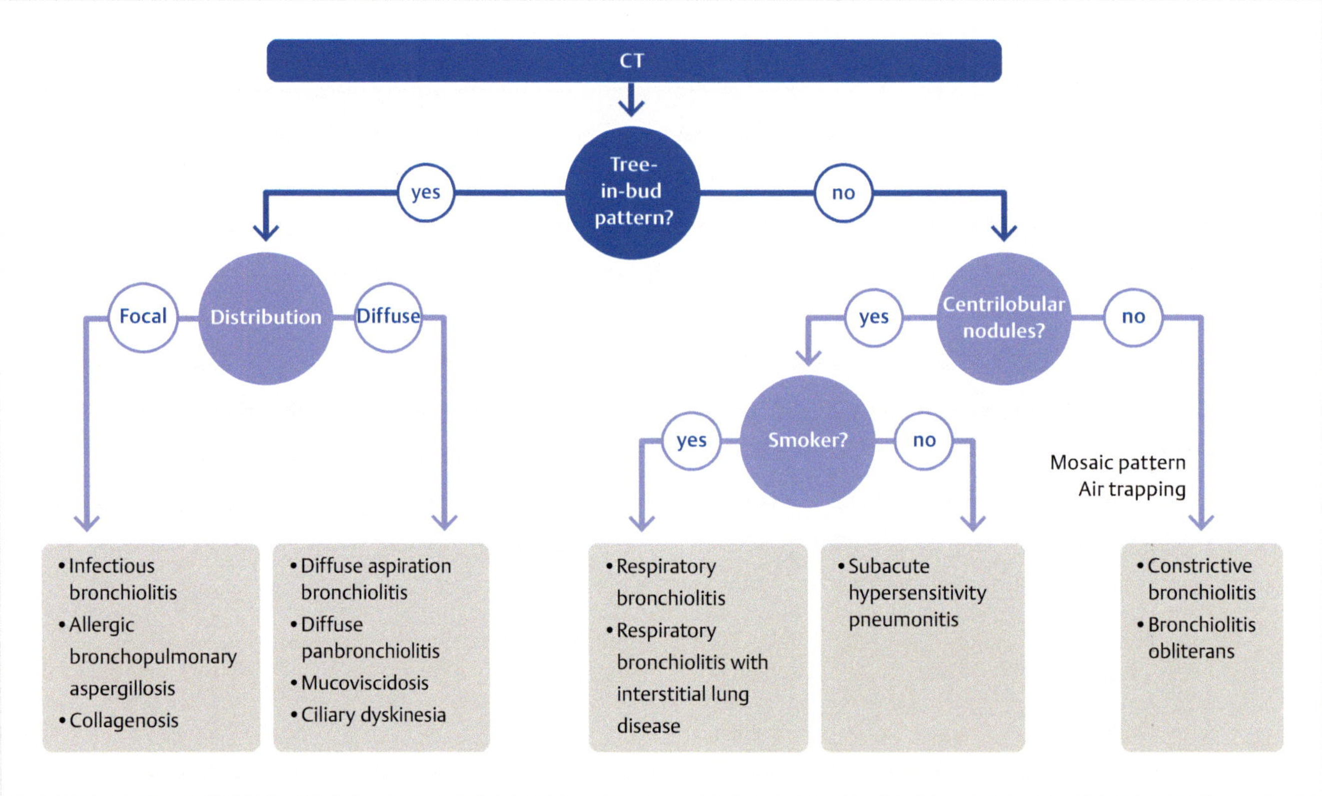

Fig. 10.16 **Diagnostic algorithm for small airway diseases.** (Reproduced with permission from Devakonda et al.[17])

10.2.1 Infectious Bronchiolitis

Bronchiolitis presents in two forms in respiratory tract infections: it occurs coincident with the infection as infectious bronchiolitis or manifests later as postinfectious bronchiolitis.

Both bacterial infections and mycobacteriosis give rise to direct imaging signs, i.e., a tree-in-bud pattern and centrilobular nodules (▶Fig. 10.17).[22]

Postinfectious bronchiolitis may occur as a sequela of infections, in particular following viral or mycoplasma pneumonia (▶Fig. 10.18). Children are affected more often than adults. Postinfectious bronchiolitis predominantly manifests as bronchiolitis obliterans and constrictive bronchiolitis. Swyer–James syndrome may develop following childhood viral pneumonia since bronchiolitis obliterans has a negative impact on the development of the diseased lung areas, in particular of the pulmonary vascular architecture.

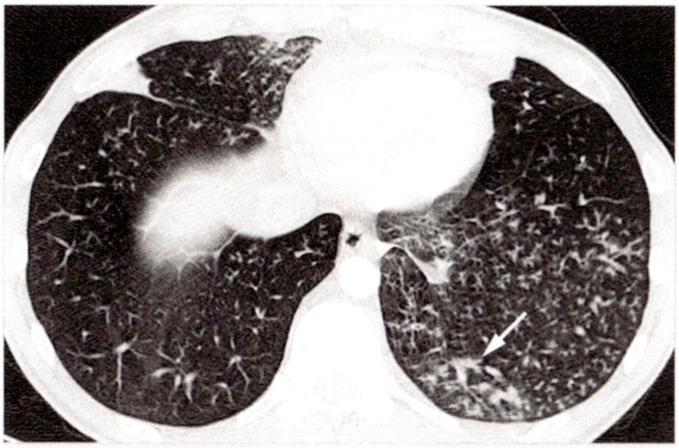

Fig. 10.17 **Infectious bronchiolitis.** CT image. Tree-in-bud pattern in the left lower lobe and small peribronchial consolidation due to bronchopneumonia of the adjacent lung tissue (*arrow*).

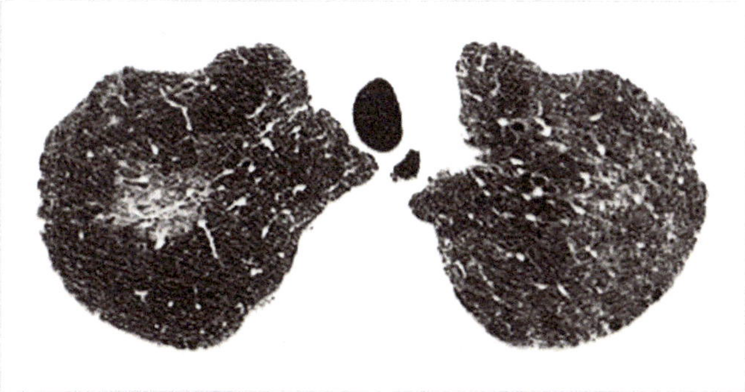

Fig. 10.18 **Postinfectious bronchiolitis obliterans.** CT image. Mosaic attenuation pattern in both upper lobes following mycoplasma pneumonia. Residual bilateral ground-glass opacities can also be identified.

10.2.2 Bronchiolitis Obliterans and Constrictive Bronchiolitis

Formerly, *bronchiolitis obliterans* was used as a collective term that encompassed various histopathologic diseases. At present, two forms are distinguished[22]:

- *Bronchiolitis obliterans in a narrower sense*: This is characterized by proliferative bronchiolitis with fibroinflammatory polyps leading to obstruction of the bronchial lumen. Often, similar polyps are found in the alveoli, giving rise to the characteristic image of organizing pneumonia.[23]
- *Constrictive (or obliterating) bronchiolitis*: This is characterized by narrowing of the small airways due to peribronchial fibrosis but does not lead to endoluminal obstruction.[23] The main causes of constrictive bronchiolitis or bronchiolitis obliterans are summarized in ▶Table 10.2. Bronchiolitis obliterans may represent chronic rejection following lung transplant or graft-versus-host disease after allogenic stem cell transplant.

The predominant imaging findings are indirect signs of bronchiolitis. Chest radiography is often normal; otherwise, diffuse hyperinflation of the lung parenchyma is observed. CT demonstrates diffusely decreased lung parenchymal density or a mosaic attenuation pattern as well as cylindrical bronchiectasis (▶Fig. 10.19). Expiratory CT scans may help establish the diagnosis if bronchiolitis obliterans is suspected: the absence of an adequate increase in lung parenchymal density in expiration is suggestive of bronchiolitis obliterans. A density difference of less than 50 HU between inspiration and expiration is deemed pathologic and indicates extensive air trapping. Often, this reduced difference in lung parenchymal density can be better visualized during a breathing cycle in dynamic CT of the ventilation cycle than in expiratory scans.

Table 10.2 Causes of bronchiolitis obliterans[19]

Causes	Examples
Postinfectious	Adenovirus
	Respiratory syncytial virus
	Influenza virus
	Mycoplasma pneumoniae
Inhalational injury	Nitrogen dioxide (silo-filler's disease)
	Sulfur dioxide
	Ammonia
	Phosgene
	Hot gases
Collagen vascular diseases	Rheumatoid arthritis
	Sjögren syndrome
Transplant recipients	Graft-versus-host disease: stem cell transplant
	Chronic rejection: lung transplant
Drug toxicity	Penicillamine
	Lomustine
Other	Inflammatory bowel disease
	Bronchiectasis, including cystic fibrosis
	Hypersensitivity pneumonitis
	Microcarcinoid tumorlets

10.2.3 Other Forms of Bronchiolitis

Involvement of the small bronchi in allergic bronchopulmonary aspergillosis may present as a diffuse tree-in-bud pattern. Furthermore, there may be other findings related to allergic bronchopulmonary aspergillosis such as central bronchiectasis, mucus impaction, atelectasis, or consolidation.

Smoking-associated *respiratory bronchiolitis* is often identified as an incidental finding on imaging or histology. If impaired lung function is present, this clinical disease entity is termed respiratory bronchiolitis with diffuse parenchymal lung disease.

Diffuse aspiration bronchiolitis is seen, in particular, in elderly, bedridden patients with neurologic deficits, and occurs secondary to chronic recurrent aspiration. This disease, too, is characterized by a diffuse tree-in-bud pattern.[17]

10

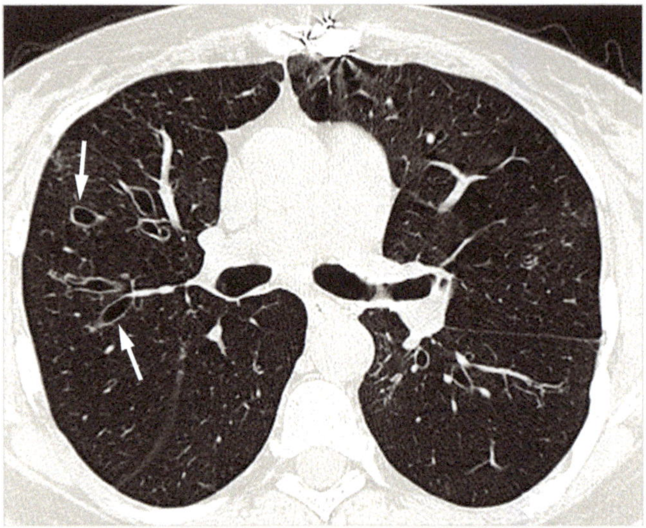

Fig. 10.19 Bronchiolitis obliterans. CT image. Diffusely decreased lung parenchymal density and cylindrical bronchiectasis (*arrows*).

Idiopathic diffuse panbronchiolitis predominantly affects persons of Japanese or Korean origin. It manifests as cough of gradual onset as well as dyspnea, and virtually always, concomitant sinusitis. On CT, a diffuse tree-in-bud pattern is seen, similar to acute infectious bronchiolitis more commonly seen in Europe. But unlike the latter, distribution is ubiquitous.[17]

Collagen vascular diseases, especially rheumatoid arthritis and Sjögren syndrome, also affect the small airways. On histology, Sjögren syndrome is characterized by follicular bronchiolitis, with lymphoid follicles identifiable in the bronchial walls.[22] The main imaging findings are centrilobular nodules and a tree-in-bud pattern, possibly combined with ground-glass opacities and bronchiectasis. It is very difficult to distinguish these findings from infectious complications on imaging. However, the latter will respond to antibiotic treatment.[17]

10.3 Summary

Tracheal stenosis is predominantly benign and usually occurs secondary to chronic pressure alteration of the tracheal wall caused by the cuff of a ventilation tube. Stenosis of the trachea or mainstem bronchi is also caused by inflammatory systemic diseases (e.g., sarcoidosis, granulomatous polyangiitis and Wegner granulomatosis, Crohn disease), infections, or trauma.

The rare *malignant tumors of the trachea* are generally squamous cell or adenoid cystic carcinomas. The associated clinical symptoms are wheezing respiration, dyspnea, dysphagia, or hemoptysis. Despite these tumors manifesting as narrowing of the tracheal lumen on radiography, they are often only retrospectively identified. Endobronchial tumors (malignant or benign, such as lipomas, papillomas, or hamartomas) and *foreign body aspiration* give rise to atelectasis or, less commonly, hyperinflation—both yielding symptoms and salient imaging findings suggestive of bronchus obstruction.

Tracheo- or bronchomalacia often manifests clinically as inspiratory stridor and may be caused by mechanical alteration from long-term intubation or trauma, chondritis, or the pressure exerted by an enlarged thyroid gland. The latter condition can often be inferred from the characteristic radiograph. Radiography and CT demonstrate large changes of airway lumina between inspiration and expiration; an expiratory doubling of the tracheal diameter is suggestive of tracheomalacia.

Inflammatory diseases of the small airways (diameter less than 2 mm) result in the following imaging signs:

- Direct signs: tree-in-bud pattern and centrilobular nodules.
- Indirect signs: mosaic attenuation pattern and diffusely decreased lung parenchymal density.

Air trapping on CT is suggestive of *bronchiolitis* and is easier to identify in expiration than in inspiration. If small airway disease is clinically suspected, inspiratory and expiratory CT scans should therefore be obtained. Infectious bronchiolitis is the most common type of bronchiolitis and is associated with predominantly direct imaging signs. Bronchiolitis obliterans and constrictive bronchiolitis produce indirect signs with air trapping and bronchiectasis. Several causes are known. Bronchiolitis obliterans often occurs as a sequela of viral or mycoplasma pneumonia. Chronic rejection after lung transplant or pulmonary graft-versus-host disease after allogenic stem cell transplant also manifests as bronchiolitis obliterans (see ▸Table 10.2).

References

[1] Kwong JS, Müller NL, Miller RR. Diseases of the trachea and main-stem bronchi: correlation of CT with pathologic findings. Radiographics 1992;12(4):645–657

[2] Prince JS, Duhamel DR, Levin DL, Harrell JH, Friedman PJ. Nonneoplastic lesions of the tracheobronchial wall: radiologic findings with bronchoscopic correlation. Radiographics 2002;22(Spec No):S215–S230

[3] Lee KS, Yoon JH, Kim TK, Kim JS, Chung MP, Kwon OJ. Evaluation of tracheobronchial disease with helical CT with multiplanar and three-dimensional reconstruction: correlation with bronchoscopy. Radiographics 1997;17(3):555–567, discussion 568–570

[4] Haghi Z, Towhidi M, Fattahi H, Lari SM. Right paratracheal air cyst (tracheal diverticulum). Respir Care 2009;54(10):1409–1411

[5] Kokkonouzis I, Haramis D, Kornezos I, Moschouris H, Katsenos S, Boucharas S. Tracheal diverticulum in an asymptomatic male: a case report. Cases J 2008;1(1):181

[6] Chen JD, Shanmuganathan K, Mirvis SE, Killeen KL, Dutton RP. Using CT to diagnose tracheal rupture. AJR Am J Roentgenol 2001;176(5):1273–1280

[7] Ambe P, Weber SA, Schauer M, Knoefel WT. Swallowed foreign bodies in adults. Dtsch Arztebl Int 2012;109(50):869–875

[8] Hitter A, Hullo E, Durand C, Righini CA. Diagnostic value of various investigations in children with suspected foreign body aspiration: review. Eur Ann Otorhinolaryngol Head Neck Dis 2011;128(5):248–252

[9] Dean CW, Speckman JM, Russo JJ. AIRP best cases in radiologic-pathologic correlation: adenoid cystic carcinoma of the trachea. Radiographics 2011;31(5):1443–1447

[10] Choplin RH, Wehunt WD, Theros EG. Diffuse lesions of the trachea. Semin Roentgenol 1983;18(1):38–50

[11] Gamsu G, Webb WR. Computed tomography of the trachea and mainstem bronchi. Semin Roentgenol 1983;18(1):51–60

[12] Onitsuka H, Hirose N, Watanabe K, et al. Computed tomography of tracheopathia osteoplastica. AJR Am J Roentgenol 1983;140(2):268–270

[13] Shepard JO, McLoud TC. Imaging the airways. Computed tomography and magnetic resonance imaging. Clin Chest Med 1991;12(1):151–168

[14] Stein MG, Gamsu G, Webb WR, Stulbarg MS. Computed tomography of diffuse tracheal stenosis in Wegener granulomatosis. J Comput Assist Tomogr 1986;10(5):868–870

[15] Wilcox P, Miller R, Miller G, et al. Airway involvement in ulcerative colitis. Chest 1987;92(1):18–22

[16] Yedururi S, Guillerman RP, Chung T, et al. Multimodality imaging of tracheobronchial disorders in children. Radiographics 2008;28(3):e29

[17] Devakonda A, Raoof S, Sung A, Travis WD, Naidich D. Bronchiolar disorders: a clinical-radiological diagnostic algorithm. Chest 2010;137(4):938–951

[18] Hwang JH, Kim TS, Lee KS, et al. Bronchiolitis in adults: pathology and imaging. J Comput Assist Tomogr 1997;21(6):913–919

[19] Hansell DM. Small airways diseases: detection and insights with computed tomography. Eur Respir J 2001;17(6):1294–1313

[20] Myers JL, Colby TV. Pathologic manifestations of bronchiolitis, constrictive bronchiolitis, cryptogenic organizing pneumonia, and diffuse panbronchiolitis. Clin Chest Med 1993;14(4):611–622

[21] Worthy SA, Müller NL. Small airway diseases. Radiol Clin North Am 1998;36(1):163–173

[22] Burgel PR, Bergeron A, de Blic J, et al. Small airways diseases, excluding asthma and COPD: an overview. Eur Respir Rev 2013;22(128):131–147

[23] Ryu JH, Myers JL, Swensen SJ. Bronchiolar disorders. Am J Respir Crit Care Med 2003;168(11):1277–1292

Chapter 11

Pleural Diseases

11 Pleural Diseases

11.1 Pneumothorax

Note

A pneumothorax is a pathologic accumulation of air in the pleural space which, because of the intrinsic elasticity of the lung, leads to separation of the visceral pleura from the parietal pleura.

The various causes of pneumothorax are summarized in ▶Table 11.1. Spontaneous pneumothorax is differentiated from traumatic, including iatrogenic, pneumothorax.

Small pneumothoraces are often asymptomatic or cause sudden chest pain. Larger pneumothoraces may additionally give rise to dyspnea. A small pneumothorax usually resolves spontaneously within a few days and in general requires no treatment but must be monitored. More rapid absorption of the pleural air is achieved through oxygen insufflation. A chest tube is needed for *larger pneumothoraces.*

Tension pneumothorax is a special form of pneumothorax (▶Fig. 11.1) in which a valve mechanism caused by the air leak in the visceral pleura allows air to escape from the lung into the pleural space in inspiration but not to return to the lung in expiration. This leads to a progressive pressure increase in the affected hemithorax. Mediastinal displacement toward the unaffected side and a low-riding diaphragm on the affected side are seen on chest radiography. Clinically, there is rapid onset of hypotension, tachycardia, dyspnea, and cyanosis. This dramatic situation stems from several pathophysiologic components[4]:

- Loss of ipsilateral, negative intrapleural pressure.
- Mediastinal displacement to the contralateral side with compression of the intrathoracic superior vena cava and kinking at the transition of the inferior vena cava to the right atrium.
- Reduced venous blood return to the heart because of the two aforementioned mechanisms, in turn giving rise to right heart failure.
- Onset of atelectasis with an ensuing increase in the pulmonary shunt volume, leading to hypoxemia, which may result in depression of the respiratory center.

Emergency pressure relief of the affected hemithorax through chest tube placement is needed for newly diagnosed tension pneumothorax. Immediate puncture of the pleural space with an adequately long cannula may help bridge the time until a definitive treatment with chest tube is possible.

11.1.1 Imaging Findings

The radiographic findings of pneumothorax will depend on the imaging position (▶Table 11.2).

The most important criterion for a *standing radiograph* is the ability to identify the visceral pleura, which has separated from the parietal pleura, as a fine linear opacity (▶Fig. 11.3). The

Table 11.1 Causes of pneumothorax[1,2]

Cause	Examples
Spontaneous	• Primary spontaneous pneumothorax (no underlying pulmonary disease): – Bullae or other emphysematous changes – Visceral pleura porosity[2,3] • Secondary spontaneous pneumothorax (with underlying pulmonary disease): – Airway diseases (chronic obstructive pulmonary disease, cystic fibrosis, asthma) – Lung infections (*Pneumocystis jirovecii* pneumonia, necrotizing pneumonia, tuberculosis) – Diffuse parenchymal lung diseases (idiopathic pulmonary fibrosis, sarcoidosis, Langerhans cell histiocytosis, lymphangioleiomyomatosis) – Collagen vascular diseases (rheumatoid arthritis, scleroderma, ankylosing spondylitis) – Malignant tumors (lung cancer, sarcoma, metastasis) • Catamenial pneumothorax (in thoracic endometriosis)
Traumatic	• Penetrating chest trauma • Displaced rib fracture with rupture of the visceral pleura
Iatrogenic	• Transthoracic lung biopsy • Placement of a central venous catheter (subclavian vein) • Thoracentesis • Transbronchial lung biopsy • Pleural biopsy • Positive pressure ventilation • Chest operations

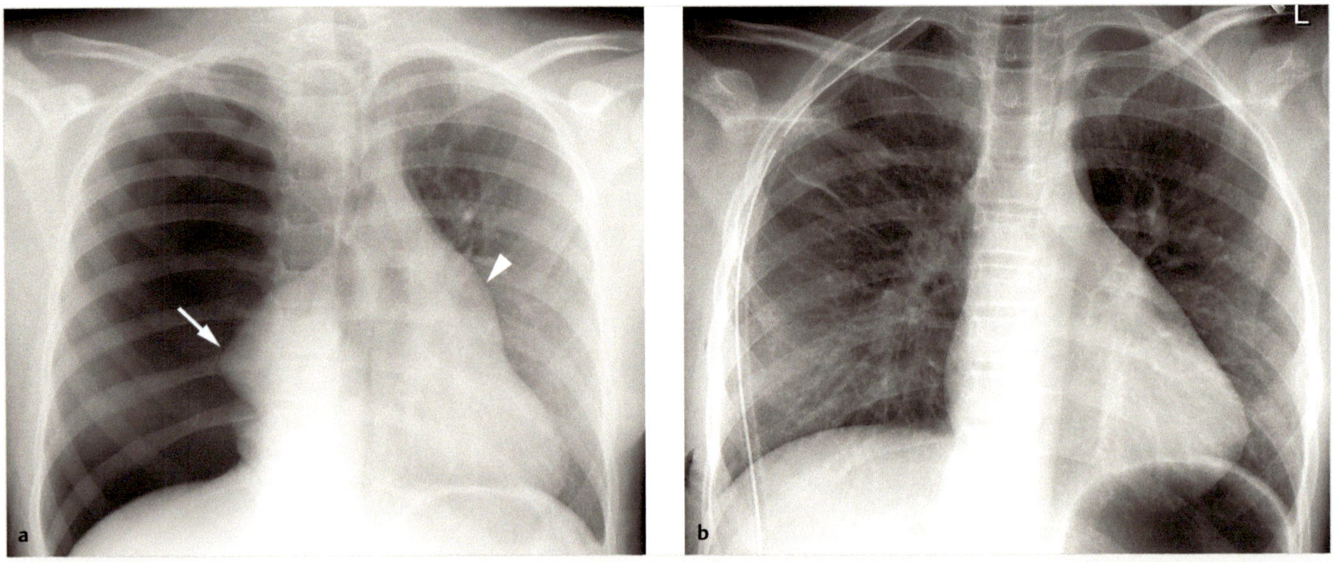

Fig. 11.1 Tension pneumothorax. Radiographs. **(a)** Baseline findings with atelectasis of the right lung (*arrow*), mediastinal displacement to the left and prominent pulmonary trunk as sign of right heart strain (*arrowhead*). **(b)** Normalization of findings following chest tube placement.

space between this line and the chest wall is a more radiolucent and, in general, avascular area (exception: pneumothorax presenting as a backdrop anterior or posterior to the fully inflated lung lobe). Lung adhesions to the chest wall may occur.

Note

Expiratory radiographs as customarily obtained in the past for diagnostic imaging of pneumothorax have no relevant diagnostic advantages over those obtained in inspiration.[5,6] Furthermore, expiratory radiographs hamper diagnostic exploration of pulmonary opacities (e.g., lung contusions in suspected traumatic pneumothorax) and make it harder to compare previous or follow-up inspiratory images. Therefore, inspiratory radiographs should, generally, be used for diagnostic imaging of pneumothorax.

Because the patient is lying down, *supine radiographs* result in an anterior pleural air collection that hampers direct detection of a visceral pleural line since often the lung abuts the lateral chest wall. Hence, diagnosis is based on indirect signs of air in the pleural space as presented in ▶Table 11.2.

Table 11.2 Projection radiography findings of pneumothorax

Standing PA radiograph	Supine PA radiograph
Visible pleural line	Heart border and mediastinum sharply delineated
Increased radiolucency between lung and chest wall	Increased radiolucency of one lung
Vasculature cannot be identified between the lung and chest wall	More radiolucent, broader and lower costophrenic angle (deep sulcus sign, ▶Fig. 11.2)

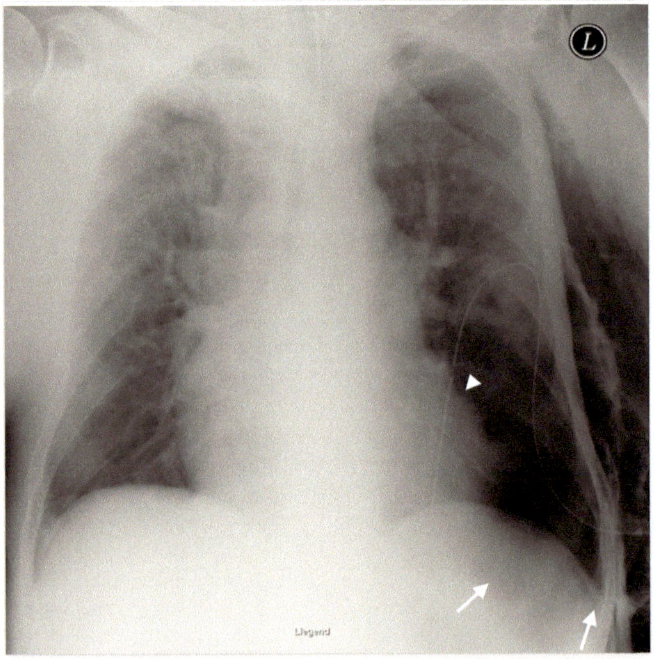

Fig. 11.2 Pneumothorax. Radiograph, supine position. Compared with the right side, increased radiolucency of the left lung, more clearly delineated left heart border (*arrowhead*) and more radiolucent as well as lower left costophrenic angle–deep sulcus sign (*arrows*). Besides, chest tube on the left.

Computed tomography (CT) has greater sensitivity than radiography for diagnosis of smaller pneumothoraces. It is even able to reliably detect pneumothorax in cases where the radiograph was inconclusive, e.g., because of chest wall emphysema. CT often provides additional information on the etiology of spontaneous pneumothorax and in many cases contributes to diagnosis and differential diagnosis of pulmonary causes (▶Fig. 11.4). The indications for CT are listed in ▶Table 11.3.

11.1.2 Differential Diagnosis

In the presence of bullous pulmonary emphysema, it may be difficult to reliably differentiate between an *emphysematous bulla and* pneumothorax since both entities manifest as an avascular space. CT is useful in such cases; to that effect, the visceral pleura should be identified to differentiate between a pleural (pneumothorax) and subpleural (emphysematous bulla) location of the air.

Skin folds can mimic pneumothorax on supine radiographs, less commonly on standing radiographs (▶Fig. 11.5). The key criteria for this *pseudopneumothorax* are vascular structures between the presumed pleural line and chest wall as well as disappearance of the presumed pleural line in the middle of the lung or its extension beyond the border of the hemithorax.

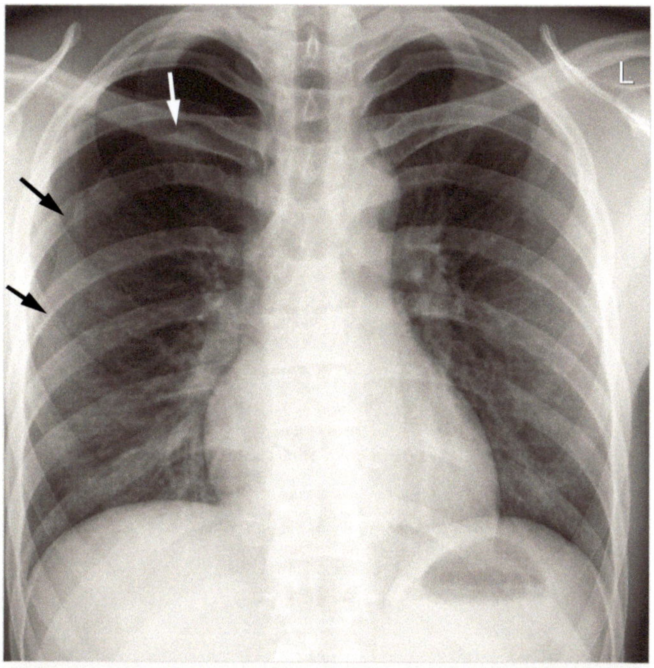

Fig. 11.3 Spontaneous pneumothorax. Radiograph. Visible pleural line, consistent with the visceral pleura (*arrows*). Between the pleural line and chest wall a more radiolucent and avascular space.

Table 11.3 CT indication for pneumothorax[7]

Indications	Remarks
Primary spontaneous pneumothorax	CT is generally not indicated for first-time pneumothorax; it can be useful for recurrent pneumothorax or clinically suspected underlying pulmonary disease that cannot be identified on a radiograph
Secondary and catamenial pneumothorax	CT is generally not indicated for first-time pneumothorax; it can be useful for recurrent pneumothorax, for persistent air leak with drainage or for preoperative management
Traumatic pneumothorax	CT is usually performed in any case as part of the diagnostic trauma work-up; however, in the presence of isolated rib fractures, pneumothorax requiring treatment can be reliably excluded with a radiograph
Iatrogenic pneumothorax	No CT indication

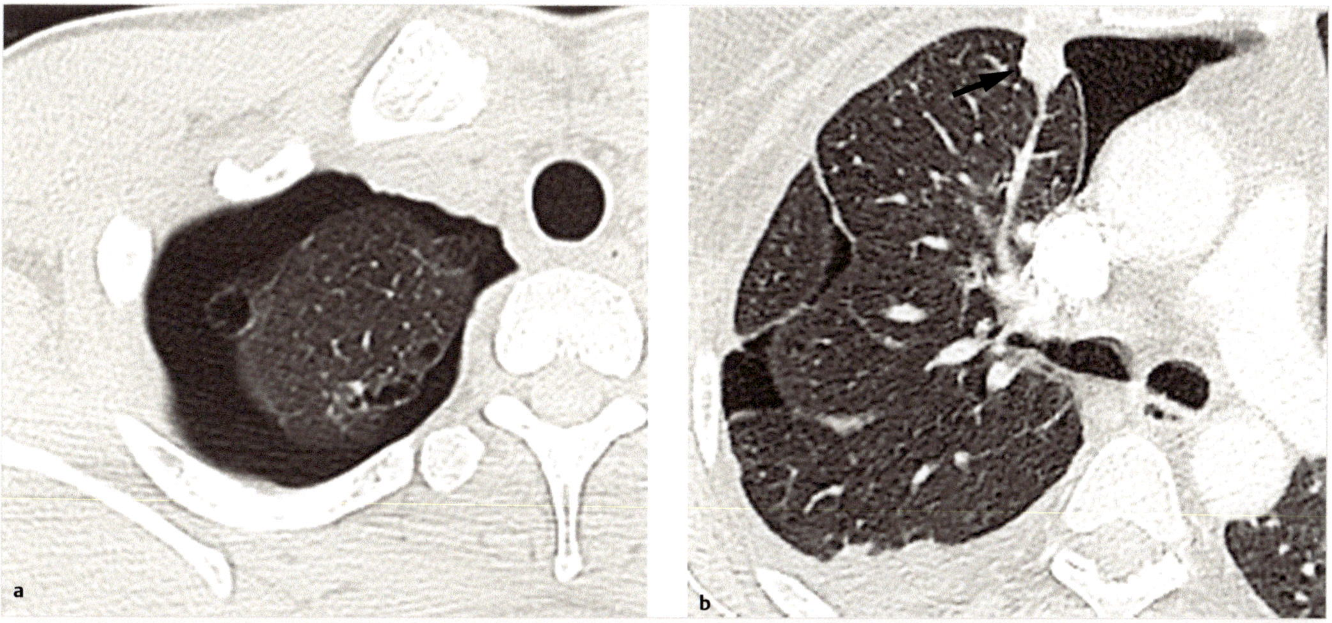

Fig. 11.4 Spontaneous pneumothorax. Examples of causes to be diagnosed on CT. **(a)** Right apical emphysematous bullae (same patient as in ▶Fig. 11.3). **(b)** Catamenial pneumothorax with pleural-based endometriosis nodule (*arrow*). Besides, minor pleural effusion.

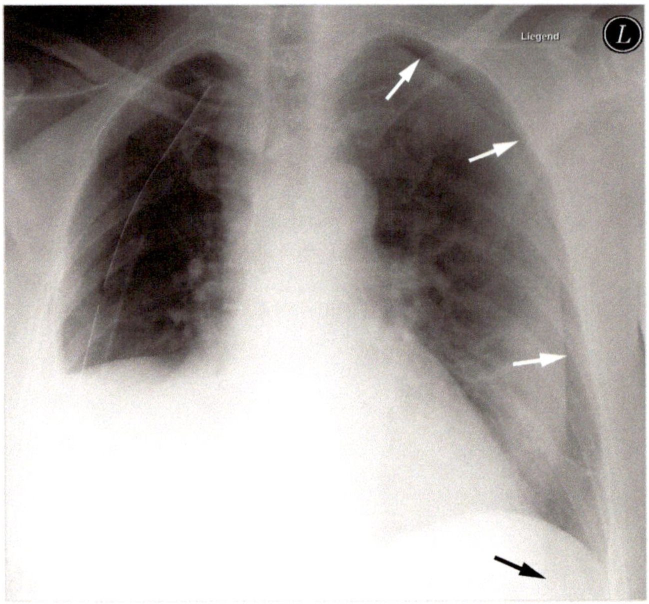

Fig. 11.5 Left pseudopneumothorax (skin fold). Radiograph, supine position. Line running in caudal direction superior to the diaphragmatic contour (*arrows*), mimicking a pleural line. Besides, chest tube after right lower lobe resection.

11.2 Pleural Effusion

Pleural effusions are caused by many pathologic conditions (▶Table 11.4). A distinction is made between transudates and exudates on the basis of their origin. Transudates stem from passive filtration of serous fluid into the pleural space, whereas exudates derive from secretion of protein-rich fluid. This distinction can be made through simple laboratory tests of pleural fluid. The effusion is classified as an exudate if at least one of the following criteria is met[8]:

- A pleural fluid-to-serum protein ratio greater than 0.5.
- A pleural fluid-to-serum lactate dehydrogenase level (LDH) ratio greater than 0.6.
- A pleural fluid LDH of more than two-thirds of maximum normal serum LDH.

Likewise, other fluids (e.g., blood, pus, or chyle) manifest as pleural effusion on imaging.

Cross-sectional imaging, particularly ultrasound, is most sensitive for detection of pleural effusion. Lateral radiographs demonstrate pleural effusions larger than 50 mL, which are initially seen as opacification of the posterior costodiaphragmatic angle. Pleural effusions larger than 100 mL are visible on posteroanterior (PA) radiographs in the lateral costodiaphragmatic angle. Because of geometric projection conditions, pleural effusions appear meniscus-shaped in standing radiographs (▶Fig. 11.6).

In supine radiographs, pleural effusion is located posterior to the lungs and is distributed more or less evenly in the chest cavity, thus causing only diffusely reduced radiolucency of the affected hemithorax. Even several hundred milliliters of pleural effusion can be overlooked in supine radiographs.

Table 11.4 Pathogenesis of pleural effusion[9]

Mechanism		Examples
Elevated fluid secretion into the pleural cavity	Increased interstitial fluid in the lung	Congestive left heart failure, pneumonia, pulmonary embolism
	Elevated intravascular pressure in the pleura	Congestive left heart failure Congestive right heart failure Superior vena cava syndrome
	Elevated capillary permeability	Pleuritis
	Elevated protein content of pleural fluid	Pulmonary edema, hemothorax
	Reduced pressure in the pleural space	Atelectasis
	Increased fluid in the peritoneum	Ascites, peritoneal dialysis
	Rupture of the thoracic duct	Chylothorax
	Rupture of thoracic blood vessels	Hematothorax
Reduced pleural fluid absorption	Obstruction of parietal pleura lymph drainage	Malignant tumor, lymphoma
	Elevated systemic venous pressure	Congestive right heart failure, superior vena cava syndrome

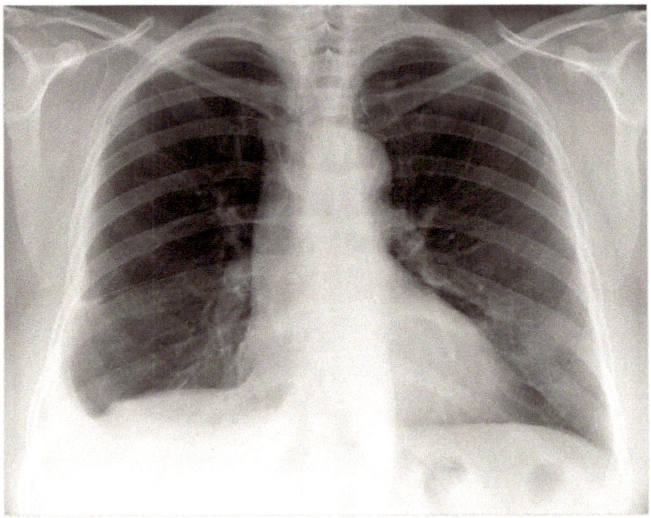

Fig. 11.6 Right pleural effusion. Radiograph. Meniscus-shaped opacity of the right lateral costophrenic angle.

A subpulmonary pleural effusion occasionally mimics a high-riding diaphragm and can be suspected if the highest point of the diaphragm is located lateral to its middle. Isolated interlobular effusions sometimes present as well-defined oval pulmonary opacities on radiography. These are known as "vanishing tumors" since they tend to migrate and disappear within a few days.

11.3 Pleural Empyema

Pleural empyema is an infection of the pleural cavity usually manifesting as pathologic pleural fluid collection. This is often caused by pneumonia, with the infection spreading secondarily into the pleural space, giving rise to an independent disease process. Less commonly, pathogens use other portals of entry, for example, a perforated lung tumor in the pleural space, following chest injury or as a complication of a surgical procedure. Pleural empyema is distinguished from a noninfected pleural effusion through laboratory analysis of the pleural fluid.[10] A summary of the criteria used to differentiate between pleural empyema and noninfected pleural effusion is given in ▶Table 11.5. The most commonly implicated pathogens are gram-negative bacteria as well as *Staphylococcus aureus* and anaerobes.[11] Tuberculosis, too, can give rise to pleural empyema. The continuous development of a chest wall abscess from a pleural empyema is known as "empyema necessitatis" (or "empyema necessitans"), which is often but not exclusively seen in mycobacterial infection.

Pleural empyema consists of three phases[10]:

- *Exudative phase*: In the visceral pleura, the inflammatory process leads to increased capillary permeability, and consecutively to exudation of protein-rich fluid into the pleural space causing an exudative pleural effusion. There is still no sign of pleural thickening.
- *Fibrinopurulent phase*: In the later course, inflammatory cells and neutrophils migrate into the pleural fluid, and fibrin is deposited on the pleural surfaces, causing thickening of the visceral and parietal pleura.
- *Organizing phase*: Fibroblast activity and capillary neogenesis lead to collagen deposition and ingrowth of granulation tissue on the pleural surfaces, and subsequent pleural fibrosis. This reaction can be very intense and lead to development of extensive pleural thickening.

Treatment is tailored to the cause and stage of pleural empyema. The underlying cause is treated whenever possible. The specific treatment for pleural empyema in the exudative phase usually consists of chest tube placement and appropriate antibiotic treatment. More advanced pleural empyema, in particular in the presence of pleural thickening, requires surgical decortication.

The imaging findings correlate to these three phases.[10] In the exudative phase, it is impossible to radiologically distinguish empyema from noninfected effusion. However, if pleural effusion has occurred secondary to pneumonia, the following constellation of findings suggests parapneumonic empyema:

- A large pleural effusion that occurs, with delay, after pneumonia.
- Persistently high or increasing clinical and laboratory signs of inflammation, despite pneumonia having already resolved.
- Deterioration of the patient's general condition after initial improvement.

In the fibrinopurulent phase, thickening and contrast enhancement of the visceral and parietal pleura can usually be clearly identified on CT (▶Fig. 11.7). This suggests empyema and is known as a *split pleura sign*.[12] The pleural fluid collection is often lentiform. Radiography may show that the pleural effusion is not free flowing but rather appears encapsulated and localized.

The organizing phase is characterized by increasing thickening of the pleural layers on CT. The empyema may exhibit higher CT density values than water. Septa can be visualized well on ultrasound, at times also on CT (▶Fig. 11.8).

Often, in addition to the findings associated with pleural empyema, its cause can also be identified on imaging, e.g., an adjacent pulmonary consolidation in parapneumonic empyema or a necrotic disintegrating tumor that has penetrated into the pleural space (see ▶Fig. 11.7).

Differentiation of pleural empyema from a lung abscess may be challenging. An acute angle between the pulmonary consolidation and visceral pleura points to an abscess (▶Fig. 11.9); furthermore, on CT lung abscesses are usually more rounded and exhibit a thicker, contrast-enhancing wall.[13] A noninfected pleural effusion cannot be distinguished on imaging from an incipient pleural empyema in the exudative phase. In such cases, thoracentesis will help make that distinction as per the criteria listed in ▶Table 11.5.

Table 11.5 Differentiation between pleural empyema and noninfected pleural effusion in a fluid sample obtained from thoracentesis.[10] One positive criterion suffices for diagnosis of pleural empyema

Parameter	Pleural empyema	Simple pleural effusion
pH	< 7.2	≥ 7.2
Glucose	< 40 mg/dL	≥ 40 mg/dL
^{LDH}**Effusion**/^{LDH}**serum**	> 0.6 or LDH > two-thirds of normal serum level	≤ 0.6 or LDH ≤ two-thirds of normal serum level
Detection of bacteria in culture or on microscopy	+	–
Purulence	+	–
Neutrophils in effusion	+	–

Abbreviation: LDH, lactate dehydrogenase.

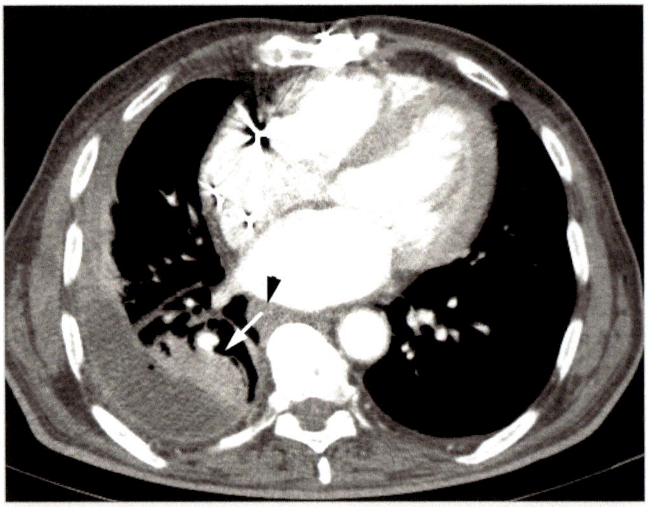

Fig. 11.7 **Right posterior parapneumonic pleural empyema.** CT image. Thickened parietal and visceral pleura with contrast enhancement (split pleura sign). This is caused by pneumonia of the right lower lobe (*arrow*) with reactive mediastinal lymphadenopathy (*arrowhead*). Besides, left pleural thickening with small calcifications.

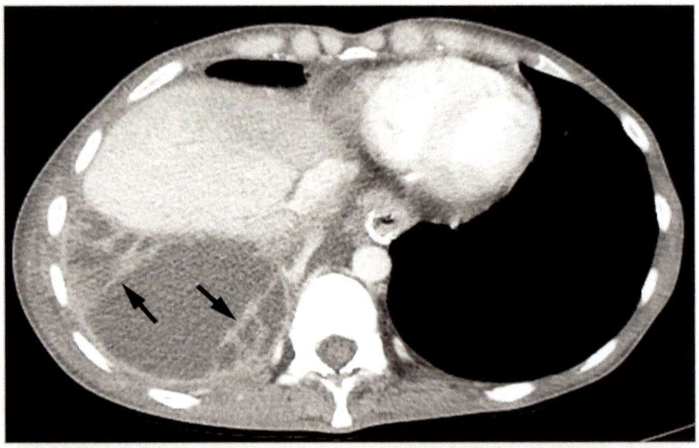

Fig. 11.8 **Right posterior chronic pleural empyema.** CT image. Thickened parietal and visceral pleura and prominent septa within empyema (*arrows*).

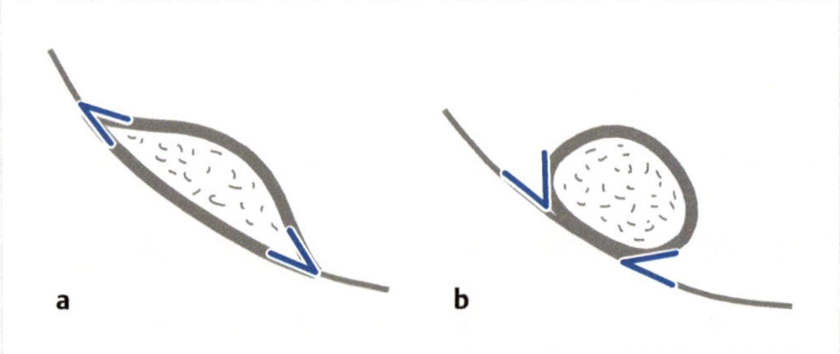

Fig. 11.9 **Differentiation between pleural and intrapulmonary findings.** Schematic diagram. **(a)** Pleural empyema: thickened parietal and visceral pleura, acute angle (*blue markings*). **(b)** Lung abscess: thick-walled lung abscess, obtuse angle (*blue markings*).

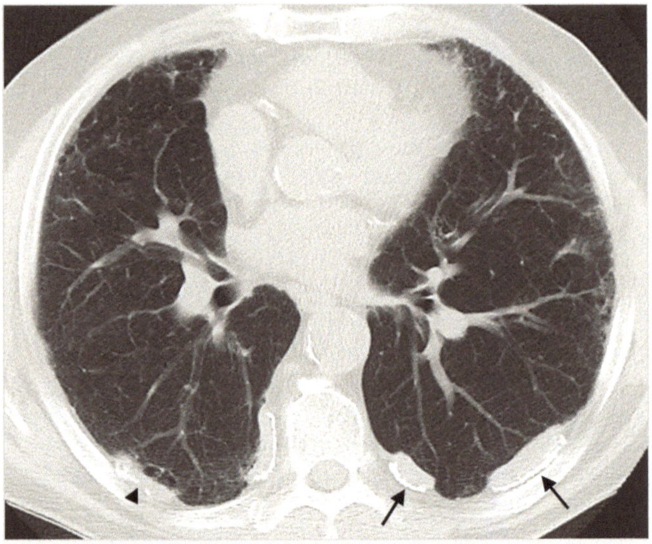

Fig. 11.10 **Pleural plaques.** CT image. Left parietal, table mountain-like calcified pleural plaques (*arrows*) and right visceral pleural thickening with adjacent opacities of lung parenchyma (*arrowhead*). Furthermore, bilateral subpleural intralobular lines consistent with asbestosis.

11.4 Pleural Fibrosis

11.4.1 Pleural Plaques

Discrete areas of hyaline or calcified fibrosis, usually located in the parietal pleura, are known as pleural plaques. These predominantly affect the costal and diaphragmatic, less often the mediastinal, pleura. A characteristic finding is their anterolateral distribution along the costal pleura in the middle lung zones and paravertebral distribution in the lower zones.[14]

At least 80% of all pleural plaques are attributable to asbestos exposure. Likewise, parietal pleural plaques are the most common asbestos-induced pathologic changes in the body. They have a typical latency period of more than 20 years following exposure. Based on their CT morphology, distinctions are made based on whether pleural plaques exhibit a table mountain-like appearance. Other appearances include thickening at the level of the pleura or spindle-shaped thickening of the parietal pleura. These findings are considered less specific to asbestos exposure than the table mountain-like appearance. Whereas parietal pleural plaques can be clearly delineated from the lung tissue, adjacent pulmonary opacities can be seen in the region of visceral pleural thickening (see Section 11.4.2) (▶Fig. 11.10). These findings, too, have lower specificity for asbestos exposure.[15]

Note

Asbestos-induced pleural and pulmonary findings:

- Bilateral, calcified parietal pleural plaques:
  - Table mountain-like.
  - Not table mountain-like.
- Unilateral, calcified parietal pleural plaques: table mountain-like.
- Bilateral noncalcified, parietal pleural plaques:
  - Table mountain-like.
  - Not table mountain-like.
- Unilateral, calcified parietal pleural plaques: not table mountain-like.
- Unilateral, noncalcified parietal pleural plaques:
  - Table mountain-like.
  - Not table mountain-like.
- Visceral pleural thickening.
- Rounded atelectasis.
- Pleural effusion.

The presentation order reflects declining specificity of the findings for asbestos exposure.[15]

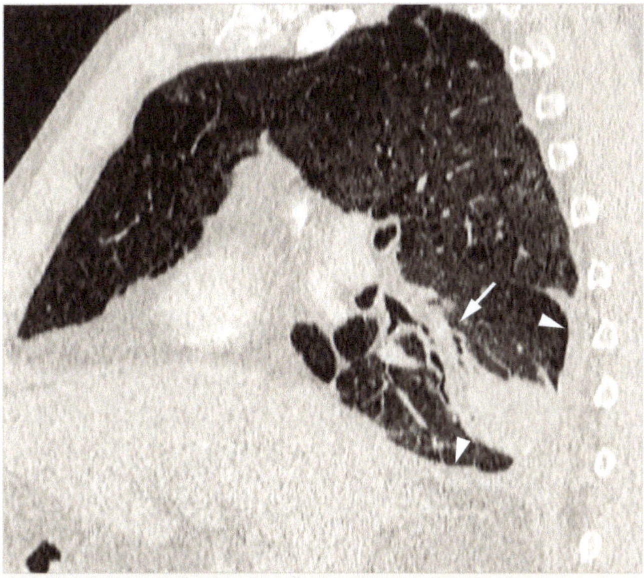

Fig. 11.11 Pleural thickening (*arrowheads*) and rounded atelectasis with hilipetal lines resembling a comet tail (*arrow*). CT image, sagittal.

The implications of pleural plaques for diagnosis and evaluation of occupational lung diseases are described in detail in Chapter 18.

11.4.2 Pleural Thickening

Pleural thickening reflects remnants of resolved pleuritis. The underlying inflammation usually originates in the lung. Pleural thickening is observed in up to 10% of postmortem examinations.[16] Extensive pleural thickening can cause restricted lung function.

Common causes of pleural thickening are shown in ▸Table 11.6. Bilateral pleural thickening is suggestive of asbestos exposure even if the radiograph does not show any other findings. Often, the pleural plaques serving as diagnostic pointers are seen only on CT.

Radiography and CT demonstrate diffuse pleural thickening. It may be difficult in individual cases to differentiate pleural thickening from pleural effusion on radiography. If clinically indicated, ultrasound or a radiograph in lateral decubitus position can help distinguish effusion from solid pleural thickening. Usually, pleural thickening is more radiolucent than pleural effusion on a PA radiograph since it has less sagittal extension.

Extensive pleural thickening involving the visceral pleura may result in hypoaeration of the adjacent lung parenchyma, a condition known as *rounded atelectasis*. An almost triangular, pleura-based consolidation with smooth margins can be seen on imaging. Characteristic hilipetal linear opacities, resembling a comet tail, are often seen on CT and are suggestive of rounded atelectasis (▸Fig. 11.11).

Pleural thickening tends to calcify. Bilateral *calcifications* are expected, in particular, in association with asbestos exposure, whereas unilateral calcifications are more common in chronic pleural empyema, calcified tuberculous pleurisy, or resolved hemothorax.

For differential diagnosis, benign pleural thickening must be distinguished from pleural carcinosis or pleural mesothelioma (see below). A typical feature of benign pleural thickening is the smooth surface without any nodular solid components and no contrast enhancement on CT.

Table 11.6 Common causes of pleural thickening[16]

Cause	Comments
Pneumonia	Status post pleuritis, often following resolved pneumonia
Tuberculosis	Status post tuberculous pleuritis, calcified tuberculous pleurisy, usually with extensive calcification
Asbestos exposure	Status post asbestos pleuritis, hyalinosis complicata; pleural plaques, often bilateral, serve as additional diagnostic pointers
Chest trauma	Status post hemothorax; ipsilateral, old rib fractures or pulmonary scarring are additional diagnostic pointers
Surgery	Postoperative following cardiac surgery, partial lung resection, decortication or pleurodesis

11.5 Pleural Tumors

The obtuse angle criterion may be useful for differentiation between a pleural and an intrapulmonary peripheral tumor (see ▸Fig. 11.9). Pleural tumors generally have obtuse angles, whereas intrapulmonary tumors originating from the pleura have acute angles. But as an exception to that, certain portions of large pleural tumors do have an acute angle but not across their entire circumference (see ▸Fig. 11.19).

11.5.1 Lipoma

Pleural lipomas originate from the fatty tissue of the parietal pleura deep to the mesothelium and extend into the pleural space and the extrapleural tissue. They are slow-growing soft, encapsulated, fat-containing benign lesions. Occasionally, lipomas also present at the diaphragm, in particular in the posterolateral portion (▸Fig. 11.12). They are usually asymptomatic incidental findings. Rarely, there is unproductive cough, back pain, and exertional dyspnea, especially in association with large lipomas.[17,18]

On radiography, lipomas manifest as relatively radiolucent opacities (▸Fig. 11.13a) that can become extremely large. On CT, lipomas can be seen as smoothly marginated, pleural-based masses that exhibit homogeneous fat-equivalent density of about −100 HU (▸Fig. 11.13b).[18]

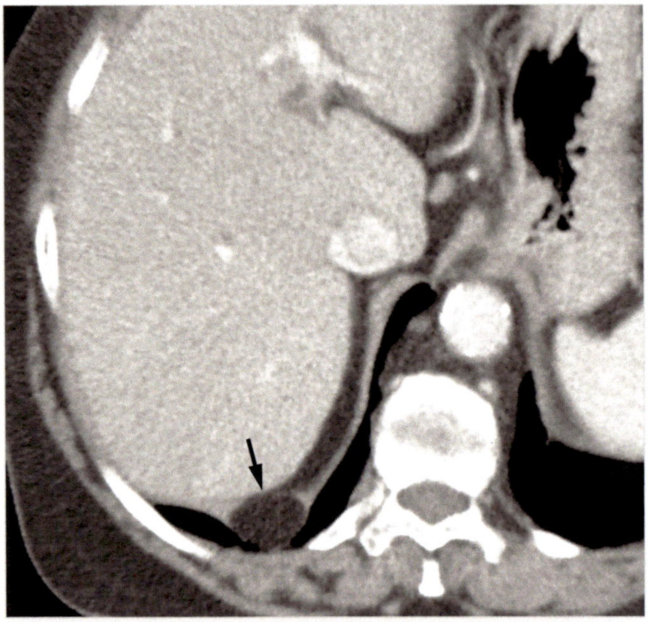

Fig. 11.12 Lipoma originating from the diaphragm (*arrow*). CT image.

When located close to the diaphragm, diaphragmatic hernias which also exhibit fat density on CT should be included in differential diagnosis (Morgagni and Bochdalek hernias).[17]

11.5.2 Pleural Mesothelioma

Mesothelioma is a rare malignant tumor that usually originates from the pleura, less commonly from the pericardium or peritoneum. Up to 90% of pleural mesotheliomas are caused by asbestos exposure.[16] Asbestos was used on a large scale in the construction industry, in particular in the 1960s and 1970s. Since the latency period between asbestos exposure and development of a clinically manifest tumor can be several decades, an increased incidence of pleural mesotheliomas can still be expected even though industrial asbestos use has been banned in many countries.

In general, the tumor clinically manifests with dyspnea, chest pain, cough, and weight loss. The parietal and visceral pleura may be affected by the tumor, and it often invades the adjacent structures of the chest wall and diaphragm. The median survival of only 12 months after diagnosis underlines the poor prognosis of pleural mesotheliomas.[19]

Often, the first manifestation of pleural mesothelioma on imaging is a unilateral pleural effusion, possibly with concomitant chest pain. In early stages, no imaging modality is able to visualize the tumor (▸Fig. 11.14). Therefore, thoracoscopy should be performed to explore a unilateral pleural effusion of unknown etiology. Later stages exhibit isolated solid pleural tumor nodules (▸Fig. 11.15) or diffuse irregular pleural thickening (▸Fig. 11.16). Often, the tumor spreads by direct

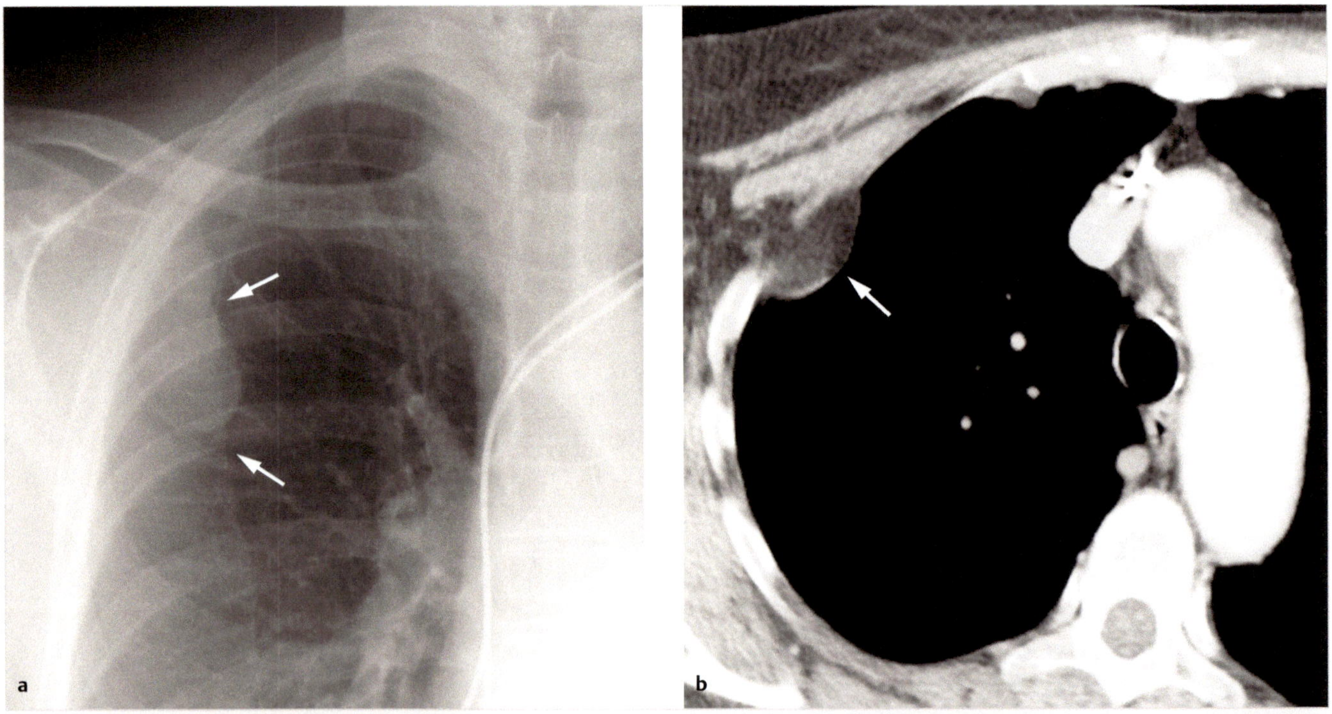

Fig. 11.13 Pleural lipoma (*arrows*). (a) Magnified section of radiograph. **(b)** CT image.

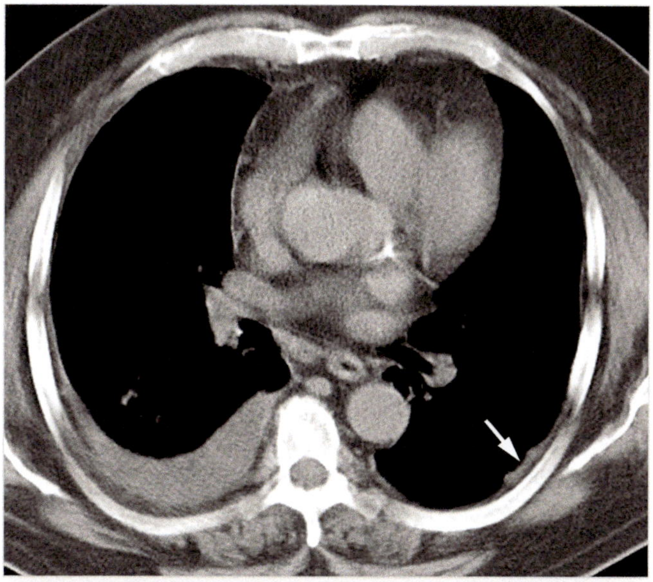

Fig. 11.14 Right pleural mesothelioma CT image. Only right pleural effusion, no evidence of solid tumor manifestations. Besides, left parietal pleural plaque in association with benign asbestos-induced pleural disease (*arrow*).

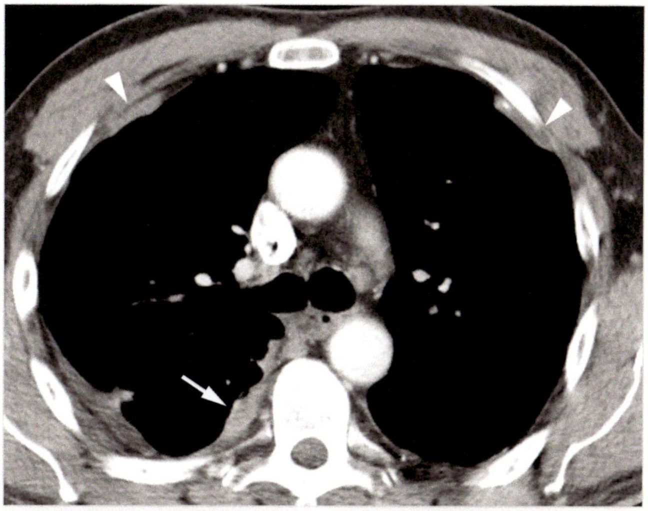

Fig. 11.15 Right pleural mesothelioma. CT image. Right posterior (*arrow*) contrast-enhanced tumor nodule and minor right pleural effusion. Besides, bilateral parietal pleural plaques in association with benign asbestos-induced pleural disease (*arrowheads*).

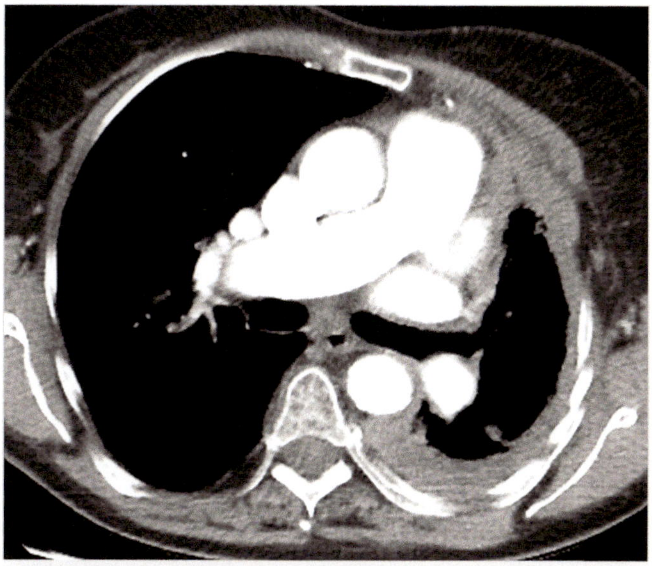

Fig. 11.16 Left pleural mesothelioma. CT image. Diffuse solid, contrast-enhancing tumor of the left pleura, resulting in considerable shrinkage of the left hemithorax.

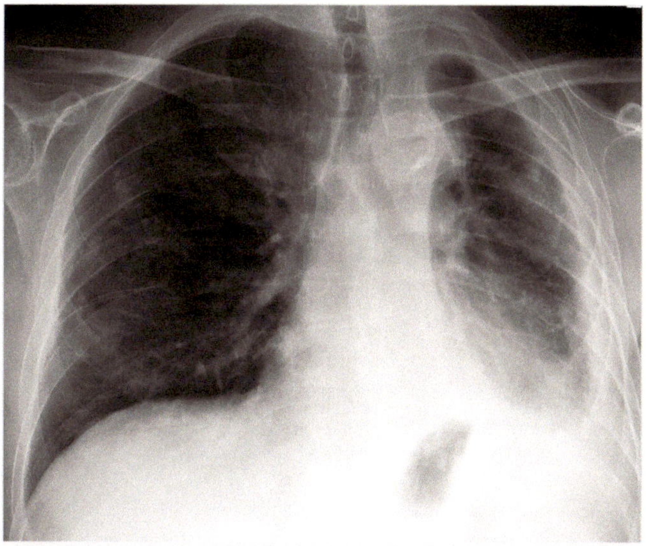

Fig. 11.17 Left pleural mesothelioma. Radiograph. Considerable volume loss of the left hemithorax and diffuse left pleural thickening.

extension into the surrounding structures, growing transdiaphragmatically into the abdominal cavity.[19] This tumor entity is characterized by pronounced fibrotic shrinkage, and at times, with considerable volume loss of the affected hemithorax (► Fig. 11.17). While asbestos causes the vast majority of pleural mesotheliomas, pleural plaques are visible only in 20% of cases.[20]

Note

Pleural mesothelioma tends to grow along any needle tracts of earlier percutaneous biopsy or along the course of a previous chest tube.[21] Irradiation of these tracts is aimed at preventing further tumor growth along this course.[22]

II

CT imaging of the chest and the entire abdomen (including the pelvis) is needed for staging of pleural mesothelioma. The TNM system presented in ▶Table 11.7 is used; the tumor stage is derived as shown in ▶Table 11.8. In individual cases, MRI yields valuable information on local tumor extension, in particular on the presence and extent of invasion of surrounding structures, such as the chest wall, mediastinum, and diaphragm.[19]

Treatment response is usually monitored with CT using a modified version of the RECIST criteria (modified RECIST [Modified Response Evaluation Criteria in Solid Tumors]): tumor thickness is measured at two sites on three axial CT slices.[24]

A reduced volume of the affected hemithorax is used for differential diagnosis of pleural mesothelioma versus pleural carcinosis. By contrast, pleural carcinosis usually results in increased volume due to the presence of solid tumors and pleural effusion.

Table 11.7 Clinical TNM staging of pleural mesotheliomas[23]

Descriptors	Definitions
T descriptor (tumor extension)	
T1	
• T1a	Tumor limited to the ipsilateral parietal ± mediastinal ±diaphragmatic pleura; no involvement of the visceral pleura
• T1b	Tumor involving the ipsilateral parietal ± mediastinal ±diaphragmatic pleura with scattered foci of tumor also involving the visceral pleura
T2	Tumor involving each of the ipsilateral pleural surfaces (parietal, visceral, mediastinal, diaphragmatic) with extension into the diaphragmatic muscle and/or extension of tumor from visceral pleura into the underlying pulmonary parenchyma
T3	Describes locally advanced but potentially resectable tumor involving all of the ipsilateral pleural surfaces (parietal, visceral, mediastinal, diaphragmatic) with at least one of the following features: • involvement of the endothoracic fascia • extension into the mediastinal fat • solitary, completely resectable focus of tumor extending into the soft tissues of the chest wall • nontransmural involvement of the pericardium
T4	Describes locally advanced technically unresectable tumor involving all of the ipsilateral pleural surfaces (parietal, visceral, mediastinal, diaphragmatic) with at least one of the following features: • Diffuse extension or multifocal masses of tumor in the chest wall, with or without associated rib destruction • Direct transdiaphragmatic extension of tumor to the peritoneum • Direct extension of tumor to the contralateral pleura • Direct extension of tumor to one or more mediastinal organs • Direct extension of tumor into the spine • Tumor extending through to the internal surface of the pericardium with or without a pericardial effusion; or tumor involving the myocardium
N descriptor (lymph node metastasis)	
NX	Regional lymph nodes cannot be assessed
N0	No regional lymph node metastases
N1	Metastases in the ipsilateral bronchopulmonary or hilar lymph nodes
N2	Metastases in the subcarinal or the ipsilateral mediastinal lymph nodes, including the ipsilateral internal mammary nodes
N3	Metastases in the contralateral mediastinal, contralateral internal mammary, ipsilateral, or contralateral supraclavicular lymph nodes
M descriptor (distant metastasis)	
MX	Presence of distant metastases cannot be assessed
M0	No distant metastasis
M1	Distant metastasis present

11.5.3 Solitary Fibrous Pleural Tumor

Like pleural mesotheliomas, solitary fibrous (pleural) tumors (SFTs) are of mesenchymal origin and can develop in both the parietal and visceral pleura. Around half of SFTs have a pedicle. The vast majority of tumors are every large when diagnosed. This tumor is found particularly in elderly patients, but SFTs are often asymptomatic. Typical symptoms may include dyspnea, chest pain, and cough. Three-quarters of SFTs are found on histology to be benign, and one-quarter malignant.[25] Initially benign SFTs may undergo secondary malignancy, especially recurrent tumors. The prognosis for complete tumor resection is generally favorable but malignant SFTs can metastasize.

On imaging, SFTs usually present as a well-defined, often lobulated mass in the lower half of the thorax; when located in basal chest regions, they can mimic a high-riding diaphragm (▶Fig. 11.18). Pleural effusion may occur in association with both malignant and benign SFTs. On CT, large SFTs, unlike their smaller counterparts, exhibit inhomogeneous density, and at times calcifications can be identified in the mass (▶Fig. 11.19). Usually, the presence of a pedicle cannot be visualized on CT. Chest wall invasion is rare; nor is lymphadenopathy expected in association with SFT. Large SFTs frequently give rise to compression atelectasis of the surrounding lung tissues but do not invade these. It is impossible to reliably distinguish between benign and malignant SFTs on imaging; a surgical specimen is needed to that effect.[25]

Table 11.8 Tumor stages of pleural mesotheliomas based on the TNM tumor formula[23]

Stages	T	N	M
IA	T1a	N0	M0
IB	T1b	N0	M0
II	T2	N0	M0
III	T3	N0	M0
	T1–3	N1	M0
	T1–3	N2	M0
IV	T4	N0	M0
	Any T	N3	M0
	Any T	Any N	M1

11.5.4 Pleural Carcinosis

Numerous malignant primary tumors can cause pleural carcinosis[14,26,27]:

- Lung cancer, in particular, pulmonary adenocarcinoma.
- Breast cancer.
- Thymic carcinoma.
- Ovarian cancer.
- Pancreatic cancer.
- Thyroid cancer.
- Gastrointestinal cancer.
- Renal cell carcinoma.

Pleural carcinosis is much more common than primary malignant pleural tumors. The tumor cells are spread either by direct extension, via the pleural cavity, hematogenously or along the pleural lymphatic system.[14]

The most common manifestation of pleural carcinosis on radiography is usually a unilateral pleural effusion, which may be very large. Solid, pleural-based masses can be identified as hemispherical, pleural-based opacities.

CT is more sensitive than radiography in visualizing solid tumors and smaller pleural effusions. In addition to the effusion, it shows diffuse pleural thickening (▶Fig. 11.20) or isolated to multiple, pleural-based, contrast-enhancing masses (▶Fig. 11.21). Occasionally, only solid pleural tumors and no effusion may be observed (▶Fig. 11.22).

Differential diagnosis includes pleural mesothelioma; sometimes, it is not possible to distinguish between pleural

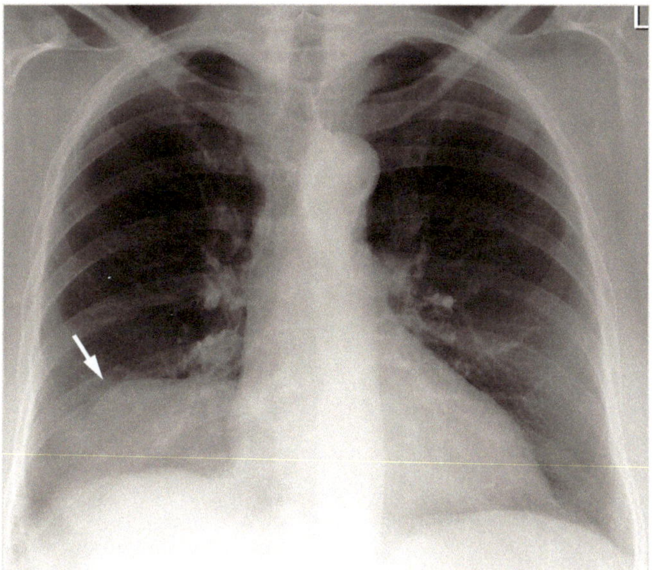

Fig. 11.18 Solitary fibrous pleural tumor. Radiograph. Right basal, smoothly marginated mass (*arrow*), mimicking a high-riding diaphragm.

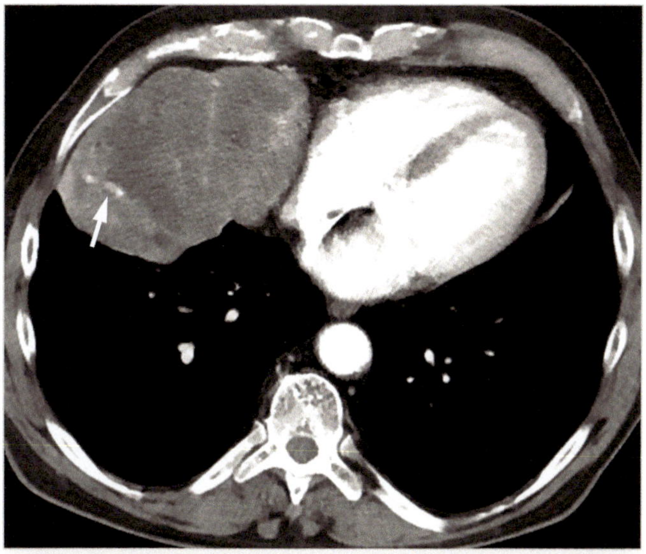

Fig. 11.19 Solitary fibrous pleural tumor. CT image. Smoothly marginated, lobulated pleural mass of inhomogeneous density and with small calcifications (*arrow*).

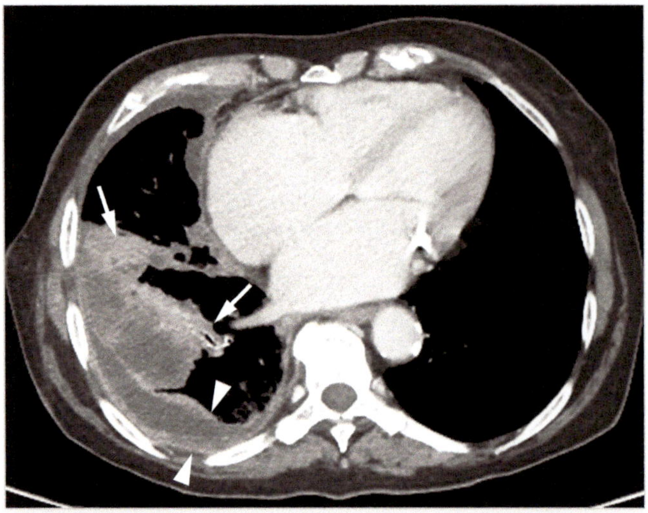

Fig. 11.20 Right pleural carcinosis. CT image. Minor pleural effusion and diffuse thickening of the parietal and visceral pleura (*arrowheads*). Besides, lung cancer in the right lower lobe with extensive necrosis (*arrows*).

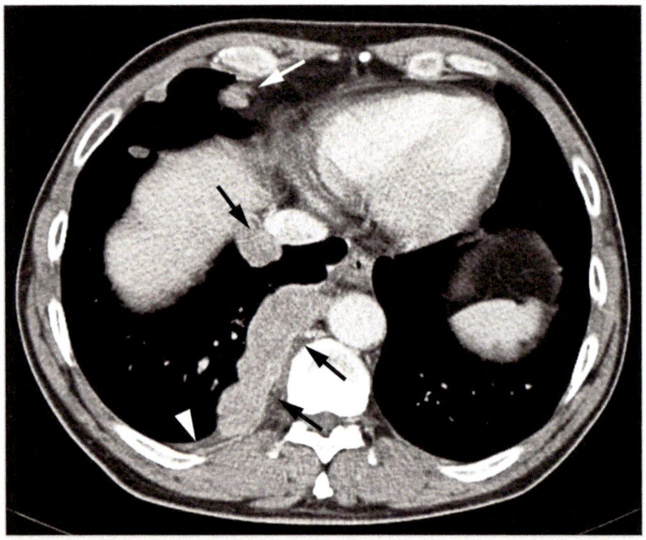

Fig. 11.22 Right pleural carcinosis. CT image. Multiple, pleural-based, contrast-enhanced masses (*arrows*), but almost no pleural effusion (*arrowhead*).

mesothelioma and pleural carcinosis on radiography, or on CT.[28] Whereas mesothelioma is associated with volume loss of the affected hemithorax, pleural carcinosis usually has a space-occupying effect due to the pleural effusion. Furthermore, the patient history often reports an extrapleural primary tumor. If no solid pleural tumor manifestations can be demonstrated even on CT, differential diagnosis includes all diseases associated with unilateral pleural effusion.

11.6 Summary

Pneumothorax is diagnosed on inspiratory radiographs; expiratory images should not be obtained. It is easier to identify pneumothorax in a standing than in a supine radiograph; the diagnostic criteria are presented in ▶Table 11.2. In terms of

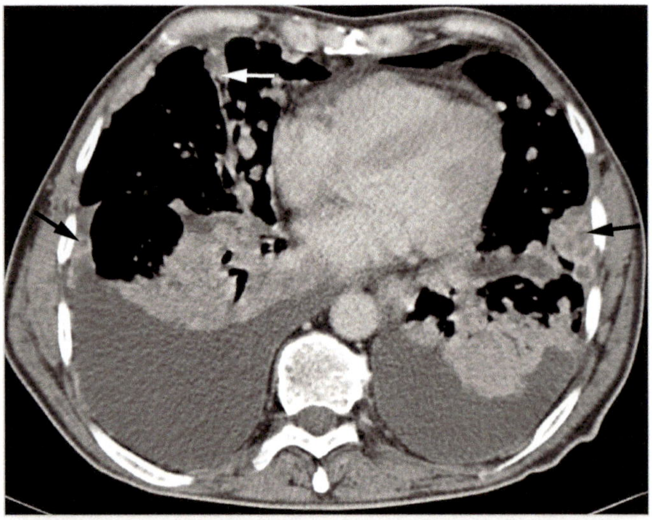

Fig. 11.21 Bilateral pleural carcinosis. CT image. Large bilateral pleural effusions and multiple pleural tumor nodules (*arrows*). Besides, lung metastasis.

causality, spontaneous pneumothorax is differentiated from traumatic and iatrogenic pneumothorax. Spontaneous pneumothorax can present as a primary condition without underlying disease or secondarily to pulmonary disease (see ▶Table 11.1). In general, CT is indicated for recurring pneumothorax or suspected underlying pulmonary disease.

Tension pneumothorax is caused by a valve mechanism of the air leak in the visceral pleura. This allows air to escape from the lung into the pleural space in inspiration but not to return to the lung in expiration, thus leading to a progressive pressure increase in the pleural space. Since it constitutes an acute, life-threatening situation, emergency pressure relief of the pleural space with chest tube placement is needed. Imaging demonstrates mediastinal displacement to the contralateral side and an ipsilateral, low-riding diaphragm.

Numerous pathologic conditions give rise to *pleural effusion* (see ▶Table 11.4). Diagnostic imaging is not able to reliably differentiate a transudate, caused by increased filtration of fluids, from an exudate resulting from fluid secretion into the pleural space. Other fluids (blood, pus, chyle), too, manifest as pleural effusion on imaging.

Pleural empyema is an infection of the pleural cavity usually occurring in parapneumonic settings. Other causes include malignant tumors that have invaded the pleural space, postsurgical complications, or penetrating chest injuries. Pleural empyema consists of three phases:

- *Exudative phase:* pleural effusion, which may not be free flowing but rather appears discrete; still no evidence of pleural thickening.
- *Fibrinopurulent phase:* purulent pleural effusion, on CT thickening and contrast enhancement of the visceral and parietal pleura (split pleura sign).
- *Organizing phase:* increased organization of septate empyema may be visible on ultrasound and on CT; development of a pleural thickening.

Empyema drainage and antibiotic treatment are effective only in the early phases; surgical decortication is needed for later stages.

At least 80% of all pleural plaques result from exposure to asbestos several decades previously. The implications of pleural plaques for diagnosis of occupational lung diseases are presented in Chapter 18.

Pleural thickening may remain after pleural inflammatory processes have been resolved and is visible on radiography and CT. Bilateral, in some cases calcified, pleural thickening is often seen in association with asbestos exposure, but also in other diseases. Unilateral calcifications can be expected in settings of chronic pleural empyema, calcified tuberculous pleurisy, or resolved hemothorax. Rounded atelectasis with a characteristic appearance on radiography may develop in the lung parenchyma adjacent to the pleural thickening.

Secondary malignant tumors of the pleura (*pleural carcinosis*) are much more common than primary tumors (pleural mesothelioma, solitary fibrous pleural tumor). Pleural carcinosis manifests as pleural effusion as well as nodular or diffuse thickening of the pleural layers; both components are also seen as isolated entities. In general, an effusion exerts a space-occupying effect. In that respect, it differs from the less common malignant pleural mesothelioma that tends to result in loss of volume of the affected hemithorax.

Pleural mesotheliomas are almost always caused by asbestos exposure and have a poor prognosis. The first manifestation is often a large unilateral pleural effusion. In the more advanced stages, parietal and visceral pleural masses, which can invade surrounding structures, are additionally seen on imaging. The TNM classification system used for pleural mesotheliomas is presented in ▶Table 11.7, and the staging system in ▶Table 11.8.

A less common primary pleural tumor, benign *lipoma*, is easily diagnosed on CT thanks to its fat content.

Solitary fibrous pleural tumor may be very large by the time of diagnosis. It is not possible on imaging to reliably differentiate between the common benign and the less common malignant form. An originally benign solitary fibrous pleural tumor tends to undergo secondary malignant transformation if not completely resected.

References

[1] Haynes D, Baumann MH. Pleural controversy: aetiology of pneumothorax. Respirology 2011;16(4):604–610

[2] Noppen M, De Keukeleire T. Pneumothorax. Respiration 2008;76 (2):121–127

[3] Noppen M, Stratakos G, Verbanck S, D'Haese J, Meysman M, Vincken W. Fluorescein-enhanced autofluorescence thoracoscopy in primary spontaneous pneumothorax. Am J Respir Crit Care Med 2004;170(6):680–682

[4] Roberts DJ, Leigh-Smith S, Faris PD, et al. Clinical manifestations of tension pneumothorax: protocol for a systematic review and meta-analysis. Syst Rev 2014;3:3

[5] Bradley M, Williams C, Walshaw MJ. The value of routine expiratory chest films in the diagnosis of pneumothorax. Arch Emerg Med 1991;8(2):115–116

[6] Seow A, Kazerooni EA, Pernicano PG, Neary M. Comparison of upright inspiratory and expiratory chest radiographs for detecting pneumothoraces. AJR Am J Roentgenol 1996;166(2):313–316

[7] Baumann MH, Strange C, Heffner JE, et al; AACP Pneumothorax Consensus Group. Management of spontaneous pneumothorax: an American College of Chest Physicians Delphi consensus statement. Chest 2001;119(2):590–602

[8] Light RW, Macgregor MI, Luchsinger PC, Ball WC Jr. Pleural effusions: the diagnostic separation of transudates and exudates. Ann Intern Med 1972;77(4):507–513

[9] Na MJ. Diagnostic tools of pleural effusion. Tuberc Respir Dis (Seoul) 2014;76(5):199–210

[10] Kuhlman JE, Singha NK. Complex disease of the pleural space: radiographic and CT evaluation. Radiographics 1997;17(1):63–79

[11] Armstrong P. Imaging of Diseases of the Chest. 2nd ed. St. Louis, MO: Mosby; 1995

[12] Kraus GJ. The split pleura sign. Radiology 2007;243(1):297–298

[13] Evans AL, Gleeson FV. Radiology in pleural disease: state of the art. Respirology 2004;9(3):300–312

[14] Jeong YJ, Kim S, Kwak SW, et al. Neoplastic and nonneoplastic conditions of serosal membrane origin: CT findings. Radiographics 2008;28(3):801–817, discussion 817–818, quiz 912

[15] Kraus T, Borsch-Galetke E, Elliehausen HJ, et al. Examples for asbestos-related findings in HRCT - criteria for the assessment of causal relationships in surveillance programmes and medical expert opinion [in German] Pneumologie 2010;64(1):37–44

[16] Fischer J. Diagnostik und Begutachtung asbestbedingter Berufskrankheiten: Interdisziplinäre S2-Leitlinie der Deutschen Gesellschaft für Pneumologie und Beatmungsmedizin und der Deutschen Gesellschaft für Arbeitsmedizin und Umweltmedizin (11.12.2010). Available at: http://www.awmf.org/uploads/tx_szleitlinien/002-038l_S2k-Diagnostik_Begutachtung_asbestbedingter_Berufskrankheiten_2010-abgelaufen.pdf

[17] Gaerte SC, Meyer CA, Winer-Muram HT, Tarver RD, Conces DJ Jr. Fat-containing lesions of the chest. Radiographics 2002;22(Spec No):S61–S78

[18] Politis J, Funahashi A, Gehlsen JA, DeCock D, Stengel BF, Choi H. Intrathoracic lipomas. Report of three cases and review of the literature with emphasis on endobronchial lipoma. J Thorac Cardiovasc Surg 1979;77(4):550–556

[19] Wang ZJ, Reddy GP, Gotway MB, et al. Malignant pleural mesothelioma: evaluation with CT, MR imaging, and PET. Radiographics 2004;24(1):105–119

[20] Leung AN, Müller NL, Miller RR. CT in differential diagnosis of diffuse pleural disease. AJR Am J Roentgenol 1990;154(3):487–492

[21] Metintaş M, Ozdemir N, Işiksoy S, et al. CT-guided pleural needle biopsy in the diagnosis of malignant mesothelioma. J Comput Assist Tomogr 1995;19(3):370–374

[22] Boutin C, Rey F. Thoracoscopy in pleural malignant mesothelioma: a prospective study of 188 consecutive patients. Part 1: Diagnosis. Cancer 1993;72(2):389–393

[23] Rusch VW; From the International Mesothelioma Interest Group. A proposed new international TNM staging system for malignant pleural mesothelioma. Chest 1995;108(4):1122–1128

[24] Byrne MJ, Nowak AK. Modified RECIST criteria for assessment of response in malignant pleural mesothelioma. Ann Oncol 2004;15(2): 257–260

[25] Rosado-de-Christenson ML, Abbott GF, McAdams HP, Franks TJ, Galvin JR. From the archives of the AFIP: Localized fibrous tumor of the pleura. Radiographics 2003;23(3):759–783

[26] Leuallen EC, Carr DT. Pleural effusion; a statistical study of 436 patients. N Engl J Med 1955;252(3):79–83

[27] Zerhouni EA, Scott WW Jr, Baker RR, Wharam MD, Siegelman SS. Invasive thymomas: diagnosis and evaluation by computed tomography. J Comput Assist Tomogr 1982;6(1):92–100

[28] O'Donovan PB, Eng P. Pleural changes in malignant pleural effusions: appearance on computed tomography. Cleve Clin J Med 1994;61(2):127–131, quiz 162

Chapter 12

Mediastinal Diseases

12 Mediastinal Diseases

12.1 Mediastinal Lymphadenopathy

> **Note**
>
> Mediastinal lymphadenopathy is present if the short diameter of the lymph node on sectional imaging is more than 10 mm. The long-axis diameter of the lymph node is not relevant for definition of lymphadenopathy.[1]

This long-standing rule has come under discussion since mediastinal lymph node stations 4R and 7 often contain normal lymph nodes larger than 10 mm. Hence, thresholds of 15 mm for station 4R and 20 mm for station 7 have been suggested.[2,3]

For hilar lymph nodes, a short-axis threshold of 3 mm is specified for the majority of lymph node stations.[1] However, that specification is based on a much earlier single publication with single-row CT.[4] In the age of thin-slice multiple-row detector CT, application of that threshold would lead to many false-positive results for hilar lymphadenopathy. A more appropriate approach is to consider a diagnosis of hilar lymphadenopathy only if there is visible evidence of pronounced lymph node enlargement on CT or MRI.

There are myriad inflammatory and malignant diseases that can potentially cause lymphadenopathy.[5] The distribution pattern of the affected lymph nodes gives insights into the underlying disease (▶Table 12.1). Both pulmonary hypertension and congestive left heart failure lead to increased fluid filtration in the pulmonary capillaries. The resultant increased lymphatic drainage from the lungs can in turn cause, generally symmetrical, hilar and mediastinal lymph node enlargement.

Homogeneous *lymph node calcification* is a sign of resolved tuberculosis. Eggshell-like lymph node calcification is seen in silicosis, coal workers' pneumoconiosis, sarcoidosis, irradiated lymphomas, and less commonly in tuberculosis (▶Fig. 12.1).

12.2 Mediastinitis

Mediastinitis is the term used to describe acute or chronic inflammation of the mediastinal structures. The acute form is almost always caused by bacteria, most commonly as an iatrogenic complication of bypass surgery or due to esophageal perforation.[6] The third most common cause is descending necrotizing inflammation from the head–neck region, usually from an odontogenic focus. Rarer causes of infection are advanced osteomyelitis, perforation of the trachea or mainstem bronchi, or hematogenous dissemination.[7,8]

Acute mediastinitis is a life-threatening condition associated with considerable mortality. The clinical manifestation includes chest pain, fever, shaking chills, and dyspnea as well as elevated inflammatory lab results. Descending mediastinitis from the neck is often recognized from neck swelling. Acute mediastinitis must be suspected if the clinical symptoms are present and mediastinal enlargement is seen on chest radiography (▶Fig. 12.2). At times, mediastinal gas bubbles may be visible. CT is the method of choice for confirmation of suspected acute mediastinitis, as well as for diagnosis of infection spread and treatment planning.

> **Note**
>
> Typical CT findings of acute mediastinitis (▶Fig. 12.3)[8]:
> - Increased density of the mediastinal fatty tissue.
> - Mediastinal gas bubbles.
> - Small mediastinal fluid collections.
> - Mediastinal lymphadenopathy.
> - Pleural effusion.
> - Pleural empyema.

Table 12.1 Typical distribution patterns of mediastinal or hilar lymphadenopathy and underlying diseases

Clinical symptoms	Typical distribution patterns of lymphadenopathy
Sarcoidosis	Bihilar and bilateral paratracheal (two-thirds of cases)
	Only bihilar, not mediastinal (one-third of cases)
	Almost always symmetrically bihilar
	Rarely, only mediastinal
	Extremely rarely, only in the posterior mediastinum
Pneumonia	Ipsilateral hilar and paratracheal
Tuberculosis	Asymmetrically or symmetrically hilar (depending on lung involvement) and paratracheal
Hodgkin disease and non-Hodgkin lymphomas	Anterior mediastinum
	Paratracheal
	Less frequently, subcarinal or symmetrically hilar
	Rarely, only hilar
Lung cancer	Asymmetrically ipsilateral hilar and paratracheal (stations 2 and 4), less often, contralateral hilar and paratracheal
	Stations 5 and 6 in primary tumors of the left upper lobe
	Station 7 in tumors of the lower lobes
Breast cancer	Along the internal thoracic vessels
	Axillary
Esophageal cancer	Paratracheal (stations 2 and 4) in primary tumors of the upper or middle third
	Supraclavicular and cervical in cervical primary tumors
	Lesser curvature of the stomach in primary tumors of the lower third
Pleural mesothelioma	Along the internal thoracic vessels
	Caudal paraspinal
	Anterior peridiaphragmatic

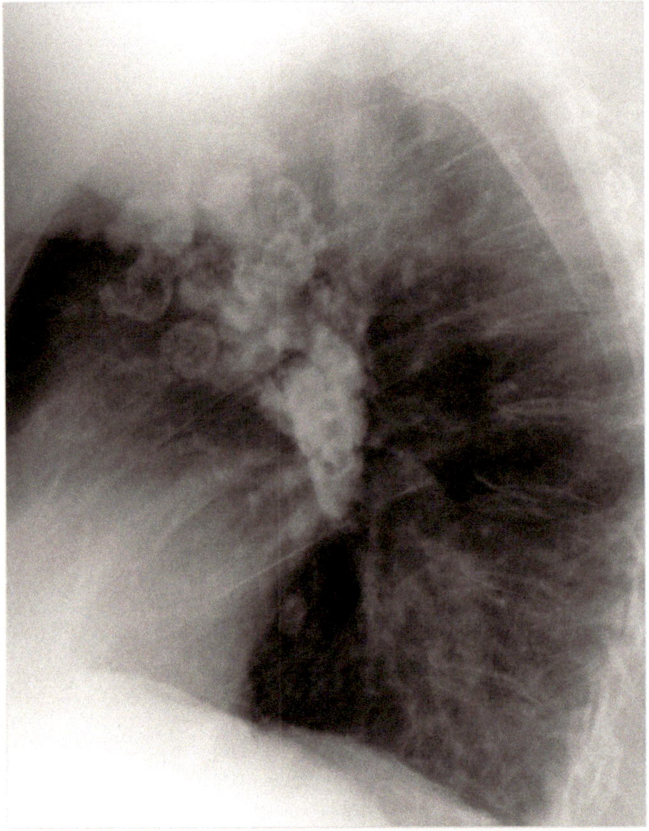

Fig. 12.1 Eggshell-like calcifications in the mediastinal and hilar lymph nodes in tuberculosis. Radiograph. Sectional magnification of a lateral image.

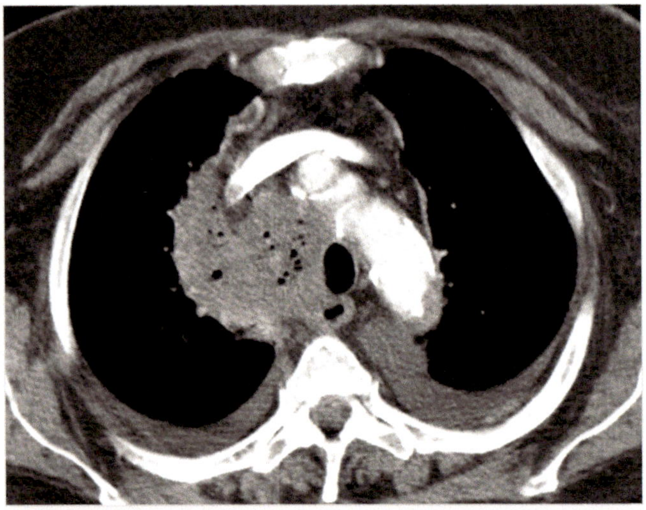

Fig. 12.3 Acute suppurative mediastinitis. CT image. Fluid-isodense mediastinal mass with gas bubbles. Small bilateral pleural effusions.

Chronic mediastinitis is divided somewhat arbitrarily into granulomatous and fibrosing or sclerosing mediastinitis. These conditions probably reflect continuing chronic infections, often caused by tuberculosis or fungi.[6,7,9] Chronic mediastinitis is also caused by numerous noninfectious diseases, such as sarcoidosis, malignancies, obstruction of the lymphatic drainage system, and autoimmune diseases.[7] Chest radiography usually shows mediastinal enlargement, including at times a hilar mass. CT characteristically visualizes a diffuse or discrete, often very extensive, mass of soft-tissue

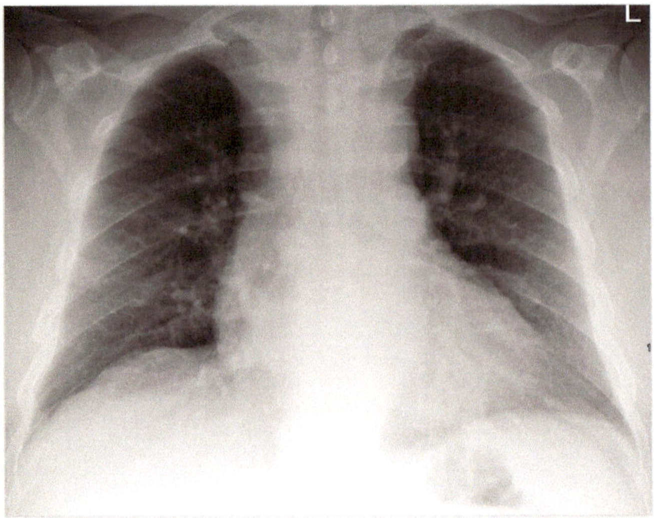

Fig. 12.2 Acute mediastinitis secondary to tracheal stenosis resection. Radiograph. Considerable enlargement and compression of the upper mediastinum.

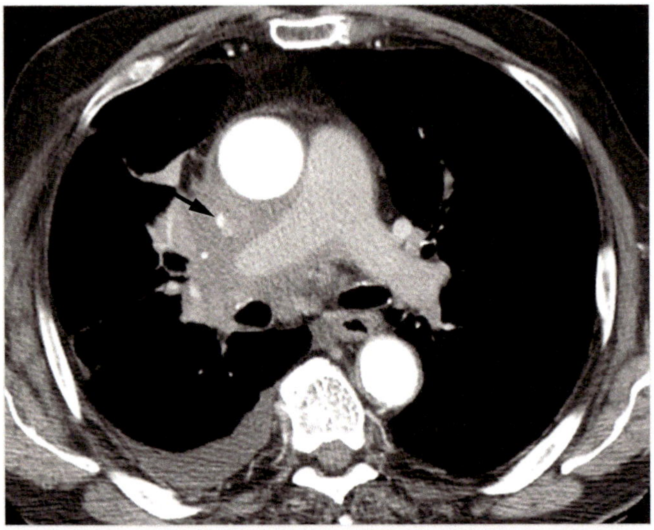

Fig. 12.4 Chronic sclerosing mediastinitis. CT image. Mediastinal and right hilar mass of soft-tissue density. High-grade stenosis of the superior vena cava (*arrow*). Small right pleural effusion.

density that can be misinterpreted as a malignant tumor or lymphoma. Calcifications may occur. Stenosis of the superior vena cava is a typical clinical manifestation and easily identified on CT (▶ Fig. 12.4).

12.3 Pneumomediastinum

The characteristic feature of pneumomediastinum is free air surrounding the mediastinal structures. Pneumomediastinum is caused by the following[8,10,11]:

- Blunt or penetrating chest injury.
- Esophageal perforation.
- Perforation of the trachea or mainstem bronchi.
- Pneumothorax.
- Positive pressure ventilation.
- Transmission of pulmonary interstitial emphysema.
- Acute mediastinitis with gas-producing bacteria.
- Cocaine consumption.

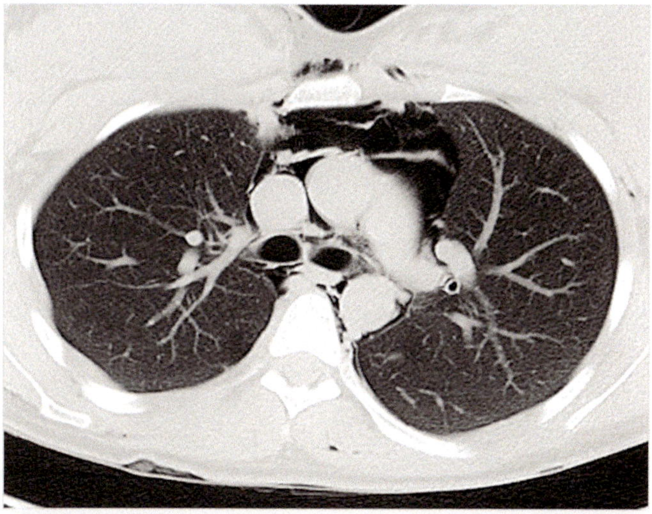

Fig. 12.5 Pneumomediastinum secondary to tear in the left mainstem bronchus. CT image. Furthermore, minor chest wall emphysema.

- Asthma attack.
- Spontaneous onset, in particular in young adults (cough, vomiting, physical exertion).

Spontaneous pneumomediastinum is a special form of pneumomediastinum usually observed in young adults and which has a benign course and does not require any particular treatment.[11] In around two-thirds of cases, pneumomediastinum can be diagnosed from the chest radiograph, showing characteristic linear radiolucent areas in the mediastinum. CT is pathognomonic (▶Fig. 12.5).

Tension pneumomediastinum is a rare complication which, like tension pneumothorax, is caused by a valve mechanism resulting in increased mediastinal pressure. This can have acute, life-threatening consequences due to compression of the heart and central airways.[8]

12.4 Esophageal Tumors

Benign esophageal tumors are 50-fold less common than esophageal carcinomas. These are predominantly *leimyomas*,[12] which are intramural tumors that originate from the smooth muscle cells and exhibit hardly any circumferential growth. They can become very large and gradually cause progressive dysphagia. On CT and MRI, they manifest as smoothly marginated and homogeneous masses. Occasionally, calcifications are seen.[13]

Duplication cysts, the second most common benign masses, become symptomatic already in childhood. On sectional imaging, the typical features of a fluid-filled cyst can be identified. These are filled with air if they communicate with the esophagus.[13]

In the vast majority of cases, the most common malignant tumor of the esophagus, *esophageal carcinoma*, is found on histology to be a squamous cell carcinoma or adenocarcinoma (▶Fig. 12.6). Smoking and alcohol abuse are the main risk factors for esophageal carcinoma. This tumor mainly affects men aged 60 to 70 years. It has a poor prognosis, with a 5-year survival of around 10%.[13] Staging is the main focus of imaging in esophageal carcinoma. CT and PET-CT are required to rule out distant metastasis as well as for evaluation of invasion of surrounding structures. Only endosonography is able to evaluate tumor extension within the esophagus; it is also superior to other cross-sectional imaging techniques for detection of lymph node metastasis. The tumor stage can be derived from the TNM staging classification (▶Table 12.2). For some stages, histologic grading is also used in addition to the imaging findings (▶Table 12.3). Tumor contact with the aorta of more than one-quarter of the vascular circumference (over 90°) is considered a criterion for probable aortic invasion.[14]

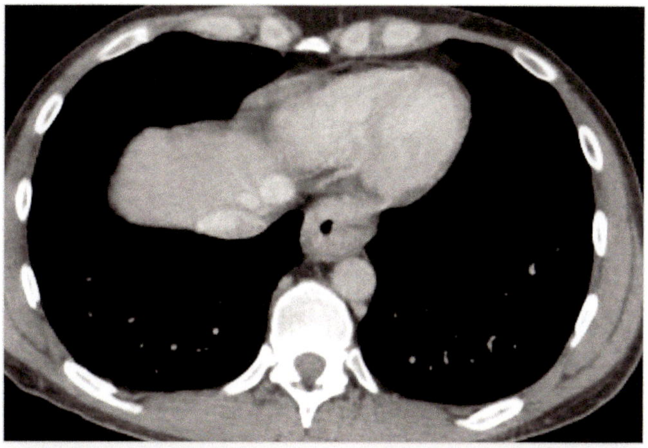

Fig. 12.6 Esophageal carcinoma. CT image. Circular wall thickening of the distal esophagus. No identifiable invasion of surrounding structures.

12.5 Mediastinal Tumors and Tumor-Like Masses

Anatomic assignment of mediastinal masses to a mediastinal compartment is useful for differential diagnosis. This allows for considerable narrowing of differential diagnoses (▶Table 12.4). Another important consideration is the CT density. Cystic masses can often be reliably identified. Presence of intratumoral fat on CT also serves as a diagnostic pointer. Masses of low density (cysts, fat-containing structures) are discussed in the following sections, followed by solid tumors, i.e., tumors of soft-tissue density.

12.5.1 Mediastinal Masses of Low Density

Cystic Masses

Cysts have a smoothly marginated, thin wall that does not exhibit contrast enhancement or invade surrounding structures. CT density is isodense to water or somewhat more hyperdense than water, depending on their content. On MRI, they show variable signal intensity. Whereas on T2 weighting cysts generally exhibit hyperintense signals similar to water, on

Table 12.2 Clinical TNM staging classification of esophageal carcinoma[15]

Descriptors	Definitions
T descriptor (tumor extension)	
TX	Primary tumor cannot be assessed
T0	No primary tumor
Tis	High-grade dysplasia
T1	Tumor invades lamina propria, muscularis mucosae or submucosa
• T1a	Tumor invades lamina propria or muscularis mucosae
• T1b	Tumor invades submucosa
T2	Tumor invades muscularis propria
T3	Tumor invades adventitia
T4	Tumor invades adjacent structures
• T4a	Resectable tumor with invasion of pleura, pericardium or diaphragm
• T4b	Unresectable tumor with invasion of other structures (aorta, vertebral body, trachea)
N descriptor (lymph node metastasis)	
NX	Regional lymph nodes cannot be assessed
N0	No regional lymph node metastasis
N1	Metastasis in 1–2 regional lymph nodes
N2	Metastasis in 3–6 regional lymph nodes
N3	Metastasis in 7 or more regional lymph nodes
M descriptor (distant metastasis)	
M0	No distant metastasis
M1	Distant metastasis

Table 12.3 Tumor stages of esophageal carcinoma based on the TNM tumor formula, taking account of histologic grading (G1 -3, GX)[15]

Stages	T	N	M	Remarks
0	Tis	N0	M0	
IA	T1	N0	M0	For G1 or GX
IB	T1	N0	M0	For G2 or G3
	T2–3	N0	M0	For G1, tumor in the lower third
IIA	T2–3	N0	M0	For G2–3, tumor in the lower third
				For G1, tumor in the upper or middle third
IIB	T2–3	N0	M0	For G2–3, tumor in the upper or middle third
	T1–2	N1	M0	
IIIA	T1–2	N2	M0	
	T3	N1	M0	
	T4a	N0	M0	
IIIB	T3	N2	M0	
IIIC	T4a	N1-2	M0	
	T4b	Any	M0	
	Any	N3	M0	
IV	Any	Any	M0	
	T	N		

T1 weighting the signal intensity may vary in accordance with the cyst content. Bronchogenic cysts are the most common cysts, followed by pericardial cysts, esophageal duplication cysts (see above), and thymic cysts. Occasionally, the shape of the often not quite rounded pericardial cysts changes over time (▶ Fig. 12.7).[18]

Mature cystic teratomas (dermoid cysts) are the most common germ cell tumors (▶Fig. 12.8). These are benign, usually asymptomatic malformation tumors diagnosed as incidental findings in young adults. They have major cystic components and may also contain the most diverse tissues(components with fat or soft-tissue density, bone, and cartilage). They are predominantly located in the anterior mediastinum, rarely in the posterior mediastinum.[19,20]

Many tumors and lymphomas undergo *cystic degeneration*, in particular when treated, and then exhibit both cystic and solid components on CT and MRI. This is the case especially for thymomas (▶Fig. 12.9), Hodgkin lymphomas, germ cell tumors, neurogenic tumors, and mediastinal lymph node metastasis.[18] Likewise, mediastinal abscesses and pancreatic pseudocysts extending into the mediastinum contain liquid components; in such cases, the clinical context suggests the diagnosis.

Masses of Fat-Equivalent Density

Detection of fat on CT in a mediastinal mass considerably narrows differential diagnosis[21]:

- *Lipomas*: smoothly marginated, benign masses of homogeneous fat density.
- *Mature cystic teratomas*(see above): these may contain fat or fluid-fat levels.
- *Teratocarcinomas*: these are rare and contain less fat and more components of soft-tissue density than benign teratomas.

Table 12.4 Assignment of solid mediastinal masses to the mediastinal compartments[16,17]

Compartment	Masses
Anterior mediastinum	• Thymic mass: thymic hyperplasia, thymic cyst, thymoma, thymic carcinoma, thymolipoma, thymic carcinoid • Lymphoma • Germ cell tumors: teratoma, seminoma, nonseminomatous germ cell tumors • Thyroid gland masses
Middle mediastinum	• Ectopic thyroid gland tissue • Lymphadenopathy (see Table 12.1) • Tracheal carcinoma • Esophageal carcinoma (see above)
Posterior mediastinum	• Neurogenic tumor • Extramedullary hematopoiesis
Upper thoracic inlet	• Goiter • Thyroid gland carcinoma • Parathyroid gland adenoma • Neurogenic tumor

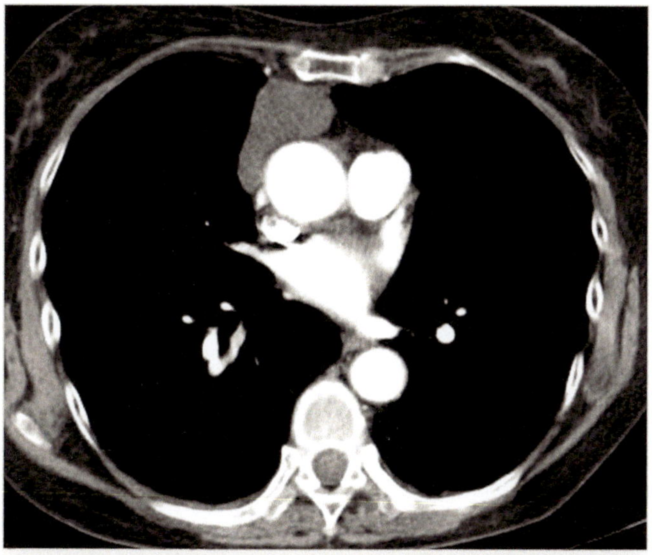

Fig. 12.7 Pericardial cyst. CT image. Smoothly marginated, cystic mass in the anterior mediastinum ventral to the ascending aorta.

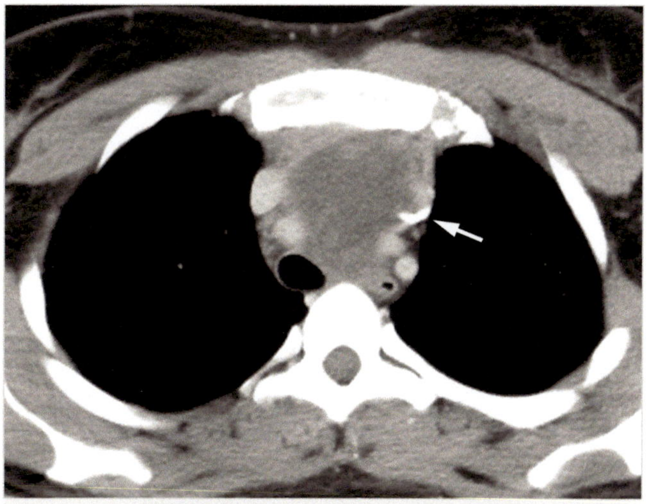

Fig. 12.8 Mature cystic teratoma. CT image. Cystic mass in the anterior and middle mediastinum with soft-tissue components in the cyst wall and small bony structure (*arrow*).

- *Thymolipomas*: These are rare, benign thymic tumors that exhibit slow growth and a combination of fat and soft-tissue density.

12.5.2 Solid Mediastinal Tumors of the Anterior Mediastinum

The majority of mediastinal masses are located in the anterior mediastinum. Four etiologies are implicated[22]:

- *Germ cell tumors* (teratomas, seminomas, and nonseminomatous germ cell tumors): The benign mature cystic teratoma was discussed in the previous section. The remaining malignant germ cell tumors are often large, sharply marginated, lobulated masses of soft-tissue density that occur in the anterior mediastinum and have no pathognomonic findings on imaging (▶ Fig. 12.10). Calcifications and hypodense components may be seen.[20]
- *Thymic tumors*: Benign thymic cysts and thymolipomas as well as cystic thymomas were discussed in the previous section. Thymomas exhibit highly variable biological behavior.[23] Smoothly marginated, encapsulated tumors (▶ Fig. 12.11) have a slow growth, whereas invasive thymomas and thymic

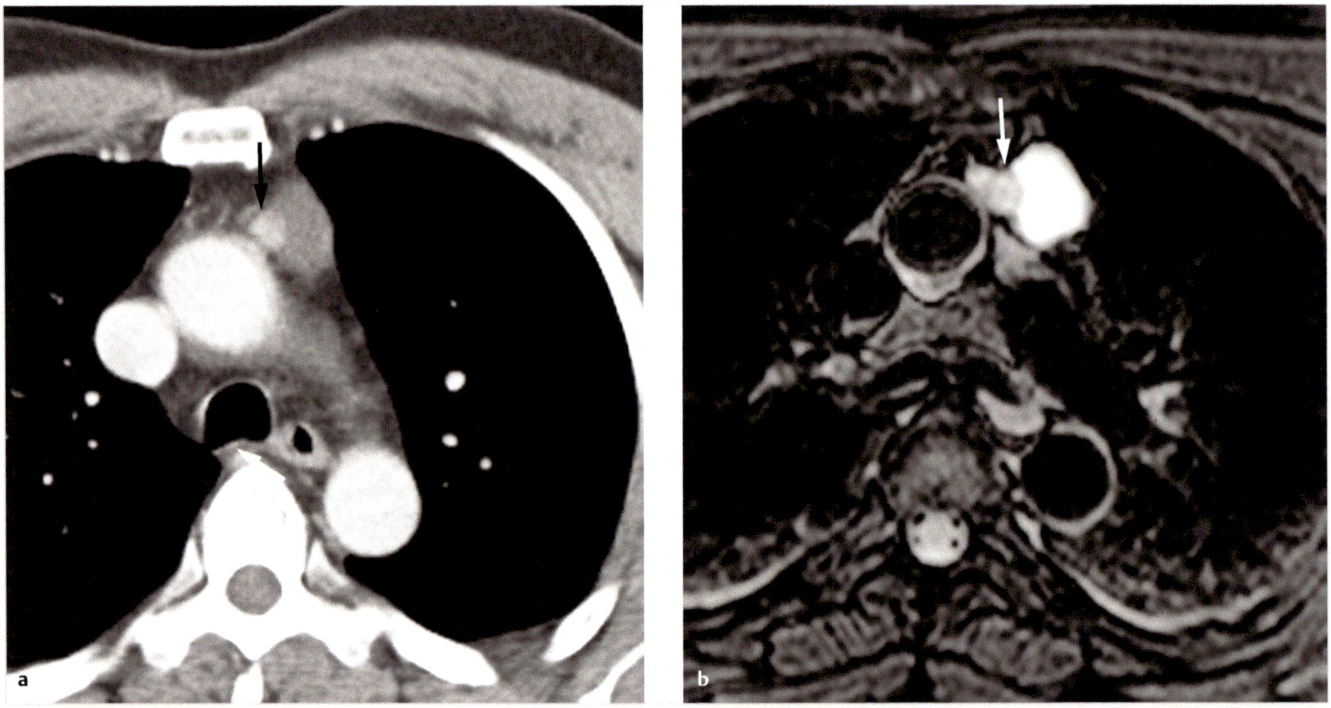

Fig. 12.9 Cystic thymoma. (a) CT image. Large cystic and small soft-tissue component (*arrow*). **(b)** MRI, T2w image with fat saturation. The soft-tissue component of the thymoma can also be identified (*arrow*).

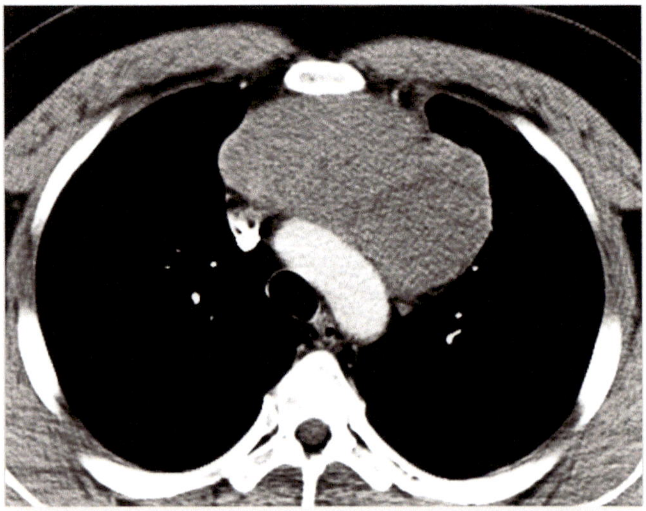

Fig. 12.10 Malignant, nonseminomatous germ cell tumor. CT image. Large, smoothly marginated, lobulated mass in the anterior mediastinum.

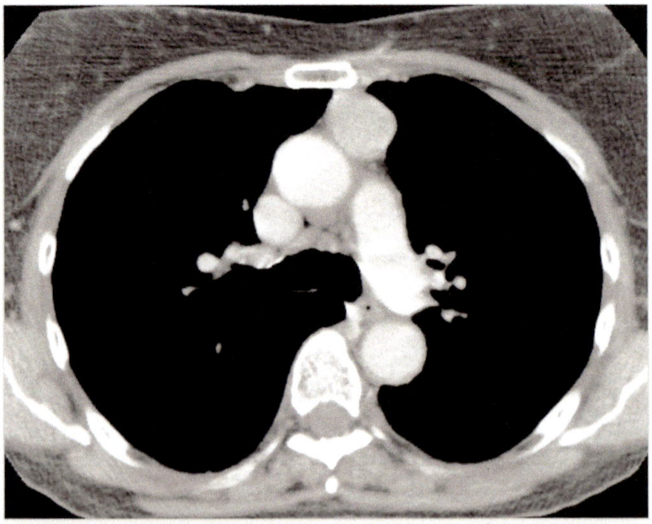

Fig. 12.11 Masaoka stage 1 thymoma. CT image. Smoothly marginated mass of the anterior mediastinum.

carcinomas (▶Fig. 12.12) are rapidly growing invasive tumors with a poorer prognosis. Staging was formerly based on Masaoka[24]; recently, a TNM stage system has been proposed[25] (▶Table 12.5). The histologic subtypes cannot be reliably distinguished on imaging; however, vascular invasion is suggestive of a thymic carcinoma.[26] Thymic carcinoids are relatively aggressive tumors with a poorer prognosis than other carcinoids.[16,27] On CT they appear as large, often inhomogeneous, masses of the anterior mediastinum which are highly vascularized in some parts (▶Fig. 12.13). Thymic hyperplasia does not constitute, in a strict sense, a thymic tumor but rather contains normal thymic tissue, often presenting as a stress reaction of the body to various causes (corticoid treatment or chemotherapy, surgery, radiotherapy, etc.) and is then known as *thymic rebound.*

- *Lymphomas*: Both Hodgkin disease and non-Hodgkin lymphomas occur predominantly in the anterior mediastinum, less commonly in other mediastinal compartments (see ▶Table 12.1). It is not possible to reliably distinguish between the various histologic types on imaging. Mediastinal lymphomas may become very large and are known as *bulky disease* if the cross-sectional diameter of the mass is more than 10 cm or more than one-third of the cross-sectional diameter of the thorax. Hodgkin disease tends to invade the anterior upper lobe segments of the lung, predominantly of the left lung (▶Fig. 12.14). Lymphoma staging is carried out in accordance with ▶Table 12.6.

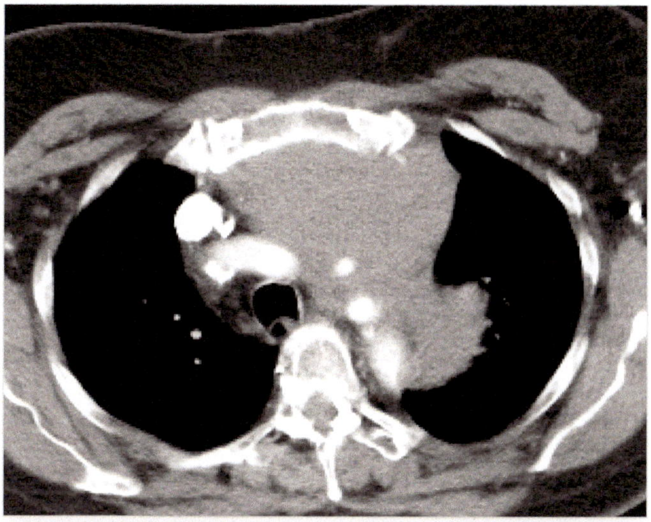

Fig. 12.12 Thymic carcinoma. CT image. Large, homogeneous mass with diffuse mediastinal invasion and encasement of the supra-aortic arteries.

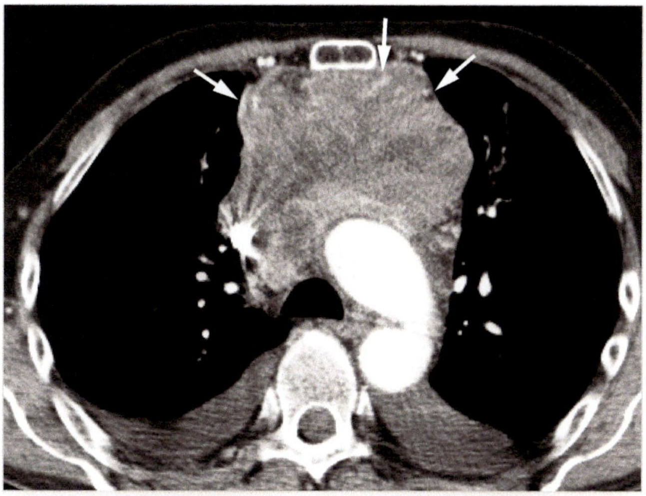

Fig. 12.13 Thymic carcinoid. CT image. Inhomogeneous mass in the anterior mediastinum, highly vascularized in the ventral aspect (*arrows*).

Table 12.5 Tumor stages of esophageal carcinoma based on the TNM tumor formula[25]

Descriptors	Definitions
T descriptor (tumor extension)	
T1	
• T1a	Encapsulated or unencapsulated, with or without extension into mediastinal fat
• T1b	Extension into mediastinal pleura
T2	Involvement of pericardium
T3	Involvement of lung, brachiocephalic vein, superior vena cava, chest wall, phrenic nerve, hilar (extrapericardial), pulmonary vessels
T4	Involvement of aorta, arch vessels, main pulmonary artery, myocardium, trachea, or esophagus
N descriptor (lymph node metastasis)	
N0	No nodal involvement
N1	Involvement of anterior (perithymic) nodes
N2	Involvement of deep intrathoracic or cervical nodes
M descriptor (distant metastasis)	
M0	No metastatic pleural, pericardial, or distant sites
M1	
• M1a	Separate pleural or pericardial nodule(s)
• M1b	Pulmonary intraparenchymal nodule or distant organ metastasis

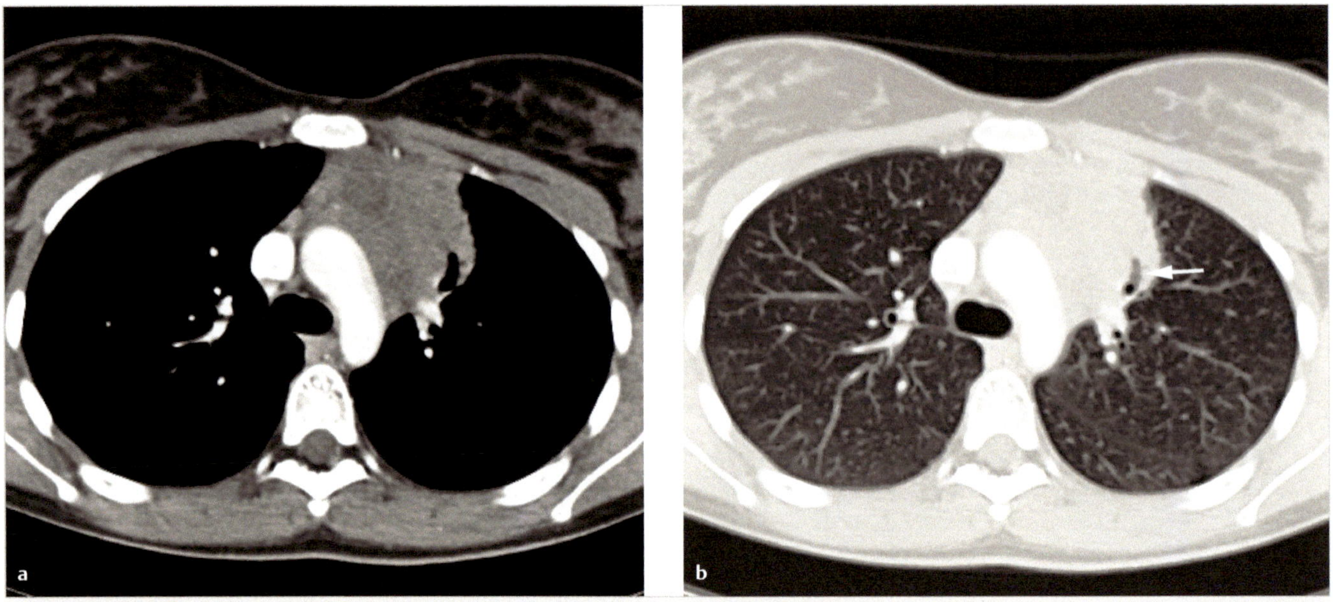

Fig. 12.14 **Hodgkin disease.** CT images. **(a)** Soft-tissue window: large mass in the anterior mediastinum. **(b)** Lung window: identifiable invasion of the left anterior upper lobe segment; the segment bronchus (*arrow*) is encased by the mass.

Table 12.6 Ann Arbor classification of lymphomas[28]

Stage	Description
I	Involvement of a single lymphatic node region (I) or of a single extralymphatic organ or site (I_E)
II	Involvement of two or more lymph node regions on the same side of the diaphragm (II) or localized involvement of extralymphatic organ or site and of one or more lymph node regions on the same side of the diaphragm (II_E).
III	Involvement of lymph node regions on both sides of the diaphragm (III), which also may be accompanied by localized involvement of extralymphatic organ or site (III_E) or by involvement of the spleen (III_S) or both (III_{SE}).
IV	Diffuse or disseminated involvement of one or more extralymphatic organs or tissues, with or without associated lymph node enlargement
Additional information:	
• A	No general symptoms
• B	General symptoms: fever (> 38°C), weight loss (> 10% within the preceding 6 months), night sweats

- *Thyroid gland masses*: Ectopic thyroid gland tissue may be found in the anterior mediastinum; however, their paratracheal location in the middle mediastinum is more common (see below). Thyroid gland tumors are found predominantly in the upper thoracic inlet. Compared with normal thyroid gland tissue, thyroid gland carcinomas are hypodense masses that invade surrounding structures at more advanced stages.

The Middle Mediastinum

The following tumors are found in the middle mediastinum:

- *Lymphomas*: These may develop in the middle mediastinum, albeit less commonly than in the anterior mediastinum.

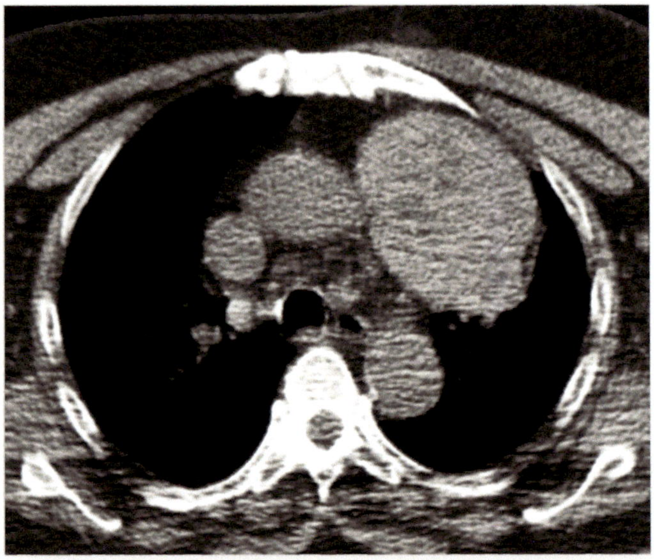

Fig. 12.15 Ectopic thyroid gland tissue in the anterior and middle mediastinum. CT image, unenhanced examination. Compared with the vessels and muscles, slightly hyperdense, inhomogeneous mass.

- *Tracheal tumors*: See Section 10.1.
- *Esophageal tumors*: See Section 12.4.
- Cysts: Bronchogenic cysts, pericardial cysts, and esophageal duplication cysts.
- *Intrathoracic goiter, ectopic thyroid gland tissue*: A smoothly marginated mass that appears hyperdense even on unenhanced CT (▶ Fig. 12.15) is suggestive of ectopic thyroid gland tissue. This may appear inhomogeneous and usually exhibits intense contrast enhancement (▶ Fig. 12.16). Retrosternal goiter manifests similarly but it is continuous with the thyroid gland.

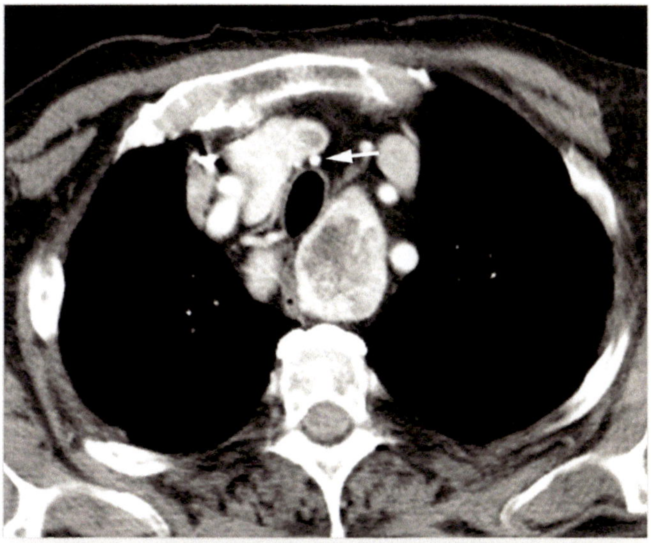

Fig. 12.16 Ectopic thyroid gland tissue in the middle mediastinum. CT image. Following IV contrast administration, considerable inhomogeneous enhancement of the left paratracheal mass similar to the right-sided, retrosternal goiter also displayed (*arrow*).

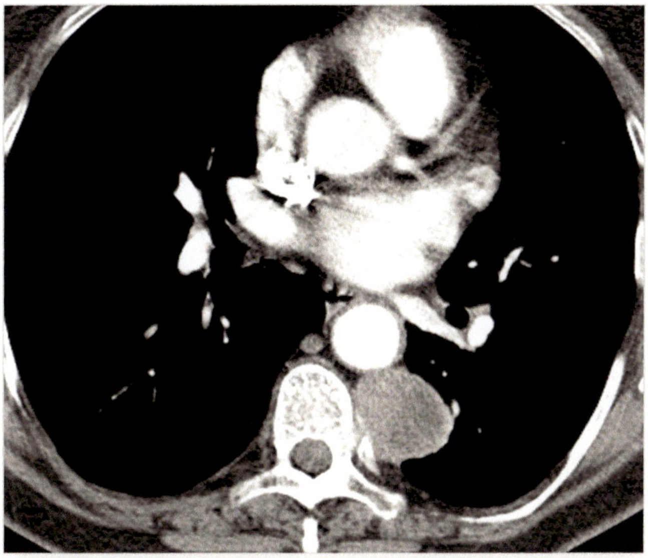

Fig. 12.17 Benign schwannoma in the posterior mediastinum. CT image. Smoothly marginated, paravertebral mass.

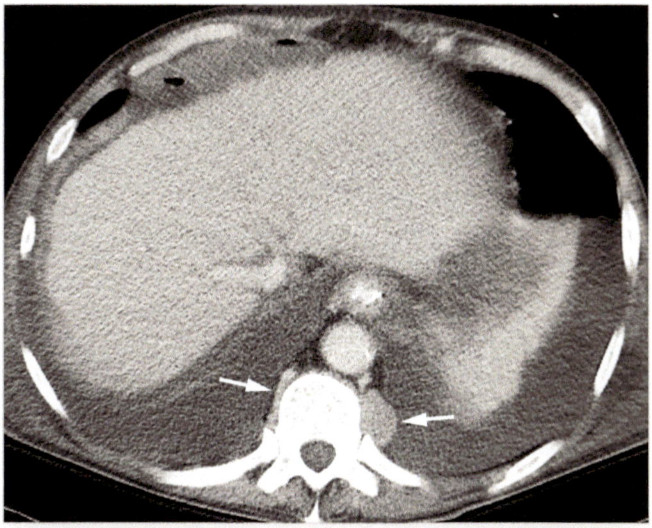

Fig. 12.18 Extramedullary hematopoiesis. CT image. Bilateral, paravertebral masses of soft-tissue density (*arrows*). Furthermore, bilateral pleural effusions with compression atelectasis of the left lower lobe.

The Posterior Mediastinum

The tumors occurring in the posterior mediastinum are predominantly neurogenic tumors, of which 80% are benign.[17] Differentiation of the various histologic types is not possible on imaging:

- *Schwannomas* are the most common benign neurogenic tumors (▶Fig. 12.17) and are encapsulated. By contrast, *neurofibromas* are unencapsulated.
- *Malignant schwannomas and neurofibromas*: The aforementioned tumors can become malignant. Neurogenic fibrosarcomas also occur.
- *Tumors of the autonomic nervous system*: These are also found in the posterior mediastinum. Their spectrum ranges from benign ganglioneuroma through ganglioneuroblastoma to malignant neuroblastoma occurring in children.

Furthermore, *extramedullary hematopoietic tissue* can develop in the posterior mediastinum, especially in association with hematologic systemic diseases. Extramedullary hematopoiesis usually manifests as bilateral, paravertebral masses of soft-tissue density (▶Fig. 12.18).

12.6 Summary

Mediastinal lymphadenopathy may be caused by myriad inflammatory and malignant diseases. The lymphadenopathy distribution pattern often gives insights into the underlying disease (see ▶Table 12.1). Mediastinal lymphadenopathy is present if the short-axis diameter of the lymph node is more than 10 mm. Eggshell-like calcifications of mediastinal lymph nodes are seen, in particular, in sarcoidosis, silicosis, and coal workers' pneumoconiosis as well as in association with lymphomas secondary to radiotherapy.

Acute mediastinitis is a life-threatening bacterial infection of the mediastinum. This is frequently of iatrogenic etiology, usually presenting after cardiac surgery or esophageal perforation. Descending necrotizing infections from an odontogenic focus are the third most common cause of disease. Chest radiography usually demonstrates mediastinal enlargement. CT is used for diagnosis confirmation as well as for monitoring infection spread and for treatment planning.

There are several causes of *pneumomediastinum* (trauma, perforation of the esophagus or tracheobronchial system, positive pressure ventilation, etc.). Spontaneous pneumomediastinum in young adults has a benign course and requires no specific treatment. Tension pneumomediastinum is caused by a valve mechanism and can develop into an acute, life-threatening condition.

II

By far, the most common esophageal tumor is *esophageal carcinoma*. CT is used for staging and assessment of any extraesophageal tumor extension as well as for monitoring for distant metastasis. Furthermore, endosonography is used for evaluation of tumor extension within the esophagus and for monitoring for lymph node metastasis. Staging is based on the TNM system presented in ▶Table 12.2.

Cystic masses of the mediastinum are quite common. These are predominantly bronchogenic cysts, pericardial cysts, thymic cysts, and esophageal duplication cysts.

Mature cystic teratomas (dermoid cysts) are characterized by their cystic components as well as their most diverse tissues which on CT may exhibit fat or soft-tissue density; they frequently also contain bony structures. This heterogeneous composition in combination with fat detection is pathognomonic.

Masses of the anterior mediastinum are of four principle types:

- *Germ cell tumors*: benign, mature cystic teratomas, malignant teratomas, seminomas, and nonseminomatous germ cell tumors
- *Thymic tumors*: thymomas, thymic carcinomas, thymolipomas, thymic carcinoids.
- *Lymphomas.*
- *Thyroid gland masses*: goiter, ectopic thyroid gland tissue, thyroid gland carcinoma.

Cystic masses are mainly found in the *middle mediastinum*, in addition to tumors of the trachea and esophagus, lymphomas, and thyroid gland masses.

Neurogenic tumors are the most common masses found in the *posterior mediastinum*. Reliable differentiation of the various histologic types (e.g., schwannoma, neurofibroma, neurogenic fibrosarcoma, ganglioneuroma, ganglioneuroblastoma, neuroblastoma) is not possible on imaging. Extramedullary hematopoiesis may present in association with hematologic systemic diseases, manifesting as one or more paravertebral masses in the posterior mediastinum.

Tumors occurring in the *upper thoracic inlet* are usually thyroid gland and parathyroid gland masses as well as neurogenic tumors.

References

[1] Hansell DM, Bankier AA, MacMahon H, McLoud TC, Müller NL, Remy J. Fleischner Society: glossary of terms for thoracic imaging. Radiology 2008;246(3):697–722

[2] Schmidt AF Jr, Rodrigues OR, Matheus RS, Kim JduU, Jatene FB. Mediastinal lymph node distribution, size and number: definitions based on an anatomical study. J Bras Pneumol 2007;33(2):134–140

[3] Ziyade S, Pinarbasili NB, Ziyade N, et al. Determination of standard number, size and weight of mediastinal lymph nodes in postmortem examinations: reflection on lung cancer surgery. J Cardiothorac Surg 2013;8:94

[4] Remy-Jardin M, Duyck P, Remy J, et al. Hilar lymph nodes: identification with spiral CT and histologic correlation. Radiology 1995; 196(2):387–394

[5] Sharma A, Fidias P, Hayman LA, Loomis SL, Taber KH, Aquino SL. Patterns of lymphadenopathy in thoracic malignancies. Radiographics 2004;24(2):419–434

[6] Athanassiadi KA. Infections of the mediastinum. Thorac Surg Clin 2009;19(1):37–45, vi

[7] Akman C, Kantarci F, Cetinkaya S. Imaging in mediastinitis: a systematic review based on aetiology. Clin Radiol 2004;59(7):573–585

[8] Katabathina VS, Restrepo CS, Martinez-Jimenez S, Riascos RF. Nonvascular, nontraumatic mediastinal emergencies in adults: a comprehensive review of imaging findings. Radiographics 2011;31(4):1141–1160

[9] Rossi SE, McAdams HP, Rosado-de-Christenson ML, Franks TJ, Galvin JR. Fibrosing mediastinitis. Radiographics 2001;21(3):737–757

[10] Alnas M, Altayeh A, Zaman M. Clinical course and outcome of cocaine-induced pneumomediastinum. Am J Med Sci 2010;339(1):65–67

[11] Caceres M, Ali SZ, Braud R, Weiman D, Garrett HE Jr. Spontaneous pneumomediastinum: a comparative study and review of the literature. Ann Thorac Surg 2008;86(3):962–966

[12] Seremetis MG, Lyons WS, deGuzman VC, Peabody JW Jr. Leiomyomata of the esophagus. An analysis of 838 cases. Cancer 1976;38(5):2166–2177

[13] Lewis RB, Mehrotra AK, Rodriguez P, Levine MS. From the radiologic pathology archives: esophageal neoplasms: radiologic-pathologic correlation. Radiographics 2013;33(4):1083–1108

[14] Picus D, Balfe DM, Koehler RE, Roper CL, Owen JW. Computed tomography in the staging of esophageal carcinoma. Radiology 1983;146(2):433–438

[15] National Comprehensive Cancer Network. Clinical practice guidelines in oncology. Esophageal and esophagogastric junction cancers (excluding the proximal 5 cm of the stomach) V.2.2013. (06.09.2013). Available at: http://www.nccn.org/professionals/physician_gls/pdf/esophageal.pdf. Accessed October 22, 2015

[16] Quint LE. Imaging of anterior mediastinal masses. Cancer Imaging 2007;7 Spec No A:S56–S62

[17] Duwe BV, Sterman DH, Musani AI. Tumors of the mediastinum. Chest 2005;128(4):2893–2909

[18] Jeung MY, Gasser B, Gangi A, et al. Imaging of cystic masses of the mediastinum. Radiographics 2002;22(Spec No):S79–S93

[19] Patel IJ, Hsiao E, Ahmad AH, Schroeder C, Gilkeson RC. AIRP best cases in radiologic-pathologic correlation: mediastinal mature cystic teratoma. Radiographics 2013;33(3):797–801

[20] Rosado-de-Christenson ML, Templeton PA, Moran CA. From the archives of the AFIP. Mediastinal germ cell tumors: radiologic and pathologic correlation. Radiographics 1992;12(5):1013–1030

[21] Gaerte SC, Meyer CA, Winer-Muram HT, Tarver RD, Conces DJ Jr. Fat-containing lesions of the chest. Radiographics 2002;22(Spec No):S61–S78

[22] Rankin S. [(18)F]2-fluoro-2-deoxy-D-glucose PET/CT in mediastinal masses. Cancer Imaging 2010;10 Spec no A:S156–S160

[23] Benveniste MFK, Rosado-de-Christenson ML, Sabloff BS, Moran CA, Swisher SG, Marom EM. Role of imaging in the diagnosis, staging, and treatment of thymoma. Radiographics 2011;31(7):1847–1861, discussion 1861–1863

[24] Masaoka A, Monden Y, Nakahara K, Tanioka T. Follow-up study of thymomas with special reference to their clinical stages. Cancer 1981;48(11):2485–2492

[25] Detterbeck FC, Stratton K, Giroux D, et al; Staging and Prognostic Factors Committee. Members of the Advisory Boards. Participating Institutions of the Thymic Domain. The IASLC/ITMIG Thymic Epithelial Tumors Staging Project: proposal for an evidence-based stage classification system for the forthcoming (8th) edition of the TNM classification of malignant tumors. J Thorac Oncol 2014;9(9, Suppl 2):S65–S72

[26] Jeong YJ, Lee KS, Kim J, Shim YM, Han J, Kwon OJ. Does CT of thymic epithelial tumors enable us to differentiate histologic subtypes and predict prognosis? AJR Am J Roentgenol 2004;183(2):283–289

[27] Rosado de Christenson ML, Abbott GF, Kirejczyk WM, Galvin JR, Travis WD. Thoracic carcinoids: radiologic-pathologic correlation. Radiographics 1999;19(3):707–736

[28] Carbone PP, Kaplan HS, Musshoff K, Smithers DW, Tubiana M. Report of the Committee on Hodgkin's Disease Staging Classification. Cancer Res 1971;31(11):1860–1861

Chapter 13

Diseases of the Chest Wall and Diaphragm

13 Diseases of the Chest Wall and Diaphragm

13.1 Infection

Chest wall infections originate in place or are transmitted from the intrathoracic space. Bacterial inflammation is usually accompanied by pain and clinically manifest inflammatory symptoms. Imaging is only needed if there is clinical suspicion of involvement of the bones or intrathoracic compartments. CT is valuable for diagnostic exploration of any intrathoracic transmission of infection, while MRI lends itself to investigation of osteomyelitis.

If severe local findings are in contrast to a mild clinical presentation, the possibility of a *tuberculous abscess* should be considered. This results from per continuitatem spread of tuberculous pleuritis and is known as "empyema necessitans" (or "empyema necessitates"). The resultant tuberculous chest wall abscesses may be very large (▶Fig. 13.1).

13.2 SAPHO Syndrome

At times, palmoplantar pustulosis of the skin as well as severe acne are seen in association with characteristic skeletal findings, in particular in the chest wall. The acronym "SAPHO syndrome" was coined to denote this combination of synovitis, acne, palmoplantar pustulosis hyperostosis, and osteitis.

The clinical presentation reflects the combination of psoriasis, spondyloarthritis, and sterile multifocal osteomyelitis. The etiology is unknown. The vast majority of the osseous changes are observed in the anterior upper chest wall, especially in the sternocostoclavicular region. There may additionally be arthritis of the adjacent joints. Other findings such as osteosclerosis of one or several vertebral bodies or sacroiliitis may be present.[1]

Imaging demonstrates sclerosis and bulging of the medial ends of the clavicle and first rib as well as similar changes in the manubrium sterni (*sternocostoclavicular hyperostosis*, ▶Fig. 13.2). Often, erosions or ankylosis of the sternoclavic-

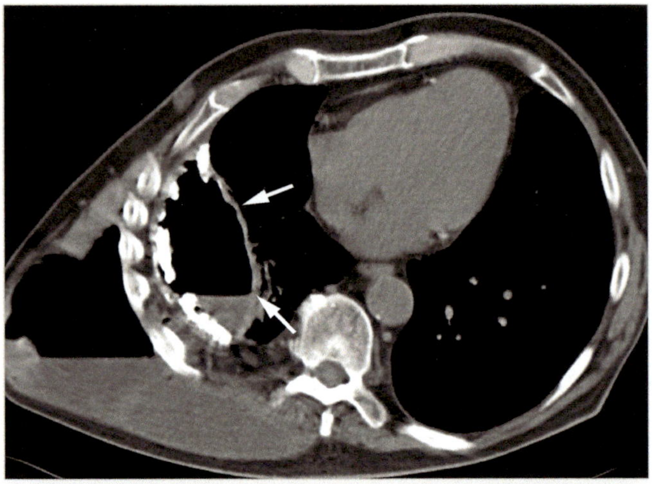

Fig. 13.1 Tuberculous chest wall abscess. CT image. Transmission of inflammation from the pleural space (*arrows*) in a case of tuberculous pleuritis, known as "empyema necessitans."

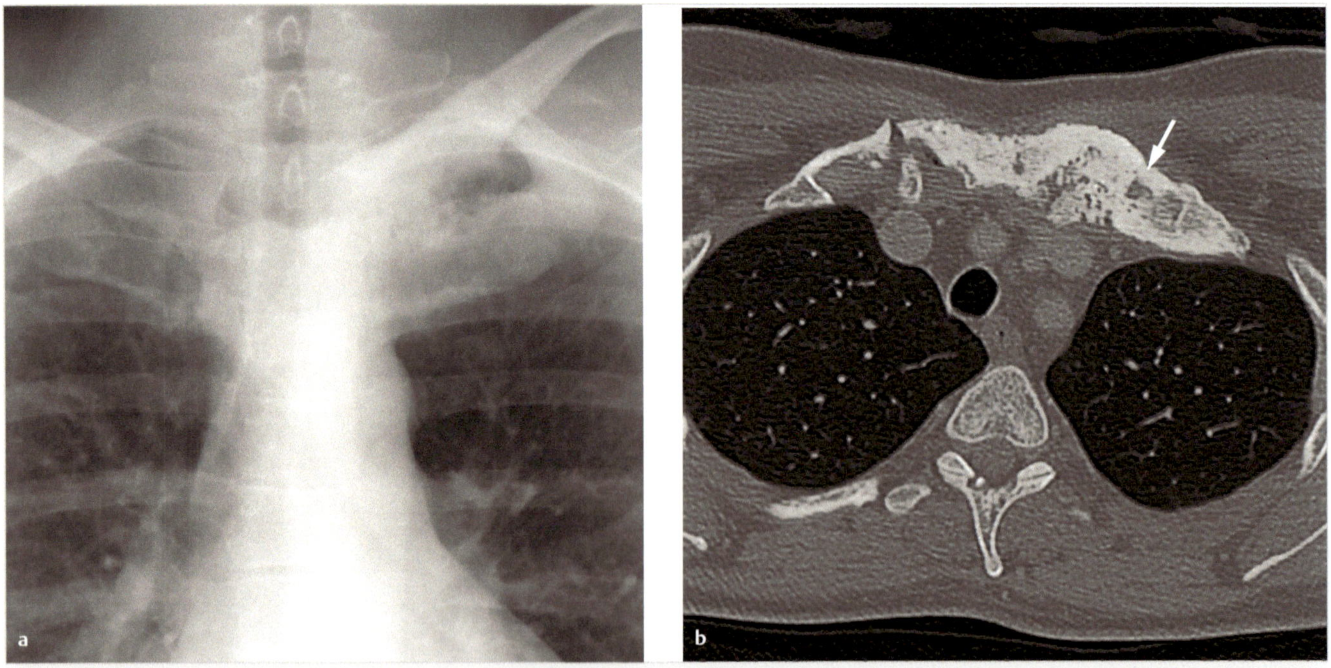

Fig. 13.2 SAPHO syndrome. Typical sternocostoclavicular hyperostosis. **(a)** Radiograph, sectional magnification. Increased sclerosis and bulging of the left medial end of the clavicle and first rib compared to the contralateral side; furthermore, sclerosis of the manubrium sterni. **(b)** CT image. In addition to increased sclerosis, small erosions can be identified in the sternocostal joint (*arrow*).

ular joints are identified in addition to abnormal ossification on CT.[2]

While the imaging findings are quite specific, they are not pathognomonic. Diagnosis is hampered in the absence of characteristic skin changes; these may have manifested several years previously.

> **Note**
>
> Differential diagnosis of SAPHO syndrome:
> - Osteomyelitis.
> - Paget's disease.
> - Avascular necrosis (osteonecrosis) of the clavicle.
> - Malignant bone tumors:
>   - Osteosarcoma.
>   - Ewing sarcoma.
>   - Metastasis.

At times, biopsy cannot be avoided for diagnosis confirmation.[1]

13.3 Tumors of the Chest Wall

The tumors described below are not specific to the chest wall but rather can occur anywhere in the entire musculoskeletal system. A guide to differentiate frequent benign from malignant tumors is given in ▶Table 13.1.

13.3.1 Benign Tumors

Benign tumors of the chest wall often exhibit characteristic imaging findings as presented in ▶Table 13.2. Typically, they are slowly growing and mostly asymptomatic. In particular, unlike the malignant tumors described in the following section, they do not cause pain of any significance.

Lipomas (see ▶Fig. 13.3) appear homogeneously fatty on CT and MRI. They occur in the chest wall both intramuscular and in the subcutaneous fat. In the latter setting, it is sometimes hardly possible to identify them on imaging despite evident clinical findings.

Fibrous dysplasia is monostotic in three-quarters of cases and polyostotic in one-quarter (see ▶Fig. 13.4). There is fusiform bulging and deformation of the affected bones, usually a rib, less commonly the clavicle. Amorphous calcifications are often observed on CT.[3]

Osteochondroma, a relatively common benign bone tumor, has a characteristic pedicled bony prominence (see ▶Fig. 13.5). The cartilage cap is best visualized on MRI; when the osteochondroma is oriented intrathoracically, it can also be seen on CT as a bony overlay of soft-tissue density.

Aneurysmal bone cysts are usually found in young adults. Their predilection sites in the chest wall are the posterior vertebral structures of the thoracic spine. Imaging demonstrates expansive osteolysis with cortical thinning.[3]

Giant cell tumors also occur in the same age group, affecting especially the sternum, clavicles, and ribs. Eccentric expansive osteolysis with cortical thinning is seen on imaging. Fluid–fluid levels are less common than in aneurysmal bone cysts.[3]

Table 13.1 Benign and malignant tumors of the chest wall

Benign tumors	Malignant tumors
• Lipoma • Neurogenic tumors: schwannoma, neurofibroma, ganglioneuroma, paraganglioma • Cavitary hemangioma • Benign bone tumors: fibrous dysplasia, osteochondroma, aneurysmal bone cyst, giant cell tumor	• Soft-tissue sarcomas • Chondrosarcoma • Osteosarcoma • Ewing sarcoma • Lymphomas • Myeloma • Malignant fibrous histiocytoma • Malignant nerve sheath tumors • Aggressive fibromatosis • Metastasis

Table 13.2 Guide to differential diagnosis of benign tumors of the chest wall[3]

Imaging findings	Tumor entities
Fat density on CT	Lipoma (▶Fig. 13.3)
Calcifications:	
• Skeletal:	
– Variable contour	Fibrous dysplasia (▶Fig. 13.4)
– Cartilage cap	Osteochondroma (▶Fig. 13.5)
• Extraskeletal, speckled	Cavitary hemangioma
Cortical thinning, fluid–fluid levels	Aneurysmal bone cyst, giant cell tumor
Smoothly marginated tumor, rib erosion, extraosseous localization	Schwannoma (▶Fig. 13.6) or neurofibroma
Located at costochondral transition	Osteochondroma (see ▶Fig. 13.5)
Paravertebral localization	Neurogenic tumor

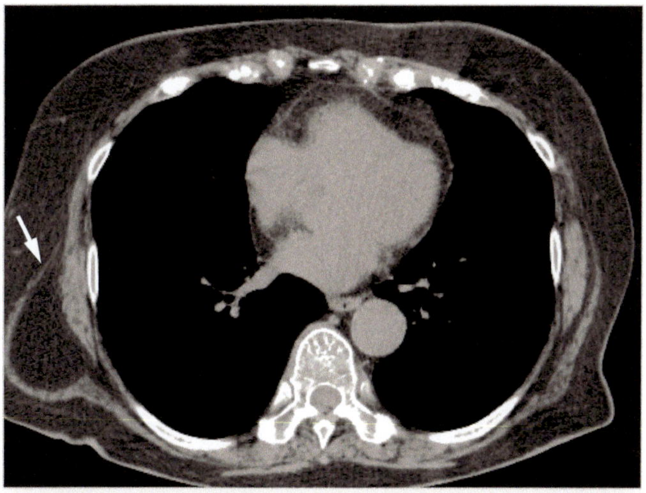

Fig. 13.3 Lipoma of the chest wall (*arrow*). CT image.

13.3.2 Malignant Tumors

Some malignant soft-tissue and bone tumors exhibit characteristic imaging findings, thus narrowing differential diagnosis (▶Table 13.3). A specific diagnosis of soft-tissue tumors, in particular, can usually only be made through invasive biopsy. However, in many cases imaging allows for differentiation from benign tumors.

> **Note**
>
> Unlike benign, generally asymptomatic, tumors, malignant tumors usually manifest clinically through pain.

Chondrosarcomas, the most common malignant bone tumors of the chest wall, have two age peaks (20 and over 50 years). A characteristic feature, which, however, is not always present, are the chondroid matrix calcifications identifiable especially on CT (see ▶Fig. 13.7). The tumors exhibit heterogeneous, in particular peripheral, contrast enhancement.[4]

Osteosarcomas rarely occur in the thorax and are usually found in young adults. The ribs, scapulae, and clavicles may be affected. They are more commonly associated with lymphogenous and hematogenous metastasis than other osteosarcomas, thus explaining the poorer prognosis of these chest wall tumors.[4]

Liposarcomas involve the chest wall only in very few cases. As fat-isodense tumors, it is very difficult to distinguish highly differentiated liposarcomas from lipomas on CT, while poorly differentiated liposarcomas have higher density, making them similar to solid tumors.

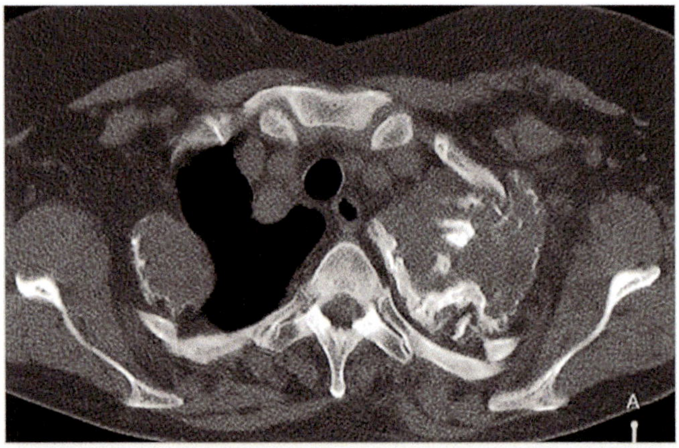

Fig. 13.4 Bilateral polyostotic fibrous dysplasia. CT image. Fusiform bulging of the ribs and considerable deformity, especially on the left.

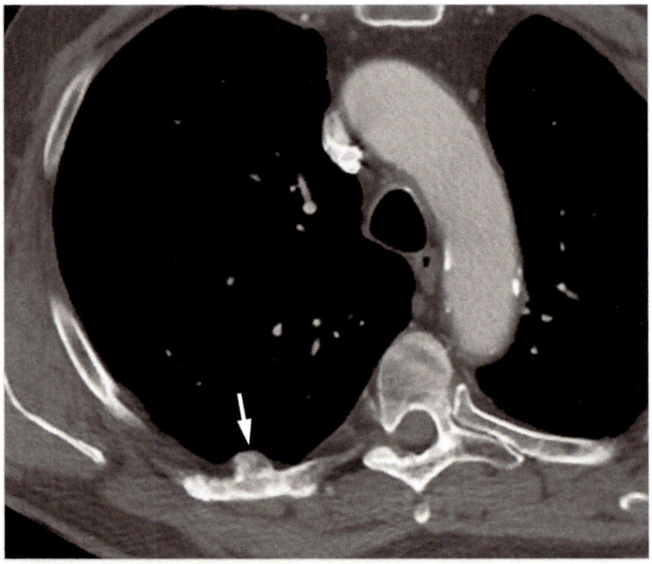

Fig. 13.5 Osteochondroma of a rib (*arrow*). CT image. Intrathoracically oriented, pedicled bony prominence.

Table 13.3 Guide to differential diagnosis of malignant tumors of the chest wall[4]

Imaging findings	Tumor entities
Fat component	Liposarcoma
Calcifications:	
• Skeletal:	
– Rings and arcs	Chondrosarcoma (▶Fig. 13.7)
– Speckled or flocculent	Chondrosarcoma
– Centrally dense	Osteosarcoma
• Extraskeletal: heterogeneous	Neuroblastoma or ganglioneuroblastoma
Diffuse osteolytic change	Multiple myeloma (▶Fig. 13.8)
Eccentric growth (children and young adults)	Ewing sarcoma (▶Fig. 13.9)
Fluid–fluid levels and calcifications (adolescents and young adults)	Synovial sarcoma
Infiltrative growth	Malignant lymphomas (▶Fig. 13.10) Aggressive fibromatosis
Nonspecific findings	• Leio- and rhabdomyosarcoma • Malignant fibrous histiocytoma • Malignant nerve sheath tumor (▶Fig. 13.11) • Soft-tissue metastasis

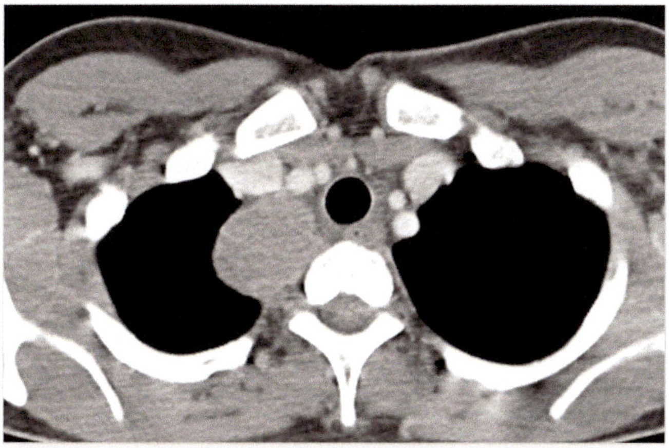

Fig. 13.6 **Schwannoma.** CT image. Smoothly marginated, right paravertebral mass with marked contrast enhancement.

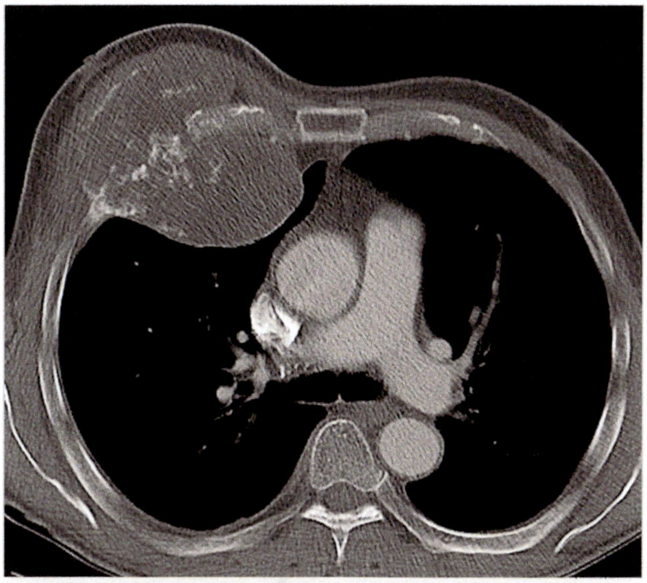

Fig. 13.7 **Chondrosarcoma of an anterior rib.** CT image. Large mass with chondroid matrix calcifications.

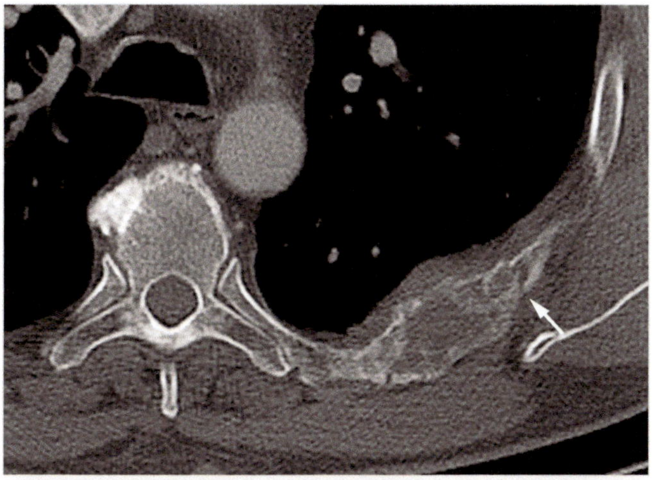

Fig. 13.8 **Plasmacytoma.** CT image. Bulging of a rib and osteolysis conferring a punched-out appearance. Nondisplaced pathologic fracture at the lateral margin of the lesion (*arrow*).

Solitary or multiple myeloma predominantly affects patients aged 50 to 70 years. Extraosseous myeloma is a mass of soft-tissue density that has no characteristic features. Bone myelomas cause osteolysis, conferring a punched-out appearance on the bones (see ▶Fig. 13.8) which are negative at scintigraphic bone scans.

Ewing sarcoma is found predominantly in children and young adults. It occurs as a solitary mass with an eccentric growth pattern or as multiple masses. Ewing sarcomas usually exhibit a space-occupying growth pattern (see ▶Fig. 13.9) and can spread by direct extension to the lung.

Malignant lymphomas are seen as enlargement of multiple lymph nodes or as a diffuse mass with an invasive growth pattern (see ▶Fig. 13.10). The typical age of disease onset is 60 years.

Aggressive fibromatosis (or desmoid tumor) is a relatively common disease mainly affecting adolescents and young adults. The infiltrative soft-tissue tumor exhibits an intermediate proliferative tendency. Aggressive fibromatosis does not metastasize, and even spontaneous regression may occur. Two growth patterns can be observed: an infiltrative pattern most common in adolescents and a nodular pattern, predominantly in adults. The lesions are usually confined to the musculature and adjacent fascia; nerves and blood vessels may be encased. On T1w MR imaging, the tumor has a signal intensity of less than or equal to that of muscle; on T2w images, an intermediate signal intensity is most common but a wide range of signal intensities can occasionally be observed.[4]

13.4 Diaphragmatic Paresis

The diaphragm, the primary respiratory muscle, is innervated by the phrenic nerve. Diaphragmatic dysfunction causes frequent respiratory problems. Depending on the residual function, the following terms are used to denote the reduction in active diaphragmatic motion:

- *Diaphragmatic paralysis*: complete loss of active motion.
- *Diaphragmatic paresis*: force reduction but still active motion.

Myriad causes affecting the entire neuromuscular excitation pathway are known (▶Table 13.4); however, often no cause can be elucidated (*idiopathic diaphragmatic paresis*).

Unilateral diaphragmatic paresis either is asymptomatic or is diagnosed due to exertional dyspnea. More rarely, bilateral diaphragmatic paresis is involved, inevitably causing symptoms since the auxiliary respiratory muscles are unable to compensate for diaphragmatic malfunction. This may result in respiratory failure.

A high-riding diaphragm seen on radiography demonstrates its functional loss (▶Fig. 13.12). Fluoroscopy or dynamic MRI sequences are used to investigate diaphragmatic motion.[6,7,8] MRI has the advantage of being able to present a three-dimensional view of diaphragmatic motion. A disadvantage is the supine position during MRI examination, causing alteration in the mechanics of breathing compared with fluoroscopy examination conducted while the patient is in the upright position.

13

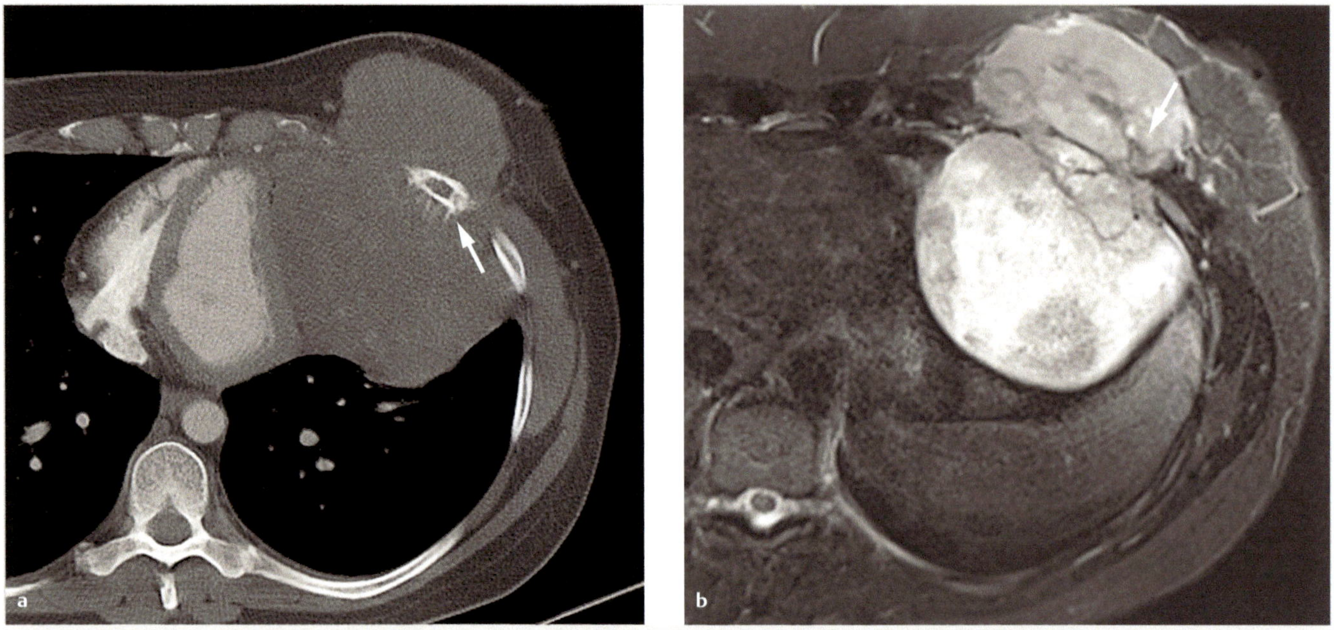

Fig. 13.9 Ewing sarcoma. Tumor with eccentric growth causing considerable lung compression. **(a)** CT image. Large soft-tissue tumor, osteolysis of the implicated rib and sunburst-like periosteal reaction (*arrow*). Compression of the left ventricle. **(b)** MRI, T2w image with fat saturation. Soft-tissue tumor with expansive growth and inhomogeneous signal hyperintensity.

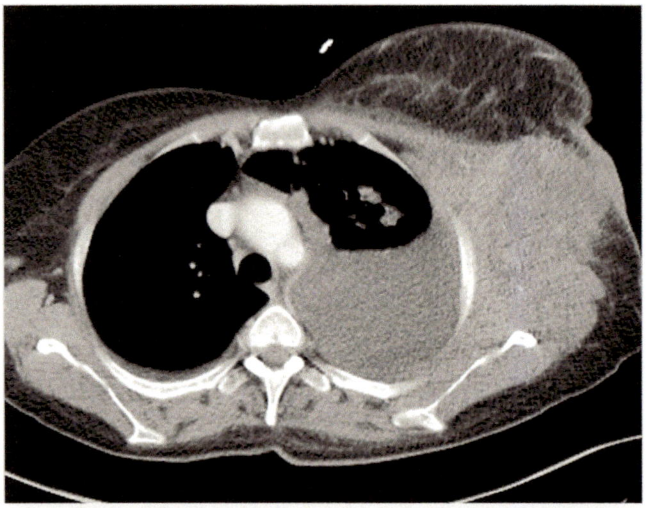

Fig. 13.10 Malignant lymphoma. CT image. Large, soft-tissue tumor with an invasive growth pattern in the left chest wall. Impaired lymphatic drainage of the left breast with increased density of fatty tissue due to edema. Large left pleural effusion.

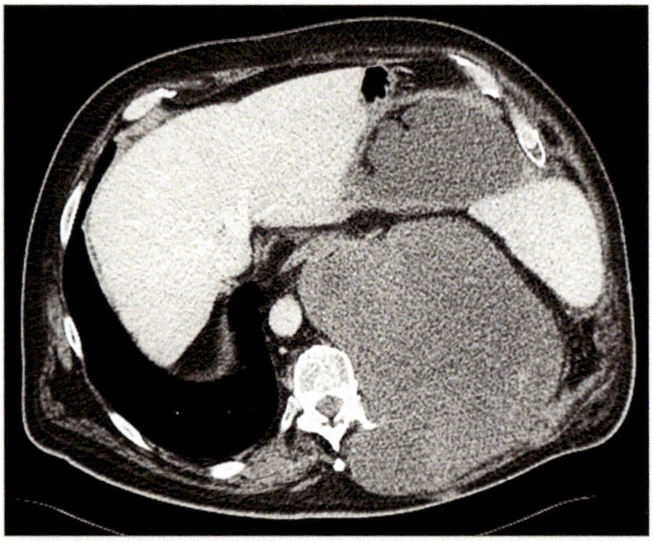

Fig. 13.11 Malignant nerve sheath tumor. CT image. Large left paravertebral, space-occupying mass.

A diaphragmatic respiratory excursion of over 4 cm is considered normal. A smaller excursion is suggestive of paresis. Complete absence of identifiable active diaphragmatic respiratory motion is consistent with paralysis, which is often accompanied by *paradoxical motion (diaphragmatic paradox)*. During inspiration the healthy diaphragm generates negative pressure in the thorax causing the paralytic diaphragm to move upward. During expiration the pressure conditions are reversed, and the paralytic diaphragm moves downward. As such, the diseased diaphragm moves opposite to the normal directions of the healthy diaphragm(▶Fig. 13.13).

Table 13.4 Causes of diaphragmatic paresis[5]

Cause	Examples
Isolated dysfunction of the phrenic nerve	• Surgical trauma • Blunt chest trauma • Tumor infiltration of the phrenic nerve • Radiotherapy • Aortic aneurysm • Goiter
Central nervous system disorders	• Cervical spondylosis • Cervical spine trauma • Cervical spine tumor • Transverse myelitis • Syringomyelia • Multiple sclerosis • Amyotrophic lateral sclerosis • Poliomyelitis • Spinal muscular atrophy • Viral diseases
Peripheral nervous system disorders	• Herpes zoster • Borreliosis • Guillain–Barré syndrome • Diabetic neuropathy • Toxins
Neuromuscular junction disorders	• Myasthenia gravis • Lambert-Eaton syndrome • Toxins
Myopathies	• Spinal muscular atrophy • Collagen vascular diseases: – Systemic lupus erythematosus – Mixed connective tissue disease – Dermatomyositis • Malnutrition • Hypo- or hyperthyroidism • Amyloidosis • Corticosteroids

The term *eventration* refers to congenital thinning of the diaphragm, giving rise to discrete bulging (known as a "diaphragmatic hump"), generally affecting the anteromedial segment of the right diaphragm.[9] This constitutes an usually asymptomatic incidental finding.

13.5 Diaphragmatic Hernia

Congenital diaphragmatic hernias have two predilection sites[5,10]:

- *Anterior → Morgagni hernia* (▶ Fig. 13.14): Incomplete fusion of the transverse ligament with the anterior chest wall leads to a right-sided anterior opening through which the abdominal structures can herniate upward. This hernia type is relatively rare.
- *Posterior → Bochdalek hernia* (▶ Fig. 13.15): Failure of fusion of the transverse septum with the intercostal muscles gives rise to a posterior opening in the diaphragm. Bochdalek hernias account for over 90% of all congenital hernias and occur predominantly on the left side. On lateral chest radiography, they typically manifest as smoothly marginated, hemispherical opacity in the posterior costophrenic angle.

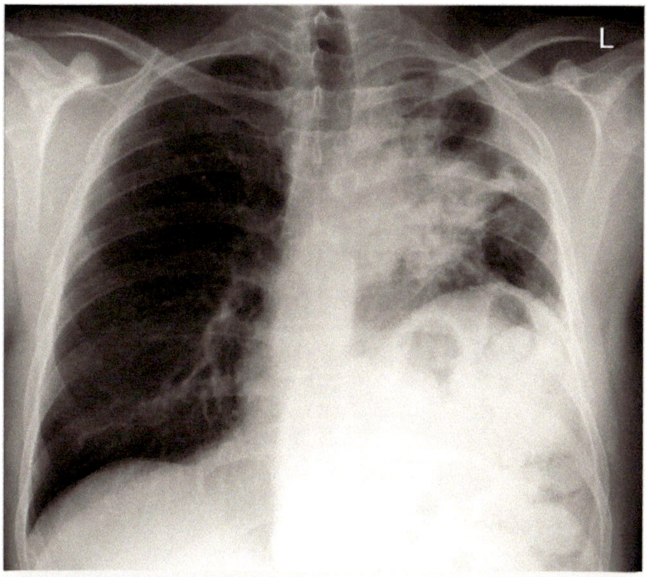

Fig. 13.12 Left diaphragmatic paresis secondary to tumor invasion of the left phrenic nerve. Radiograph. Left high-riding diaphragm and left central lung cancer.

Acquired diaphragmatic hernias affecting the esophageal hiatus are known as hiatal hernias (▶ Fig. 13.16). Parts of the stomach are displaced upward into the chest cavity, chiefly because of the cardia of the stomach sliding upward (axial sliding hernia), less commonly the cardia slides beside the esophagus (paraesophageal hernia). The term "upside-down stomach" denotes supradiaphragmatic displacement of almost the entire stomach (▶ Fig. 13.17). Often, larger hiatal hernias can be identified on chest radiographs as air-containing structures in the inferior middle mediastinum, sometimes in association with air-fluid levels. They are often diagnosed by chance in elderly persons.

Traumatic diaphragmatic hernias are discussed in Section 15.1.5.

13.6 Deformities of the Chest Wall

The *funnel chest* (pectus excavatum) is the most common congenital deformity of the chest wall with an incidence of 0.10 to 0.25% of all births.[11] It results from too fast and uncoordinated growth of the caudal rib cartilage. This pushes the sternum posteriorly, causing the rib cartilage to project

13

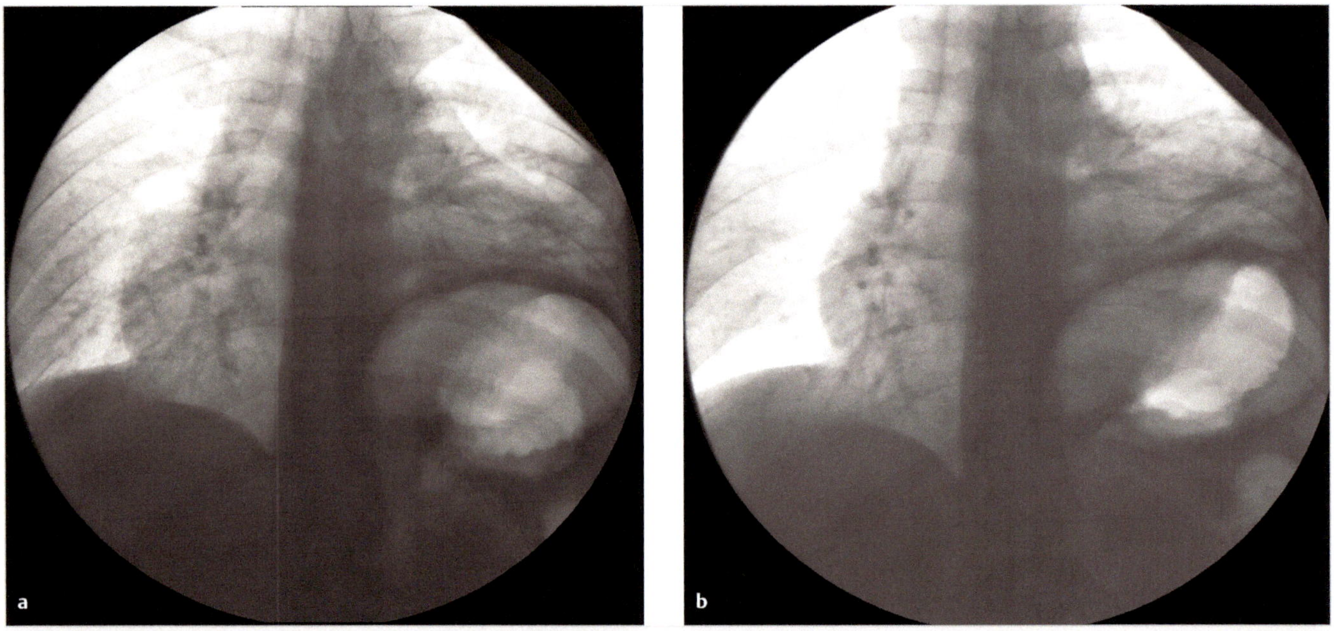

Fig. 13.13 **Left diaphragmatic paralysis. Fluoroscopy images.** Paradoxical motion of the left diaphragmatic. **(a)** Expiratory image. **(b)** Inspiratory image: the left diaphragm is higher than in expiration.

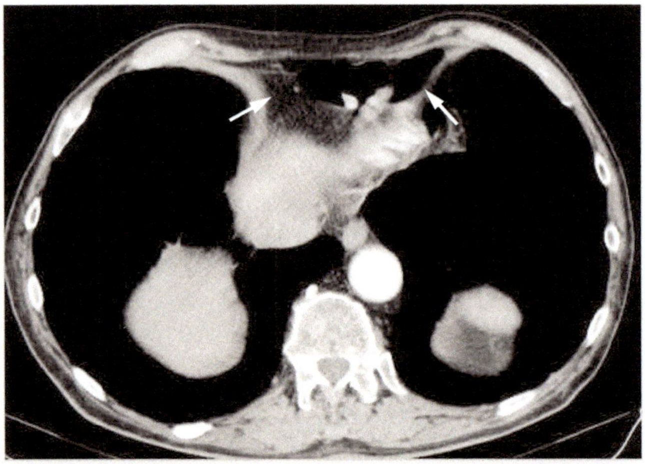

Fig. 13.14 **Morgagni hernia.** CT image. Parts of the transverse colon and mesenterial fat can be identified anterior to the heart (*arrows*).

anterior to the sternum (▶Fig. 13.18).[12] On rare occasions, this deformity is associated with certain syndromes (Marfan syndrome, Ehlers–Danlos syndrome, congenital heart diseases). A funnel chest is usually asymptomatic; it may also result in a slightly compromised physical performance because of displacement of the heart and lungs. Corrective surgery may be indicated in such cases, as sometimes resorted to for cosmetic reasons.[2] To that effect, the sternum is fractured and elevated with a metal bracket (▶Fig. 13.19). Sectional imaging (CT or MRI) is useful for preoperative management.

In the *pigeon chest* (pectus carinatum), the sternum is displaced anteriorly, unlike in the funnel chest (▶Fig. 13.20). With an incidence of 1:1,500 births, this is less common than the funnel chest and is associated with scoliosis in one-third of cases. Often, it leads to reduced physical strength and exertional dyspnea which can be considerably improved through corrective surgery.[2]

Cervical ribs, which are asymptomatic in the vast majority of cases, are found in around 0.5% of the population. Occasionally, they compress vessels and nerves supplying the arm in the upper thoracic outlet. This causes pain, hand swelling, or thoracic outlet syndrome. Cervical ribs can generally be clearly identified on posteroanterior radiographs. CT is able to directly visualize compression of vascular structures.

13.7 Summary

Occasionally, sectional imaging is needed to explore the extent of *chest wall infections*. MRI is superior to CT in identifying bone involvement (osteomyelitis). CT usually suffices for demonstration or exclusion of involvement of intrathoracic compartments. Large chest wall abscesses with relatively few symptoms should call to mind tuberculous empyema necessitans.

SAPHO syndrome, a rare disease of rheumatoid etiology, is sometimes associated with psoriasis. It results in characteristic skin efflorescences (palmoplantar pustulosis, severe acne) and highly specific skeletal radiographic findings of the upper thoracic outlet (sternocostoclavicular hyperostosis).

Both multiple benign and malignant *tumors* occur in the chest wall. The specific tumor type can be diagnosed on imaging

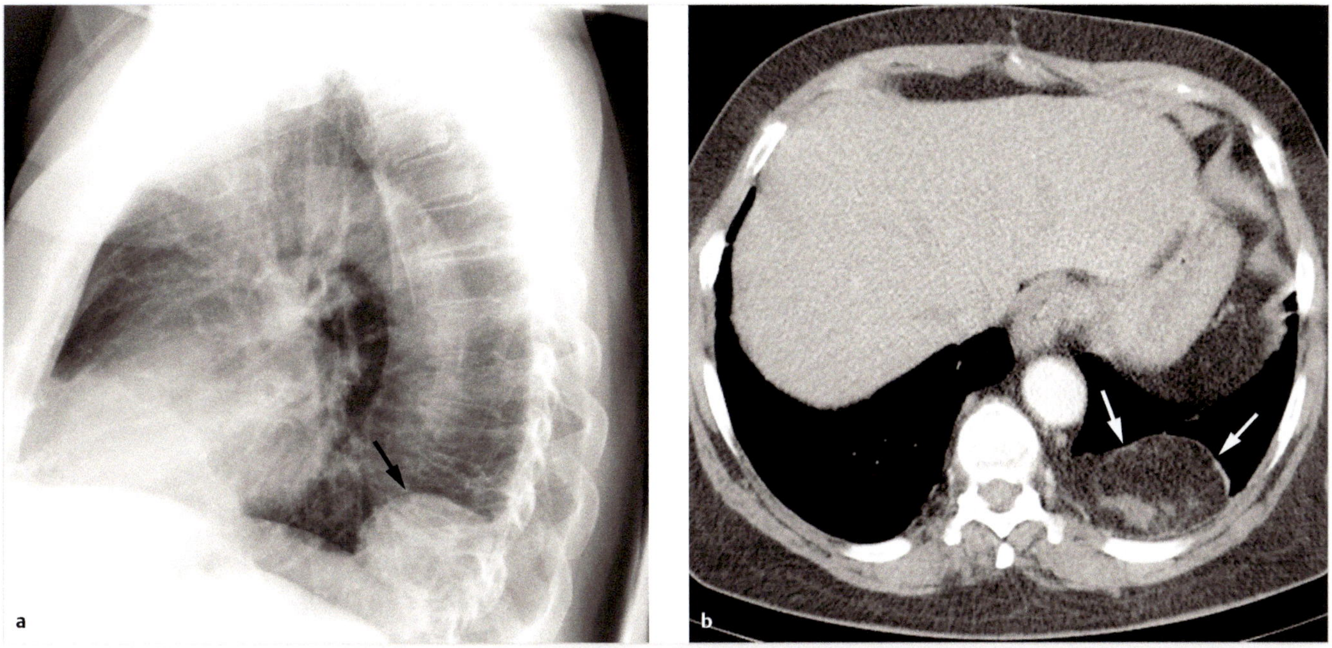

Fig. 13.15 Bochdalek hernia. (a) Radiograph, sectional magnification. Smoothly marginated, hemispherical opacity in the left posterior costophrenic angle (*arrow*). **(b)** CT image. Left posterior herniation of abdominal fat (*arrows*).

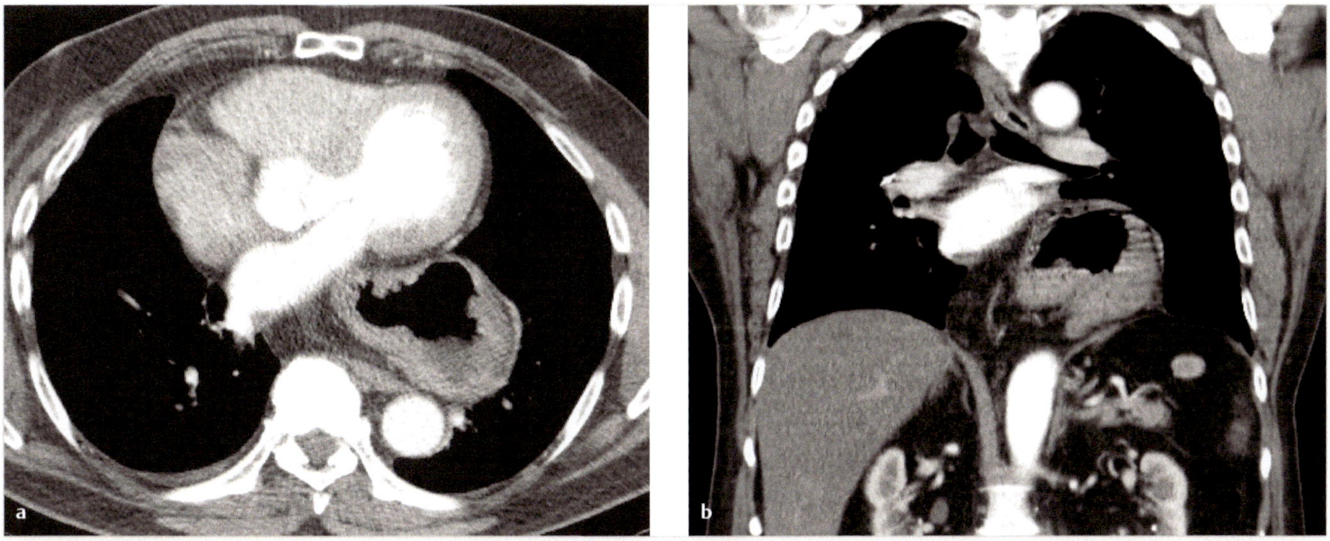

Fig. 13.16 Hiatal hernia. Intrathoracic herniation of parts of the stomach through the esophageal hiatus **(a)** CT axial. **(b)** CT coronal.

only for a few tumor entities, e.g., lipoma. However, differentiation between probably benign and malignant tumors is possible in most cases (see ▸Table 13.2 and ▸Table 13.3).

Numerous causes of *diaphragmatic paresis* are known (see ▸Table 13.4), but it is often idiopathic. A high-riding diaphragm and reduced diaphragmatic motion (less than 4 cm) on dynamic examination (fluoroscopy or MRI) are suggestive of diaphragmatic paresis. Complete diaphragmatic paralysis differs from incomplete diaphragmatic paresis through its complete absence of active motion and paradoxical diaphragmatic motion.

Diaphragmatic hernias are classified as congenital (often posterior Bochdalek hernia, less common anterior Morgagni hernia) and acquired hernias (hiatal hernias: paraesophageal and hiatal sliding hernias, traumatic diaphragmatic hernias).

Funnel chest is the most common *congenital deformity of the sternum.* This results in posterior displacement of the lower part of the sternum. Less common is the pigeon chest causing anterior displacement of the sternum. *Cervical ribs,* usually an incidental finding, are rarely symptomatic but can cause thoracic outlet syndrome or compression of nerves in the brachial plexus.

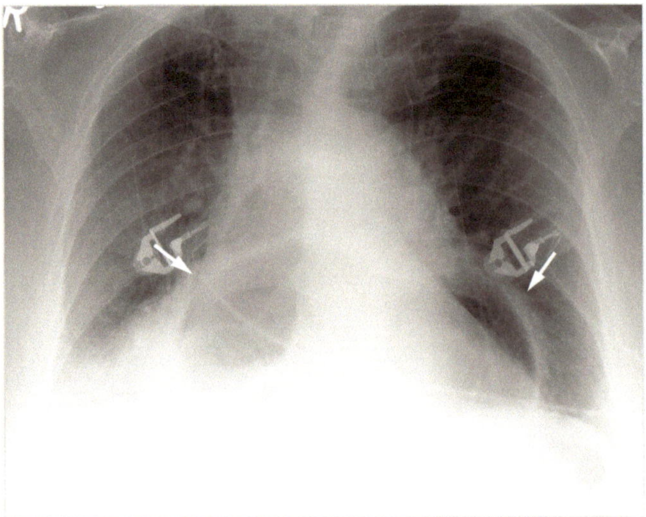

Fig. 13.17 **Upside-down stomach.** Radiograph. Large, smoothly marginated, air-containing retrocardial structure (*arrows*), consistent with a herniated stomach.

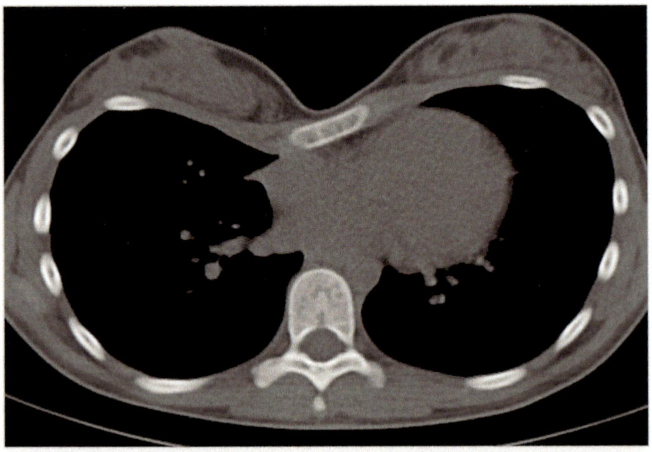

Fig. 13.18 **Funnel chest.** CT image. Posterior displacement of the sternum and displacement of the heart toward the left.

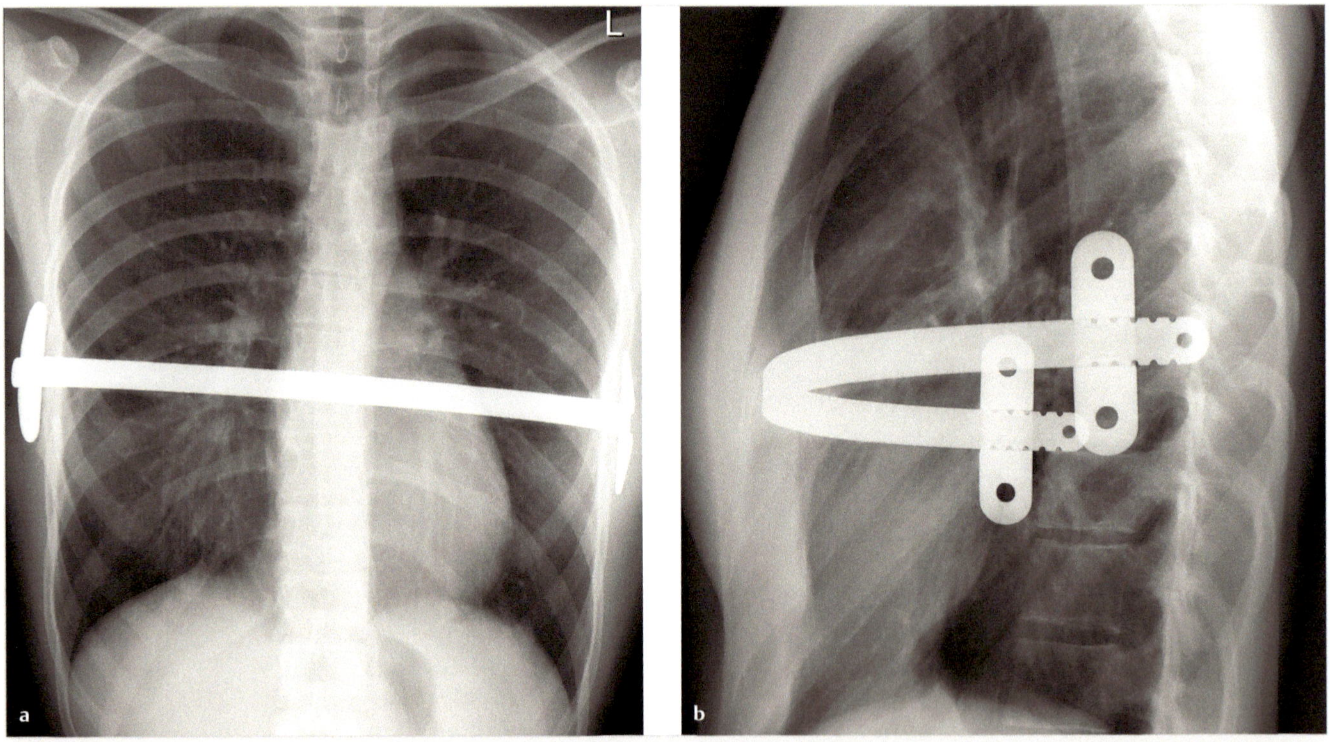

Fig. 13.19 **Corrective surgery of funnel chest.** Radiographs. Same female patient as in ▶Fig. 13.18. The sternum has been elevated by means of the metal bracket inserted into the chest wall. **(a)** Posteroanterior image. **(b)** Lateral image, sectional magnification.

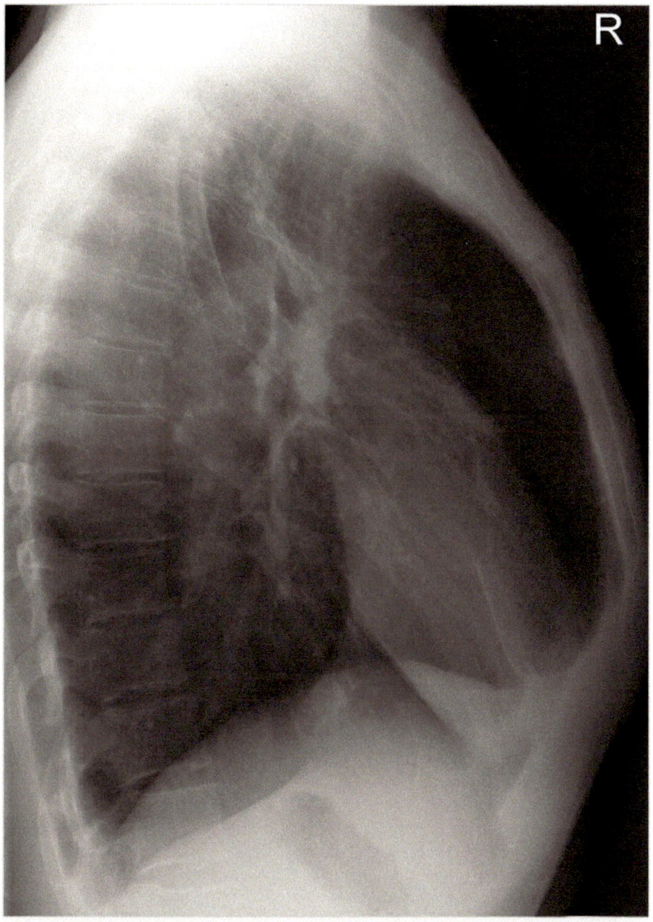

Fig. 13.20 Pigeon chest. Radiograph, lateral.

References

[1] Cotten A, Flipo RM, Mentre A, Delaporte E, Duquesnoy B, Chastanet P. SAPHO syndrome. Radiographics 1995;15(5):1147–1154

[2] Restrepo CS, Martinez S, Lemos DF, et al. Imaging appearances of the sternum and sternoclavicular joints. Radiographics 2009;29(3):839–859

[3] Tateishi U, Gladish GW, Kusumoto M, et al. Chest wall tumors: radiologic findings and pathologic correlation: part 1. Benign tumors. Radiographics 2003;23(6):1477–1490

[4] Tateishi U, Gladish GW, Kusumoto M, et al. Chest wall tumors: radiologic findings and pathologic correlation: part 2. Malignant tumors. Radiographics 2003;23(6):1491–1508

[5] Nason LK, Walker CM, McNeeley MF, Burivong W, Fligner CL, Godwin JD. Imaging of the diaphragm: anatomy and function. Radiographics 2012;32(2):E51–E70

[6] Gierada DS, Curtin JJ, Erickson SJ, Prost RW, Strandt JA, Goodman LR. Diaphragmatic motion: fast gradient-recalled-echo MR imaging in healthy subjects. Radiology 1995;194(3):879–884

[7] Kiryu S, Loring SH, Mori Y, Rofsky NM, Hatabu H, Takahashi M. Quantitative analysis of the velocity and synchronicity of diaphragmatic motion: dynamic MRI in different postures. Magn Reson Imaging 2006;24(10):1325–1332

[8] Unal O, Arslan H, Uzun K, Ozbay B, Sakarya ME. Evaluation of diaphragmatic movement with MR fluoroscopy in chronic obstructive pulmonary disease. Clin Imaging 2000;24(6):347–350

[9] Yeh HC, Halton KP, Gray CE. Anatomic variations and abnormalities in the diaphragm seen with US. Radiographics 1990;10(6):1019–1030

[10] Taylor GA, Atalabi OM, Estroff JA. Imaging of congenital diaphragmatic hernias. Pediatr Radiol 2009;39(1):1–16

[11] Creswick HA, Stacey MW, Kelly RE Jr, et al. Family study of the inheritance of pectus excavatum. J Pediatr Surg 2006;41(10):1699–1703

[12] Jeung MY, Gangi A, Gasser B, et al. Imaging of chest wall disorders. Radiographics 1999;19(3):617–637

Chapter 14

Vascular Diseases

14 Vascular Diseases

14.1 Diseases of the Pulmonary Arteries

14.1.1 Acute Pulmonary Embolism

Venous thromboembolism is one of the most common cardiovascular diseases. It comprises two clinical disease entities: deep vein thrombosis, usually in the legs, and pulmonary embolism, with the latter having a more severe course for the patient. The spectrum of clinical manifestations ranges from lethal circulatory collapse to asymptomatic incidental findings. Several predisposing factors increase the risk of venous thromboembolism, e.g., major trauma, surgery, fractures of the lower limbs, spinal injuries, and malignant tumors. For younger women, the main risk factor is oral contraception.

The typical symptoms of pulmonary embolism include dyspnea of sudden onset, pleuritic chest pain, or retrosternal pain as well as cough. Hemoptysis, fever, or syncope occurs less commonly. In one-quarter of cases, signs of deep vein thrombosis of the leg can also be detected. Hypoxemia in arterial blood gas analysis is suggestive of pulmonary embolism, but it is seen only in around half of cases. Oligosymptomatic or asymptomatic pulmonary embolism is not uncommon.

The pathophysiologic mechanism of pulmonary embolism is generally based on impaired right heart function due to an increased right ventricular afterload. The resultant dilation of the right ventricle causes tricuspid valve insufficiency. At the same time, the rising wall tension of the right ventricular muscle cells activates neurohormones, triggering a myocardial inflammatory reaction. The resultant increase in myocardial oxygen demand leads to myocardial ischemia which, in turn, reduces heart muscle contractility. The now reduced right ventricular stroke volume decreases the left ventricular preload. The left ventricular blood volume drops, causing a lowered systemic blood pressure. Declining coronary perfusion exacerbates right ventricular ischemia. The interaction of these pathophysiologic processes culminates in cardiogenic shock and death.[1]

The choice of treatment is based on the early mortality risk. Two strategies are available: an aggressive approach with thrombolysis (interventional thrombus fragmentation) or a less aggressive one with thromboendarterectomy and anticoagulation treatment. The former is associated with a higher complication rate, in particular bleedings. A simple initial risk stratification determines the adequate diagnostic and therapeutic strategy (▶Table 14.1).[1,2]

The widely used score systems illustrated in ▶Table 14.2 and ▶Table 14.3 have only moderate discriminatory power for assessment of the clinical probability of pulmonary embolism. Two-thirds of all patients with a score consistent with a high clinical probability do indeed have a pulmonary embolism. However, 10% of patients with a low probability are also revealed to have an embolism. D-dimer testing considerably increases the discriminatory power of the diagnostic algorithm for patients with a low or intermediate probability. Therefore, before resorting to computed tomography pulmonary angiography (CTPA), this laboratory parameter is measured for hemodynamically stable patients who do not have a high probability of pulmonary embolism.

Chest radiography no longer plays any role in diagnostic imaging of suspected pulmonary embolism. Radiography is unable to directly visualize the embolism, relying instead on indirect findings: platelike atelectasis, pleural-based consolidations consistent with pulmonary infarction (so-called Hampton hump), pleural effusion, oligemia (Westermark sign), prominent central pulmonary arteries, or a high-riding diaphragm.[7]

CTPA has now supplanted the formerly common ventilation/perfusion (VQ) scan and is currently the imaging modality of choice in settings of clinically suspected pulmonary embolism. On CTPA, the embolism is directly visualized as an intravascular contrast filling defect (▶Fig. 14.1). Already a large-scale study conducted quite some time ago predominantly with four-row CT scanners demonstrated a high accuracy for that technique, with a sensitivity of 83% and specificity of 96%.[8] More modern CT scanners will undoubtedly have higher sensitivity.

Table 14.1 Diagnostic and therapeutic strategy relative to the early mortality risk[1]

Diagnosis/treatment	High early mortality risk	No high early mortality risk
Definition	Shock or hypotension[a]	No shock, no hypotension
Diagnosis	CTPA, if this is immediately available, otherwise echocardiography (dilation of the right ventricle?)	For high clinical probability (see ▶Table 14.2): primary CTPA For low/intermediate clinical probability (see ▶Table 14.2): • D-dimer test • For positive D-dimer test: CTPA
Treatment	Primary reperfusion (thrombolysis, interventional or surgical recanalization)	Anticoagulation

Abbreviation: CTPA, computed tomography pulmonary angiography.
[a]Systolic blood pressure below 90 mm Hg or drop of at least 40 mm Hg for at least 15 min if this was not caused by new onset arrhythmia, hypovolemia, or sepsis.

14

II

Table 14.2 Clinical Wells score for assessment of clinical probability of pulmonary embolism[1]

Wells score	Points (original version[3])	Points (simplified version[4])
Previous pulmonary embolism or deep vein thrombosis	1.5	1
Heart rate ≥ 100/min	1.5	1
Surgery or immobilization within the past 4 weeks	1.5	1
Hemoptysis	1	1
Active cancer	1	1
Clinical signs of deep vein thrombosis	3	1
Alternative diagnosis less likely than pulmonary embolism	3	1
Clinical probability		
Three-level score:		
• Low probability	0–1	
• Intermediate probability	2–6	
• High probability	≥ 7	
Two-level score:		
• Pulmonary embolism unlikely	0–4	0–1
• Pulmonary embolism likely	≥ 5	≥ 2

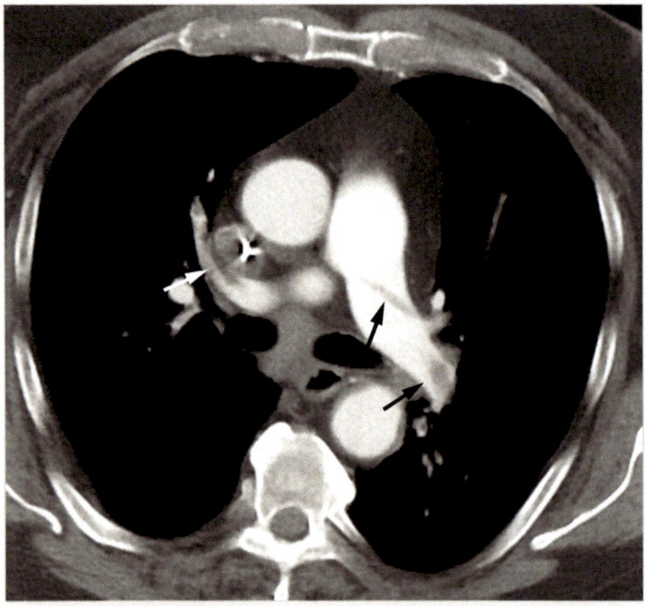

Fig. 14.1 Acute pulmonary embolism. CT image. Contrast filling defects in the central pulmonary arteries (*arrows*).

Furthermore, CT provides additional information. An enlarged right ventricle indicates right heart strain of prognostic relevance. To that effect, the cross-sectional diameter (short axis) of the right (RV) and left ventricle (LV) is measured on the axial

Table 14.3 Revised Geneva score for assessment of clinical probability of pulmonary embolism[1]

Revised Geneva score	Points (original version[5])	Points (simplified version[6])
Previous pulmonary embolism or deep vein thrombosis	3	1
Heart rate:		
• 75–94/min	3	1
• > 95/min	5	2
Surgery or fracture within the past month	2	1
Hemoptysis	2	1
Active cancer	2	1
Unilateral lower limb pain	3	1
Pain on lower limb deep venous palpation and unilateral edema	4	1
Age > 65 years	1	1
Clinical probability		
Three-level score:		
• Low probability	0–3	0–1
• Intermediate probability	4–10	2–4
• High probability	≥ 11	≥ 5
Two-level score:		
• Pulmonary embolism unlikely	0–5	0–2
• Pulmonary embolism likely	≥ 6	≥ 3

CT image; an RV/LV quotient >1 attests to right heart strain.[9,10,11] Various parameters have been proposed for assessment of right heart strain or estimation of prognosis, e.g., several score systems for determination of the thromboembolic burden or measurement of the pulmonary artery diameter, its ratio to the aortic diameter, and protrusion of the ventricular septum toward the left heart. The validity of all these values is disputed and they are probably of no prognostic relevance.[10]

Dilation of the superior vena cava or azygos vein is suggestive of congestive right heart failure, which has a poor prognosis.[10,12] IV contrast reflux into the hepatic veins is an indirect sign of tricuspid valve insufficiency. However, there is no proof of correlation with the severity of pulmonary embolism.[13]

Triangular pleural-based consolidations or ground-glass opacities (▶ Fig. 14.2) are consistent with pulmonary infarction and can occasionally be identified in patients with pulmonary embolism.

Clinical management of pulmonary embolism has to contend with two challenging constellations:

- *Isolated subsegmental pulmonary embolism*: Exclusively subsegmental localization is seen on CTPA in up to10% of all pulmonary embolisms.[14] Such findings have a low positive predictive value and high interobserver variability.[15] Their

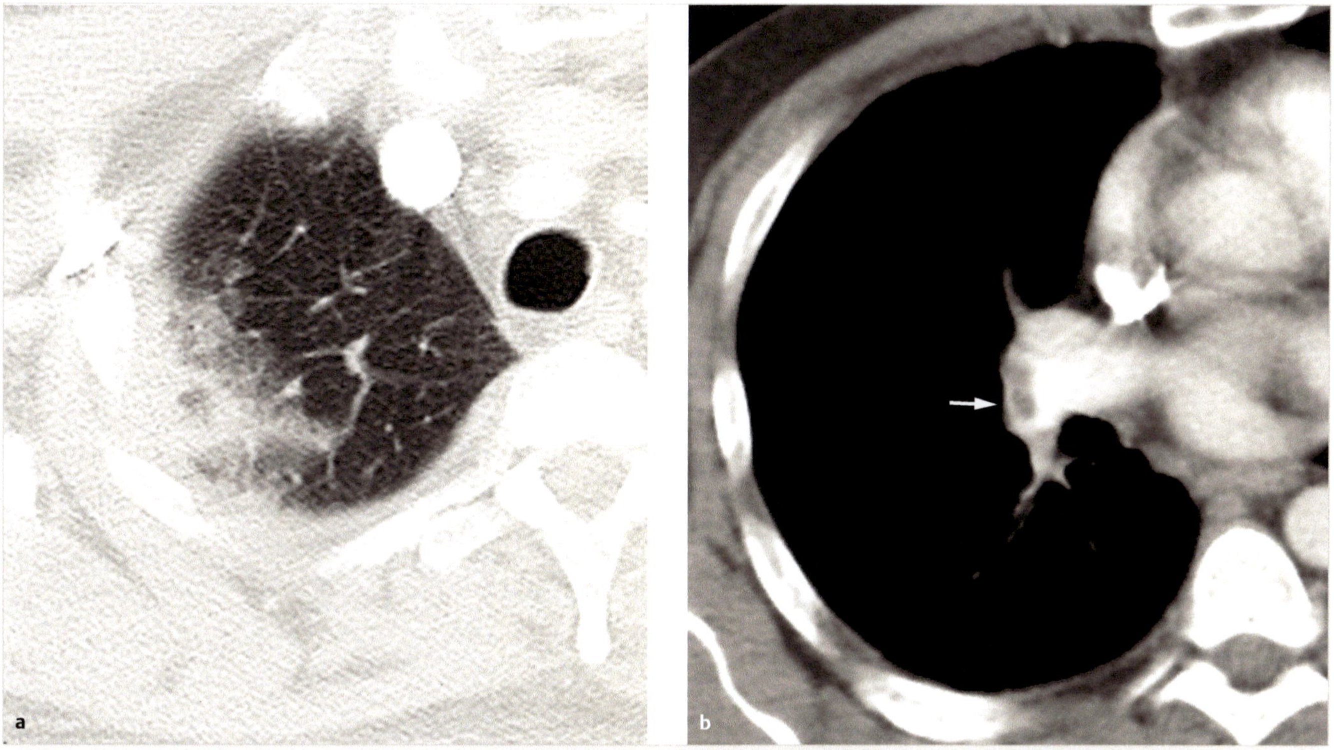

Fig. 14.2 Pulmonary infarction secondary to acute pulmonary embolism. CT images. **(a)** Pulmonary infarction: pleural-based consolidation and ground-glass opacity in the right apical upper lobe segment. **(b)** Underlying pulmonary embolism in the right upper lobe artery (*arrow*).

clinical significance depends on the extent of embolism (solitary or multiple emboli) and the underlying comorbidities. Adjunctive compression sonography of the leg veins is advisable to rule out deep vein thrombosis of the leg requiring treatment. In the event of negative compression sonography in settings of isolated subsegmental pulmonary embolism, the need for anticoagulant therapy should be considered in individual cases. To that end, the clinical probability of pulmonary embolism and the existing cardiopulmonary reserve must be weighed up against the treatment-induced bleeding risk.[1,15]

- *Asymptomatic pulmonary embolism*: Another problem emanates from completely asymptomatic pulmonary embolism incidentally identified in 1 to 2% of all CT scans.[16,17,18,19,20] Anticoagulant treatment is recommended at least for patients with a malignant tumor and central pulmonary embolism.[1,21] Study data increasingly suspect overdiagnosis of pulmonary embolism with widespread use of CTPA.[1,22,23,24,25]

Deep vein thrombosis (DVT) of the leg is the most common cause of pulmonary embolism. CT venography and compression sonography are diagnostically equivalent for detection of DVT.[26] However, preference should be given in principle to compression sonography since CT venography involves considerable radiation exposure for the patient.[1] But an exception should be made for patients whose cases are known in advance to provide insufficient ultrasound examination conditions. In such cases, CT venography can be performed at the same time as CTPA to exclude DVT.

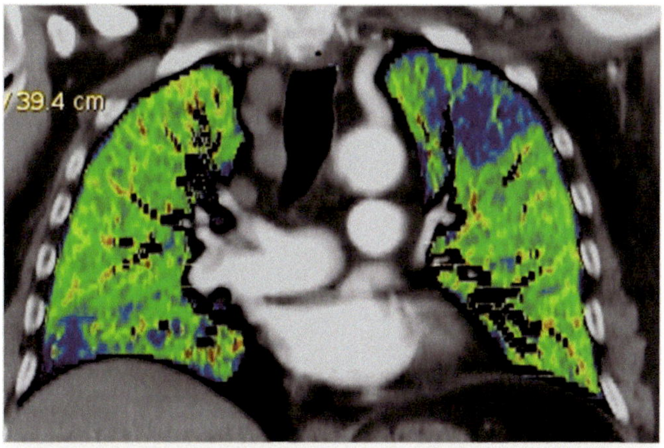

Fig. 14.3 Acute pulmonary embolism. DECT, coronal. On the iodine map (color depiction) bilateral wedge-shaped perfusion defects (*blue*). Same patient as in ▶Fig. 14.1.

Dual-energy CT (DECT) and MRI are able to directly visualize embolism-related defects in lung perfusion.[27] If CTPA is carried out as DECT, iodine maps can be generated from the CT dataset. These show the contrast distribution within the lung parenchyma and will thus demonstrate perfusion defects (▶Fig. 14.3) and provide additional information on the vascular architecture.[28] Not all embolisms identified on

CTPA are associated with a perfusion defect. The converse applies to a lesser degree, i.e., it is not possible on CTPA to find a correlate for every perfusion defect. The clinical significance of this additional information is still unclear but extensive perfusion defects are possibly associated with a poor prognosis.[29]

Simultaneously, DECT spectral imaging can enhance the vascular contrast in the pulmonary arteries. A lower virtual kV setting thus helps increase diagnostic reliability and allows for use of lower concentrated IV contrast media, if necessary.[30] At times, there may be inadequate contrast enhancement of the pulmonary arteries because of a Valsalva maneuver during the CT scan (transient interruption of contrast phenomenon[31]). Retrospective increase of vascular contrast by lowering the virtual kV setting may be helpful in such cases.

14.1.2 Chronic Thromboembolic Disease and Chronic Thromboembolic Pulmonary Hypertension

The endoluminal thrombotic emboli occurring in acute pulmonary embolism normally resolve completely within a few weeks. But if resolution is incomplete, chronic pulmonary embolism becomes established (chronic thromboembolic disease, CTED).

CT demonstrates completely occluded vessels with a smaller than normal caliber compared to the proximate blood vessels as well as sickle-shaped contrast filling defects, consistent with wall-adherent thrombi (▶Fig. 14.4). Other characteristic findings include small-caliber pulmonary arteries with wall thickening, and possibly with wall calcification, as well as intravascular webs and bands. The lung parenchyma exhibits

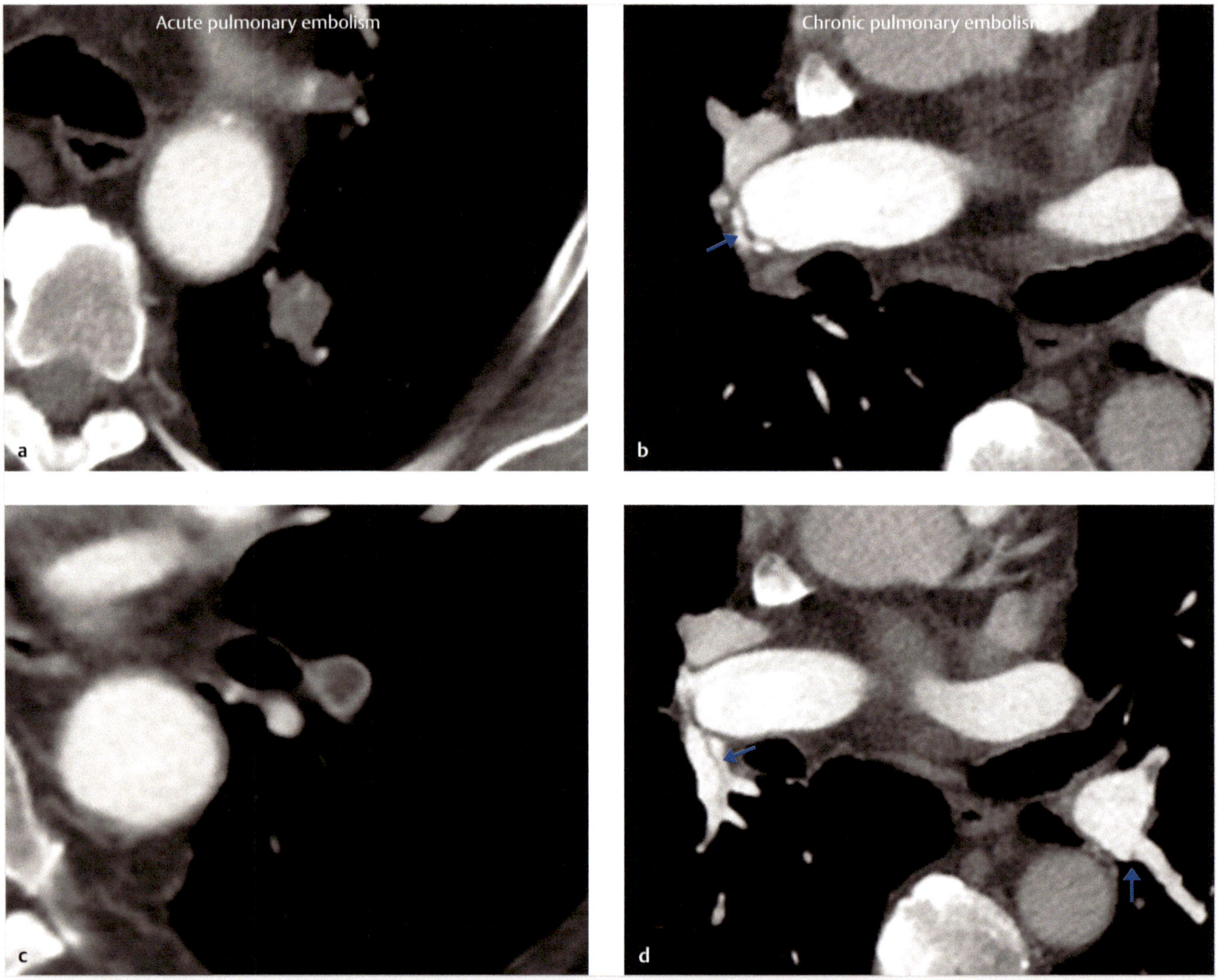

Fig. 14.4 Typical CT findings in acute and chronic pulmonary embolism. CT images. **(a)** Complete obstruction of pulmonary artery. **(b)** Central contrast filling defect. **(c)** Sickle-shaped contrast filling defects with calcifications (*arrow*). **(d)** Intraluminal webs and bands (*arrows*).

a mosaic attenuation pattern because of regional oligemia. The formation of systemic bronchial artery collaterals can be recognized from dilation of the bronchial arteries (▶ Fig. 14.5).[20,32,33]

A rare but important condition that should be included in differential diagnosis of intravascular contrast filling defects in the pulmonary arteries is *angiosarcoma*, a malignant tumor originating from the vascular wall (▶ Fig. 14.6). This is very often initially misinterpreted as chronic thromboembolic disease.[34,35,36] The most important differentiation criterion is visible extravascular lesion growth, which can be expected in angiosarcoma but not in chronic embolism.

In a small percentage of patients with symptomatic acute pulmonary embolism, persistent obstruction of the pulmonary arterial vascular bed results in the development of pulmonary hypertension (see below).[1] This is known as *chronic thromboembolic pulmonary hypertension* (CTEPH). The disease is thought to be underdiagnosed since initially it causes only nonspecific symptoms of pulmonary hypertension.[37] A considerable proportion of patients with chronic thromboembolic pulmonary hypertension have no previous reports of an acute pulmonary embolic event.

Chronic thromboembolic pulmonary hypertension is present if the following conditions have been met:

- Pulmonary arterial mean pressure of at least 25 mm Hg with pulmonary capillary wedge pressure of no more than 15 mm Hg.
- At least, one segmental pulmonary perfusion defect[38] or one instance of vascular occlusion on CT or pulmonary angiography.[1]

The only curative treatment option is pulmonary endarterectomy. The prognosis for patients who cannot undergo surgical treatment is poor. Currently, interventional balloon angioplasty of the pulmonary arteries is being investigated for some of these patients. Furthermore, vasodilators have been recently approved for conservative treatment of CTEPH.

Ventilation/perfusion (VQ) scan is considered to be the diagnostic reference standard for detection of perfusion defects.[39] A normal VQ scan virtually rules out the presence of chronic thromboembolic pulmonary hypertension eligible for surgical treatment.[40]

CTPA is unable to visualize with adequate sensitivity the vascular changes in chronic thromboembolic pulmonary hypertension but is needed to explore the feasibility of surgical treatment. DECT is able to demonstrate lung perfusion during CTPA. In the future, it could also be used to detect perfusion defects and, as such, for primary diagnosis of chronic thromboembolic pulmonary hypertension (▶ Fig. 14.7), although reliable data to that effect are not yet available.[37,41,42]

In addition to the findings of chronic thromboembolic disease described at the beginning of this chapter, chronic thromboembolic pulmonary hypertension is often accompanied by dilated bronchial arteries. Furthermore, the increased pulmonary arterial pressure causes more fluid displacement from the blood vessels into the interstitium, thus resulting in a rise in the

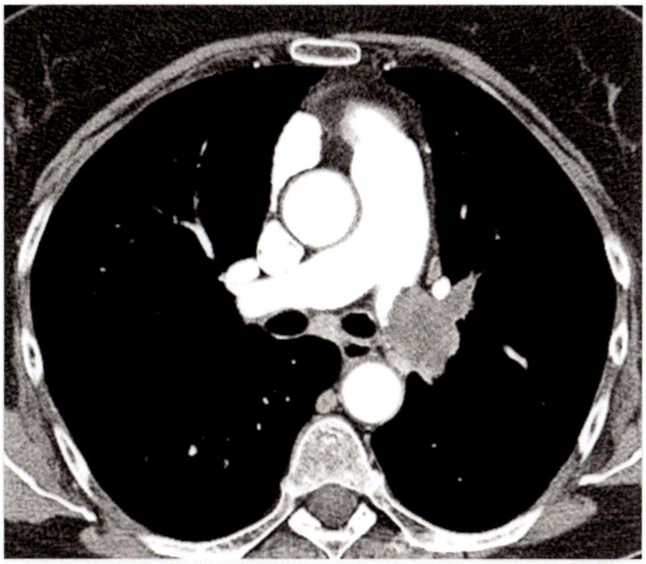

Fig. 14.6 Angiosarcoma of the left pulmonary artery. CT image.

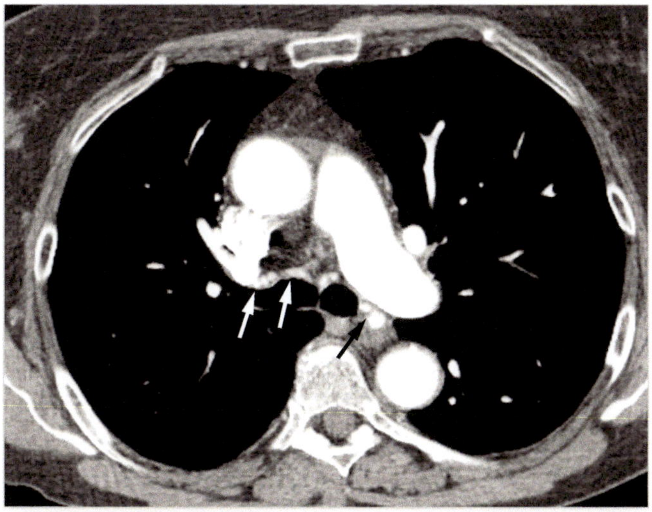

Fig. 14.5 Dilated bronchial arteries (*arrows*) in chronic thromboembolic disease CT image.

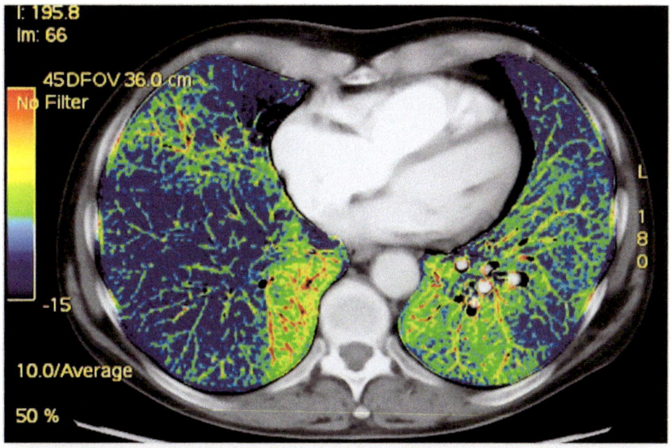

Fig. 14.7 Chronic thromboembolic pulmonary hypertension. DECT. On the iodine map (color depiction) bilateral, large areas of segmental hypoperfusion (*blue*). Furthermore, considerable narrowing of the pulmonary arteries of the right lower lobe.

amount of fluid drained via the pulmonary lymph vessels. This, in turn, often leads to enlargement of the hilar and mediastinal lymph nodes.

II

Note

CT findings in chronic thromboembolic pulmonary hypertension (CTEPH):

- Contrast filling defects (complete or sickle-shaped) in the pulmonary arteries.
- Pulmonary artery narrowing.
- Pulmonary artery wall thickening, possibly with calcification.
- Intraluminal webs and bands.
- Mosaic attenuation pattern.
- Dilated bronchial arteries.
- Mediastinal and hilar lymphadenopathy.
- On DECT, segmental perfusion defects on the iodine map.

In operable patients, additional pulmonary angiography is required for indication and planning of surgical treatment.[1,43] Pulmonary angiography is superior to cross-sectional imaging in visualizing peripheral vascular occlusion (▶Fig. 14.8).

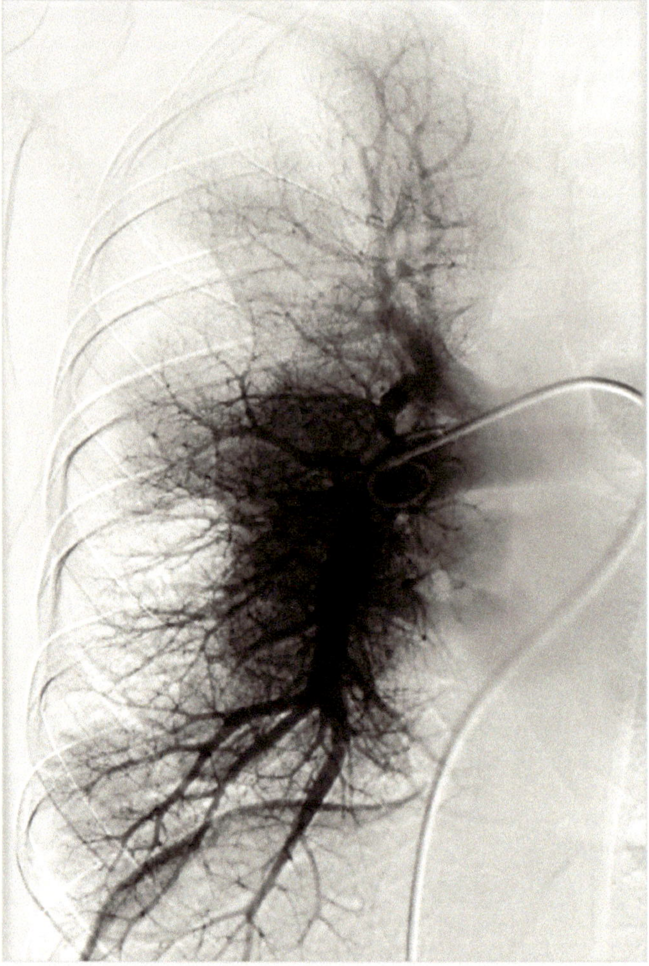

Fig. 14.8 Chronic thromboembolic pulmonary hypertension. Pulmonary angiogram. Widespread vascular blockages and wedge-shaped perfusion defects.

14.1.3 Pulmonary Hypertension

Pulmonary hypertension results from numerous diseases and pathologic states. Clinical classification of pulmonary hypertension, which was last revised in 2013 (Nice Classification), divides these conditions into five groups, as illustrated in ▶Table 14.4.

Some of the causes of pulmonary hypertension can be diagnosed on imaging, in particular lung diseases, e.g., chronic obstructive pulmonary disease (Nice Classification no. 3.1), diffuse parenchymal lung diseases (no. 3.2), chronic thromboembolic pulmonary hypertension (no. 4), and systemic diseases, such as sarcoidosis, pulmonary Langerhans cell histiocytosis, and lymphangioleiomyomatosis (no. 5.2). The secondary effects of pulmonary hypertension on the pulmonary vessels and heart can also be identified on CT. The characteristic CT findings are summarized in ▶Table 14.5.

Special imaging findings of veno-occlusive disease as well as pulmonary capillary hemangiomatosis (Nice Classification no. 1') are discussed in Section 14.2.

Visualization of lung perfusion on DECT or MRI allows limited differential diagnostic insights into the cause of pulmonary hypertension. In particular, the detection of segmental perfusion defects is characteristic of chronic thromboembolic pulmonary hypertension. In idiopathic arterial pulmonary hypertension, diffuse hypoperfusion can be identified, and in chronic obstructive pulmonary disease, the perfusion defects correlate with the extent of pathologic parenchymal lung changes (▶Fig. 14.9). In the majority of cases of chronic thromboembolic pulmonary hypertension, dilation of the bronchial arteries is observed, but this is rare in idiopathic pulmonary arterial hypertension. Peripheral pulmonary arteries of corkscrew appearance may be seen due to plexogenic arteriopathy and point to idiopathic pulmonary arterial hypertension.[45]

14.1.4 Swyer–James Syndrome

Swyer–James syndrome is caused by early childhood pulmonary infection that triggers postinfectious bronchiolitis obliterans.[46] The implicated infections are often viral or mycoplasma pneumonias. Bronchiolitis obliterans results in narrowing of the bronchiolar lumina and, accordingly, in reduced ventilation of the affected lung portions. The consecutive hypoxic pulmonary vasoconstriction reduces lung perfusion. In a developing lung, these processes lead to hypoplasia of the vascular architecture of the diseased lung portions. In general, Swyer–James syndrome becomes symptomatic only several years later, but usually still in childhood or early adolescence, when it causes recurrent pulmonary infections or nonspecific pulmonary symptoms, such as exertional dyspnea or productive cough.[47]

Table 14.4 Nice classification of pulmonary hypertension; modified from Simonneau et al[44]

Group		Diseases	
1	Pulmonary arterial hypertension	1.1	Idiopathic pulmonary arterial hypertension
		1.2	Heritable pulmonary arterial hypertension due to defects in the following genes:
		1.2.1	• BMPR2 gene
		1.2.2	• ALK-1-, ENG-, SMAD9-, CAV1-, KCNK3 genes
		1.2.3	• Unknown genetic defects
		1.3	Drug and toxin induced
		1.4	Pulmonary arterial hypertension associated with:
		1.4.1	• Connective tissue disease
		1.4.2	• HIV infection
		1.4.3	• Portal hypertension
		1.4.4	• Congenital heart diseases
		1.4.5	• Schistosomiasis
		1'	Pulmonary veno-occlusive disease and/or pulmonary capillary hemangiomatosis
		1"	Persistent pulmonary hypertension of the newborn
2	Pulmonary hypertension due to left heart disease	2.1	Left ventricular systolic dysfunction
		2.2	Left ventricular diastolic dysfunction
		2.3	Valvular disease
		2.4	Congenital or acquired left heart inflow/outflow tract obstruction and congenital cardiomyopathies
3	Pulmonary hypertension due to lung diseases and/or hypoxia	3.1	Chronic obstructive pulmonary disease
		3.2	Diffuse parenchymal lung disease
		3.3	Other pulmonary diseases with mixed restrictive and obstructive pattern
		3.4	Sleep-disordered breathing
		3.5	Alveolar hypoventilation disorders
		3.6	Chronic exposure to high altitude
		3.7	Developmental lung diseases
4	Chronic thromboembolic pulmonary hypertension		
5	Pulmonary hypertension with unclear multifactorial mechanisms	5.1	Hematologic disorders: chronic hemolytic anemia, myeloproliferative disorders, splenectomy
		5.2	Systemic disorders: sarcoidosis, pulmonary Langerhans cell histiocytosis, lymphangioleiomyomatosis
		5.3	Metabolic disorders: glycogen storage disease, Gaucher disease, thyroid disorders
		5.4	Others: tumoral obstruction, fibrosing mediastinitis, chronic renal failure, segmental pulmonary hypertension

A salient finding on chest radiography is hyperlucency and vascular rarefaction of the affected lung portions. CT additionally demonstrates a decrease in pulmonary arterial branching in the diseased areas. The findings are not necessarily confined to a single lung lobe, and at times show asymmetrical involvement of both lungs (▶Fig. 14.10). The latter is an important differential diagnostic criterion for distinguishing Swyer–James syndrome from congenital lobar emphysema. Moreover, the characteristic findings of bronchiolitis obliterans are present; air trapping and bronchiectasis can generally be identified.[48]

14.2 Diseases of the Pulmonary Veins

Pulmonary veno-occlusive disease (PVOD) is diagnosed predominantly in children and young adults, manifesting as thrombosis of the pulmonary veins and venules as well as eccentric intimal fibrosis of unknown etiology. The main clinical symptom is slowly progressive dyspnea; episodes of acute pulmonary edema or hemoptysis may present. On CT, the combination of signs of pulmonary arterial hypertension (see ▶Table 14.5) and interstitial or alveolar pulmonary edema is considered virtually pathognomonic for pulmonary veno-occlusive disease. Another conspicuous finding is the small calibers of the central pulmonary veins (▶Fig. 14.11).[45]

Pulmonary capillary hemangiomatosis (PCH) is a rare clinical disease entity, causing pulmonary arterial hypertension and, like pulmonary veno-occlusive disease, is associated with normal pulmonary venous pressure. Proliferation of capillaries in the alveolar walls is seen on histology. Pulmonary capillary hemangiomatosis appears to be associated with several diseases but its cause continues to be unknown. Imaging demonstrates multiple, well-defined ground-glass nodules. Unlike in pulmonary veno-occlusive disease, there is no evidence of interlobar septal thickening. Signs of pulmonary arterial hypertension are usually present (see ▶Table 14.5).[49]

Table 14.5 CT findings of pulmonary hypertension[45]

Pulmonary arterial hypertension	Pulmonary venous hypertension
• Dilation of the central pulmonary arteries • Abrupt tapering of the peripheral pulmonary arteries • Right ventricular hypertrophy • Right ventricular and atrial enlargement • Dilation of bronchial arteries • Mosaic attenuation pattern • Mediastinal or hilar lymphadenopathy	• Interstitial and alveolar pulmonary edema • Findings of pulmonary arterial hypertension

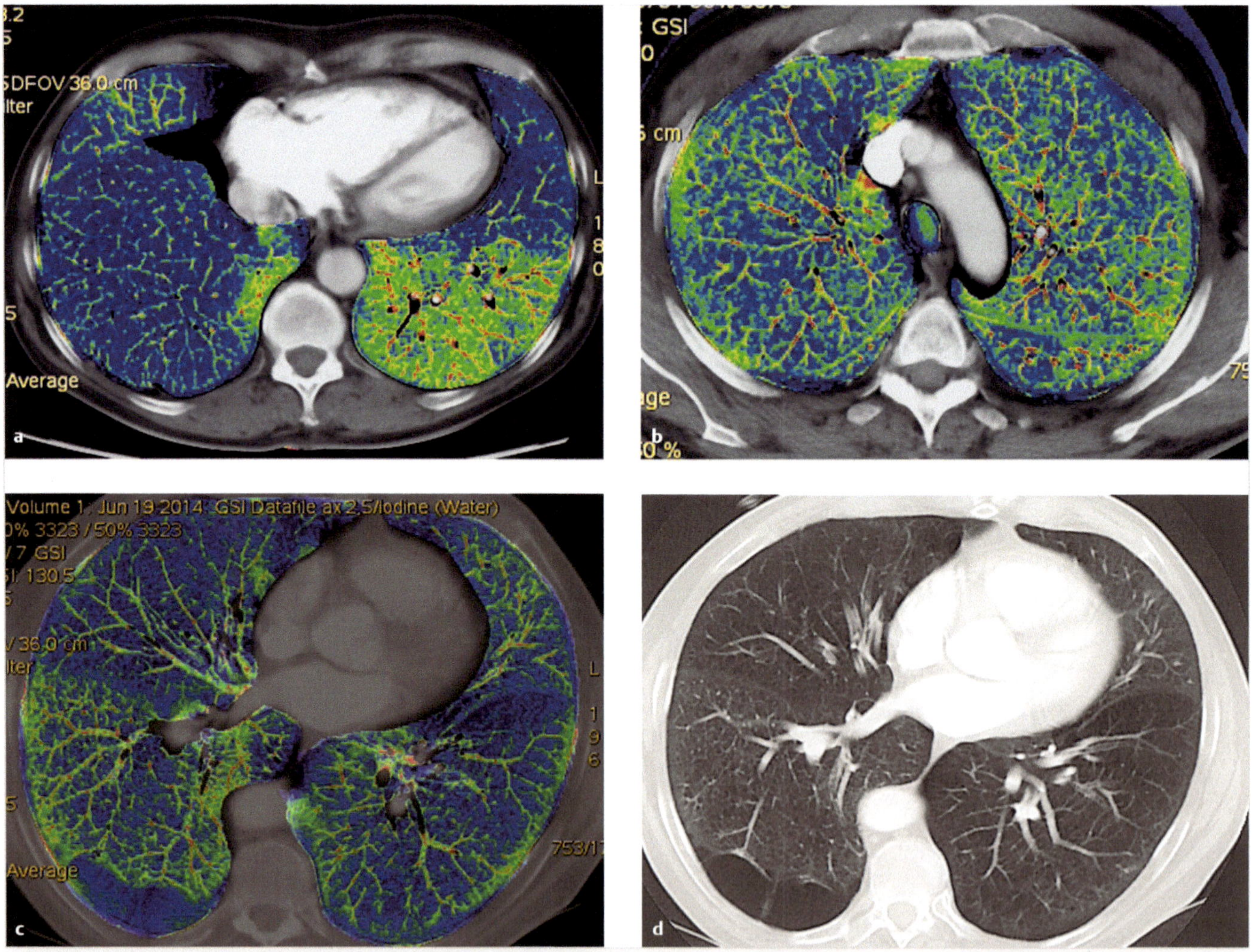

Fig. 14.9 **Pulmonary hypertension.** DECT. Differential diagnosis of various types of pulmonary hypertension. **(a)** Iodine map. Chronic thromboembolic pulmonary hypertension with segmental perfusion defects. **(b)** Iodine map. Idiopathic arterial pulmonary hypertension with diffuse hypoperfusion. **(c)** Iodine map. Pulmonary emphysema with perfusion defects in the emphysematous areas. Corresponding lung window in **d. (d)** Lung window. Pulmonary emphysema with bullae in the right lower lobe. Same slice as in **c.**

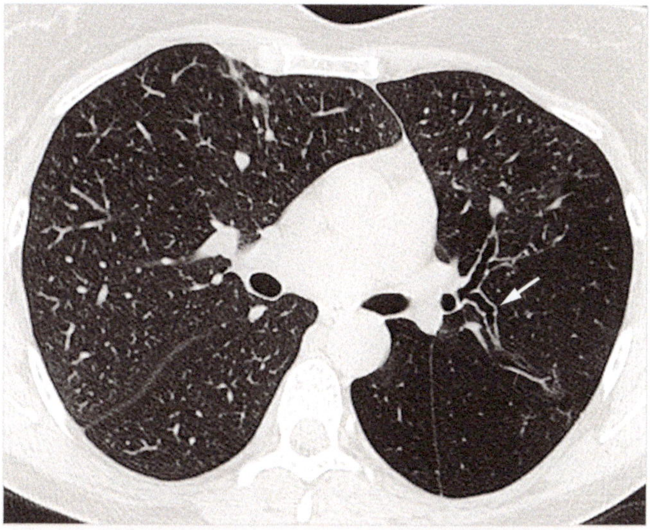

Fig. 14.10 Swyer–James syndrome. CT image. Reduced density of the left upper lobe and the left apical lower lobe segment, small-caliber and rarefied vessels of the left lung, and cylindrical bronchiectasis (*arrow*).

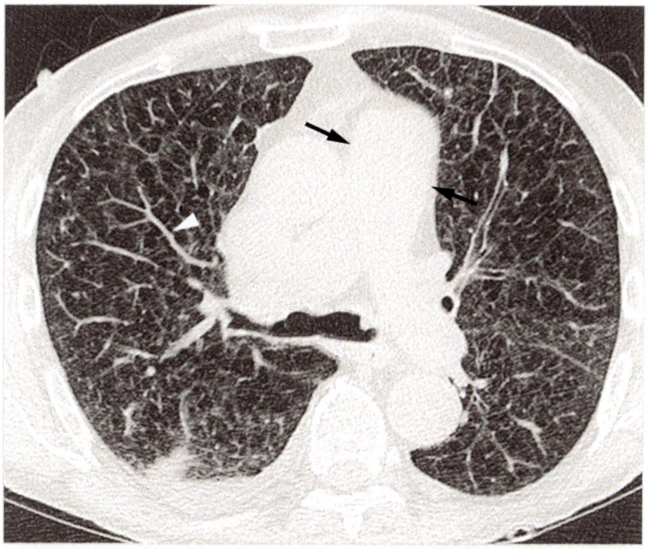

Fig. 14.11 Pulmonary veno-occlusive disease. CT image. Ubiquitous interlobular septal thickening, very narrow pulmonary veins (*arrowhead*), dilated pulmonary trunk (*arrows*), and minor bilateral pleural effusion.

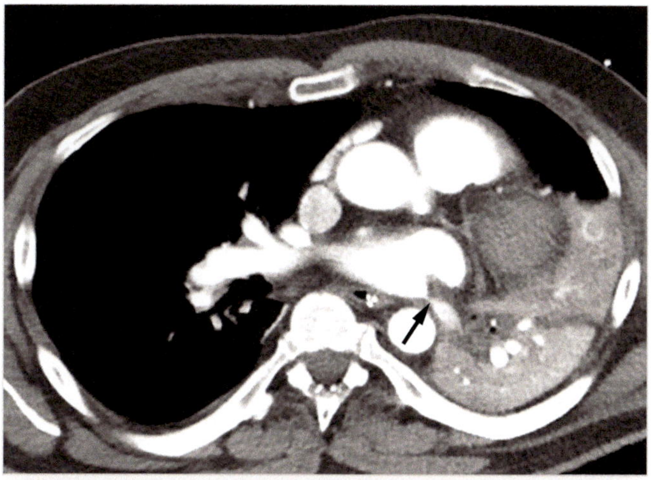

Fig. 14.12 Central stenosis of the left lower pulmonary vein (*arrow*) as postinterventional complication of pulmonary vein isolation. CT image. Furthermore, left lower lobe atelectasis due to extensive left hilar collateral circulation (not depicted).

Pulmonary vein isolation is a minimally invasive cardiac intervention used to treat idiopathic and paroxysmal atrial fibrillation. *Central pulmonary vein stenosis* may occur as a postinterventional complication, leading to the development of collateral circulation and hydrostatic pulmonary edema in the lung portions drained by the stenotic vein (▶Fig. 14.12).

14.3 Diseases of the Aorta and Major Arteries

14.3.1 Acute Aortic Syndrome

Acute aortic syndrome is a life-threatening emergency medical condition necessitating immediate diagnosis and urgent treatment. The main symptoms are acute chest pain or pain along the spinal column, especially between the scapulae. Other symptoms include hemodynamic instability, hypotension, tachycardia, and syncope. Arterial hypertension is an important predisposing factor.

Computed tomography angiography (CTA), ideally with ECG gating, is absolutely indicated as the method of choice. In individual cases adjunctive MRI or transesophageal echocardiography may be required.[50] Based on the imaging findings, several diseases with similar clinical presentation can be differentiated. These are discussed in the following sections (▶Fig. 14.13).[51]

Heart attack and pulmonary embolism are other clinical differential diagnoses that can be excluded by means of appropriate examination protocols, as assured by high-performance CT scanners ("triple-rule-out" CT).[53] The undifferentiated use of such protocols in settings of acute chest pain in clinical routine is disputed. One counterargument is the associated high radiation exposure.[54]

Aortic Dissection

The most common cause of acute aortic syndrome is aortic dissection. Because of a tear in the aortic intima, the blood surges through a "false" lumen between the intima and media and reenters the aortic lumen ("true" lumen) via another more distal intimal tear. A distinction is made between acute and chronic dissection depending on the duration of the symptoms, with chronic dissection lasting for at least 2 weeks.

The Stanford classification distinguishes two types of aortic dissection in accordance with the location[52]:

- *Type A dissection*: involvement of the ascending aorta and aortic arch.
- *Type B dissection*: involvement of the descending aorta distal to the origin of the left subclavian artery.

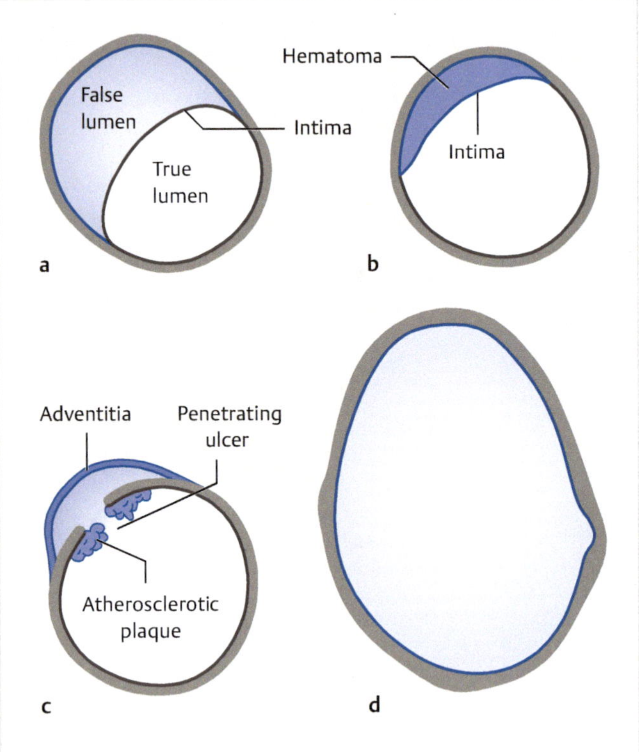

Fig. 14.13 Diseases that can cause acute aortic syndrome. Schematic diagram.[52] **(a)** Aortic dissection. **(b)** Intramural hematoma. **(c)** Penetrating atherosclerotic ulcer. **(d)** Aortic aneurysm.

Whereas type A dissection requires emergency surgical repair, chronic type B dissection is treated conservatively provided that there are no ischemic complications. There are established interventional radiology techniques for acute type B and for some type A dissections.[50]

Occasionally, deposition of intimal calcification can be identified on the inside of the aorta even on unenhanced CT. CTA visualizes the true and false lumen separated by the intima (▶Fig. 14.14). The false lumen occasionally contains narrow areas of lower density consistent with frayed portions of the media, thus helping to differentiate it from a true lumen.

In settings of a thrombosed false lumen, differential diagnosis versus other aortic diseases is difficult, especially intramural hematoma and thrombosed aortic aneurysm. An aortic dissection has a characteristic spiral-shaped configuration which can help to distinguish it from a wall hematoma or parietal thrombus of an aortic aneurysm. The latter two entities tend to remain in the same position relative to the aortic circumference along their entire proximal to distal extension.

Note

Several artefacts can mimic an intima in the vascular lumen, in particular streak artefacts caused by highly concentrated IV contrast in the central veins and pulsation artefacts on non-ECG synchronized images. An awareness of these artefacts and appropriate contrast-material timing reduces the risk of false-positive results on CTA.[55]

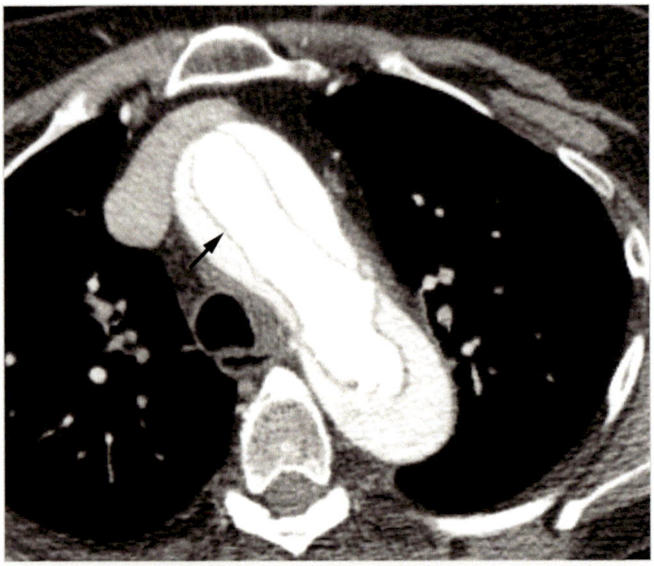

Fig. 14.14 Stanford type A dissection. CT image. Detached intima (*arrow*) in aortic arch.

Intramural Hematoma

Intramural hematoma is caused by rupture of the vasa vasorum in the aortic wall. This results in a hematoma in the aortic wall but without necessarily creating a portal of entry into the aortic intima. It accounts for around 10% of acute aortic syndromes. As for aortic dissection, it is defined in accordance with the Stanford classification relative to its location.

Unenhanced CT is able to visualize a wall hematoma as a sickle-shaped, hyperdense structure in the aorta. Following IV contrast administration, the intramural hematoma persists as unenhanced wall thickening.

Penetrating Atherosclerotic Ulcer

In settings of atherosclerosis, plaques that may ulcerate develop. Ulceration involving deeper layers of the aortic wall and causing a medial hematoma is known as a penetrating atherosclerotic ulcer.[56] Ongoing disease progression gives rise to a saccular aortic aneurysm or the wall defect directly causes—less commonly—a covered or open rupture. Open rupture is generally fatal. Elderly patients with severe atherosclerosis are particularly at risk. Often, concomitant aortic aneurysms are found at other locations.

On CT, contrast accumulation can be identified outside the aortic lumen. The most salient finding is dilation of the contrast-enhanced lumen with a relatively small entry of generally no more than 2 cm. The ruptured ulcer cannot be distinguished from a ruptured aortic aneurysm (▶Fig. 14.15).

Symptomatic Aortic Aneurysm

The term "aneurysm" is used to describe dilation of the lumen by more than 5 cm of the ascending and by more than 4.5 cm of the descending aorta or dilation of the aortic diameter by more than 50% of the normal diameter size for the corresponding age group.[57] Most thoracic aortic aneurysms are

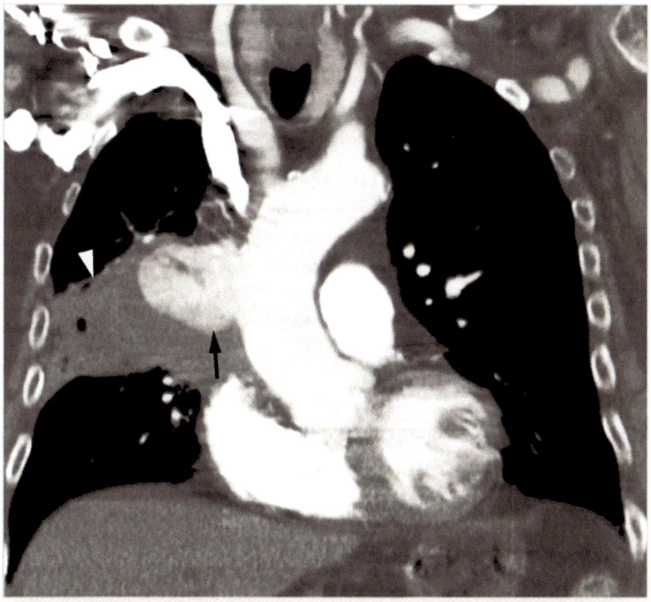

Fig. 14.15 Covered rupture into the right lung of a penetrating atherosclerotic ulcer (*arrow*). CT image, coronal. Clinical hemoptysis. The consolidation in the right lung is consistent with pulmonary hemorrhage (*arrowhead*).

of atherosclerotic etiology; less commonly, they are linked to other diseases of the aorta, e.g., connective tissue diseases such as Marfan syndrome as well as infectious or noninfectious aortitis.[58] A fusiform true aneurysm affecting all three aortic wall layers (intima, media, and adventitia) is the most common form. Perforation of the vascular wall results in an extravascular hematoma, a so-called spurious aneurysm. This is rarely seen in the thoracic aortic and is almost always iatrogenic.

Most thoracic aortic aneurysms do not cause any symptoms. A rapid increase in size, an impending rupture, or already occurred (usually covered) rupture creates an unstable state constituting acute aortic syndrome. The rupture risk is significantly increased for an ascending aorta diameter of 6 cm or more and for a descending aorta diameter of 7.2 cm or more.[50,58] Likewise, a diameter increase of more than 5 mm per year is associated with a higher rupture risk.[59]

There is a risk of overestimating the aortic diameter on CTA axial slices since often the slice is not positioned orthogonal to the longitudinal diameter of the aorta. Therefore, the diameter should be measured on multiplanar reformatted slices perpendicular to the aortic axis.[60] The frequent parietal wall thrombi can be identified as contrast filling defects (▸Fig. 14.16).

14.3.2 Vasculitis of the Great Vessels

Vasculitis of the small and medium arteries presents, inter alia, in the lung parenchyma. The aorta and pulmonary arteries are often implicated in vasculitis of the great vessels. The cause of the vasculitis discussed here is unknown but is thought to be linked to autoimmune mechanisms. Hence, immunosuppressive therapy is administered to treat these diseases.

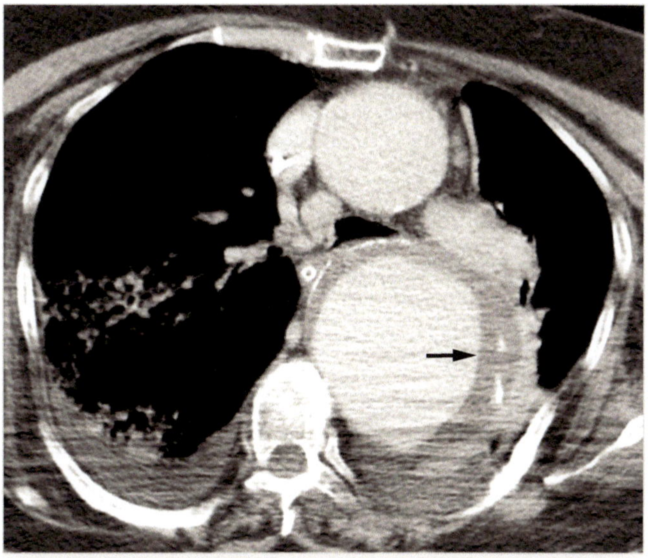

Fig. 14.16 Atherosclerotic aortic aneurysm of the descending aorta. CT image. Wall thrombi can be identified as contrast filling defects in the aortic lumen (*arrow*).

The involvement of the pulmonary arteries with development of vasculitic aneurysms is seen most frequently in *Behçet's disease*. In addition, CT shows intraluminal thrombi and triangular consolidation which risk being misinterpreted as venous thromboembolism.[61]

Takayasu arteritis is a systemic arteritis affecting especially the aorta and its branches. Involvement of the pulmonary arteries causes pulmonary hypertension in more than half of cases.[61]

Giant cell arteritis cannot be distinguished from Takayasu arteritis on imaging. Pulmonary hypertension is less common.[61] Aortitis is present in the majority of cases, manifesting as wall thickening on CT and MRI (▸Fig. 14.17). Characteristic findings include stenosis, thrombi, and vascular occlusion, as well as aneurysms.[62,63] On MRI signal changes in the aortic wall are observed additionally, in particular hyperintense signal on T2w sequences (▸Fig. 14.18). Arteritis of the great vessels can be demonstrated with greater sensitivity on PET as increased tracer uptake, even if other imaging modalities do not yet show any abnormality.

14.4 Summary

Acute pulmonary embolism is associated with a broad spectrum of clinical manifestations ranging from sudden death to asymptomatic incidental findings. The choice of diagnostic methods and treatment is based on the early mortality risk:

- In case of hypotension or shock, CTPA or, as a substitute, echocardiography is performed immediately. Treatment is aimed at primary recanalization of the vessels affected by embolic occlusion.
- For hemodynamically stable patients with a high probability of pulmonary embolism, CTPA is first carried out. If there is a low or intermediate probability, D-dimer testing

14

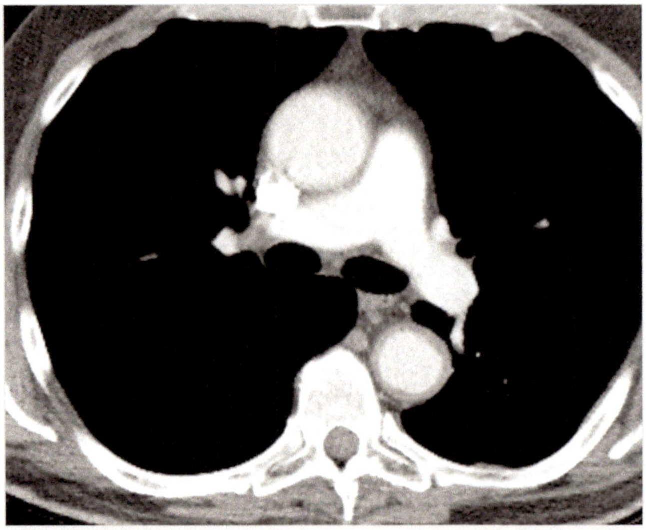

Fig. 14.17 Giant cell arteritis. CT image. Wall thickening of descending aorta.

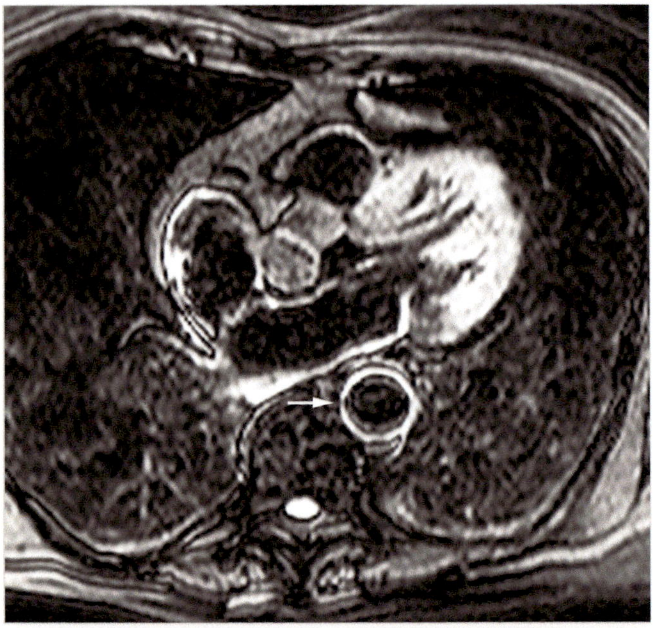

Fig. 14.18 Giant cell arteritis. T2w MRI sequence with fat saturation. Increased signal intensity of the aortic wall (*arrow*).

is performed first, followed by CTPA if the test was positive. Treatment consists of anticoagulation.

To estimate the clinical probability, several validated score systems are available and are chosen in accordance with local preferences (see ▸Table 14.2 and ▸Table 14.3). The extent of right heart strain determines the prognosis for pulmonary embolism. CTPA is able to directly visualize dilation of the right ventricle and thus contributes to estimation of prognosis.

Clinical management of isolated subsegmental and unsuspected incidental pulmonary embolism is problematic; overdiagnosis is thought to occur. In individual cases, the benefits of anticoagulant therapy must be weighed against the bleeding risk. At least patients with malignant disease and central pulmonary embolism should receive treatment even if it is asymptomatic.

A small percentage of acute pulmonary embolisms do not undergo complete resolution, instead giving rise to *chronic thromboembolic disease* with a risk of onset of pulmonary hypertension (chronic thromboembolic pulmonary hypertension). Diagnostic criteria are based on the presence of pulmonary hypertension (pulmonary arterial mean pressure of at least 25 mm Hg and pulmonary capillary wedge pressure no more than 15 mm Hg) and evidence of at least one segmental perfusion defect on imaging (reference standard: ventilation/perfusion [VQ] scan).

The Nice classification divides the causes of *pulmonary hypertension* into five groups (see ▸Table 14.4):

- Pulmonary arterial hypertension.
- Pulmonary hypertension secondary to left heart diseases.
- Pulmonary hypertension secondary to lung diseases and/or hypoxia.
- Chronic thromboembolic pulmonary hypertension.
- Pulmonary hypertension with unclear multifactorial mechanisms.

Some of the causes of pulmonary hypertension can be diagnosed on imaging (chronic obstructive pulmonary disease, diffuse parenchymal lung diseases, chronic thromboembolic pulmonary hypertension, and systemic diseases, such as sarcoidosis). Characteristic findings for pulmonary arterial hypertension are dilation of the central pulmonary arteries and right heart enlargement (see ▸Table 14.5); in the less common pulmonary venous hypertension (e.g., resulting from veno-occlusive disease), interstitial, and possibly alveolar, pulmonary edema is seen additionally.

Swyer–James syndrome develops as a sequela of early childhood pneumonia with postinfectious bronchiolitis obliterans causing hyperinflation of the affected lung parenchyma and hypoplasia of the pulmonary vessels.

Acute aortic syndrome is a life-threatening condition; the most salient clinical symptom is chest pain of sudden onset. Four causes with partially overlapping features cannot be differentiated clinically but can be differentiated with CTA as the imaging method of choice:

- *Aortic dissection*: Because of an intimal tear a second—false—aortic lumen is formed between the intima and media. On CTA the false lumen may be seen to be filled with contrast or is thrombosed. The Stanford classification distinguishes:
  - Type A dissection (proximal to the origin of the left subclavian artery): surgical emergency.
  - Type B dissection (distal to the origin of the left subclavian artery): conservative treatment, in particular for chronic dissection, or endovascular therapy with stent-graft placement.
- *Intramural hematoma*: Intramural rupture of the vasa vasorum leads to an aortic wall hematoma without intimal tear. On unenhanced CT, a sickle-shaped area of hyperdensity in the aorta can be identified.
- *Penetrating atherosclerotic ulcer*: An atherosclerotic ulcer penetrates into the deep aortic wall layers where it forms

a wall hematoma. Later, this can develop into a sacciform aortic aneurysm, and may also rupture.
- *Unstable aortic aneurysm*: Aortic aneurysms with a growth rate of more than 5 mm per year are considered unstable and prone to rupture; that also applies to large aortic aneurysms.

Vasculitis of the great vessels, in particular Takayasu arteritis and giant cell arteritis, often affects the aorta and its branches. It manifests on CT and MRI as wall thickening, stenosis, vascular occlusion, and wall thrombosis. Imaging is unable to differentiate the individual disease entities. The involvement of the pulmonary arteries often results in pulmonary hypertension.

References

[1] Konstantinides SV, Torbicki A, Agnelli G, et al; Task Force for the Diagnosis and Management of Acute Pulmonary Embolism of the European Society of Cardiology (ESC). 2014 ESC guidelines on the diagnosis and management of acute pulmonary embolism. Eur Heart J 2014;35(43):3033–3069, 3069a–3069k

[2] Abrahams-van Doorn PJ, Hartmann IJC. Cardiothoracic CT: one-stop-shop procedure? Impact on the management of acute pulmonary embolism. Insights Imaging 2011;2(6):705–715

[3] Wells PS, Anderson DR, Rodger M, et al. Derivation of a simple clinical model to categorize patients probability of pulmonary embolism: increasing the models utility with the SimpliRED D-dimer. Thromb Haemost 2000;83(3):416–420

[4] Gibson NS, Sohne M, Kruip MJHA, et al; Christopher study investigators. Further validation and simplification of the Wells clinical decision rule in pulmonary embolism. Thromb Haemost 2008;99(1):229–234

[5] Le Gal G, Righini M, Roy PM, et al. Prediction of pulmonary embolism in the emergency department: the revised Geneva score. Ann Intern Med 2006;144(3):165–171

[6] Klok FA, Mos ICM, Nijkeuter M, et al. Simplification of the revised Geneva score for assessing clinical probability of pulmonary embolism. Arch Intern Med 2008;168(19):2131–2136

[7] Worsley DF, Alavi A, Aronchick JM, Chen JT, Greenspan RH, Ravin CE. Chest radiographic findings in patients with acute pulmonary embolism: observations from the PIOPED Study. Radiology 1993;189(1):133–136

[8] Stein PD, Fowler SE, Goodman LR, et al; PIOPED II Investigators. Multidetector computed tomography for acute pulmonary embolism. N Engl J Med 2006;354(22):2317–2327

[9] Contractor S, Maldjian PD, Sharma VK, Gor DM. Role of helical CT in detecting right ventricular dysfunction secondary to acute pulmonary embolism. J Comput Assist Tomogr 2002;26(4):587–591

[10] Ghaye B, Ghuysen A, Bruyere PJ, D'Orio V, Dondelinger RF. Can CT pulmonary angiography allow assessment of severity and prognosis in patients presenting with pulmonary embolism? What the radiologist needs to know. Radiographics 2006;26(1):23–39, discussion 39–40

[11] Lim KE, Chan CY, Chu PH, Hsu YY, Hsu WC. Right ventricular dysfunction secondary to acute massive pulmonary embolism detected by helical computed tomography pulmonary angiography. Clin Imaging 2005;29(1):16–21

[12] Ghaye B, Ghuysen A, Willems V, et al. Severe pulmonary embolism:pulmonary artery clot load scores and cardiovascular parameters as predictors of mortality. Radiology 2006;239(3):884–891

[13] Collomb D, Paramelle PJ, Calaque O, et al. Severity assessment of acute pulmonary embolism: evaluation using helical CT. Eur Radiol 2003;13(7):1508–1514

[14] Carrier M, Righini M, Wells PS, et al. Subsegmental pulmonary embolism diagnosed by computed tomography: incidence and clinical implications. A systematic review and meta-analysis of the management outcome studies. J Thromb Haemost 2010;8(8):1716–1722

[15] Stein PD, Goodman LR, Hull RD, Dalen JE, Matta F. Diagnosis and management of isolated subsegmental pulmonary embolism: review and assessment of the options. Clin Appl Thromb Hemost 2012;18(1):20–26

[16] Farrell C, Jones M, Girvin F, Ritchie G, Murchison JT. Unsuspected pulmonary embolism identified using multidetector computed tomography in hospital outpatients. Clin Radiol 2010;65(1):1–5

[17] Jia CF, Li YX, Yang ZQ, Zhang ZH, Sun XX, Wang ZQ. Prospective evaluation of unsuspected pulmonary embolism on coronary computed tomographic angiography. J Comput Assist Tomogr 2012;36(2):187–190

[18] Palla A, Rossi G, Falaschi F, Marconi L, Pistolesi M, Prandoni P. Is incidentally detected pulmonary embolism in cancer patients less severe? A case-control study. Cancer Invest 2012;30(2):131–134

[19] Sahut D'Izarn M, Caumont Prim A, Planquette B, et al. Risk factors and clinical outcome of unsuspected pulmonary embolism in cancer patients: a case-control study. J Thromb Haemost 2012;10(10):2032–2038

[20] Wittram C, Maher MM, Yoo AJ, Kalra MK, Shepard JA, McLoud TC. CT angiography of pulmonary embolism: diagnostic criteria and causes of misdiagnosis. Radiographics 2004;24(5):1219–1238

[21] Kearon C, Akl EA, Comerota AJ, et al. Antithrombotic therapy for VTE disease: antithrombotic therapy and prevention of thrombosis. Chest 2012;141:e419S–e494S

[22] Anderson DR, Kahn SR, Rodger MA, et al. Computed tomographic pulmonary angiography vs ventilation-perfusion lung scanning in patients with suspected pulmonary embolism: a randomized controlled trial. JAMA 2007;298(23):2743–2753

[23] Tsai J, Grosse SD, Grant AM, Hooper WC, Atrash HK. Trends in in-hospital deaths among hospitalizations with pulmonary embolism. Arch Intern Med 2012;172(12):960–961

[24] Wiener RS, Schwartz LM, Woloshin S. Time trends in pulmonary embolism in the United States: evidence of overdiagnosis. Arch Intern Med 2011;171(9):831–837

[25] Wiener RS, Schwartz LM, Woloshin S. When a test is too good: how CT pulmonary angiograms find pulmonary emboli that do not need to be found. BMJ 2013;347:f3368

[26] Goodman LR, Stein PD, Matta F, et al. CT venography and compression sonography are diagnostically equivalent: data from PIOPED II. AJR Am J Roentgenol 2007;189(5):1071–1076

[27] Frechen D, Krüger S, Paetsch I, et al. Pulmonary perfusion imaging: new insights into functional consequences of pulmonary embolism using a multicomponent cardiovascular magnetic resonance imaging protocol. J Am Coll Cardiol 2012;60(22):2335–2337

[28] Kang MJ, Park CM, Lee CH, Goo JM, Lee HJ. Dual-energy CT: clinical applications in various pulmonary diseases. Radiographics 2010;30(3):685–698

[29] Bauer RW, Frellesen C, Renker M, et al. Dual energy CT pulmonary blood volume assessment in acute pulmonary embolism - correlation with D-dimer level, right heart strain and clinical outcome. Eur Radiol 2011;21(9):1914–1921

[30] Remy-Jardin M, Pontana F, Faivre JB, et al. New insights in thromboembolic disease. Radiol Clin North Am 2014;52(1):183–193

[31] Bernabé-García JM, García-Espasa C, Arenas-Jiménez J, Sánchez-Payá J, de la Hoz-Rosa J, Carreres-Polo JO. Has "respiratory coaching" before deep inspiration an impact on the incidence of transient contrast interruption during pulmonary CT angiography? Insights Imaging 2012;3(5):505–511

[32] Castañer E, Gallardo X, Ballesteros E, et al. CT diagnosis of chronic pulmonary thromboembolism. Radiographics 2009;29(1):31–50, discussion 50–53

[33] Ley S, Ley-Zaporozhan J, Pitton MB, et al. Diagnostic performance of state-of-the-art imaging techniques for morphological assessment of vascular abnormalities in patients with chronic thromboembolic pulmonary hypertension (CTEPH). Eur Radiol 2012;22(3):607–616

[34] Bhagwat K, Hallam J, Antippa P, Larobina M. Diagnostic enigma: primary pulmonary artery sarcoma. Interact Cardiovasc Thorac Surg 2012;14(3):342–344

[35] Kauczor HU, Schwickert HC, Mayer E, Kersjes W, Moll R, Schweden F. Pulmonary artery sarcoma mimicking chronic thromboembolic disease: computed tomography and magnetic resonance imaging findings. Cardiovasc Intervent Radiol 1994;17(4):185–189

[36] Kim JB, Kim SH, Lim SY, et al. Primary angiosarcoma of the pulmonary trunk mimicking pulmonary thromboembolism. Echocardiography 2010;27(2):E23–E26

[37] Wirth G, Brüggemann K, Bostel T, Mayer E, Düber C, Kreitner KF. Chronic thromboembolic pulmonary hypertension (CTEPH) - potential role of multidetector-row CT (MD-CT) and MR imaging in the diagnosis and differential diagnosis of the disease. RoFo Fortschr Geb Rontgenstr Nuklearmed 2014;186(8):751–761

[38] Hoeper MM, Mayer E, Simonneau G, Rubin LJ. Chronic thromboembolic pulmonary hypertension. Circulation 2006;113(16):2011–2020

[39] Fedullo P, Kerr KM, Kim NH, Auger WR. Chronic thromboembolic pulmonary hypertension. Am J Respir Crit Care Med 2011;183(12):1605–1613

[40] Wilkens H, Lang I, Blankenburg T, et al. Chronic thromboembolic pulmonary hypertension—a position paper [in German]. Dtsch Med Wochenschr 2014;139(Suppl 4):S155–S165
[41] Ameli-Renani S, Rahman F, Nair A, et al. Dual-energy CT for imaging of pulmonary hypertension: challenges and opportunities. Radiographics 2014;34(7):1769–1790
[42] Dournes G, Verdier D, Montaudon M, et al. Dual-energy CT perfusion and angiography in chronic thromboembolic pulmonary hypertension: diagnostic accuracy and concordance with radionuclide scintigraphy. Eur Radiol 2014;24(1):42–51
[43] Sugiura T, Tanabe N, Matsuura Y, et al. Role of 320-slice CT imaging in the diagnostic workup of patients with chronic thromboembolic pulmonary hypertension. Chest 2013;143(4):1070–1077
[44] Simonneau G, Gatzoulis MA, Adatia I, et al. Updated clinical classification of pulmonary hypertension. J Am Coll Cardiol 2013;62(25, Suppl):D34–D41
[45] Grosse C, Grosse A. CT findings in diseases associated with pulmonary hypertension: a current review. Radiographics 2010;30(7):1753–1777
[46] Swyer PR, James GC. A case of unilateral pulmonary emphysema. Thorax 1953;8(2):133–136
[47] Wasilewska E, Lee EY, Eisenberg RL. Unilateral hyperlucent lung in children. AJR Am J Roentgenol 2012;198(5):W400–14
[48] Hansen M, Kauczor HU, Pascher EW, Mildenberger P. Swyer-James-Syndrom: Darstellung mit der hochauflösenden Computertomographie. RoFo Fortschr Geb Rontgenstr Nuklearmed 1996; 165(5):499–501
[49] Frazier AA, Franks TJ, Mohammed TL, Ozbudak IH, Galvin JR. From the Archives of the AFIP: pulmonary veno-occlusive disease and pulmonary capillary hemangiomatosis. Radiographics 2007;27(3):867–882
[50] Hallinan JTPD, Anil G. Multi-detector computed tomography in the diagnosis and management of acute aortic syndromes. World J Radiol 2014;6(6):355–365
[51] Abbas A, Brown IW, Peebles CR, Harden SP, Shambrook JS. The role of multidetector-row CT in the diagnosis, classification and management of acute aortic syndrome. Br J Radiol 2014;87(1042):20140354
[52] Castañer E, Andreu M, Gallardo X, Mata JM, Cabezuelo MA, Pallardó Y. CT in nontraumatic acute thoracic aortic disease: typical and atypical features and complications. Radiographics 2003;23(Spec No):S93–S110
[53] Halpern EJ. Triple-rule-out CT angiography for evaluation of acute chest pain and possible acute coronary syndrome. Radiology 2009;252(2):332–345
[54] Ayaram D, Bellolio MF, Murad MH, et al. Triple rule-out computed tomographic angiography for chest pain: a diagnostic systematic review and meta-analysis. Acad Emerg Med 2013;20(9):861–871
[55] Batra P, Bigoni B, Manning J, et al. Pitfalls in the diagnosis of thoracic aortic dissection at CT angiography. Radiographics 2000;20 (2):309–320
[56] Chung JW, Park JH, Im JG, Chung MJ, Han MC, Ahn H. Spiral CT angiography of the thoracic aorta. Radiographics 1996;16(4):811–824
[57] Posniak HV, Olson MC, Demos TC, Benjoya RA, Marsan RE. CT of thoracic aortic aneurysms. Radiographics 1990;10(5):839–855
[58] Booher AM, Eagle KA. Diagnosis and management issues in thoracic aortic aneurysm. Am Heart J 2011;162(1):38–46.e1
[59] Prescott-Focht JA, Martinez-Jimenez S, Hurwitz LM, et al. Ascending thoracic aorta: postoperative imaging evaluation. Radiographics 2013;33(1):73–85
[60] Bean MJ, Johnson PT, Roseborough GS, Black JH, Fishman EK. Thoracic aortic stent-grafts: utility of multidetector CT for pre- and postprocedure evaluation. Radiographics 2008;28(7):1835–1851
[61] Marten K, Schnyder P, Schirg E, Prokop M, Rummeny EJ, Engelke C. Pattern-based differential diagnosis in pulmonary vasculitis using volumetric CT. AJR Am J Roentgenol 2005;184(3):720–733
[62] Chung JW, Kim HC, Choi YH, Kim SJ, Lee W, Park JH. Patterns of aortic involvement in Takayasu arteritis and its clinical implications: evaluation with spiral computed tomography angiography. J Vasc Surg 2007;45(5):906–914
[63] Jacquier A, Chabbert V, Vidal V, et al. [Imaging of the thoracic aorta in adults: when, how and why?] J Radiol 2004;85(6 Pt 2):854–869

Chapter 15

Chest Trauma

15 Chest Trauma

In European countries, blunt chest trauma is significantly more common than penetrating chest trauma (e.g., gunshot or stab wounds). Two-thirds of all blunt chest injuries are caused by road traffic accidents, with a mortality rate of up to 25%.[1]

Whole-body CT is the mainstay imaging modality in emergency polytrauma management. The image reconstruction speed of modern CT scanners is fast enough to provide the entire image dataset for clinical decision-making within a very short time. Therefore, CT has now supplanted radiography of the chest and pelvis for management of hemodynamically stable polytrauma patients.[2,3]

Nonetheless, chest radiography continues to have its place for hemodynamically unstable patients. It is easier to perform than CT, if necessary, even during ongoing resuscitation, and is able to demonstrate a number of important findings (e.g., tension pneumothorax, large hemothorax, malpositioned implants).[2]

For CT, intravenous contrast injection is needed to detect vascular injuries and rupture of parenchymatous organs. Sagittal image reconstructions are useful for accurate diagnosis of spinal injuries. With volume rendering technique (VRT) even complex bone fractures can be quickly and clearly visualized.

15.1 Blunt Chest Trauma

15.1.1 Lung Parenchyma

Almost one of every two patients with blunt chest trauma has *lung contusions*. This involves alveolar hemorrhage and interstitial edema in the region of the greatest mechanical impact on the lung parenchyma (coup and, possibly, contrecoup). CT demonstrates ill-defined ground-glass opacities of variable density, which may evolve to consolidations (▶ Fig. 15.1). At times, massive contusions trigger adult respiratory distress syndrome. Lung contusions resolve within a few days. Conversely, persistent pulmonary opacities are suggestive of another cause, such as infection, aspiration, blood clot, or atelectasis.

Lung lacerations result from rupture of the lung tissue. They may be solitary or multiple. Air-filled cavities are consistent with pneumatoceles, whereas consolidations are caused by hematomas. A combination of these two types with fluid-fluid levels is possible (▶ Fig. 15.2). Pneumatoceles generally resolve with parenchymal scarring within 1 to 3 weeks.[4]

Aspiration pneumonia manifests within the first day of injury as pulmonary opacity. It is typically located in the posterior portions of the lower lobes.

15.1.2 Mediastinum

Pneumomediastinum is suggestive of a rupture of the trachea, esophagus, or central, mediastinal bronchi. Occasionally, acute life-threatening tension pneumomediastinum occurs. On chest radiography, pneumomediastinum may be misinterpreted as pneumothorax if air is seen only beneath the mediastinal pleura and no other mediastinal air collections are visible.[2] The risk of misinterpretation is much lower on CT. Pneumomediastinum often spreads to adjacent compartments, causing cervical and thoracic soft-tissue emphysema (▶ Fig. 15.3).

Tracheobronchial ruptures are relatively rare. They very often involve the right mainstem bronchus. The resultant posterior displacement of the collapsed lung is known as "fallen lung sign." Tracheal tears usually occur in the lower tracheal at the transition from the cartilaginous to the membranous part (▶ Fig. 15.4).

Rupture of the esophagus is rarely seen in its thoracic part since the dorsal location confers good protection. The cervical esophagus is more commonly affected. Thoracic esophageal rupture is associated with a mortality rate of 90%, generally because of acute mediastinitis.[4]

Many vascular injuries involve the thoracic aorta. By contrast, the other mediastinal vessels are rarely implicated. It has been estimated that around three-quarters of all patients with aortic rupture do not reach the hospital alive; likewise, the mortality

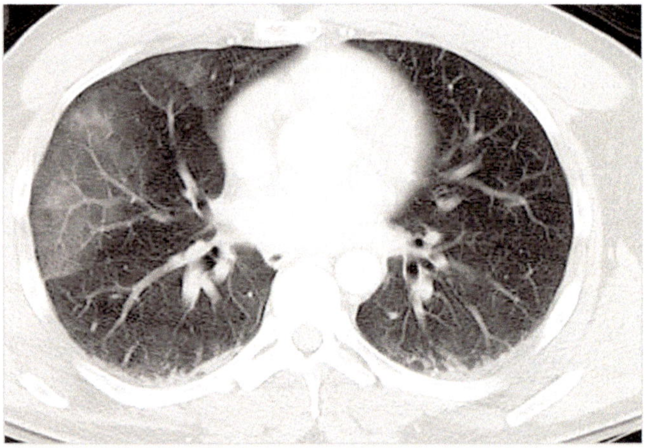

Fig. 15.1 Lung contusion. CT image. Ill-defined ground-glass opacities in the right upper lobe. Furthermore, moderate dependent opacities in the posterior lower lobes.

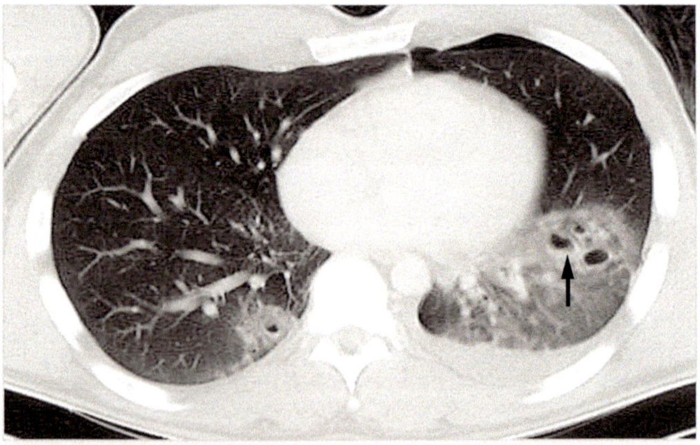

Fig. 15.2 Lung lacerations. CT image. Cystic structures (pneumatoceles) in both lower lobes, one with a small air-blood level (*arrow*). Besides, small left pneumothorax, small left pleural effusion and lung contusions.

rate within the first 24 hours in the hospital is considerable.[5,6] *Aortic injuries* are classified into four types or severity grades[7,8]:

- *Type I*: intimal tear.
- *Type II*: intramural hematoma.
- *Type III*: pseudoaneurysm.
- *Type IV*: rupture.

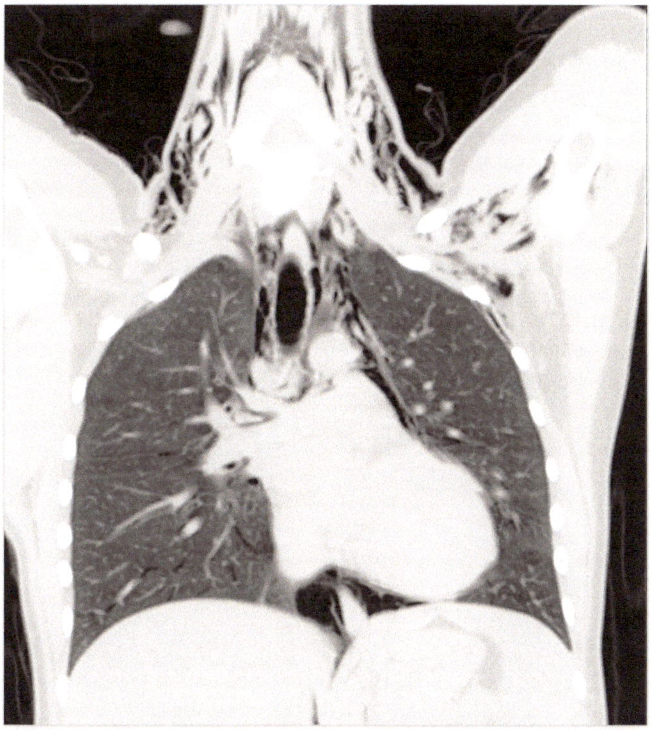

Fig. 15.3 Pneumomediastinum and cervical soft-tissue emphysema following injury to the left mainstem bronchus. CT, coronal MPR.

Detection of a mediastinal hematoma on CT is suggestive of aortic injury (▶Fig. 15.5). Tears in the vascular wall, thrombi in the aortic lumen, pseudoaneurysm (▶Fig. 15.6), and contrast extravasation secondary to rupture can be directly visualized. Contour discontinuity, a double aortic lumen, or pseudocoarctation are seen additionally. The latter term describes the abrupt tapering of the aortic lumen distal to the left subclavian artery compared with the ascending aorta.[3] Around 90% of aortic injuries occur in the anteromedial portion of the aortic isthmus distal to the origin of the left subclavian artery[9] because at this site the ligamentum arteriosum fixes in place the aortic arch. While type I aortic injuries (intimal tear) need only conservative therapy, emergency treatment is recommended for the other types, preferentially with endovascular stent-graft placement.[8] For hemodynamically unstable patients, it is

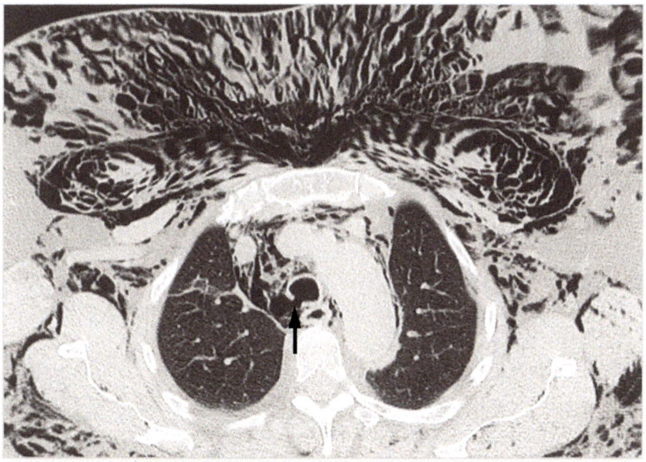

Fig. 15.4 Tracheal rupture. CT image. Defect at the transition from the cartilaginous to the posterior membranous part of the trachea (*arrow*). Resultant mediastinal emphysema and massive thoracic soft-tissue emphysema.

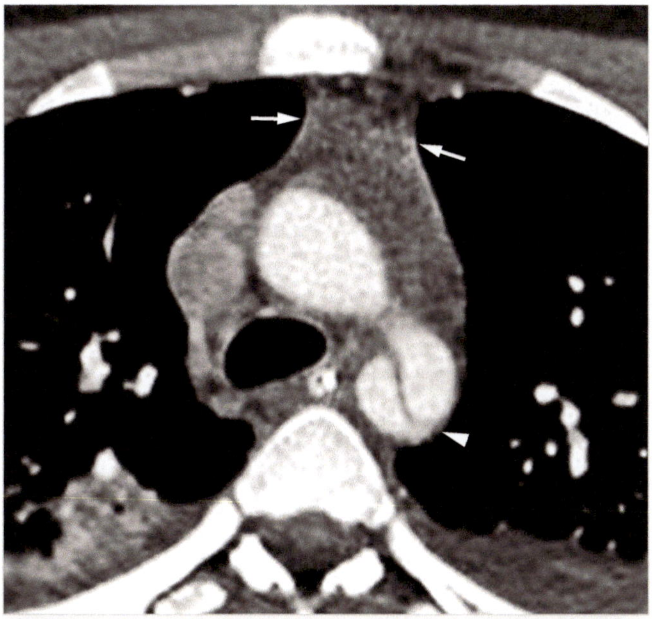

Fig. 15.5 Mediastinal hematoma. CT image. Retrosternal structure of soft-tissue density (*arrows*). Furthermore, pseudoaneurysm of the descending aorta (*arrowhead*).

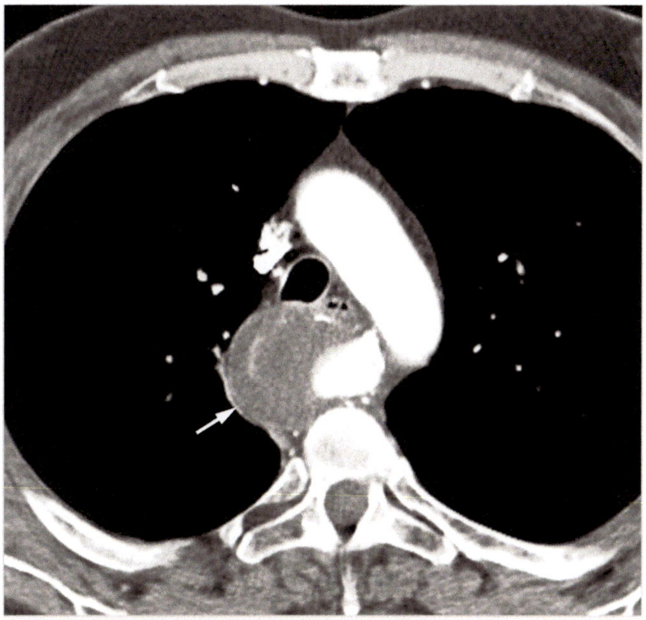

Fig. 15.6 Large, partially thrombosed, aortic pseudoaneurysm (*arrow*). CT image.

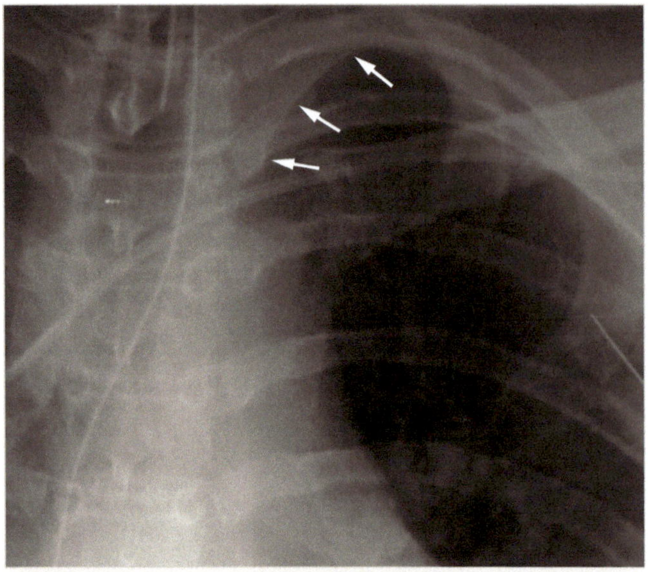

Fig. 15.7 **Apical cap in aortic rupture.** Radiograph, sectional magnification. Smoothly marginated, left apical extrapleural opacity of soft-tissue density (*arrows*).

important that aortic injury be diagnosed based on the radiography findings (▶Fig. 15.7), as presented in Table 15.1. Negative chest radiography just about rules out aortic rupture (predictive value 96–98%).[7,10]

Venous bleeding is associated with a high mortality rate and can cause hemopericardium and cardiac (also called pericardial) tamponade. Other diagnostic pointers are venous thrombosis or venous occlusion, vascular irregularities, hematomas, and contrast extravasation.[13]

Pneumopericardium, a rare condition, can like tension pneumomediastinum quickly become life threatening due to rising pressure. Esophageal rupture and pleuropericardial fistulas are potential causes.[3]

Table 15.1 Signs of aortic injury on radiography[10,11,12]

Signs	Validity
Abnormal aortic arch contour	Sensitivity 53–100%, Specificity 21–63%
Mediastinal enlargement	Sensitivity 53–100%, Specificity 15–60%
Apical cap	Sensitivity 9–63%, Specificity 75–96%
Enlarged paratracheal stripes	
Enlarged paraspinal lines	Sensitivity 2–12%, Specificity 97–99%
Caudally displaced left mainstem bronchus	Sensitivity 1–4%
Aortopulmonary window opacity	Negative predictive value 83–86%
Tracheal displacement	

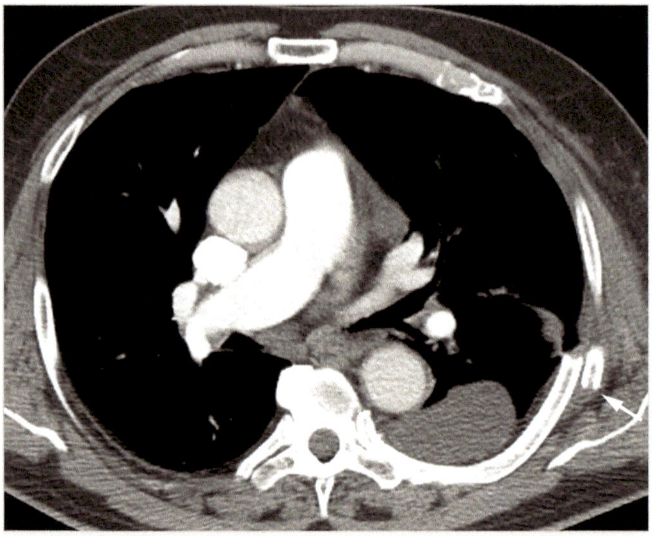

Fig. 15.8 Left hemothorax secondary to rib fracture (*arrow*). CT image. Pleural muscle-isodense fluid collection.

15.1.3 Pleural Space

Around 30 to 50% all patients with blunt chest trauma develop *hemothorax*, a blood collection in the pleural space. On CT, it appears similar to a pleural effusion but with a higher density of 35 to 70 HU (▶Fig. 15.8).

Pneumothorax is discussed in detail in Section 11.1. Fragments from rib fractures can damage the visceral pleura and cause pneumothorax. This is seen in around 30 to 40% of all blunt chest injuries and can be an acute life-threatening condition in case of tension pneumothorax. Up to three-quarters of all pneumothoraces cannot be reliably identified on chest radiography and are only be detected on CT.[14] Iatrogenic pneumothorax is not uncommon since chest tubes are often placed in preclinical emergency care. Malpositioning of a chest tube in the lung parenchyma (▶Fig. 15.9) creates a bronchopleural fistula which may cause persistent pneumothorax.

15.1.4 Trunk Wall

Rib fractures, in particular of the 4th to 8th rib, are seen in around half of all patients with blunt chest trauma. Fractures of the 1st to 3rd rib are indicative of high-energy trauma, which may involve the brachial plexus and subclavian vessels. Fractures of the 8th to 11th rib are often seen in association with upper abdominal injuries.[3] An unstable thorax is present if at least three ribs are fractured at two or more locations (▶Fig. 15.10).

Sternum fractures, which are less common, are caused in the vast majority of cases by road traffic accidents, often in association with lung, heart, or spinal injuries.[3] Clavicular and scapular fractures are relatively common.

Only around 3% of blunt chest injuries involve *injury to the thoracic spine*. In a large percentage of cases, there is also spinal

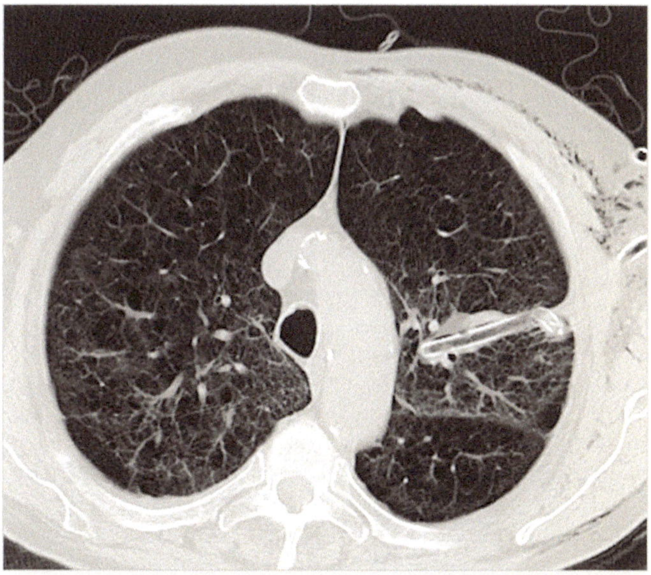

Fig. 15.9 Malpositioned chest tube in the lung parenchyma of the left upper lobe. Besides, minor chest wall emphysema. CT image.

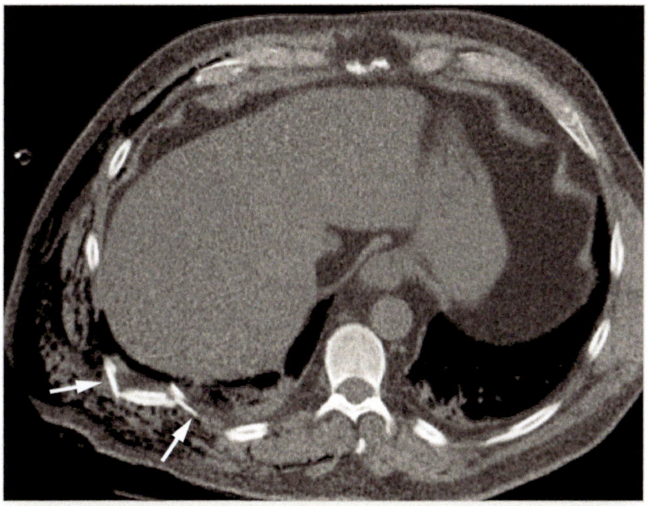

Fig. 15.10 Multifragmentary fracture of the ribs (*arrows*). CT image. Resultant unstable thorax. Furthermore, chest wall emphysema.

cord injury, in particular at the level of the 9th to 11th thoracic vertebra.[15]

Chest wall hematomas either develop secondary to chest call injury or are iatrogenic, for example, after chest tube placement. *Soft tissue emphysema* usually has its origin in rupture of the tracheobronchial system or in pneumothorax, rarely in esophageal rupture.

15.1.5 Diaphragm

Traumatic diaphragmatic hernias or diaphragmatic ruptures are often overlooked on a radiograph. On CT, herniated abdominal structures can be directly visualized in the thorax (▶Fig. 15.11). In many cases, the posterolateral portion of the left diaphragm is affected; intrathoracic herniation of the stomach is usually seen.

> **Note**
>
> Traumatic diaphragmatic hernias can be easily confused with a pre-existing Bochdalek hernia. Diaphragmatic discontinuity due to a Bochdalek hernia is rarely seen before age 40 years. It is usually young people who experience blunt chest trauma. Therefore, distinguishing between Bochdalek hernia and diaphragmatic rupture is often only possible on the basis of the patient's age.[16]

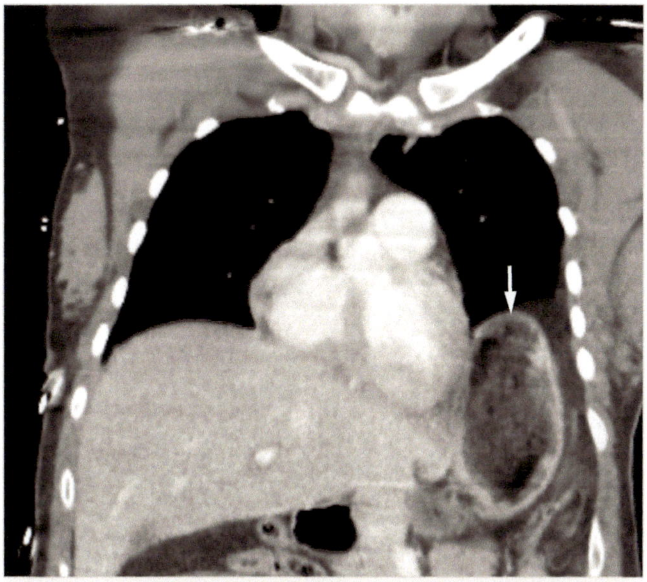

Fig. 15.11 Left, traumatic diaphragmatic hernia. CT, coronal MPR. Herniation of the stomach and abdominal fat into the left hemithorax (*arrow*).

15.2 Penetrating Chest Trauma

Compared with blunt chest trauma (see above), the incidence of the injuries described for penetrating chest trauma varies in accordance with the mechanism of injury. Lung lacerations occur in principle more often. Because vascular and parenchymal injuries are usually present, bleeding in the pleural and pericardial

15

II

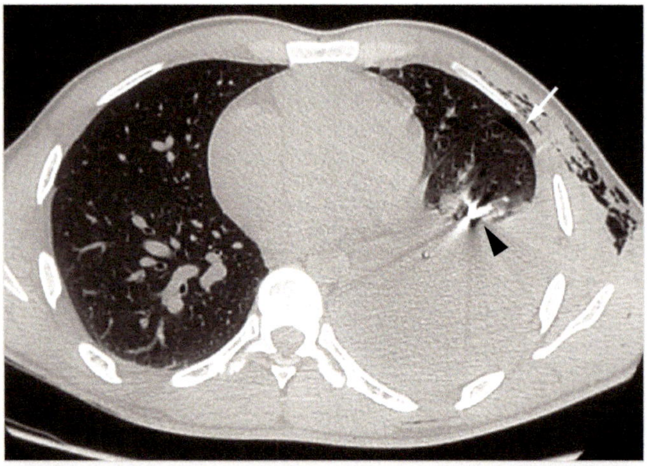

Fig. 15.12 Thoracic gunshot wound. CT image. Projectile in the left lower lobe (*arrowhead*). Large left hemothorax, besides, small left pneumothorax (*arrow*). Minor chest wall emphysema.

Table 15.2 Radiographic differential diagnoses of mediastinal enlargement following chest trauma

Traumatic/ nontraumatic	Differential diagnoses
Traumatic	• Mediastinal hematoma • Traumatic aortic pseudoaneurysm • Aortic rupture • Other arterial injury • Venous bleeding • Sternal fracture • Vertebral body fracture • Lung contusion adjacent to mediastinum
Incidental (non-traumatic)	• Mediastinal lipomatosis • Thymus (in children, adolescents) • Mediastinal tumor • Shallow inspiration depth

cavity is regularly observed (▶Fig. 15.12). Pneumothorax is common if the pleural cavity had been opened, in particular in settings of concomitant lung injury. The spectrum of cardiac injuries ranges from pericardial laceration, with or without heart dislocation (posterior heart displacement), through coronary artery injury to defects in the cardiac muscle, papillary muscles and cardiac valves.[17]

CT has high sensitivity for detection of pathologic air and blood collections and is useful for reconstruction of the penetration tract, which is of relevance for surgical repair.[17]

15.3 Summary

Blunt chest trauma is more common than penetrating injuries in European countries. The first diagnostic measure undertaken for hemodynamically unstable patients is usually radiography of the chest and pelvis; for stable patients, CT is the mainstay imaging modality.

Table 15.3 CT signs of aortic injury

Direct/indirect	Findings
Direct	• Contour discontinuity • Intimal tear • Intramural hematoma • Pseudoaneurysm • Double aortic lumen • Pseudocoarctation • Thrombus in the aortic lumen • Contrast extravasation
Indirect	• Mediastinal hematoma

Lung contusions are the most common form of pulmonary injury and resolve within a few days. *Lung lacerations* result from rupture of the lung tissue, giving rise to pneumatoceles, hematomas, or a combination of both. They resolve within 1 to 3 weeks with scar formation. Aspiration pneumonia is another cause of pulmonary opacity. This is predominantly seen in the posterior portions of the lower lobes. It may undergo suppuration and is then difficult to differentiate from a pneumatocele.

Various injuries and nontraumatic events can cause mediastinal enlargement on radiographs (▶Table 15.2). The most important cause in trauma patients, *mediastinal hematoma*, is suggestive of vascular injury.

CT is able to directly visualize *aortic injury* (▶Table 15.3). Depending on the degree of severity, an intimal tear, intramural hematoma, pseudoaneurysm, or contrast extravasation is seen. Intimal tears are treated conservatively, while higher grade aortic injuries require emergency treatment, preferentially with endovascular stent-graft placement.

A *diaphragmatic rupture* is sometimes difficult to diagnose on radiography. Diagnostic pointers are a high-riding diaphragm or obliteration of the diaphragmatic contour. On CT, a diaphragmatic rupture is usually easy to detect but should not be confused with pre-existing Bochdalek hernia.

Pneumothorax is common in chest trauma. Injury to the trachea or mediastinal bronchi causes pneumomediastinum. Less commonly, pneumomediastinum has its origin in interstitial emphysema associated with lung parenchymal injuries or esophageal rupture.

References

[1] Miller LA. Chest wall, lung, and pleural space trauma. Radiol Clin North Am 2006;44(2):213–224, viii

[2] Oikonomou A, Prassopoulos P. CT imaging of blunt chest trauma. Insights Imaging 2011;2(3):281–295

[3] Palas J, Matos AP, Mascarenhas V, Herédia V, Ramalho M. Multidetector computer tomography: evaluation of blunt chest trauma in adults. Radiol Res Pract 2014;2014:864369

[4] Moore AV, Putnam CE, Ravin CE. The radiology of thoracic trauma. Bull N Y Acad Med 1981;57(4):272–292

[5] Arthurs ZM, Starnes BW, Sohn VY, Singh N, Martin MJ, Andersen CA. Functional and survival outcomes in traumatic blunt thoracic aortic injuries: An analysis of the National Trauma Databank. J Vasc Surg 2009;49(4):988–994

[6] Jamieson WRE, Janusz MT, Gudas VM, Burr LH, Fradet GJ, Henderson C. Traumatic rupture of the thoracic aorta: third decade of experience. Am J Surg 2002;183(5):571–575

[7] Azizzadeh A, Keyhani K, Miller CC III, Coogan SM, Safi HJ, Estrera AL. Blunt traumatic aortic injury: initial experience with endovascular repair. J Vasc Surg 2009;49(6):1403–1408
[8] Lee WA, Matsumura JS, Mitchell RS, et al. Endovascular repair of traumatic thoracic aortic injury: clinical practice guidelines of the Society for Vascular Surgery. J Vasc Surg 2011;53(1):187–192
[9] Alkadhi H, Wildermuth S, Desbiolles L, et al. Vascular emergencies of the thorax after blunt and iatrogenic trauma: multi-detector row CT and three-dimensional imaging. Radiographics 2004;24(5):1239–1255
[10] Mirvis SE, Bidwell JK, Buddemeyer EU, Diaconis JN, Pais SO, Whitley JE. Imaging diagnosis of traumatic aortic rupture. A review and experience at a major trauma center. Invest Radiol 1987;22(3):187–196
[11] Gavelli G, Canini R, Bertaccini P, Battista G, Bnà C, Fattori R. Traumatic injuries: imaging of thoracic injuries. Eur Radiol 2002;12(6):1273–1294
[12] Marnocha KE, Maglinte DD. Plain-film criteria for excluding aortic rupture in blunt chest trauma. AJR Am J Roentgenol 1985;144(1):19–21
[13] Holly BP, Steenburg SD. Multidetector CT of blunt traumatic venous injuries in the chest, abdomen, and pelvis. Radiographics 2011;31 (5):1415–1424
[14] Ball CG, Kirkpatrick AW, Feliciano DV. The occult pneumothorax: what have we learned? Can J Surg 2009;52(5):E173–E179
[15] Costantino M, Gosselin MV, Primack SL. The ABC's of thoracic trauma imaging. Semin Roentgenol 2006;41(3):209–225
[16] Van Hise ML, Primack SL, Israel RS, Müller NL. CT in blunt chest trauma: indications and limitations. Radiographics 1998;18(5):1071–1084
[17] Co SJ, Yong-Hing CJ, Galea-Soler S, et al. Role of imaging in penetrating and blunt traumatic injury to the heart. Radiographics 2011;31(4):E101–E115

Chapter 16

Diagnostic Imaging of the Chest in Intensive Care Medicine

16 Diagnostic Imaging of the Chest in Intensive Care Medicine

16

16.1 Indications for Chest Radiography in Intensive Care Medicine

The value of daily routine chest radiography for each patient in an intensive care unit has long been a contentious issue. A recent meta-analysis did not find any advantage for daily chest radiography compared with clinically indicated chest radiography.[1] Therefore, the use of daily routine chest radiography in the intensive care unit has now been abandoned.[1,2,3,4,5]

In its appropriateness criteria, the American College of Radiology lists the relevant indications, as illustrated in ▶Table 16.1.

16.2 Detection and Malposition of Implanted Devices

16.2.1 Tracheal Tubes

The distal end of the endotracheal tube should be positioned 4 to 6 cm above the tracheal bifurcation (▶Fig. 16.1). Movement of the head leads to downward or upward positioning of the tube by approximately 2 cm.[6] Malposition of the endotracheal tube is common, but with widespread variation in the incidence reported in the literature (2–46%). Only in a minority of cases is this clinically suspected.[5] Therefore, radiography is warranted to confirm correct tube position after insertion. The distal end of the tube is usually placed too low in one of the two mainstem bronchi or too high. Less often, the endotracheal tube is positioned in the esophagus. If so, the tube does not follow the tracheal contour on chest radiography.

> **Note**
>
> Certain clinical situations require separate lung ventilation. This is generally the case in lung surgery. The tip of the double lumen endotracheal tube is placed in one mainstem bronchus and the tube ventilates the other lung via a side hole. Such a finding should not be misinterpreted as tube malposition.

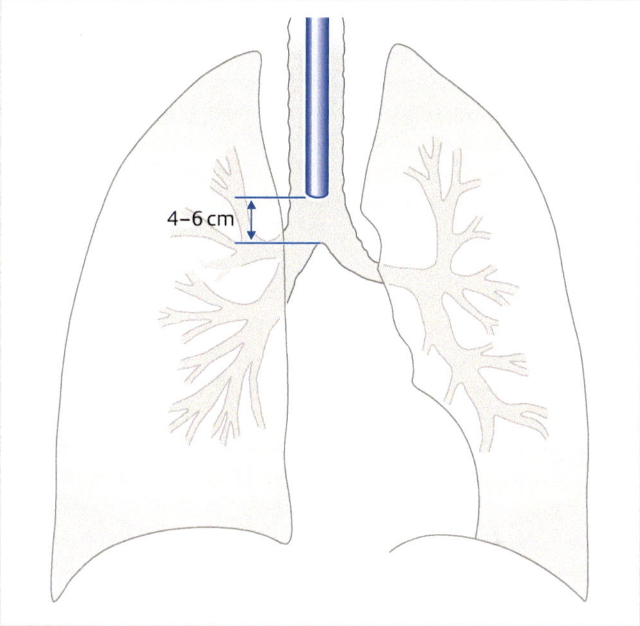

Fig. 16.1 Correct position of a tracheal tube. Schematic diagram.

Table 16.1 Indications for chest radiography for intensive care unit patient[5]

Indications	Appropriateness criteria[a]
Admission to intensive care unit	7
Stable patient, no change in clinical status	3
Patient with clinical worsening	9
Post-insertion of tube or catheter	9
Post-chest tube removal	5[b]

[a] Appropriateness criteria:
1–3 = Usually not appropriate
4–6 = May be appropriate
7–9 = Usually appropriate
[b] Data are largely based on studies of patients following cardiothoracic surgery and are not generalizable.

16.2.2 Central Venous Catheters

Ideally, the tip of a central venous catheter is located just above the opening of the superior vena cava into the right atrium (▶Fig. 16.2). On chest radiography, it corresponds to a position of approximately 4 cm below the tracheal bifurcation. Too low placement in the right atrium can cause cardiac dysrhythmia and mechanical irritation of the tricuspid valve.

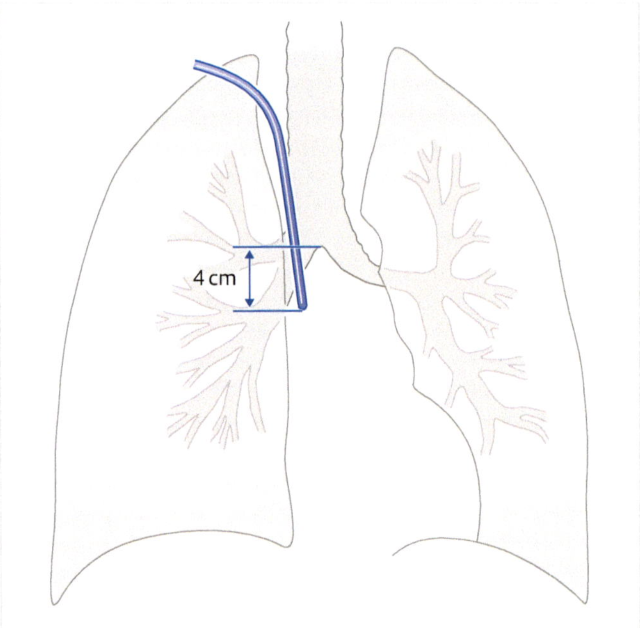

Fig. 16.2 Correct position of a central venous catheter. Schematic diagram.

Malposition is seen in around 10% of central venous catheters (▶Fig. 16.3). Puncture-related pneumothoraces are less common at a rate of up to 6%, and occur most often with the subclavian approach.[6] Hence, radiography is indicated immediately after insertion. If extravascular catheter position is suspected, instillation of a few milliliters of contrast media is recommended for verification of extra- or intravascular placement. New onset pleural effusion and rapidly progressive mediastinal widening are signs of extravascular line placement. If the catheter is not seen to be positioned exactly at the right mediastinal border but is observed instead to run in the direction of the aortic arch, intra-arterial position should be suspected. This can be confirmed or excluded through blood gas analysis of a sample taken from the catheter.

16.2.3 Pulmonary Artery Catheters (Swan-Ganz Catheter)

The tip of a pulmonary artery catheter is normally positioned in the right pulmonary artery (▶Fig. 16.4). Correct placement in the pulmonary artery is verified by registration of the pressure curve, thus largely precluding any relevant malpositioning. But malpositioning can be expected if a characteristic pulmonary artery pressure curve cannot be recorded during placement. Chest radiography is used for documentation of an often clinically suspected malposition and helps to correct this. Chest radiography is always indicated immediately after catheter insertion to confirm correct position and exclude pneumothorax.

Central placement of the catheter tip in the proximal pulmonary trunk can irritate the pulmonary valve because of catheter pulsation. A very peripheral catheter position, usually well into

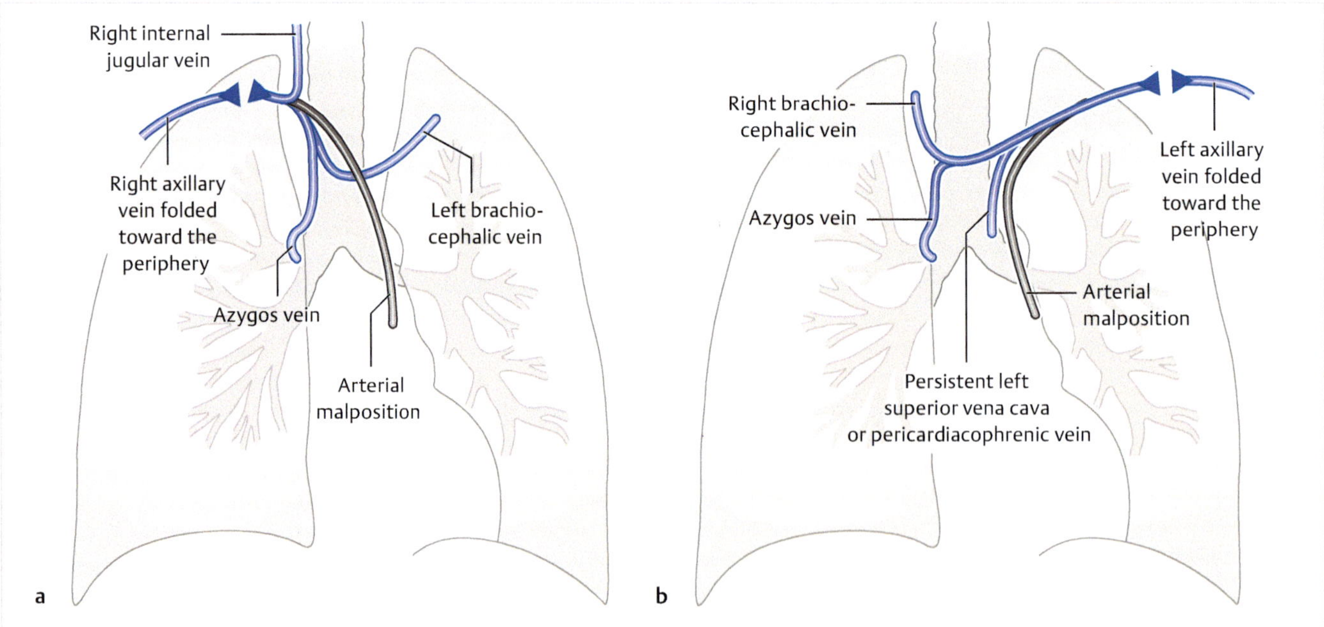

Fig. 16.3 Typical malpositions of central venous catheters. Schematic diagram. **(a)** For right-sided placement. **(b)** For left-sided placement.

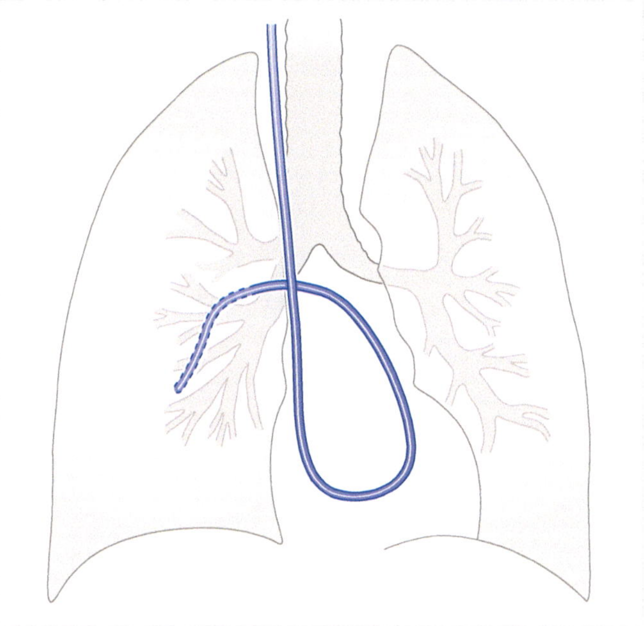

Fig. 16.4 Correct position of a pulmonary artery catheter. Schematic diagram. *Dotted line*: wedge position.

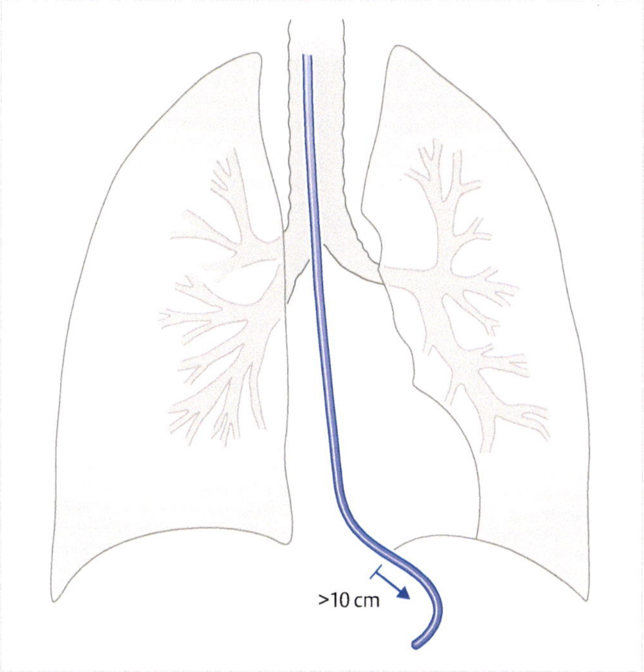

Fig. 16.5 Correct position of a nasogastric tube. Schematic diagram.

the right lower lobe artery, corresponds to the measurement position for the pulmonary capillary wedge pressure, known as the *wedge position*. After measurement, the catheter is usually pulled back again into a central pulmonary artery.

16.2.4 Nasogastric Tubes

Nasogastric tubes usually have side holes which are several centimeters distant from the tip. Therefore, a nasogastric tube should be positioned at least 10 cm below the diaphragm to prevent reflux into the esophagus as well as aspiration (▶ Fig. 16.5). Placement of the nasogastric tube tip in the esophagus is the most common malposition. There are many reasons for this:

- The tube is not advanced far enough.
- The tube was placed correctly initially but was then dislodged upward.
- The tube is reverted in the esophagus.

The nasogastric tube may, on rare occasions, enter the tracheobronchial tree. Because of the potentially severe complications, the correct infradiaphragmatic tube position must be confirmed radiographically at least before infusing nutrient solutions.

> **Note**
>
> Some nasogastric tubes are only faintly radiopaque and are difficult to detect on chest radiography, in particular in the upper abdomen. Changing the window settings or gray scale inversion may help locate the tube tip. In the worst case scenario, the nasogastric tube must be rendered visible through instillation of a few milliliters of contrast media.

16.2.5 Chest Tubes

Chest tubes are widely used in thoracic surgery and are placed under visual control; hence, malposition is not expected in this setting. Moreover, chest tube placement is a routine procedure in the intensive care unit and preclinical emergency medicine. In the latter setting, tube malposition occurs in approximately 10% of cases.[7,8,9] Therefore, chest radiography is recommended for chest tubes inserted on the intensive care unit setting to exclude malposition and pneumothorax and to verify the effectiveness of the drainage function. Persistent air fistula through the chest tube suggests a tube malposition in the lung parenchyma; CT is superior to chest radiography at visualizing or excluding this condition.

Complications occur relatively rarely during chest tube removal. Occasional pneumothorax is usually clinically suspected and only rarely constitutes an unexpected finding on chest radiography. Therefore, routine radiography is not mandatory after chest tube removal.[5,10]

16.2.6 Intra-Aortic Balloon Pump

An intra-aortic balloon pump (IABP) is implanted in patients with severe left ventricular failure to support cardiac pump function. A long balloon inserted via the femoral artery into the aorta always inflates in diastole, thus pumping blood from the aorta into the periphery. The balloon deflates again in systole. The IABP itself is usually not visualized on chest radiography; at most, only a small metallic marker is identified at the proximal tip of the balloon which should be positioned just distal

II

to the origin of the left subclavian artery from the aortic arch. Accordingly, the marker is projected between the middle and lower third of the aortic notch (▶Fig. 16.6). A too-high location of the balloon presents a risk of occlusion of the left subclavian artery, while in the worst case scenario too-low placement may cause intestinal ischemia due to occlusion of the origins of the large abdominal arteries.

16.2.7 Other Implanted Devices

Artificial hearts are classified as follows in accordance with their support function:

- Left ventricular assist devices (LVAD).
- Right ventricular assist devices (RVAD).
- Biventricular assist devices (BiVAD).

Their visualization on chest radiography depends on the specific type of device. The location of the connections should always be compared with previous radiographs to exclude device dislocation.

The same applies for temporary or permanent *cardiac pacemakers* and *implantable cardioverter defibrillators* (ICD aggregates). They undergo functional testing when implanted; hence, immediate postinterventional images can serve as a reference for correct location of the implanted devices.

Extracorporeal lung assist device (ECMO, extracorporeal membrane oxygenation) is placed under echocardiographic guidance. The catheters which can be identified on chest radiography vary according to the system used.[11] Follow-up chest radiography is used to ensure there is no dislocation of the implanted devices.

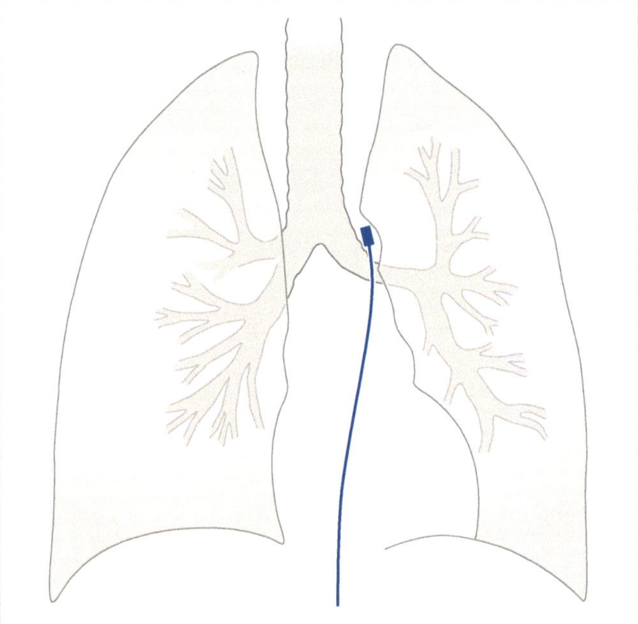

Fig. 16.6 Correct position on an intra-aortic balloon pump. Schematic diagram.

16.3 Typical Findings in Intensive Care Unit Patients

Atelectasis is the most common cause of lung opacities on the chest radiographs of intensive care unit (ICU) patients. Two-thirds of all atelectases affect the left lower lobe, followed by the right lower lobe and the right upper lobe.[12] There are several reasons for atelectasis:

- Bronchial obstruction due to mucus or blood.
- Compression because of a pleural effusion or cardiomegaly.
- Relaxation due to pneumothorax.
- Tracheal tube malposition.
- The patient's persistent supine position.

Radiographic signs of atelectasis include consolidation that can result in a loss of the contour of the diaphragm or the heart (▶Fig. 16.7). At times, large areas of atelectasis exhibit signs of volume loss with mediastinal shift and displacement of pulmonary fissures (on supine radiographs only the right minor fissure is visible) and bundling of pulmonary structures. Enlarging pulmonary opacity seen in a persisting atelectasis is suggestive of bacterial superinfection.[6]

Section 5.2 describes the challenges of radiographic differential diagnosis of hospital-associated *pneumonia* in mechanically ventilated patients (see also ▶Table 5.4).

Many ventilation schemes include a positive end-expiratory pressure (*PEEP*). This leads to aeration of atelectases, including microatelectasis, and reduction of pulmonary edema due to changed pressure relations in the lung parenchyma. This results in an improved appearance of the chest radiograph, with less pathologic lung opacities, such as edema or atelectasis. However, PEEP ventilation does not improve the underlying pathologic conditions. Therefore, when interpreting the

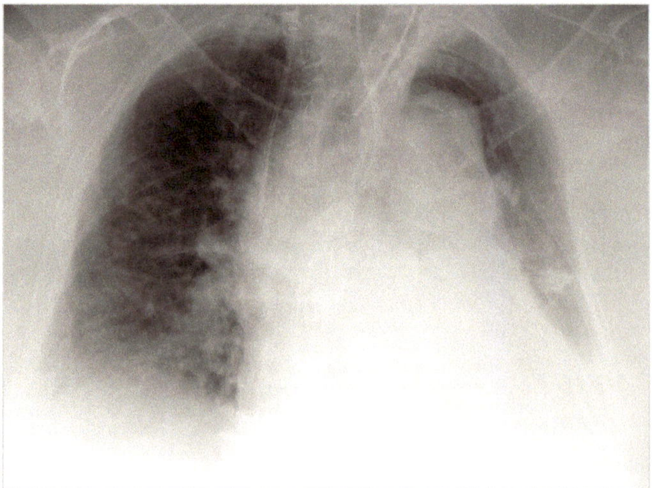

Fig. 16.7 Atelectasis in an obese patient. Radiograph, supine image. Left lower lobe atelectasis due to cardiomegaly: opacity of the retrocardiac space and blurring of the left diaphragm. Furthermore, partial atelectasis of the right lower lobe, blurring of the lateral portion of the right diaphragm.

radiographs of mechanically ventilated patients, the following guiding rule should be borne in mind "PEEP paints a pretty picture!" (▶Fig. 16.8).

Patients receiving high-pressure ventilation have an increased risk for *barotrauma* of the lungs; imaging demonstrates interstitial emphysema, pneumomediastinum, or pneumothorax. There are several causes of pleural effusions in intensive care unit patients.

16.4 Congestive Heart Failure

> **Note**
>
> The term congestive heart failure describes the heart's inability to pump sufficiently to maintain an adequate blood flow to the organs (forward failure) or involves congestion of blood before the heart (backward failure).

Depending on the ventricle affected, a distinction is made between left-sided and right-sided congestive heart failure, each with its own clinical and radiographic manifestations. A combination of both types may be seen; this is known as *global congestive heart failure* with overlapping findings of left-sided and right-sided congestive heart failure. A common feature is usually cardiomegaly.

The vascular pedicle width(▶Fig. 16.9) is a useful differential diagnostic parameter, especially for assessment of the time course. Congestive heart failure generally causes widening of the vascular pedicle. The vascular pedicle width is essentially determined by the caliber of the superior vena cava, thus permitting evaluation of the volume status of the central veins: an increase of the vascular pedicle width by 1 cm roughly corresponds to a 2-liter increase of the circulating blood volume .[13]

16.4.1 Left-sided Congestive Heart Failure

Diagnosis of left-sided congestive heart failure is one domain of radiology. Chest radiography is able to visualize pathologic changes (▶Table 16.2) even before there is clinical evidence of manifest congestive heart failure. Initially, the failing left ventricle causes increased pressure and volume in the left atrium. This directly affects the pulmonary veins which dilate because of the resultant pulmonary venous pressure increase. Consequently, the pulmonary capillary pressure increases. In accordance with the Starling equation, fluid is displaced out of the capillaries and into the interstitium, causing interstitial pulmonary

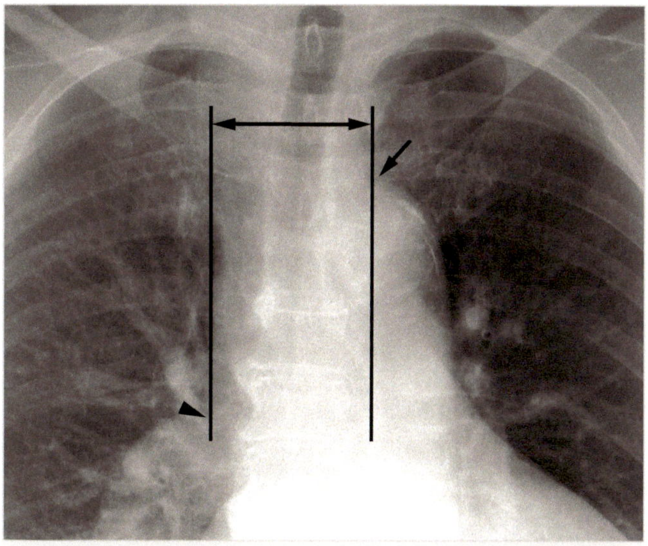

Fig. 16.9 Measurement of the vascular pedicle width. Radiograph. The width is measured horizontally between two points (normal value 43–53 mm): between the origin of the left subclavian artery at the aortic arch (*arrow*) and the intersection of the right mainstem bronchus with the superior vena cava (*arrowhead*).

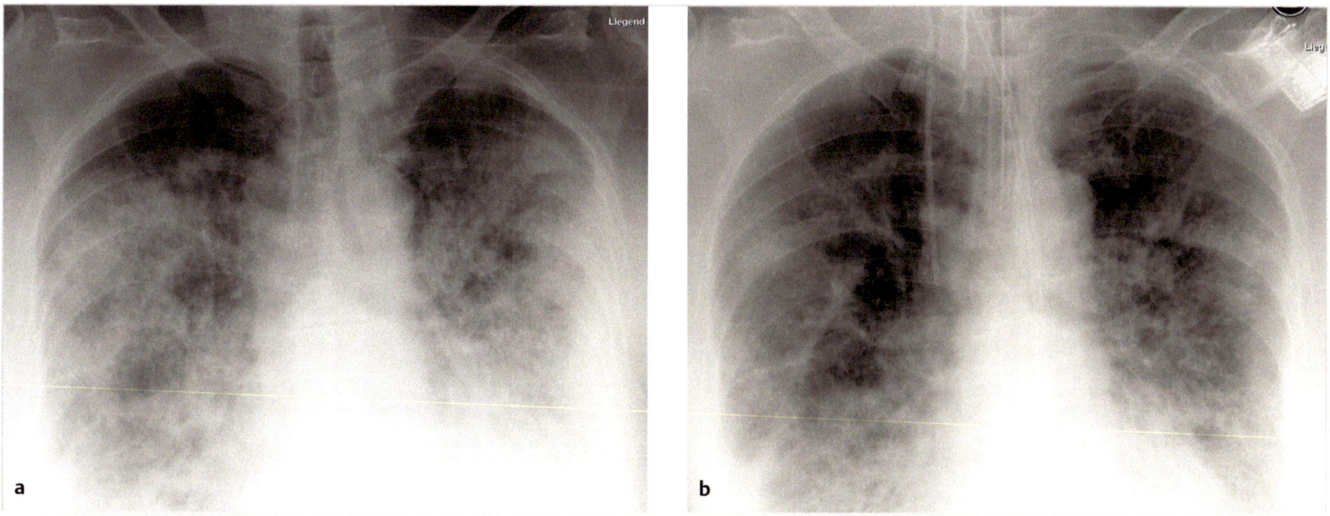

Fig. 16.8 Impact of positive pressure ventilation on chest radiography. Patient with lung fibrosis and pneumonia. **(a)** Before intubation. **(b)** After intubation and with PEEP ventilation (12 cm H_2O). No change in clinical status, markedly improved radiolucency of the lungs on chest radiography.

Table 16.2 Radiologic findings in left-sided congestive heart failure

Pathomechanisms	Radiographic signs on supine image
Backward failure of the left heart	
Dilation of the left atrium	Widening of the tracheal bifurcation
Pulmonary venous pressure increase	
Dilation of the pulmonary veins	Right upper lobe vein > 4 mm
Pulmonary capillary pressure increase	
Fluid displacement into the interstitium	Interstitial pulmonary edema
Fluid displacement into the alveoli	Alveolar pulmonary edema

edema. Alveolar pulmonary edema later occurs once the fluid absorption capacity of the interstitium has been exhausted.

A *pleural effusion* arises from the visceral pleura. Because of pulmonary edema, the pulmonary lymph drainage system is overloaded and unable to drain the interstitial pulmonary fluid, resulting in transudation of the fluid through the visceral pleura into the pleural space.

Occasionally, *pulmonary blood flow redistribution* from the base of the lung toward the apex can be identified on erect radiographs. Normally, the basal lung regions are better perfused than the apical parts. Onset of pulmonary edema is also first noted in the basal portions. The interstitial fluid prolongs the oxygen diffusion path. The reduced oxygen partial pressure in the blood causes hypoxic pulmonary vasoconstriction in the basal lung; consequently, blood flow to the apical regions unaffected by vasoconstriction is increased. This phenomenon cannot be identified on supine radiographs since the distribution of pulmonary blood flow differs from that seen in the upright position.

16.4.2 Right-Sided Congestive Heart Failure

Right-sided congestive heart failure is usually clinically evident before chest radiography shows clear pathologic changes. Peripheral edema is the main clinical manifestation of right-sided congestive heart failure; ascites and pleural effusion as well as congested veins may also be identified. The principle radiographic sign of right-sided congestive heart failure seen on chest radiography is a pleural effusion. The increased pressure in the systemic veins results in increased capillary fluid filtration via the serous membranes into the body cavities. Hence, unlike in left-sided congestive heart failure, the pleural effusion arises from the parietal pleura in right-sided congestive heart failure. Widening of the mediastinum is due to dilation of the superior vena cava; this also results in an enlarged vascular pedicle. A congested liver can cause a right-sided, high-riding diaphragm.

16.5 Pulmonary Edema

Pulmonary edema is a frequent cause for admission of a patient to the intensive care unit. Its myriad causes are summarized in ▶Table 16.3. There are two main types of pulmonary edema based on the different underlying pathophysiology determined by the Starling equation:

- *Hydrostatic edema*: The pulmonary capillary pressure is increased and the vascular wall permeability is normal; this results in fluid displacement out of the capillaries and into the interstitium, causing interstitial edema.
- *Permeability edema*: The permeability of the vascular wall is increased and the pulmonary capillary pressure is normal. Fluid flow to the alveoli is considerably faster than in hydrostatic edema causing alveolar edema; but the interstitium is less involved than in hydrostatic edema.

16.5.1 Hydrostatic Edema

Interstitial edema is the most common type of hydrostatic edema. The typical findings associated with interstitial edema on chest radiography are as follows (▶Fig. 16.10):

- Interlobular septal thickening, identified as septal lines (formerly called Kerley B lines).
- Thickening of the peribronchovascular connective tissue (bronchial cuffing), recognizable from orthogonally projected bronchi (e.g., segmental bronchi 3 and 6).
- Unsharp vascular structures due to peribronchovascular connective tissue edema.

Table 16.3 Causes of pulmonary edema

Hydrostatic edema	Permeability edema
• Left-sided congestive heart failure • Renal failure • Hyperhydration	• Sepsis • Adult respiratory distress syndrome • Inhalation noxae • Drug-induced • Altitude edema • Neurogenic • Burns

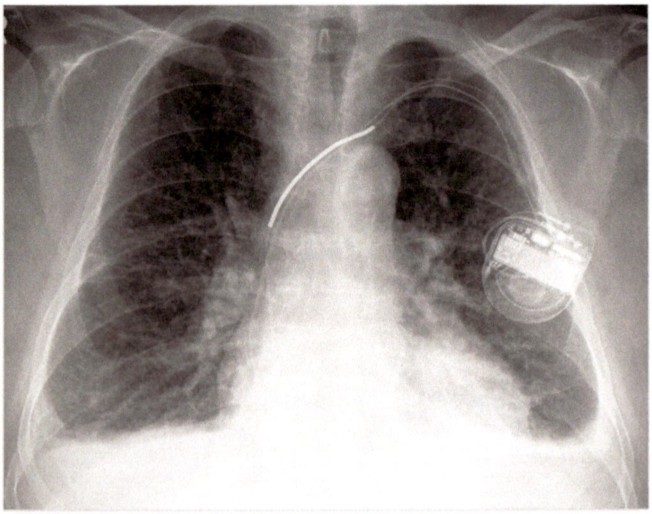

Fig. 16.10 Hydrostatic pulmonary edema in congestive heart failure. Radiograph. Bilateral interlobular septal thickening (formerly called Kerley B lines), especially in the basal lung, cardiomegaly, bilateral pleural effusions.

On CT, only interlobular septal thickening is initially seen, later followed by diffuse ground-glass opacities with a geographic distribution (▶Fig. 16.11). The latter usually orient themselves toward the lobule boundaries.

When the fluid absorption capacity of the pulmonary interstitium is exhausted, interstitial edema progresses to alveolar edema with formation of bilateral perihilar consolidations known as *batwing edema.*

Cardiogenic pulmonary edema differs in terms of its distribution from nephrogenic or hyperhydration-induced pulmonary edema. The former generally exhibits basal and perihilar predominance, while the latter has a central symmetrical distribution.[14] Widening of the *vascular pedicle* or progressive increase over time can be observed in all types. Together with cardiomegaly this constitutes a differential diagnostic criterion for differentiation versus permeability edema.

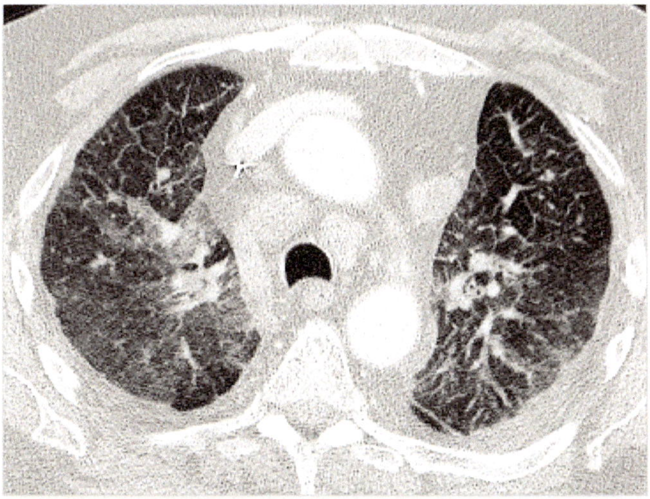

Fig. 16.11 Hydrostatic pulmonary edema in congestive heart failure. CT image. Interlobular septal thickening, bilateral ground-glass opacities, bilateral pleural effusions.

Note

In acute mitral regurgitation right upper lobe predominance for pulmonary edema is found and should not be misinterpreted as pneumonia.[6]

16.5.2 Permeability Edema

Unlike hydrostatic edema, permeability edema has no identifiable interstitial component on chest radiography. Alveolar pulmonary edema manifests on chest radiography through diffuse bilateral pulmonary opacities (▶Fig. 16.12a). On CT, bilateral, patchy ground-glass opacities and consolidations are seen (▶Fig. 16.12b).

The *vascular pedicle* is narrowed or decreased over time; this serves as a criterion for differentiation versus advanced hydrostatic edema.[6]

16.6 Adult Respiratory Distress Syndrome

Adult respiratory distress syndrome (ARDS) is defined clinically.

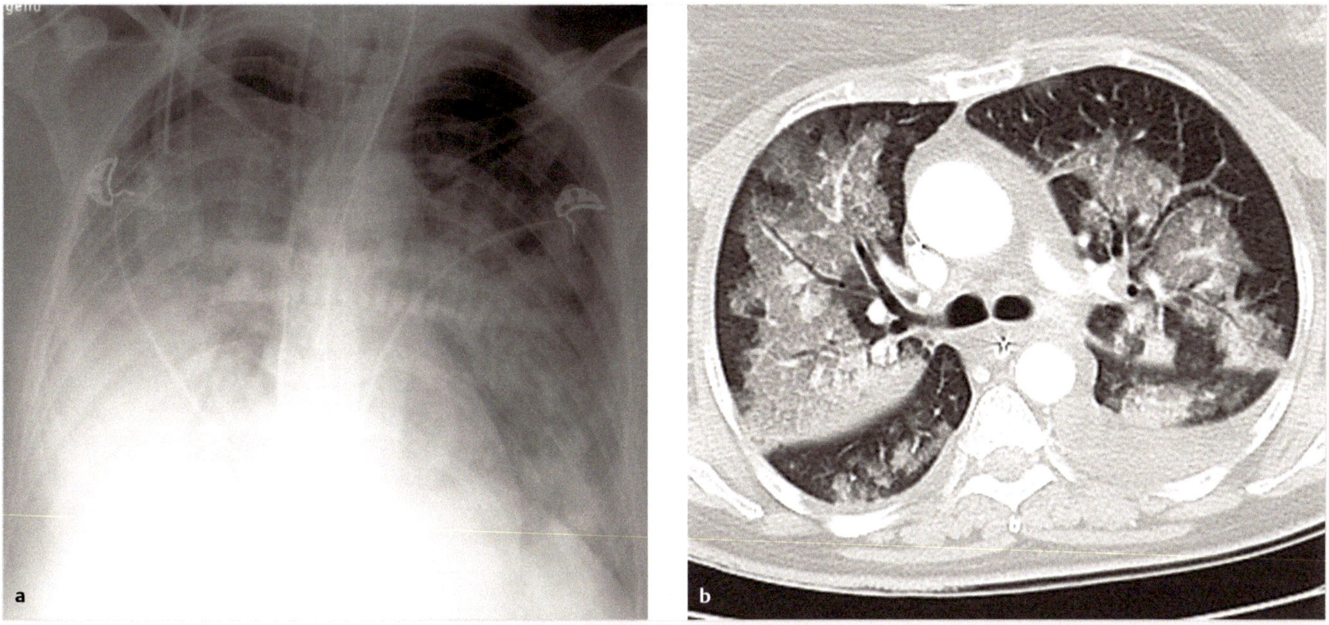

Fig. 16.12 Permeability edema. (a) Radiograph, supine image. Bilateral, diffuse pulmonary opacities. Bilateral pleural effusions. Compared with Fig. 16.10 narrow vascular pedicle. **(b)** CT image. Bilateral ground-glass opacities and consolidations. No interlobular septal thickening.

Note

Definition of adult respiratory distress syndrome as per the Berlin Definition 2011[15]:

- Onset within 1 week.
- Bilateral pulmonary opacities without any other plausible explanation.
- Respiratory failure not explained by congestive heart failure or hypervolemia.
- Oxygenation: oxygen partial pressure in arterial blood/oxygen content of the breathing air:
  - Mild adult respiratory distress syndrome: 200 to less than 300 mm Hg.
  - Moderate adult respiratory distress syndrome: 100 to less than 200 mm Hg.
  - Severe adult respiratory distress syndrome: less than 100 mm Hg.

Adult respiratory distress syndrome is triggered by the most diverse causes:

- *Pulmonary triggers*: inhalation injuries, toxic pulmonary edema, pneumonia, aspiration, lung contusion, near-drowning, fat embolism, amniotic fluid embolism, inhalation of hyperbaric oxygen.
- *Extrapulmonary triggers*: sepsis, trauma, shock, burns, pancreatitis, medication, massive blood transfusion, disseminated intravascular coagulation.

Direct or indirect pathologic cascade systems are activated in the lung, causing an exudative inflammatory reaction in the early phase. Protein influx into the alveoli deactivates the surfactant and inhibits its production. This gives rise to alveolar collapse resulting in impaired gas exchange and right-left shunts. After a few days, the inflammatory reaction is followed by a proliferative and then a fibrotic phase. Lung fibrosis occurs in the absence of restoration to the original state (*restitutio ad integrum*).

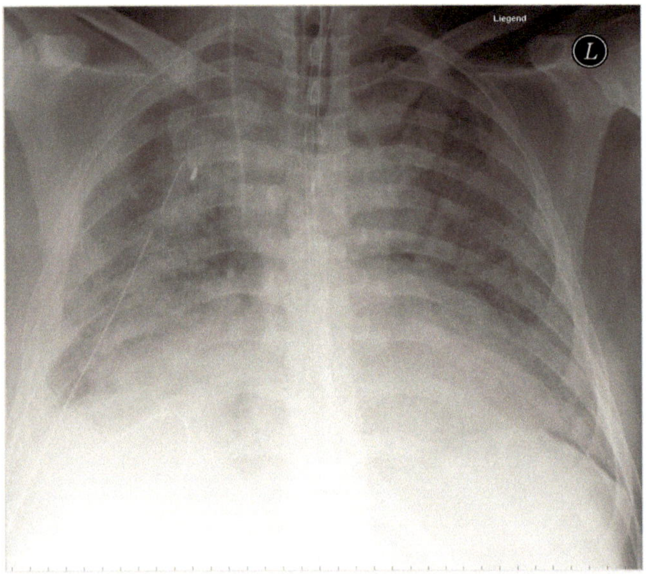

Fig. 16.13 Adult respiratory distress syndrome. Radiograph, supine image. Normal radiograph on previous day, now bilateral "white lung."

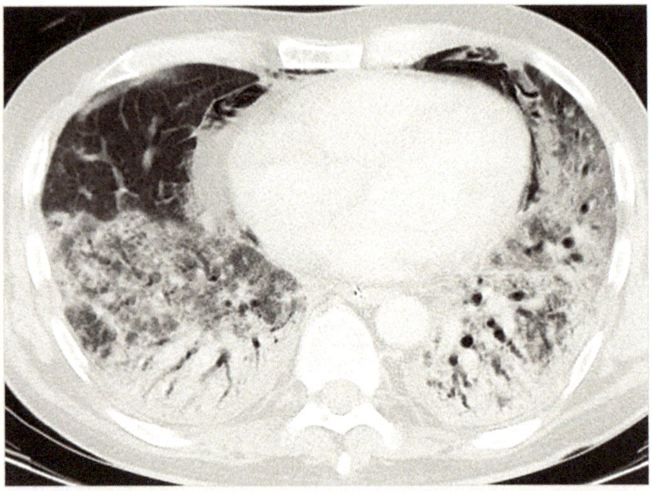

Fig. 16.14 Adult respiratory distress syndrome. CT image. Typical three-layer structure with anterior layer of normal lung tissue and posterior consolidations, with intervening ground-glass opacities.

In the early exudative phase of ARDS, bilateral pulmonary opacities are seen on radiography and are difficult to distinguish from pulmonary edema, with development of a "white lung" in severe cases (▶Fig. 16.13). On CT, a three-layer structure is typically seen, especially in extrapulmonary-induced ARDS: an anterior layer of normal lung tissue, ground-glass opacities in the center, and posterior consolidations (▶Fig. 16.14). However, these findings are less well identifiable in pulmonary ARDS.

Within 1 week, the diffuse opacities evolve to a reticular pattern which over the course of a few weeks either resolves or persists, giving rise to lung fibrosis.[6]

16.7 Summary

Chest radiography is indicated in the intensive care unit on admission of a new patient, after placement of devices (such as catheters, tubes) and in the event of worsening of the patient's clinical status. Daily routine chest radiography is not indicated when there is no change in the patient's condition.

Particular attention must be paid to ensuring correct positioning of all *implanted devices* since radiologists are better than clinicians at detecting any malpositioning. ▶Fig. 16.1, ▶Fig. 16.2, ▶Fig. 16.3, ▶Fig. 16.4, ▶Fig. 16.5, and ▶Fig. 16.6 feature schematic diagrams showing the correct position of commonly implanted devices. Moreover, all changes to the location of the implanted devices versus previous examination may be relevant and should be reported.

Most ventilation schemes include positive end-expiratory pressure (PEEP). An increased PEEP reduces atelectasis and pulmonary edema even without any change in the patient's clinical status: "PEEP paints a pretty picture."

Left-sided congestive heart failure results in *pulmonary edema* by increasing the pulmonary venous pressure. The implicated pathomechanism and resultant imaging findings are presented in Table 16.2. Like nephrogenic and hyperhydration edema, cardiogenic pulmonary edema constitutes hydrostatic edema of interstitial onset. Imaging shows interlobular septal thickening and ground-glass opacities. These are later followed by alveolar edema with bilateral central consolidations (batwing edema). Conversely, permeability edema results from myriad pathological states (see Table 16.3). Radiography demonstrates primary alveolar edema. Signs of interstitial edema are largely absent. The vascular pedicle width (see ▶Fig. 16.9) is a useful measure for differentiation between advanced hydrostatic edema and permeability edema. It is also used for assessment of the patient's hydration status on follow-up examinations. Widening of the vascular pedicle is suggestive of hydrostatic edema, while narrowing is indicative of permeability edema.

Adult respiratory distress syndrome is defined clinically and consists of an acute inflammatory reaction of the lung to the most diverse triggers, e.g., pneumonia, trauma, sepsis, shock, or burns. Radiography demonstrates acute onset, bilateral pulmonary opacities that evolve to a reticular pattern within 1 week and either resolve or progress to lung fibrosis.

References

[1] Oba Y, Zaza T. Abandoning daily routine chest radiography in the intensive care unit: meta-analysis. Radiology 2010;255(2):386–395

[2] Graat ME, Choi G, Wolthuis EK, et al. The clinical value of daily routine chest radiographs in a mixed medical-surgical intensive care unit is low. Crit Care 2006;10(1):R11

[3] Hendrikse KA, Gratama JWC, Hove Wt, Rommes JH, Schultz MJ, Spronk PE. Low value of routine chest radiographs in a mixed medical-surgical ICU. Chest 2007;132(3):823–828

[4] Reeb J, Falcoz PE, Olland A, Massard G. Are daily routine chest radiographs necessary after pulmonary surgery in adult patients? Interact Cardiovasc Thorac Surg 2013;17(6):995–998

[5] Suh RD, Genshaft SJ, Kirsch J, et al. ACR appropriateness criteria – intensive care unit patients (26.02.2015). Available at: https://acsearch.acr.org/docs/69452/Narrative/

[6] Eisenhuber E, Schaefer-Prokop CM, Prosch H, Schima W. Bedside chest radiography. Respir Care 2012;57(3):427–443

[7] Bekemeyer WB, Crapo RO, Calhoon S, Cannon CY, Clayton PD. Efficacy of chest radiography in a respiratory intensive care unit. A prospective study. Chest 1985;88(5):691–696

[8] Henschke CI, Pasternack GS, Schroeder S, Hart KK, Herman PG. Bedside chest radiography: diagnostic efficacy. Radiology 1983;149(1):23–26

[9] Strain DS, Kinasewitz GT, Vereen LE, George RB. Value of routine daily chest x-rays in the medical intensive care unit. Crit Care Med 1985;13(7):534–536

[10] Sepehripour AH, Farid S, Shah R. Is routine chest radiography indicated following chest drain removal after cardiothoracic surgery? Interact Cardiovasc Thorac Surg 2012;14(6):834–838

[11] Lee S, Chaturvedi A. Imaging adults on extracorporeal membrane oxygenation (ECMO). Insights Imaging 2014;5(6):731–742

[12] Shevland JE, Hirleman MT, Hoang KA, Kealey GP. Lobar collapse in the surgical intensive care unit. Br J Radiol 1983;56(668):531–534

[13] Ely EW, Haponik EF. Using the chest radiograph to determine intravascular volume status: the role of vascular pedicle width. Chest 2002;121(3):942–950

[14] Milne EN, Pistolesi M, Miniati M, Giuntini C. The radiologic distinction of cardiogenic and noncardiogenic edema. AJR Am J Roentgenol 1985;144(5):879–894

[15] The ARDS Definition Task Force. Acute respiratory distress syndrome. JAMA 2012:307

Chapter 17

Treatment-Related Changes

17 Treatment-Related Changes

17.1 The Postoperative Thorax

17.1.1 Partial Lung Resection

Surgical Techniques

Partial lung resection is performed for therapeutic and, less commonly, also for diagnostic purposes:

- *Diagnostic resection*: This is mostly done for histologic analysis of suspicious pulmonary nodules or for diagnosis of diffuse parenchymal lung diseases. In general, less lung tissue is removed for diagnostic purposes compared with therapeutic interventions. The technique used is usually wedge resection where a wedge-shaped piece of lung tissue measuring a few centimeters is removed with a stapler. Such methods which are not based on anatomic structures are known as *atypical resections* (▶Table 17.1).
- *Therapeutic resection*: This is usually done for surgical treatment of lung tumors and, less commonly, also for elimination of chronic inflammatory processes. It normally involves anatomic resection except in the case of metastasis surgery (see following sections): an anatomically defined part of the lung is removed, often a lung lobe (lobectomy), in contrast to the atypical resection described above. In the right lung, treatment sometimes requires the removal of two lobes: either the upper and middle lobes (upper bilobectomy) or the middle and lower lobes (lower bilobectomy). Removal of the right upper and lower lobes as bilobectomy is not technically feasible. Pneumonectomy is needed instead.

The maximum extension of the resection is determined by the size and location of the pathologic process and is limited by the expected postoperative lung function. Occasionally, the standard oncologic procedure, i.e., at least lobectomy, is not a feasible option for patients with a limited preoperative lung function. Therefore, in such cases, surgery may be confined to removal of individual lung segments (segmental resection).

Lung metastases are usually removed by means of atypical resection. Unlike in lung carcinoma, anatomic resection is generally not needed, thus ensuring that as much lung parenchyma as possible is preserved. The standard surgical procedures are wedge resection and laser resection. In the latter, a laser is used to extract the metastatic lesion including a safety margin in a virtually circular manner from the surrounding lung tissue, and the pleura is sutured to close the surgical defect.

Table 17.1 Surgical techniques in lung resection

Anatomic resection	Atypical resection
• Segmental resection • Lobectomy • Bilobectomy (upper, lower) • Pneumonectomy	• Wedge resection • Laser resection

Radiologic Findings

Anatomic Resection

Note

Radiologic findings in anatomic resection:

- Hemithorax volume loss:
  - High-riding diaphragm.
  - Mediastinal shift to the operated side.
- Lobar fissures not identifiable.
- Pleural thickening.
- Pleural cavity (generally only in the immediate postoperative phase).
- Pulmonary consolidations (in particular in segmental resection).
- Middle lobe atelectasis (in right upper lobe resection).
- Hilar enlargement (in the immediate postoperative phase).

The most salient finding on chest radiography in anatomic resection is the *volume loss* of the operated lung: the diaphragm on the operated side is somewhat higher than normal and the mediastinum has shifted slightly to the operated side (▶Fig. 17.1). There is often remarkably little noticeable volume loss in lobectomies and segmental resections because the remaining lung parenchyma completely fills the space in the chest cavity and contains comparatively more air than the contralateral side. Occasionally, apart from nonrecognition of one lobar fissure, there are virtually no signs of the previous lobectomy on chest radiography.

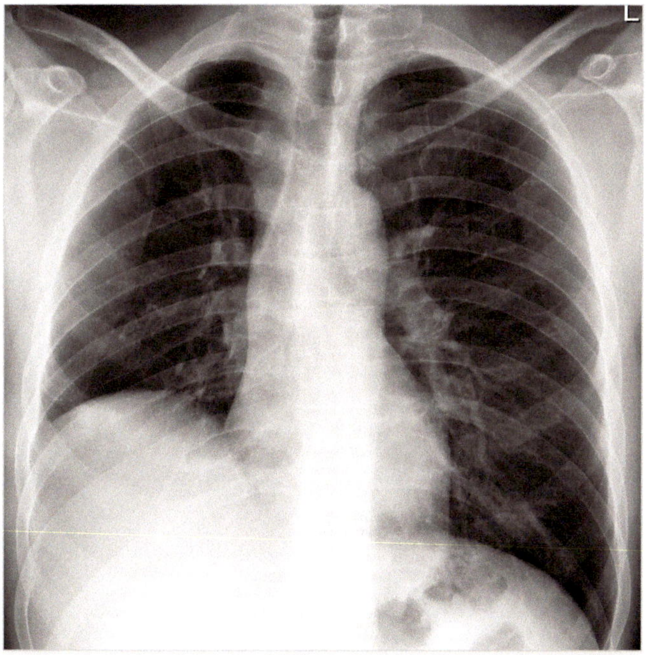

Fig. 17.1 Right lower lobe resection. Radiograph. Right high-riding diaphragm and slight mediastinal shift to the right.

II

If the remaining lung parenchyma is unable to completely fill the chest cavity, an air-containing pleural cavity is seen postoperatively. This is usually replaced within a few days by a pleural effusion that over time is converted to connective tissue, thus giving rise to a permanent pleural thickening (▶ Fig. 17.2). Rarely, the air-containing cavity persists for months or even years.

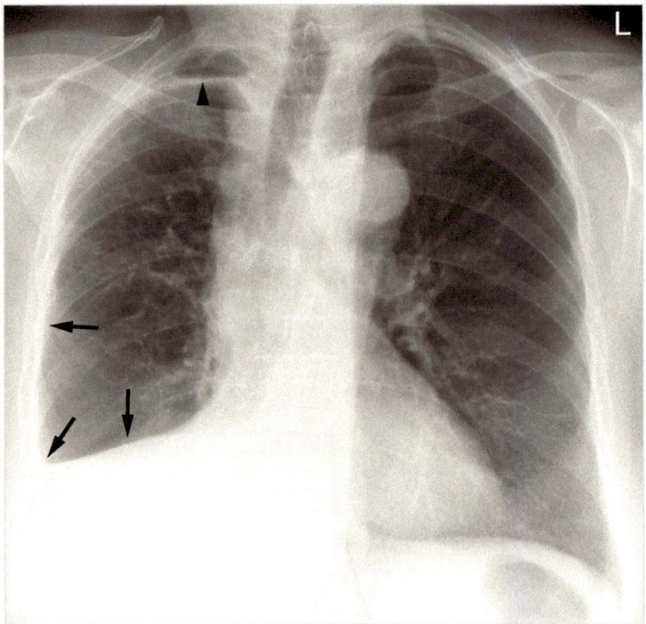

Fig. 17.2 Pleural thickening (*arrows*) after right lower lobe resection. Furthermore, persistent small, right-apical pneumothorax (*arrowhead*). Radiograph.

Whereas lobectomies and bilobectomies usually leave no radiologically discernible scars in the lung parenchyma, segmental resections are often associated with radiologic findings. Only entire lung lobes, but not segments, are separated by the visceral pleura. During lobectomy, the entire lobe can be detached virtually atraumatically from the surrounding lung parenchyma along this boundary. In contrast, segmental resection requires surgical dissection in the lung parenchyma causing identifiable consolidations in the operated lobe at the site of the resected segment (▶ Fig. 17.3).

Surgical treatment of lung carcinoma routinely includes systematic hilar and mediastinal lymphadenectomy. Occasionally, hilar enlargement is seen on the operated side in the immediate postoperative course (▶ Fig. 17.4); this resolves within a few days.

At times, a small triangular opacity based at the apex of the diaphragm can be observed following upper lobe resection. This “juxtaphrenic peak” is caused by cranial displacement of an accessory fissure or of septa associated with the pulmonary ligament.

On postoperative CT, surgical changes to the bronchial system can be identified additionally. Broncho- and angioplastic surgical techniques are needed to treat centrally located tumors or large hilar lymph node metastases. Conversancy with these techniques is useful for correct interpretation of the imaging findings. Parts of the central bronchi or vessels are resected in these procedures (known as *sleeve resections*) and a distal part of the bronchus or artery is anastomosed with the mainstem bronchus or artery, respectively For example, in right upper lobe bronchial sleeve resection, the distal mainstem bronchus, including the origin of the upper lobe bronchus as well as the proximal intermediate bronchus, is resected, and then the distal intermediate bronchus is connected to the proximal mainstem bronchus (▶ Fig. 17.5).

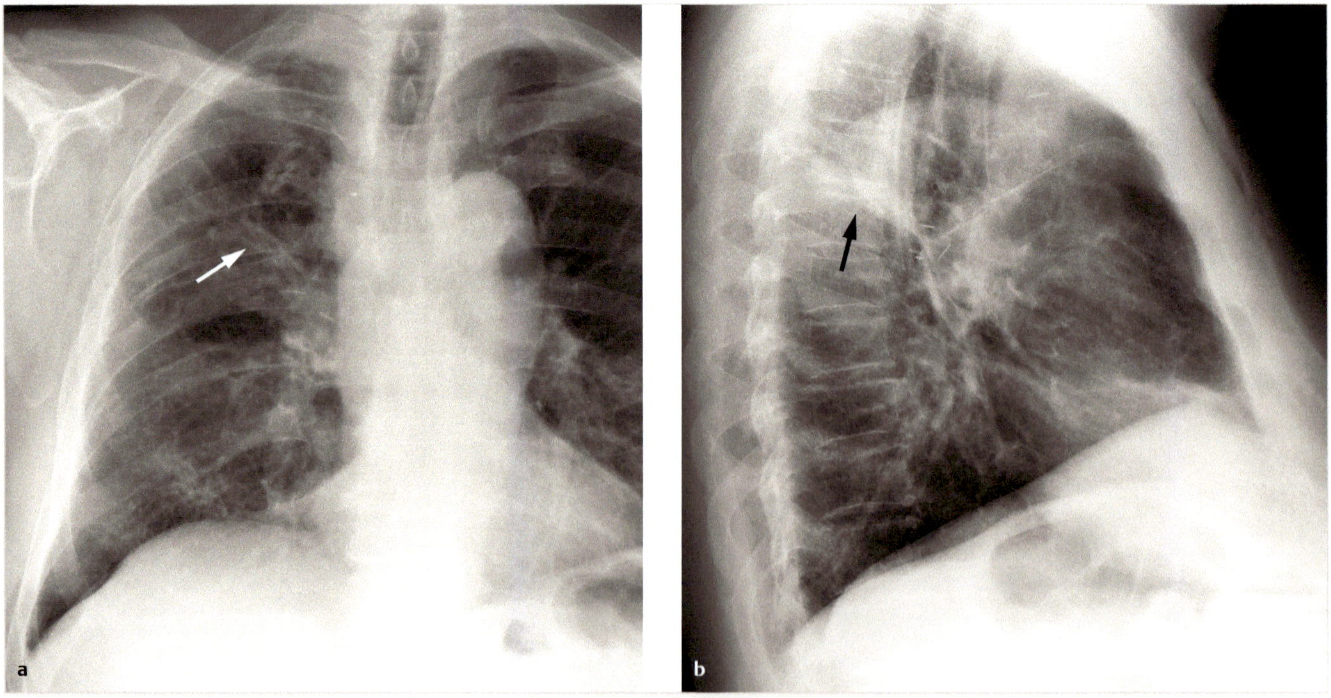

Fig. 17.3 Pulmonary consolidation following resection of the posterior right upper lobe segment (*arrows*). Radiographs. **(a)** Posteroanterior image. **(b)** Lateral image.

Atypical Resection

Note

Radiologic findings in atypical resection:

- In *wedge resection:* Linear consolidations originating from the pleura.
- In *laser resection*:
  - Rounded consolidations.
  - Juxtapleural cavities.

Wedge resections leave virtually linear consolidations in the lung parenchyma, which originate from the pleural lung surface and are usually a few centimeters long (▶Fig. 17.6). The metal clips applied with the stapler may be visible.

Laser resections leave rounded defects in the lung parenchyma. Since the visceral pleura is closed again with a suture over the resection defect, this often leads to development of pleural-based rounded, cyst-like structures. Their relatively thin wall is caused by the laser-induced coagulation necrosis of the lung parenchyma (▶Fig. 17.7). On chest radiography, such surgical defects manifest as cavities (▶Fig. 17.8), resembling lung abscesses. These normal postoperative findings after laser resection must not be misinterpreted as an infectious complication.

Wedge and laser resections are frequently combined in metastasis surgery. Hence, the sequelae of both procedures may manifest simultaneously.

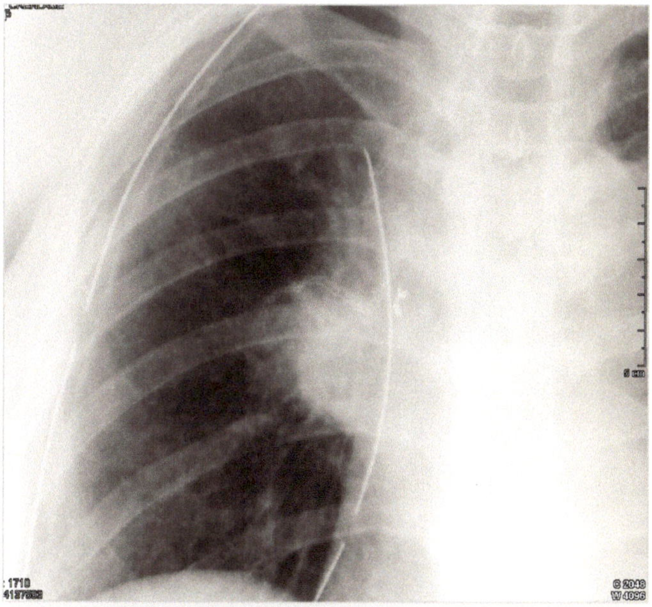

Fig. 17.4 Postoperative hilar enlargement following right upper lobe resection. Magnified section of a radiograph. Postoperative right-sided chest tubes as well as right perihilar clip chain.

Complications

General complications common for all surgical techniques are described in Chapter 17.1.8. The following are specific to partial lung resections:

Right upper lobe resections present a risk of postoperative hypoaeration of the middle lobe which now occupies the position of the resected upper lobe in the chest cavity. This causes upward displacement of the middle lobe bronchus, which normally arises in an anteroinferior direction from the intermediate

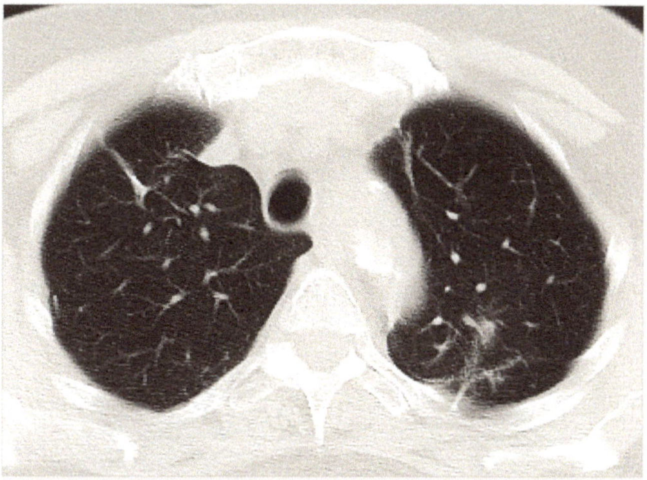

Fig. 17.6 Bilateral wedge resections. CT image. Linear, pleural-based consolidations in both upper lobes.

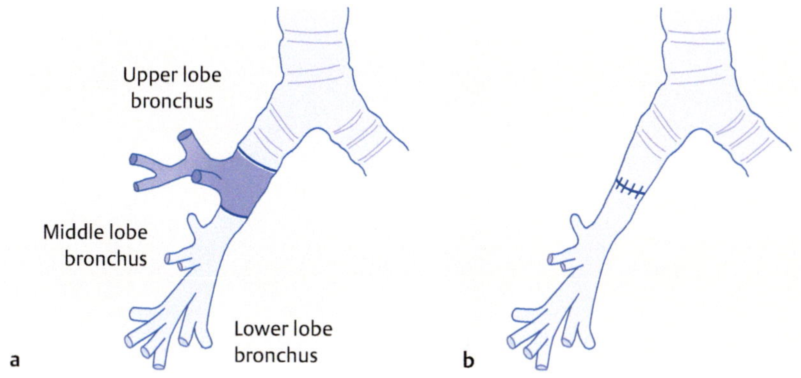

Fig. 17.5 Principle underlying bronchial sleeve resection. Schematic diagram.

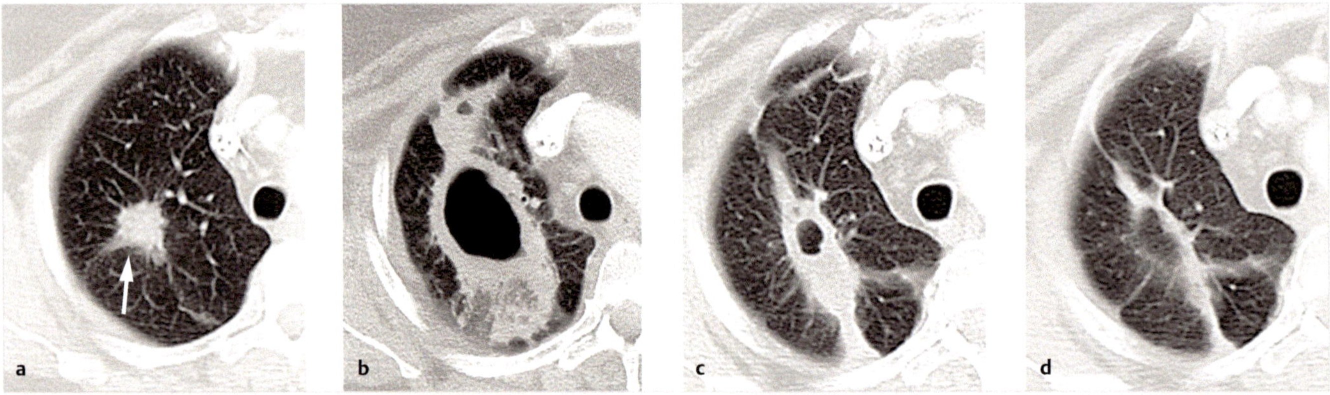

Fig. 17.7 Laser resection in right upper lobe. CT images. **(a)** Preoperative finding: metastasis in the right upper lobe (*arrow*). **(b)** Postoperative day 10: thick-walled cavity. **(c)** Third postoperative month. **(d)** Ninth postoperative month.

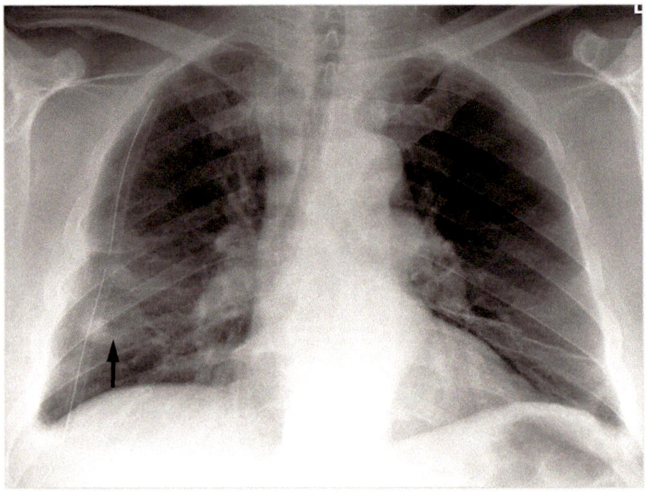

Fig. 17.8 Laser resection in right lower lobe. Radiograph. Cavity in the right lower zone (*arrow*). Postoperative right-sided chest tube.

bronchus, and can now become kinked at the site of origin. The resultant bronchial stenosis causes early postoperative *middle lobe atelectasis* (▸Fig. 17.9). If this condition persists, *middle lobe syndrome* characterized by chronic recurrent middle lobe infections can develop; in the worst case, eventual middle lobe resection is required.

17.1.2 Pneumonectomy

At times, resection of an entire lung, known as pneumonectomy, may be necessary to treat central lung carcinomas. The chest cavity is empty apart from air immediately postoperative and completely fills with fluid over the course of several weeks. Later the fluid becomes organized and transforms to connective tissue, the so-called fibroserothorax.[1] Imaging demonstrates increased radiolucency of the pneumonectomy cavity in the immediate postoperative course. The air–fluid level seen on upright chest radiography continues to rise upward over time until the entire hemithorax exhibits opacities of soft-tissue density (▸Fig. 17.10).

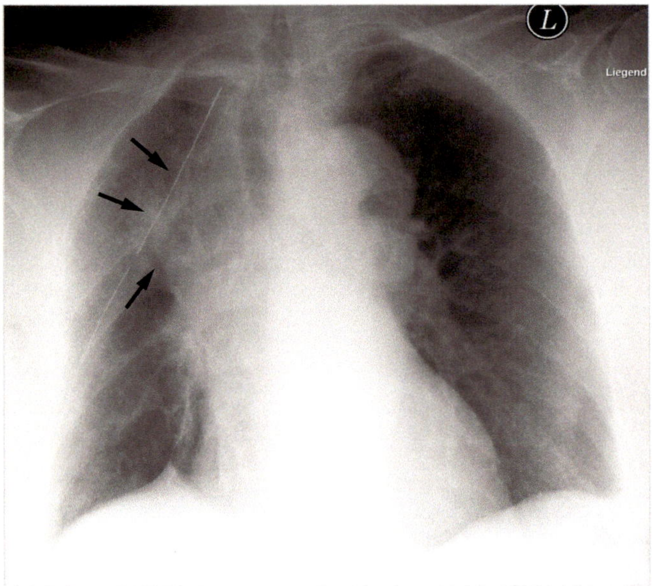

Fig. 17.9 Middle lobe atelectasis following right upper lobe resection (*arrows***).** CT image. Postoperative right-sided chest tube.

Occasionally, a smoothly marginated, paramediastinal opacity is seen in early chest radiographs lateral to the bronchial stump (▸Fig. 17.11).[2] This is consistent with a muscle or pericardial flap attached intraoperatively to the mainstem bronchus stump to prevent bronchial stump fistula.

In addition to general complications, pneumonectomy is associated with a number of specific complications now described below.[1]

Pneumonectomy causes sudden-onset hyperperfusion of the remaining lung, pulmonary arterial pressure increase, and right heart overload. Postoperative pulmonary edema is seen in up to 5% of cases. In milder cases, this demonstrates the radiographic findings of hydrostatic pulmonary edema, while in severe cases it resembles adult respiratory distress syndrome. The underlying mechanism of this deeply feared and usually fatal complication is not fully understood. It is thought to be linked to elevated hydrostatic intravascular pressure and increased capillary permeability.[1]

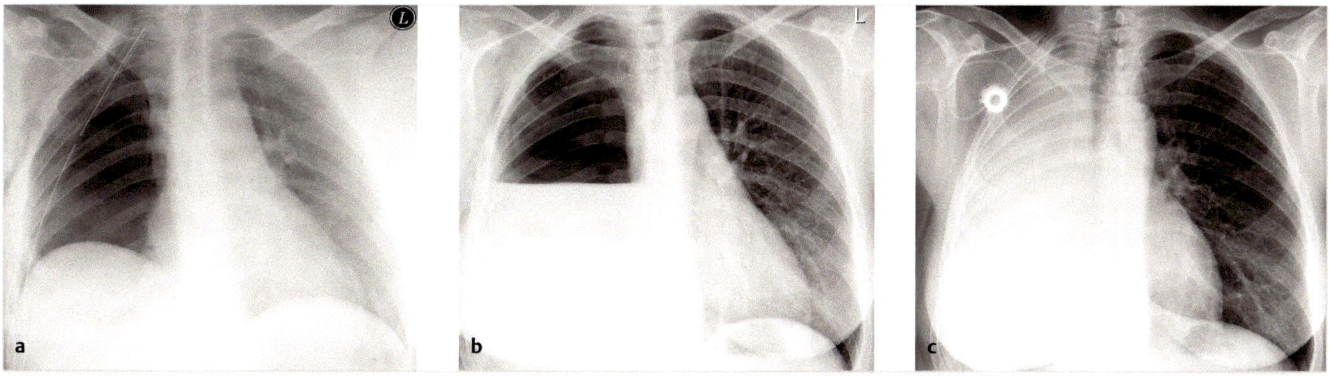

Fig. 17.10 Status post right pneumonectomy. Radiographs. **(a)** Supine image on postoperative day 1. **(b)** Upright image on postoperative day 3. **(c)** After 9 months.

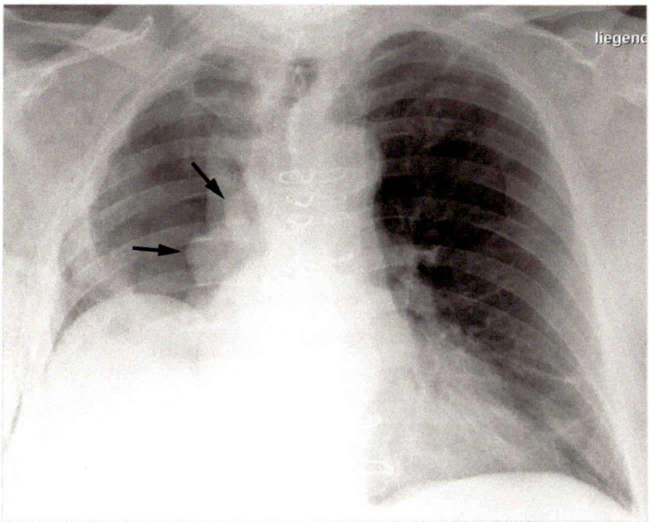

Fig. 17.11 Status post right pneumonectomy. Radiograph. Muscle flap introduced into chest cavity for coverage of the bronchial stump (*arrows*).

The sudden drop in fluid levels in the pneumonectomy cavity is suggestive of *bronchial stump leakage*, which is associated with a considerable mortality rate. Likewise, new onset of postoperative mediastinal or chest wall emphysema points to bronchial stump fistula (▶Fig. 17.12).

Postpneumonectomy syndrome typically occurs in younger patients during the first postoperative year, predominantly after right-sided pneumonectomy. Clinical symptoms include increasing exertional dyspnea, inspiratory stridor, and recurrent lung infections. The hyperexpanded lung leads to mediastinal displacement to the operated side, in turn causing ipsilateral tracheal displacement and hyperextension of the mainstem bronchus of the remaining lung (▶Fig. 17.13).

17.1.3 Surgery for Pleural Diseases

Surgery for pleural diseases is usually indicated in settings of pleural empyema, malignant tumors, or less commonly because of persistent pneumothorax.

Pleurodesis

Pleurodesis, where the pleural layers are stuck together, may be performed to treat a symptomatic malignant pleural effusion. To that effect, a chemical substance, e.g., talc, is introduced into the pleural space. The ensuing inflammatory reaction causes the parietal pleura and visceral pleura to stick together and thus prevent the development of a new large pleural effusion.

> **Note**
>
> Radiologic findings in pleurodesis:
>
> - Smooth or nodular pleural thickening.
> - Pleural talc deposits of calcific density (in talc pleurodesis).
> - Temporary pleurodesis reaction:
>   - Pulmonary consolidations.
>   - Ground-glass opacities.
>   - Coarse parenchymal bands.

On postoperative chest radiography, there is normally marked regression of pleural effusion compared with that seen prior to pleurodesis. It is crucial to ensure the absence of pleural air collections since these cause separation of the pleural layers, preventing the desired adhesion of the parietal and visceral pleura.

Around postoperative day 3 to 5, onset of a concomitant reaction of the lung parenchyma lasting around 2 weeks is sometimes seen on imaging (▶Fig. 17.14).[3] On chest radiography, progressive pulmonary opacities occur.[4] CT demonstrates coarse linear opacities and intralobular lines, ground-glass opacities, and smaller consolidations in the peripheral lung parenchyma (▶Fig. 17.15). Most of these findings will have resolved within a few weeks.

Imaging shows persistent smooth or nodular pleural thickening. On PET-CT, these areas of pleural thickening can exhibit considerable FDG uptake, hampering differential diagnosis versus pleural tumor manifestations.[5] The talc used in talc pleurodesis is often visualized on CT as deposits of calcific density in the pleural space, thus mimicking calcified pleural plaques.[6]

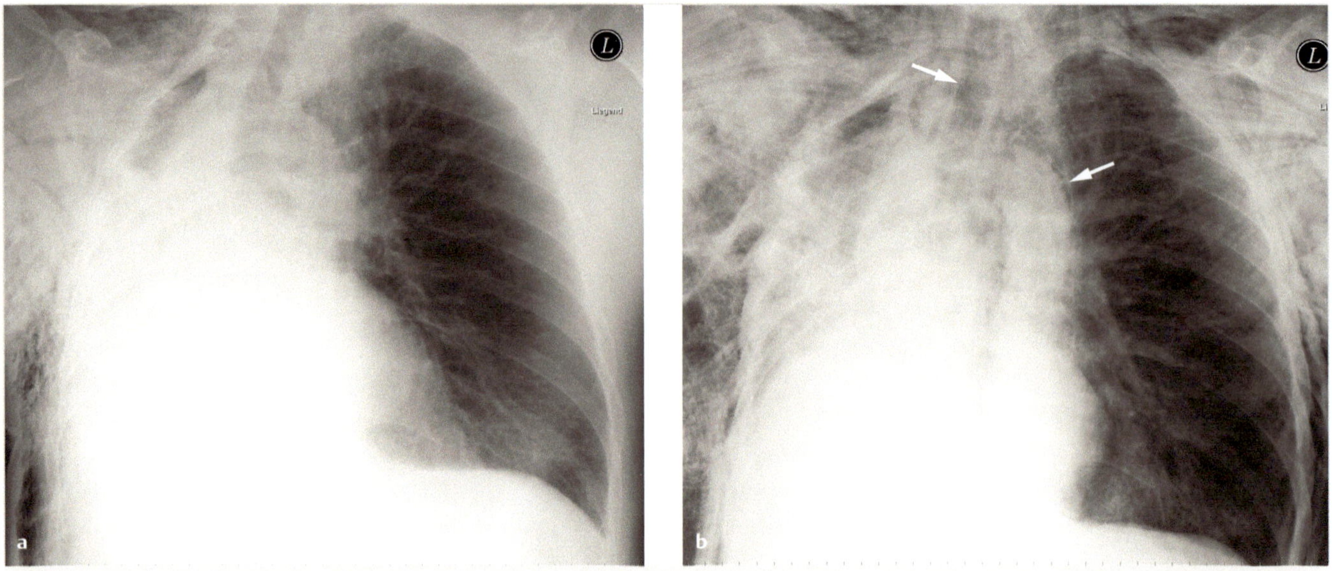

Fig. 17.12 Bronchial stump leak following right pneumonectomy. Radiographs. **(a)** Supine image on postoperative day 3: mild chest wall emphysema, otherwise normal findings following right pneumonectomy. **(b)** Supine image on postoperative day 4: massive progressive chest wall emphysema and new-onset mediastinal emphysema (*arrows*).

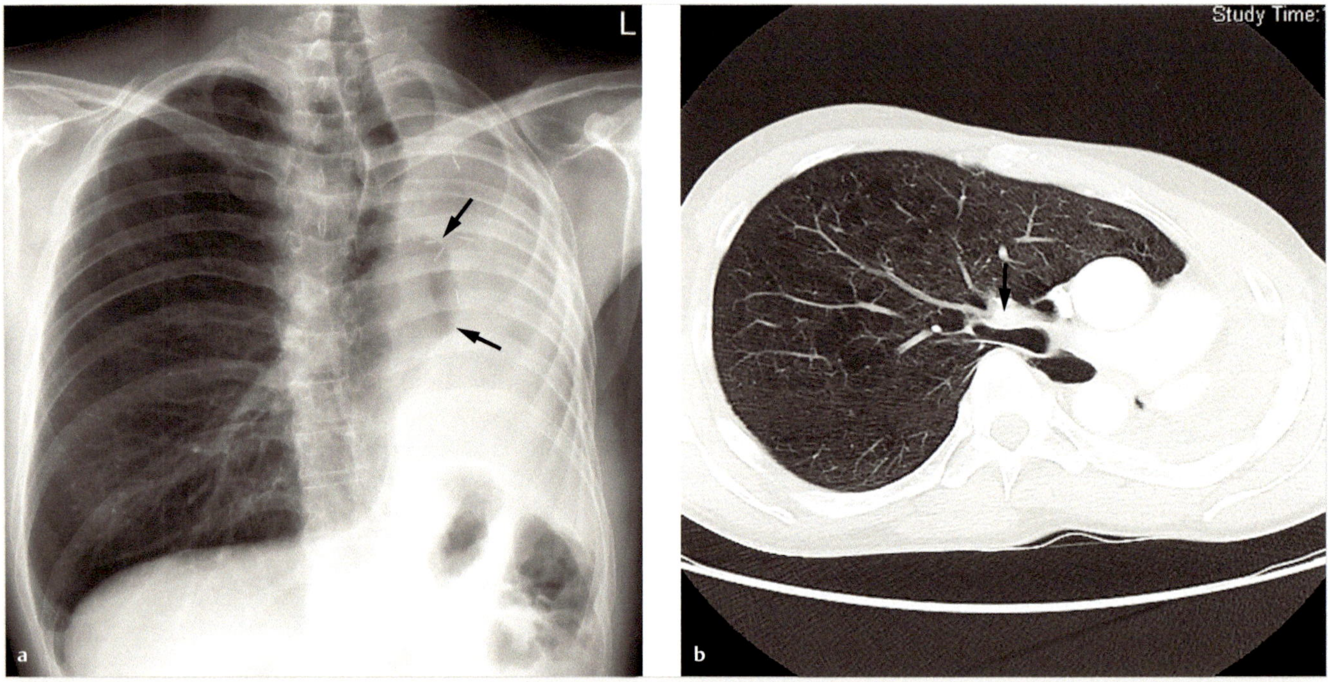

Fig. 17.13 Postpneumonectomy syndrome following left pneumonectomy. **(a)** Radiograph. Tracheal displacement to the left and anterior herniation of the right lung into the left hemithorax (*arrows*). **(b)** CT image. Hyperextension of the right mainstem bronchus located anterior to the spine (*arrow*).

Pleurectomy and Decortication

Pleurectomy, i.e., removal of the parietal pleura, is usually used for surgical treatment of pneumothorax. Lung decortication involves partial or complete removal of the visceral pleura from the lung, e.g., in pleural empyema or pleural mesothelioma. The main purpose of decortication is to remove the thickened pleura as this hampers expansion and aeration of the underlying lung.

On chest radiography and CT, it is not possible in settings of pleural enlargement to reliably distinguish between surgical sequelae, tumor, and inflammation. At times, considerable

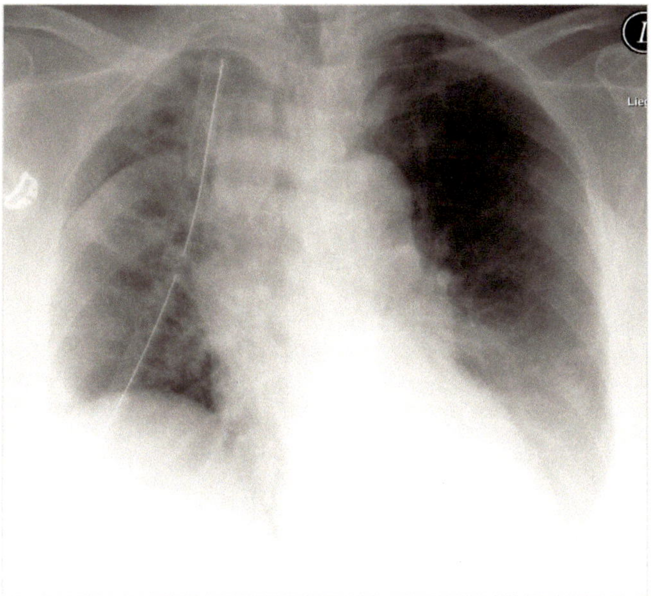

Fig. 17.14 **Pleurodesis reaction 3 days after right talc pleurodesis.** Radiograph. Diffuse consolidations and ground-glass opacities of the right lung. Postoperative right-sided chest tube.

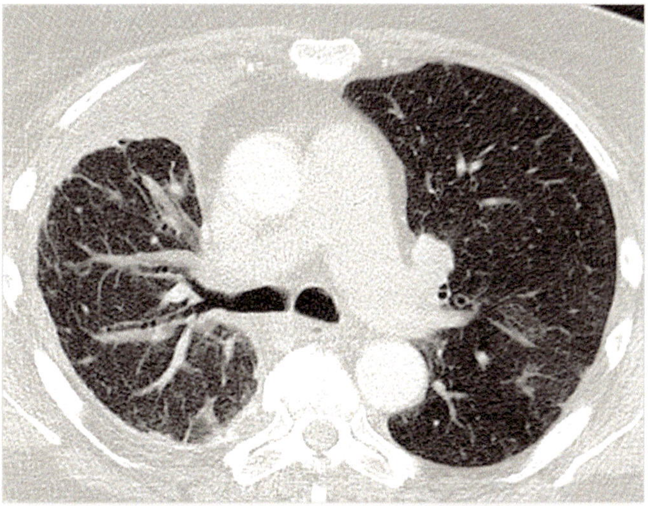

Fig. 17.15 **Pleurodesis reaction 2 weeks after right talc pleurodesis.** CT image. Diffuse pleural thickening, subpleural consolidations, mild ground-glass opacities, and coarse intralobular lines.

atelectasis of the subpleural lung tissue is seen in the immediate postoperative phase, especially after decortication. These areas of atelectasis are surgical manifestations that usually resolve within a few days.

17.1.4 Surgery for Pneumothorax

Surgical treatment of recurrent pneumothorax entails atypical resection of bullous changes in the lung parenchyma. In addition, partial pleurectomy can be performed to achieve adhesion of the pleural layers and thus prevent recurrence of pneumothorax.

The sequelae of atypical partial lung resection can be identified on imaging. This procedure is generally performed as wedge resection. Bullae are usually found at the apices of the upper and lower lobes.

The chief determinant of a successful treatment outcome is the immediate postoperative contact between the parietal and visceral pleura. Even the most minute pleural air inclusion is clinically relevant and must be meticulously sought on postoperative chest radiography. The information presented on partial lung resection and surgery for pleural diseases also applies for chest radiography after surgery for pneumothorax.

17.1.5 Lung Transplantation

Lung transplantation has become established as a treatment option for end-stage diffuse parenchymal lung diseases, chronic obstructive pulmonary disease, and pulmonary hypertension. Both single- and double-lung transplants are carried out, also in combination with heart transplantation. Imaging has an important role in follow-up of lung transplant patients for early detection of complications. These and the associated imaging findings are presented in ▶Table 17.2.

> **Note**
>
> The most dangerous complication in the first posttransplantation year is bacterial infection; later the patient's life is at risk because of chronic rejection.[7]

Opportunistic infections following organ transplantation are discussed in Section 5.3. Of particular relevance for lung transplant patients is cytomegalovirus infection. This can still manifest even months or years later, whereas the greatest risk by fungal infections is seen in the first posttransplantation weeks.

Special complications occur at different time points[8]:

- *Immediate complications* (within the first 24 h): Donor–recipient size mismatch becomes evident during or immediately after transplant surgery. Malposition of the peri- or intraoperatively inserted catheters and tubes or complications related to their placement (e.g., tube malposition as well as pneumo- or hemothorax after insertion of a central venous line) also become clinically or radiologically manifest within the first postoperative hours. Preformed antibodies to donor-specific antigens (e.g., HLA or AB0 antigens) are thought to be responsible for fulminant hyperacute rejection manifesting immediately after transplantation and leading to death.[9]
- *Early complications* (1 day to 1 week): If the donor lung was already damaged by ischemia before transplantation, reperfusion edema may occur when the donor lung is connected

Table 17.2 Radiologic features in postoperative complications of lung transplantation[8]

Complications	Radiologic features
Organ size mismatch	• Atelectasis • Hyperinflation
Reperfusion edema	• Perihilar ground-glass opacities • Bronchial wall thickening
Acute pleural complications	• Pneumothorax • Pleural effusion • Hemothorax
Dehiscence of bronchial anastomosis	• Pneumothorax • Pneumomediastinum • Chest wall emphysema
Stenosis of bronchial anastomosis	• Bronchial stenosis • Air trapping
Rejection:	
• Hyperacute	• Massive consolidations in the transplanted lung
• Acute	• Ground-glass opacities • Interlobular septal thickening • Intralobular lines
• Chronic	• Bronchiestasis • Air trapping • Mosaic attenuation pattern • Bronchial wall thickening • Centrilobular nodules • Tree-in-bud pattern
Infection:	
• *Candida* pneumonia	• Miliary pattern • Nodules • Ground-glass opacities • Consolidations
• Invasive pulmonary aspergillosis	• Angiotopic nodules • Triangular consolidations • Halo sign • Air crescent sign
• Cytomegalovirus pneumonia	• Small nodules • Ground-glass opacities • Consolidations
• Mycobacteriosis	• Miliary pattern • Ground-glass opacities • Tree-in-bud pattern • Consolidations • Pleural effusion • Lymphadenopathy
Cryptogenic organizing pneumonia Lymphoproliferative diseases	• Bilateral consolidations • Multiple nodules, consolidations • Lymphadenopathy • Pleural effusion • Interlobular septal thickening

to the recipient's vascular system. This can manifest anytime from the first hours to postoperative day 4; reperfusion edema usually resolves within 2 months but also can also persist for 6 months. On imaging, it manifests as hydrostatic pulmonary edema. Postoperative pleural effusions usually resolve within 2 weeks. Persistent pneumothorax or mediastinal or chest wall emphysema may be indicative of bronchial anastomotic leak (dehiscence).

- *Intermediate complications* (1 week to 2 months): Acute rejection generally occurs during postoperative week 2. Chest radiography demonstrates perihilar and basal opacities, interlobular septal thickening and pleural effusions.[10]

Although the CT features are nonspecific, they are suggestive of acute rejection in this clinical context. The most salient features are irregular ground-glass opacities (▶Fig. 17.16), less commonly bronchial wall thickening and interlobular septal thickening.[11] Rapid improvement of the clinical and radiologic findings in response to corticosteroid therapy is characteristic of acute rejection. The most common bronchial anastomotic complications are anastomotic leak, occurring in the first postoperative month, and anastomotic stenosis which presents in the later course (▶Fig. 17.17). The latter often develops from the former. Bacterial pneumonia, in particular with gram-negative bacteria (*Pseudomonas*, *Klebsiella*), is the most frequent infection in the first postoperative month. *Candida* pneumonia also occurs during this period.

- *Late complications* (more than 2 months posttransplantation): In addition to bronchial anastomotic stenosis, bronchomalacia also occasionally occurs in the first 4 months. This manifests as bronchial wall instability and bronchial collapse. The change in the bronchial diameter can be visualized on inspiratory and expiratory CT scans or on dynamic CT of the ventilation cycle. At least one of every two lung transplant patients is prone to cytomegalovirus infections.[12] Fungal infections are also common, in particular invasive pulmonary aspergillosis. On rare occasions, tuberculosis or atypical mycobacteriosisis seen at a later stage. Around one-quarter of all patients develop pulmonary embolisms, frequently in the transplanted lung.[8] Chronic rejection of the transplant occurs after around 6 months, manifesting as bronchiolitis obliterans syndrome. Clinical symptoms may include progressive worsening of lung function, affecting around half of all transplant recipients within 5 years and thus constituting the most important long-term complication of lung transplantation. Chronic rejection is more likely to occur in settings of previous episodes of acute rejection, active cytomegalovirus infection, and HLA incompatibility between the organ donor and recipient.[13] The most characteristic findings on CT are bronchiectasis, bronchial wall thickening, mosaic attenuation pattern, and air trapping (▶Fig. 17.18). The best predictor of chronic rejection is detection of extensive air trapping on expiratory images or on dynamic CT of the ventilation cycle.[8] Furthermore, certain diffuse parenchymal lung diseases occur in the transplanted lung, in particular, cryptogenic organizing pneumonia. Lymphoproliferative diseases usually present in the first posttransplantation year, at times even already during the first month. These are predominantly B cell disorders; Epstein–Barr virus is detected in 90% of such patients. Multiple nodules or consolidations are typically seen on chest radiography and CT, some with halo sign, less commonly also interlobular septal thickening, pleural effusions, or mediastinal lymphadenopathy.[8]

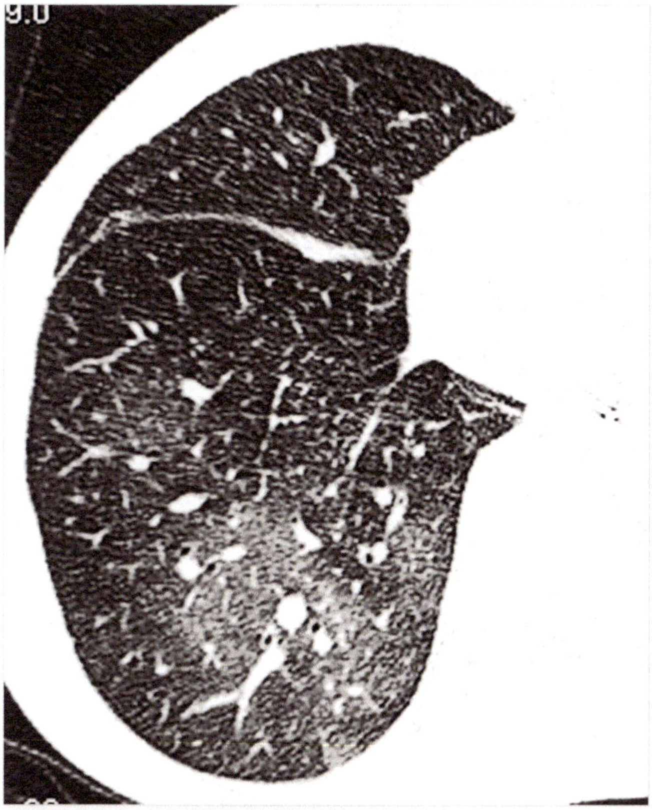

Fig. 17.16 **Acute rejection following right-sided, single-lung transplantation.** CT image. Irregular ground-glass opacities in the lower lobe of transplanted lung.

Several diseases that required lung transplantation can recur in the transplanted lung[8,14]:

- Sarcoidosis.
- Lymphangioleiomyomatosis.
- Pulmonary Langerhans cell histiocytosis.

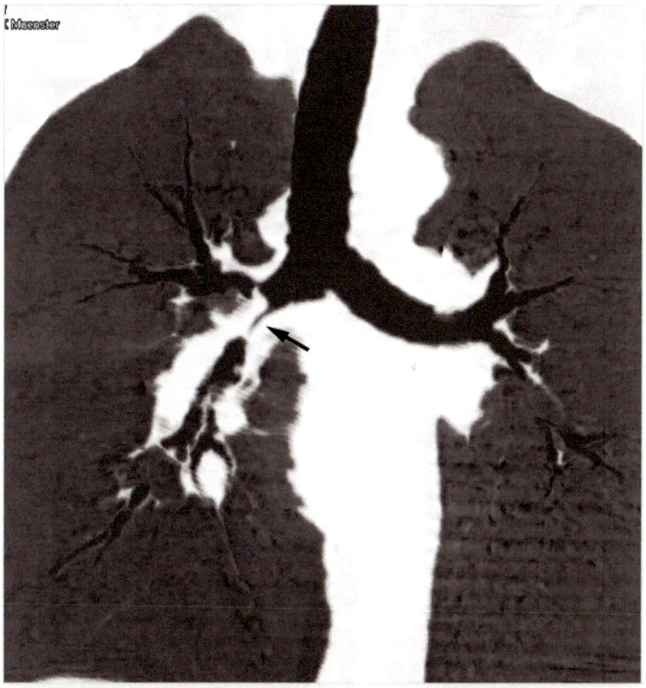

Fig. 17.17 Anastomotic stenosis (*arrow*) following right-sided, single-lung transplantation. CT, coronal MinIP.

- Talcosis.
- Diffuse panbronchiolitis.
- Pulmonary alveolar proteinosis

Sarcoidosis, in particular, recurs in one-third of lung transplant cases.[14]

Note

Continuous immunosuppressive drug therapy is needed after lung transplantation. Accordingly, the likelihood of drug-induced lung disease and opportunistic infections should be borne in mind for differential diagnosis of the imaging findings.

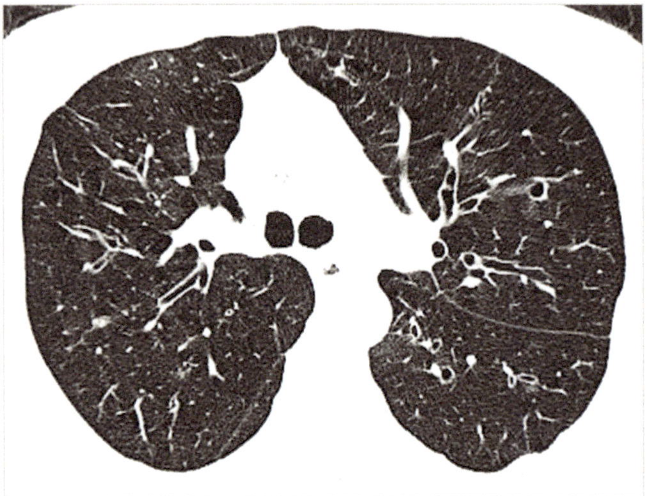

Fig. 17.18 Chronic rejection following double-lung transplantation. CT image. Cylindrical bronchiestasis, bronchial wall thickening, and mild mosaic attenuation pattern.

17.1.6 Heart Surgery

Generally, postoperative changes following heart surgery are less easily identified on chest radiography and CT compared with surgery for pulmonary or pleural diseases.

Metallic implants can be identified on chest radiography after many cardiosurgical procedures. Metal clips are seen in the anterior mediastinum especially after coronary artery bypass surgery. These are found along the course of the blood vessels used for the bypass, usually the internal thoracic artery or an interposed vein.

Artificial cardiac valves are used most frequently as a replacement for the aortic valve (▶Fig. 17.19) or mitral valve (▶Fig. 17.20). The position of a mechanical cardiac valve replacement device is easy to identify on chest radiography but a valve made of biological material is scarcely visible. Exceptions to that rule are minimally invasive biovalves inserted via a transfemoral access route or the apex of heart (transcatheter aortic valve implantation, TAVI): a metallic stent carrying the biovalve presses the existing aortic valve into the aortic wall, thus creating space for the valve replacement device (▶Fig. 17.21).

The operative access route most frequently used in heart surgery is *median sternotomy.* Its sequelae can be routinely seen on chest radiography. The sternum is stabilized with wire cerclage during closure of the surgical wound; this is done as straight wire rings or figure-8 formations (see ▶Fig. 17.20). Fractured sternal cerclages (▶Fig. 17.22) are indicative of postoperative sternal instability. Less commonly, other closure systems are used. By contrast, if sternotomy is needed for lung surgery absorbent sutures that are not visible on imaging are used for wound closure.

Heart transplantation is predominantly performed using an orthotopic procedure. Here, the diseased recipient heart is excised and the donor heart is implanted in its place. Heterotopic heart transplantation is uncommon. Here, the donor heart is placed in the right hemithorax alongside the recipient heart. This results in a considerably enlarged cardiac silhouette on

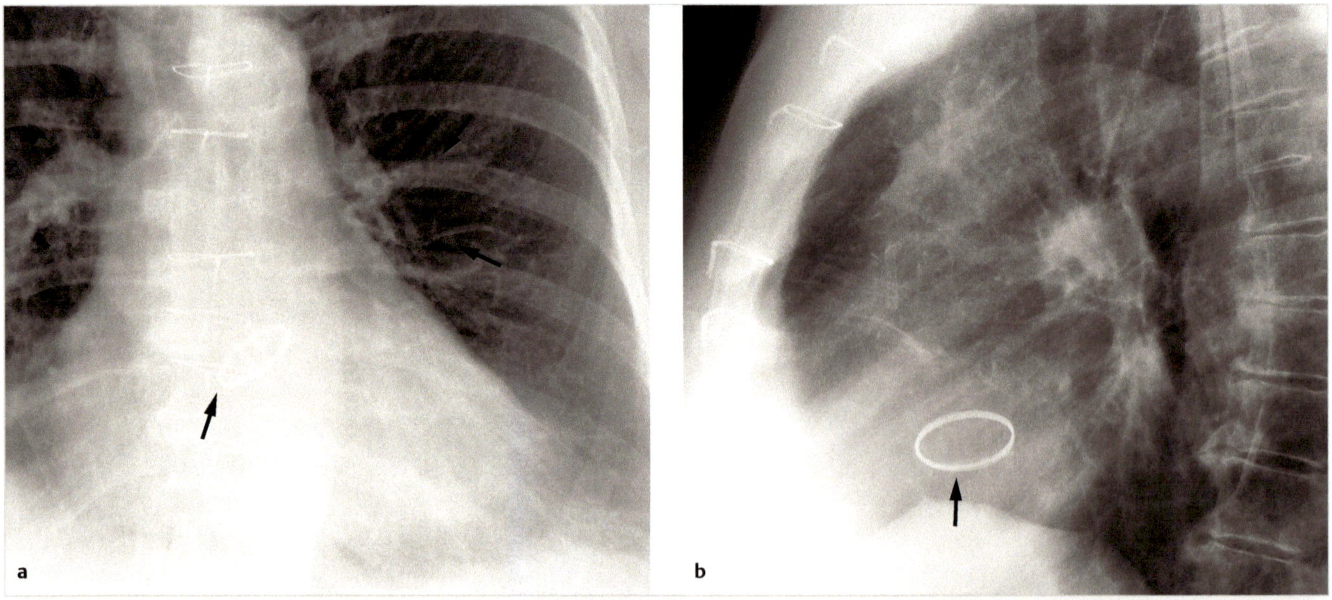

Fig. 17.19 Mechanical aortic valve replacement (*arrows*). Radiographs. **(a)** Magnified section of posteroanterior image. **(b)** Magnified section of lateral image.

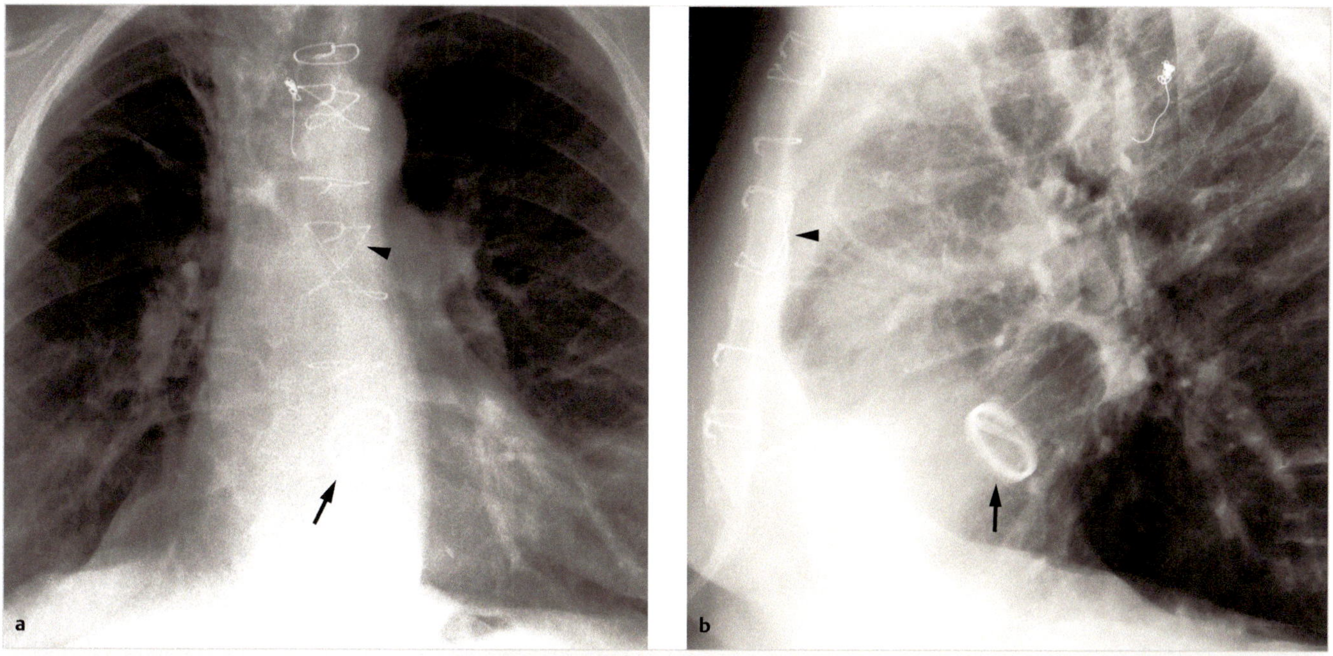

Fig. 17.20 Mechanical mitral valve replacement (*arrows*). Radiographs. Sternal cerclage following median sternotomy, partially using a figure-8 formation (*arrowhead*). Furthermore, coil in a bronchial artery. **(a)** Magnified section of posteroanterior image. **(b)** Magnified section of lateral image.

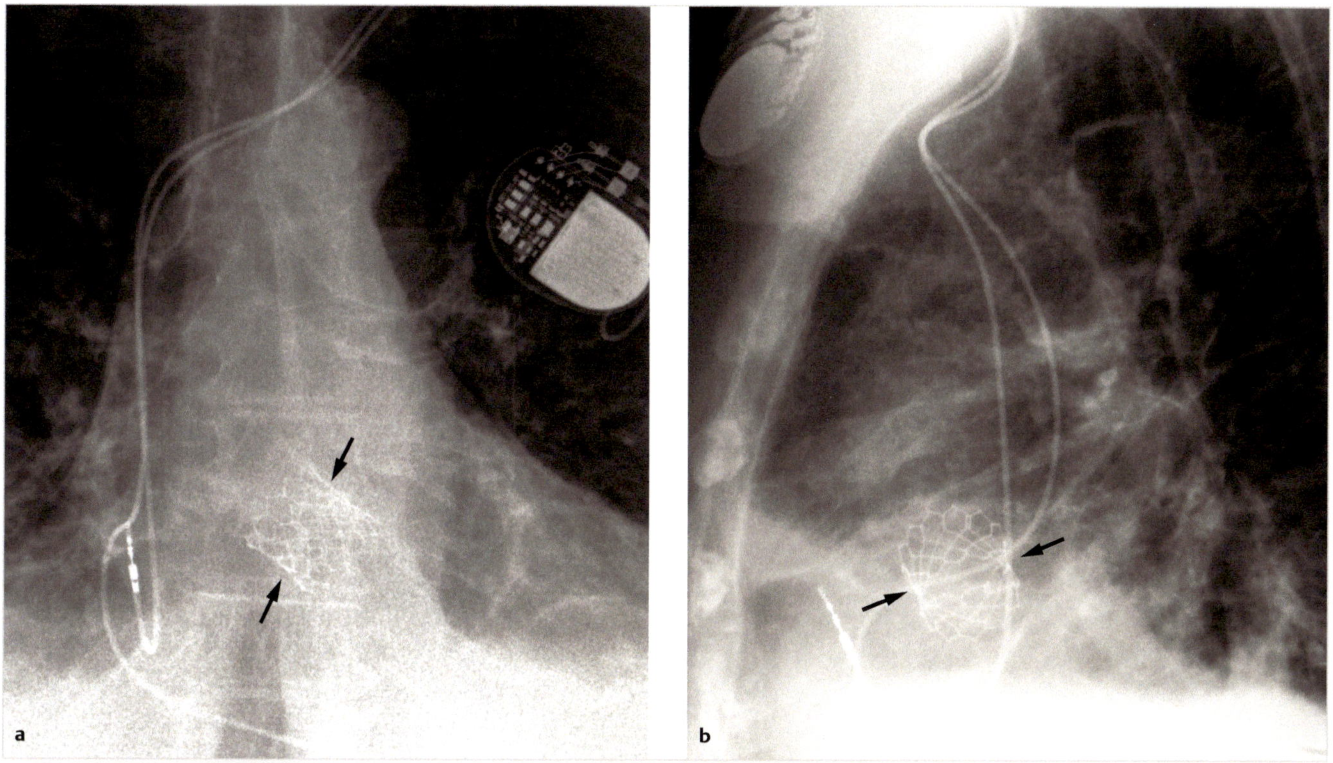

Fig. 17.21 Transfemoral aortic valve replacement. Radiographs. Valve replacement instead of aortic valve (*arrows*). Furthermore, implanted pacemaker. **(a)** Magnified section of posteroanterior image. **(b)** Magnified section of lateral image.

postoperative chest radiography and is also conducive to development of right-sided lower lobe atelectasis. The criteria normally used for evaluation of heart size measurements are no longer applicable after heart transplantation since the size of the donor heart may differ greatly in relation to the recipient chest size. The temporal course identifiable on postoperative images rather than comparison with pretransplantation images is the chief determinant for evaluation of heart size.

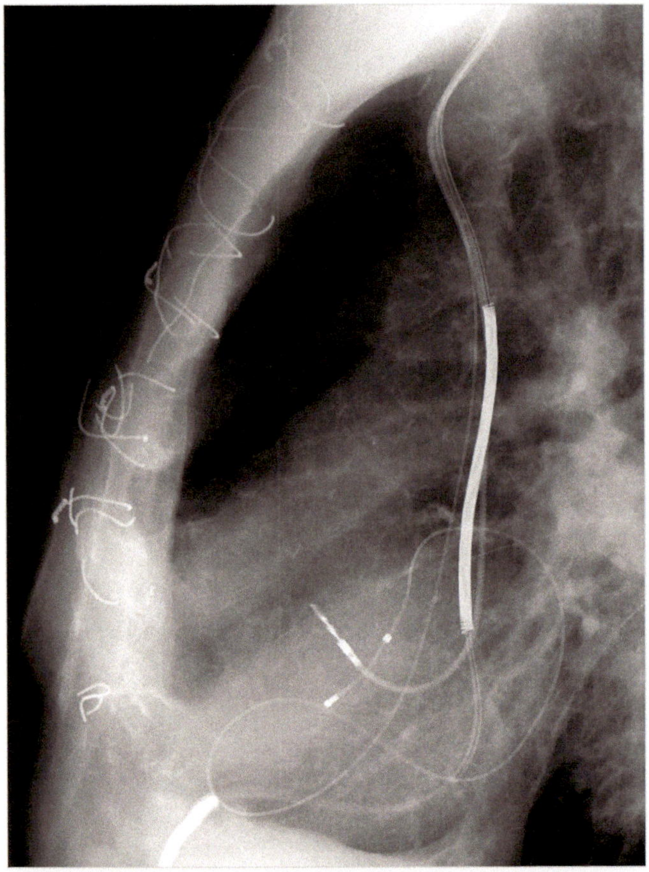

Fig. 17.22 Fractured sternal cerclages following cardiac artery bypass operation. Lateral radiograph. Furthermore, central lung cancer in the right lower lobe as well as implanted cardioverter defibrillator.

Infectious complications after heart transplantation are similar to those seen in lung transplant patients.

Chest radiographs obtained in the immediate postoperative period after heart surgery exhibit typical changes—regardless of the surgical procedure used (see also ▶Fig. 17.28).[15] These usually resolve within a few weeks.

> **Note**
>
> Typical postoperative findings after heart surgery[15]:
>
> - Enlarged cardiac silhouette.
> - Mediastinal widening.
> - Left lower lobe atelectasis (retrocardiac opacity).
> - Pleural effusion, especially on the left.
> - Pneumomediastinum.
> - Pneumothorax.
> - Pneumopericardium.
> - Chest wall emphysema.

The most salient general complications on chest radiography are hemothorax as well as hemopericardium. The latter manifests as cardiac enlargement with a "bocksbeutel" silhouette.

Dressler syndrome presents postoperatively after several weeks to months. General symptoms include fatigue and fever as well as pain in the chest and left shoulder. Imaging demonstrates pleural effusions and a pericardial effusion.[16,17]

17.1.7 Esophageal Surgery

A variety of several surgical techniques is used for treatment of esophageal cancer, less commonly also for benign esophageal motility disorders. A common principle underlying all procedures is curative resection of the esophagus and restoration of continuity of the gastrointestinal tract. To that effect, the remaining proximal esophagus or hypopharynx is anastomosed with a more distal segment of the gastrointestinal tract, usually with the stomach, at times also with a segment of the colon or the jejunum.[18] The following access routes are distinguished:

- *Transthoracic esophagectomy:* Esophageal cancer in the middle or distal third of the esophagus are resected using a right-sided thoracic and additional abdominal access route. The stomach is partially mobilized into the thorax and anastomosed with the proximal esophagus. The cranially mobilized stomach is usually positioned in the prevertebral space, less commonly in the retrosternal or right paravertebral space (▶Fig. 17.23). The anastomosis site is in the thorax.
- *Transhiatal esophagectomy:* This technique lends itself to resection of cancers of the distal third of the esophagus and does not involve opening of the chest cavity. Via an abdominal and cervical access route, the esophagus is mobilized in the entire mediastinum and then resected. Next the stomach is anastomosed with the cervical esophagus; hence the anastomosis site is in the cervical thorax.

Intraoperative *injury to the recurrent laryngeal nerve* impairs glottal closure and can cause postoperative aspiration pneumonia. *Injury to the trachea* or to the mainstem bronchi located in the mediastinum, usually to the posterior membranous part, gives rise at times to an esophagotracheal or esophagobronchial fistula.

Apart from these intraoperative and general complications, there are certain postoperative complications specific to esophagectomy[18]:

- *Anastomotic leak:* This generally manifests in the first postoperative week. Barium swallow is routinely obtained at the end of the first postoperative week to test for anastomotic tightness. Around half of anastomotic leaks are clinically inapparent and heal without any specific treatment. Fistulas leading to adjacent structures, especially to the tracheobronchial system and pleura as well as mediastinitis can occur as complications of an anastomotic leak.
- *Anastomotic stricture:* A pre-existing anastomotic leak is a predisposing factor for anastomotic stricture. The stricture can be well visualized on barium swallow. It is often formed during the healing process of the gastroesophageal anastomosis, especially in settings of previous anastomotic hypoperfusion or an anastomotic leak. Onset of an anastomotic stricture in the late postoperative period may be indicative of local tumor recurrence.
- *Chylothorax:* The thoracic duct must often be resected during esophagectomy; it can also be intraoperatively injured. On imaging chylothorax manifests as a persistent right-sided pleural effusion. By contrast, postoperative pleural effusions are more common in the contralateral hemithorax, i.e., on the left side.

- *Impaired intestinal passage:* Impaired passage through the anastomosis is suspected on detection of a fluid level in the esophagus on chest radiography. This is indicative of delayed emptying.
- *Herniation of abdominal organs into the thorax.*
- *Reflux esophagitis.*

17.1.8 General Complications of Thoracic Surgery

Secondary bleeding occurs within a few hours after surgery leading to *hemothorax*. The clinical presentation is suggestive: drainage of large amounts of bloody secretions via the chest tubes, hemodynamic instability, or a sudden drop in serum hemoglobin concentration. The clinical suspicion is confirmed on detection of extensive opacities of the operated hemithorax on chest radiography (▶Fig. 17.24).

Resection of the lung parenchyma requires one-lung ventilation with a double-lumen tube. The lung being operated on should be deflated during the surgical procedure. Hence, only the contralateral lung is ventilated intraoperatively. If there is pre-existing damage to the lung parenchyma (e.g., because of lung fibrosis or chronic obstructive pulmonary disease), one-lung ventilation can result in *barotrauma* of the contralateral lung. That presents a risk for development of unilateral adult respiratory distress syndrome (▶Fig. 17.25). This is a particularly feared complication of open lung biopsy, as performed for differential diagnosis of diffuse parenchymal lung diseases, since the fibrotic lung is especially sensitive to positive pressure ventilation.

Parenchymal air leakage or a bronchial stump leak can maintain a *bronchopleural fistula* following all types of lung resection, and manifests clinically as a persistent bubbling of air from a chest tube. Pneumothorax and persistent or even progressive chest wall emphysema are characteristic imaging findings; mediastinal emphysema may also be seen additionally but is less common (see ▶Fig. 17.12).

Postoperative infections affect the lung, pleural space, or chest wall. Most chest wall infections are clinically evident and only rarely is diagnostic imaging required. Postoperative pneumonia rarely presents before postoperative day 3 and usually involves bacterial infection.

Pleural empyema most often occurs secondary to pneumonectomy and is predominantly caused by pathogens entering the normally sterile pleural space via a leaking bronchial stump. Pleural empyema usually manifests in the early postoperative period, less commonly months later. A persistent large or increasing pleural effusion may be a radiologic sign of *pleural*

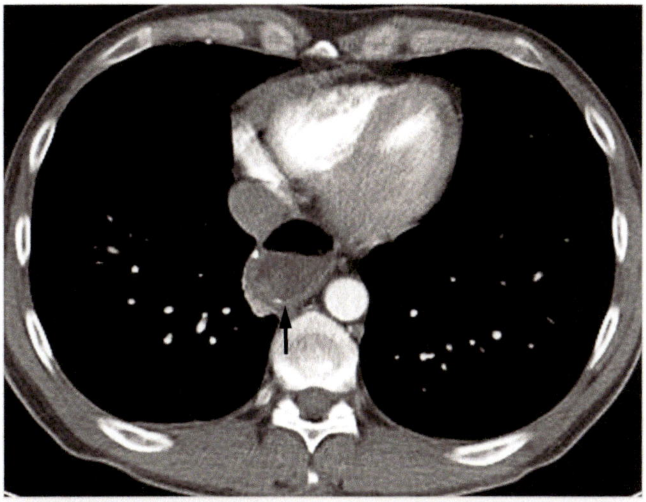

Fig. 17.23 Esophagectomy and cranial mobilization of stomach (*arrow*). CT image.

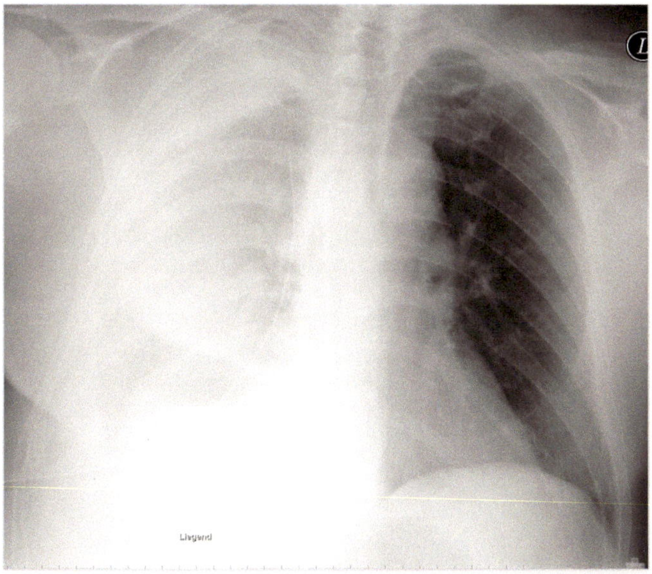

Fig. 17.24 Secondary bleeding following right upper lobe resection. Radiograph. Extensive opacity of the right hemithorax due to large amounts of pleural fluid, clinical hemothorax.

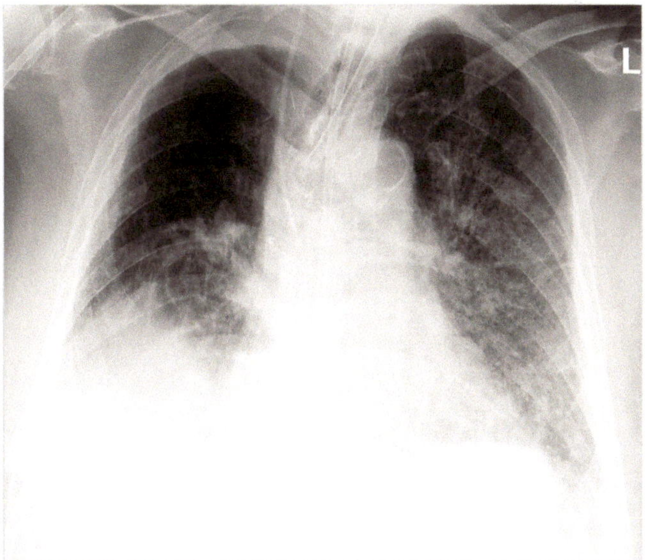

Fig. 17.25 Unilateral left adult respiratory distress syndrome following middle lobe resection. Radiograph. Extensive ground-glass opacities and reticular pattern in left lung.

empyema. Identification of pleural empyema on imaging is less easy in a pneumonectomy cavity compared with after partial lung resections. Radiologic criteria are a persistent or new-onset air–fluid level as well as an increasingly space-occupying fluid collection in the pneumonectomy cavity leading to mediastinal displacement to the nonoperated side.[19]

Surgical treatment of pleural empyema, especially in settings of bronchial stump leakage following pneumonectomy, requires creation of an open *thoracic window* to assure continuous access for cleaning the infected chest cavity (▶Fig. 17.26).

The access route via the fifth intercostal space usually used in open lung surgery requires *rib spreading*, which occasionally causes fractures to adjacent ribs. Relevant dislocation of rib fragments rarely occurs; usually, such fractures are incidental imaging findings. Occasionally, the intercostal space used for surgical access is gaping because of the defective intercostal muscles (▶Fig. 17.27), thus posing a risk of lung tissue herniation into the chest wall.

The term *gossypiboma* refers *to* a retained foreign object such as cotton materials inadvertently left behind in a body cavity during surgery. These materials are usually swabs in the case of thoracic surgery.[19] The dressing materials used in the operating room are marked with an interwoven metallic thread, unlike the dressing materials used on the wards. Hence, these can be easily identified on chest radiography (▶Fig. 17.28). On CT gossypibomas resemble tumor masses. While the pathognomonic metallic thread is of diagnostic value, it should not be mistaken for calcifications (▶Fig. 17.29).

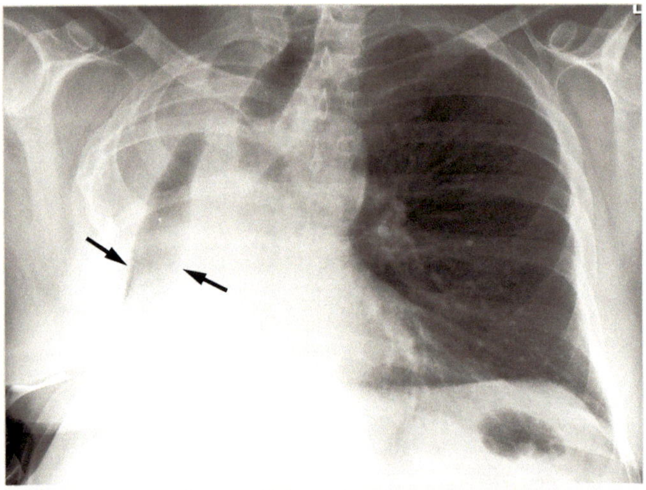

Fig. 17.26 Treatment of right pleural empyema following pneumonectomy by means of thoracic window (*arrows*). Radiograph.

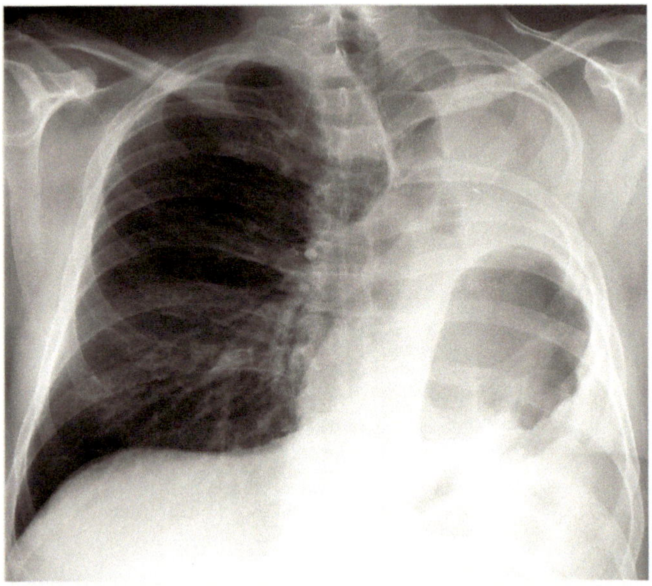

Fig. 17.27 Gaping four intercostal space following left pneumonectomy. Radiograph.

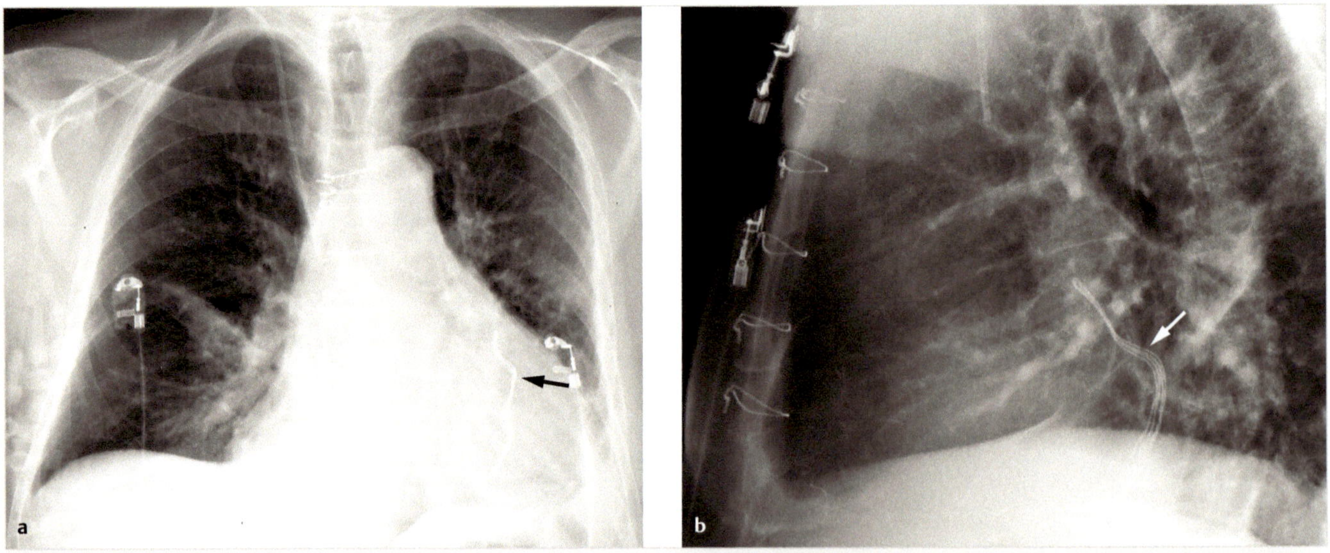

Fig. 17.28 Gossypiboma. Radiographs. Swab with interwoven metallic thread in the retrocardiac pericardial sac (**a, b,** *arrows*) following cardiac artery bypass surgery. Furthermore, postoperative cardiomegaly and left pleural effusion. **(a)** Posteroanterior image. **(b)** Magnified section of lateral image.

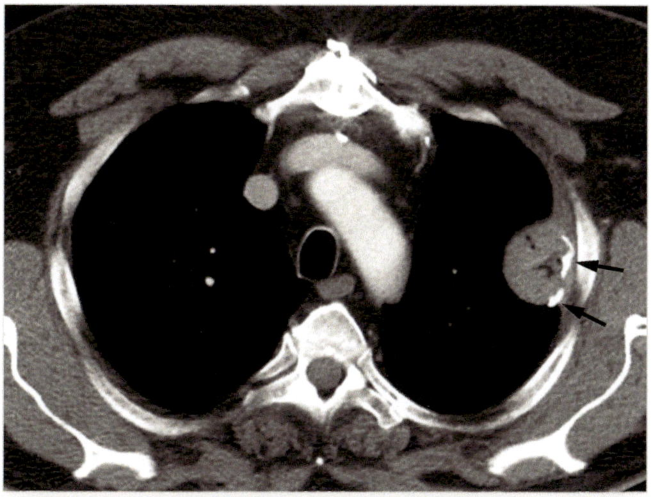

Fig. 17.29 Gossypiboma following cardiac artery bypass surgery. CT image. Pleura-based mass in left chest. The pathognomonic metallic threads (*arrows*) can be identified. Furthermore, sternal cerclages.

17.2 Bronchoscopic and Surgical Procedures for Treatment of Pulmonary Emphysema

Hyperinflation of the lung parenchyma during pulmonary emphysema causes exertional dyspnea with considerable adverse effects on the patient. First, it gives rise to a barrel-shaped chest deformity making the intercostal respiratory muscles less efficient. Second, because of its low-riding position, the diaphragm as the most important respiratory muscle is no longer able to generate optimal force. This further aggravates the existing dyspnea. This situation can be remedied by reducing the lung volume which in turn enhances diaphragmatic curvature and intercostal muscle efficiency. There is a wide variety of interventional bronchoscopic and surgical procedures available for lung volume reduction.

17.2.1 Bronchoscopic Procedures

17

A common procedure involves the implantation of endobronchial *valves* into the most hyperinflated lung segments or into an entire lung lobe. These one-way valves allow air to escape from the hyperinflated lung parenchyma, simultaneously preventing the entry of inhaled air into these areas and thus causing hypoaeration of the previously hyperinflated lung regions. This results in lung volume loss and improved breathing mechanics (▶ Fig. 17.30). These effects can be reversed through removal of the implanted endobronchial valves under bronchoscopic guidance.

The main reason for failure of this therapeutic concept is *collateral ventilation* from surrounding lung tissue in the valve-deflated lung regions, for example, arising from incompletely formed lobar fissures. If continuity of the fissures on thin-slice CT is less than 90%, collateral ventilation of relevance can be expected. Furthermore, balloon occlusion of the supply lobe bronchus under bronchoscopic guidance is able to detect collateral ventilation.[20]

Other bronchoscopic procedures for permanent volume loss of certain lung regions are being tested. For example, bronchial torsion of an emphysematous lobe can be achieved through implantation of elastic nitinol coils. Furthermore, steam

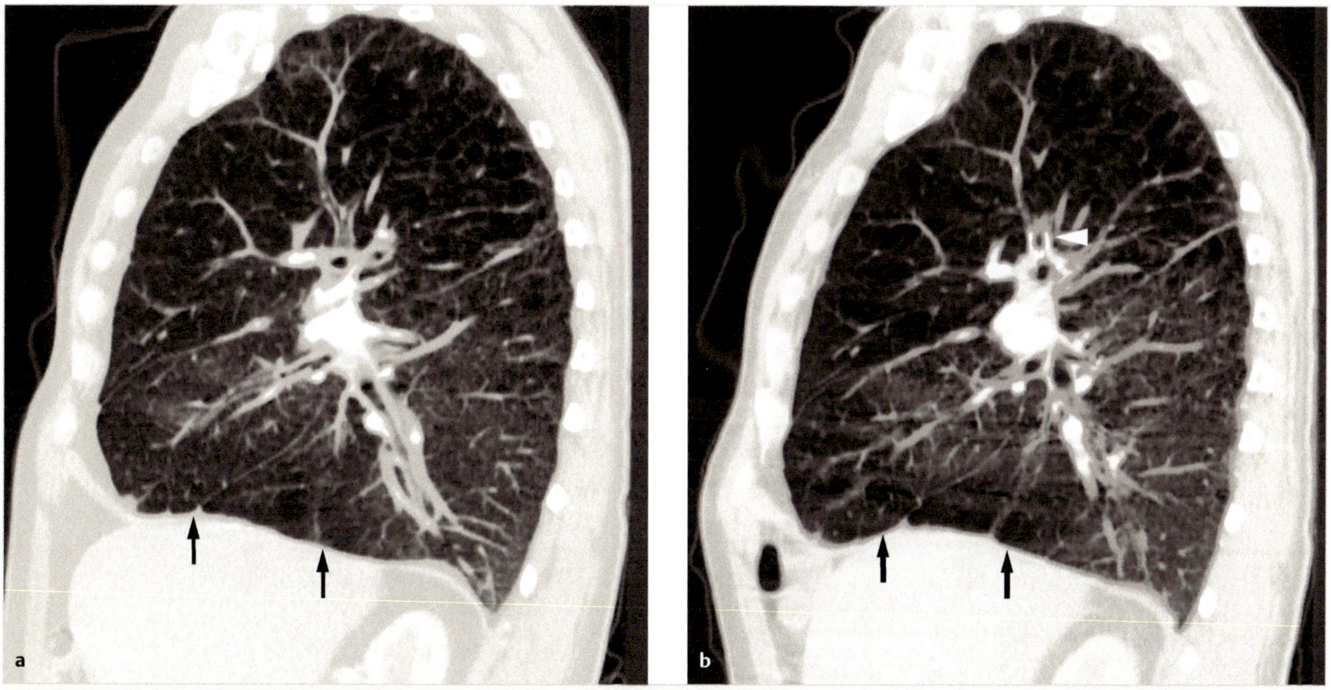

Fig. 17.30 Endobronchial valve implantation in pulmonary emphysema. CT images, sagittal MPR. **(a)** Before valve implantation: hyperinflated right upper lobe, flattened diaphragm (*arrows*) and enlarged sagittal thoracic diameter.**(b)** Following valve implantation: endobronchial valve in the right upper lobe bronchus (*arrowhead*), enhanced diaphragmatic curvature (*arrows*) and smaller sagittal thoracic diameter.

thermal ablation causes chronic fibrosis of the lung tissue in treated lung areas.[20]

17.2.2 Lung Volume Reduction Surgery

In order to reduce the enlarged lung volume, most hyperinflated lung areas can be surgically removed, usually by means of multiple atypical wedge resections. Inhomogeneous distribution of emphysema, usually most affecting the upper lobes, is a precondition for such a surgical approach. The aim is to remove diseased lung tissue while preserving relatively healthy lung regions. Like the bronchoscopic procedures, this is thought to improve the breathing mechanics.

Air leaks at the resection margins that are difficult to eliminate and persist for several days are commonly seen in the postoperative period because surgery is performed in highly vulnerable emphysematous lung tissue. Imaging findings consist of persistent postoperative pneumothorax and chest wall emphysema, less commonly also mediastinal emphysema.

Other generic complications of partial lung resection are described in previous sections.

17.3 Radiotherapy

Radiotherapy of thoracic malignancies requires radiation doses that are high enough to invariably damage the adjacent lung parenchyma. Affected lung parenchyma responds with organizing pneumonia that is commonly visible on imaging. This condition is described in the section on diffuse parenchymal lung diseases due to extrinsic noxae.

17.4 Chemotherapy

Chemotherapy is a standard treatment method in oncology. The damage caused to the bone marrow leads, depending on its intensity, to immunoincompetence of different degrees, making patients susceptible to opportunistic pulmonary infections.

The cytostatics as well as the numerous other drugs can trigger the most diverse pulmonary diseases, especially diffuse parenchymal lung diseases. Therefore, differential diagnosis of pulmonary diseases occurring in patients undergoing chemotherapy should always include drug-induced lung disease.

17.5 Stem Cell Transplantation

Stem cell transplantation is a complex method used for treatment of malignant hematologic disorders (leukemia, lymphoma, and plasmocytoma). An identical therapeutic concept designed primarily to destroy malignant cells by means of high-dose chemotherapy and whole-body irradiation is employed for all disorders. This inevitably also destroys the patient's healthy hematopoietic stem cells. Therefore, healthy stem cells are infused immediately thereafter; these are harvested from a genetically identical donor (syngenic, from identical twins), another donor (allogenic) or from the patient themself (autologous). These cells are sourced from the bone marrow (bone marrow transplantation), peripheral blood (stem cell transplantation) or the umbilical cord blood.

Since donor stem cells are transplanted in all of these procedures, *stem cell transplantation* has become established as a collective term. The term *bone marrow transplantation*, formerly used to denote one of these procedures, is now obsolete.

Appropriate immunosuppression is required after transplantation.[21]

17.5.1 Complications of Stem Cell Transplantation

This therapeutic concept makes patients very susceptible to opportunistic infections. During the first posttransplantation month, patients are particularly prone to bacterial pneumonia and pulmonary mycosis, especially invasive pulmonary aspergillosis. The principle infections in the later period are *Pneumocystis jirovecii* and cytomegalovirus pneumonia.

Moreover, this complex form of therapy presents a risk of numerous *noninfectious pulmonary complications* (▶Table 17.3). These affect the lung parenchyma, vascular endothelium, or the respiratory epithelium depending on the site of attack of the noxae. While higher incidences of virtually all these diseases are seen after stem cell transplantation, they are not specific to the latter. The only exception consists of pulmonary cytolytic thrombi (PCT),[22] a rare disease entity occurring only after allogenic stem cell transplantation: endothelial swelling of the arterial, capillary, and venous vessels triggered by an acute graft-versus-host disease (see below) leads to the formation of thrombi. Imaging visualizes this disorder as multiple nodules that are difficult to distinguish from infectious causes.[23]

Idiopathic pneumonia syndrome (IPS) is a collective term denoting the most diverse diseases. A common feature of all these disorders is that they present in stem cell transplant patients, have no infectious source, and give rise to pulmonary opacities on chest radiography.

Table 17.3 Noninfectious complications of stem cell transplantation in relation to predilection site.[22]

Predilection sites	Noninfectious complications
Lung parenchyma	• Idiopathic pneumonia syndrome • Drug-induced lung disease • Radiation pneumonitis • Eosinophilic pneumonia • Pulmonary alveolar proteinosis
Vascular endothelium	• Idiopathic pneumonia syndrome • Pulmonary veno-occlusive disease • Transfusion-related acute lung injury • Pulmonary cytolytic thrombi • Pulmonary arterial hypertension • Pulmonary thromboembolism
Respiratory epithelium	• Idiopathic pneumonia syndrome • Chronic graft-versus-host disease

> **Note**
>
> Subsumed under the term "idiopathic pneumonia syndrome" are the following diseases[22]:
> - Acute interstitial pneumonia.
> - Adult respiratory distress syndrome.
> - Capillary leak syndrome, peri-engraftment respiratory distress syndrome.
> - Diffuse alveolar hemorrhage.
> - Cryptogenic organizing pneumonia.
> - Bronchiolitis obliterans syndrome.

17.5.2 Graft-versus-Host Disease

Graft-versus-host disease (GvHD) is the term used to describe the immunologic reaction triggered by the transplanted foreign, immunocompetent cells to the cells and tissues of the transplant recipient after allogenic stem cell transplantation.

Acute graft-versus-host disease occurs after 1 month to a year, predominantly affecting the skin, gastrointestinal tract, and liver. Lung involvement is rare and manifests as mild fibrosis, cysts, and nodules.[23]

Chronic graft-versus-host disease frequently involves the lung where it gives rise to two disease entities:

- Bronchiolitis obliterans syndrome: In terms of histology, this involves constrictive bronchiolitis. Clinical symptoms include progressive dyspnea and persistent cough; increasing obstruction is detected in lung function tests. This disease entity has a poor prognosis.
- Cryptogenic organizing pneumonia: This presents in around 10% of all stem cell transplant patients. Risk factors are allogenic stem cell transplantation and other manifestations of graft-versus-host disease.[23]

Bronchiolitis obliterans syndrome as an expression of chronic graft-versus-host disease can be relatively specifically diagnosed on CT, most easily on expiratory scans or dynamic CT of the ventilation cycle (▶Fig. 17.31). The remaining disease entities described in this chapter have no pathognomonic findings. The key to correct diagnosis is multidisciplinary, in-depth discussion of the clinical and radiologic findings.

17.6 Summary

Lung Surgery

Partial lung resections are classified as anatomic (along anatomic boundaries, i.e. lobar and segmental boundaries) and atypical resections (see ▶Table 17.1).

Anatomic resections are used for surgical treatment of lung cancer. The standard oncologic procedure is removal of at least one lobe of lung and systematic mediastinal lymphadenectomy. At times, complete tumor resection necessitates more extensive surgery, such as removal of two right lung lobes (upper or lower bilobectomy) or pneumonectomy.

A common feature of all anatomic resections is the, sometimes only subtle, volume loss of the operated lung visualized on chest radiography. This may be accompanied by a high-riding diaphragm and mediastinal displacement as well as disappearance of individual interlobar fissures. Following pneumonectomy, the chest cavity now containing only air becomes filled with fluid over the course of weeks. The fluid converts to connective tissue resulting in a fibrothorax over the next months.

Diagnostic partial lung resections and metastasectomy as well as lung volume reduction surgery are usually performed as *atypical wedge resections;* laser resection is additionally used for metastasectomy. The sequelae of atypical resection and segmental resections can be identified on chest radiography as opacities in the lung parenchyma. On CT, wedge resection manifests as a virtually linear opacity extending from the pleura,

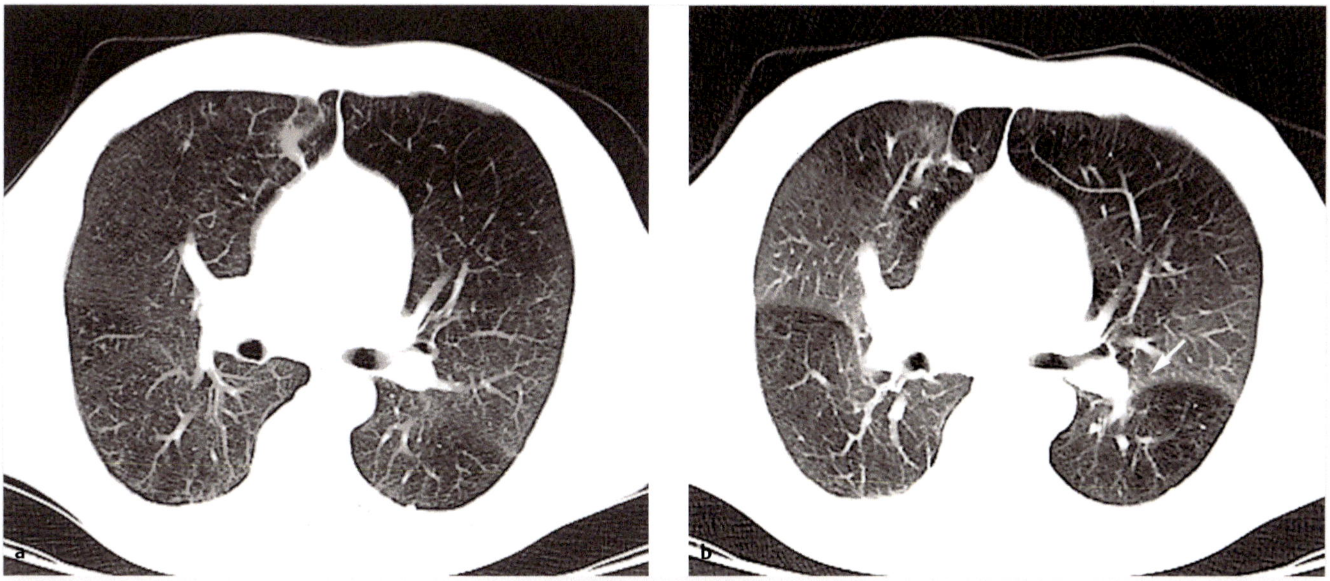

Fig. 17.31 Chronic graft-versus-host disease following stem cell transplantation due to plasmocytoma. Mosaic attenuation pattern and extensive air trapping, particularly conspicuous on the expiratory image. **(a)** Inspiratory CT image. **(b)** Expiratory CT image.

while laser resection appears as a rounded, often cavitary, opacity.

Typical postoperative *complications* of partial lung resections:

- Hemothorax (extensive opacity of the operated hemithorax).
- Air leak as well as bronchial stump leak (persistent pneumothorax, chest wall or mediastinal emphysema).
- Pneumonia.
- Pleural empyema.
- Adult respiratory distress syndrome (ARDS), may also present unilaterally on the contralateral side as ventilator-associated ARDS.

Heart Surgery

Following heart surgery, metallic implants can be identified: metallic clips along the bypass (interposed vein or left internal thoracic artery) in coronary artery bypass surgery and an implanted cardiac valve in mechanical cardiac valve replacement. Cardiac valves made of biological material are scarcely visible on chest radiography. Characteristic postoperative findings include enlargement of the cardiac silhouette, mediastinal enlargement, left pleural effusion, and left lower lobe atelectasis (retrocardiac opacities) in the immediate postoperative course.

Early postoperative complications include hemothorax and hemopericardium. The latter can be identified on chest radiography as a "bocksbeutel" shaped enlarged cardiac silhouette.

Esophagectomy

Esophagectomy is a surgical option for treatment of esophageal cancer. To that effect, part of the esophagus is resected and continuity of the digestive tract is assured through cranial mobilization of the stomach, less commonly of the jejunum, or by interposition of a segment of the colon. Two basic access routes are used: transthoracic (via a right-sided thoracotomy) as well as transhiatal (via the upper abdomen and cervical route without opening the chest cavity).

The most frequent postoperative *complication* is anastomotic leak presenting a risk of fistula formation to adjacent structures and mediastinitis. Chylothorax results from injury or resection of the thoracic duct. Anastomotic stenosis often occurs during the healing process of an anastomotic leak; onset after several months or even years may be indicative of local tumor recurrence.

Transplantation

Lung transplantations are performed as both single- and double-lung transplantations, sometimes in combination with heart transplantation (heart–lung transplantation). An overview of the imaging findings after lung transplantation is given in ▶Table 17.2. Acute rejection usually manifests in the second posttransplantation week and is characterized by bilateral ground-glass opacities. By contrast, chronic rejection presents only months or years later as bronchiolitis obliterans syndrome with extensive air trapping and bronchiestasis.

Heart transplantation is predominantly performed using an orthotopic procedure (as replacement for the diseased recipient heart), less commonly as a heterotopic procedure (the donor heart is placed in the right hemithorax alongside the recipient heart). In the latter case, there is considerable enlargement of the postoperative cardiac silhouette.

After both lung and heart transplantation, patients are at risk for *opportunistic infections*. In the first posttransplantation weeks, these are predominantly caused by bacteria and fungi; viral infections predominate in the later period, especially cytomegalovirus pneumonia.

Lymphoproliferative diseases occur in around 5% of heart and lung transplant patients. Their most salient features are multiple pulmonary nodules or consolidations, possibly with halo sign, and mediastinal lymphadenopathy. Pleural effusions and interlobular septal thickening also occur.

Radiotherapy

Radiation pneumonitis manifests as a characteristic pulmonary sequela of thoracic radiotherapy usually 4 to 12 weeks after completion of radiotherapy. It can occur in association with radiation doses from 20 Gy and is routinely observed with doses of 40 Gy.

Chemotherapy

Patients receiving systemic chemotherapy are susceptible to opportunistic pulmonary infections depending on the aggressiveness of the treatment regimen. Differential diagnosis of pulmonary symptoms should also include drug-induced lung disease.

Stem Cell Transplantation

Stem cell transplantation is a procedure used to treat malignant hematologic disorders. All malignant cells are destroyed by means of high-dose chemotherapy and whole-body irradiation. This therapy inevitably also inflicts massive and permanent damage on the hematopoietic stem cells. Therefore, it must be followed immediately by stem cell transplantation, while harvesting the stem cells from another donor (allogenic), from the patient themself (autologous) or less commonly from genetically identical donors (syngenic).

Patients undergoing this therapy become immunoincompetent in the long term and are thus at considerable risk for opportunistic infections. Noninfectious pulmonary complications are also common (see ▶Table 17.3).

The adverse reaction exhibited by transplanted immunocompetent cells against the recipient organism after allogenic stem cell transplantation is known as *graft-versus-host disease* (GvHD). Whereas acute graft-versus-host disease affects particularly the skin, gastrointestinal tract, and liver, chronic graft-versus-host disease often manifests in the lung as bronchiolitis obliterans syndrome. Its most salient features are air trapping and bronchiestasis. Findings suggestive of cryptogenic organizing pneumonia are less common.

Other infectious and noninfectious complications of stem cell transplantation have no specific imaging findings. Multidisciplinary discussion of all findings is therefore needed for correct diagnosis and therapy decision-making.

References

[1] Chae EJ, Seo JB, Kim SY, et al. Radiographic and CT findings of thoracic complications after pneumonectomy. Radiographics 2006;26(5):1449–1468

[2] Gladish GW, Rice DC, Sabloff BS, Truong MT, Marom EM, Munden RF. Pedicle muscle flaps in intrathoracic cancer resection: imaging appearance and evolution. Radiographics 2007;27(4):975–987

[3] Rossi VF, Vargas FS, Marchi E, et al. Acute inflammatory response secondary to intrapleural administration of two types of talc. Eur Respir J 2010;35(2):396–401

[4] Gill AJ, Mathur MN, Tattersall SF. Systematic response to talc pleurodesis. Am J Respir Crit Care Med 2004;169(9):1074–1075, author reply 1074–1075

[5] Kwek BH, Aquino SL, Fischman AJ. Fluorodeoxyglucose positron emission tomography and CT after talc pleurodesis. Chest 2004;125(6):2356–2360

[6] Narayanaswamy S, Kamath S, Williams M. CT appearances of talc pleurodesis. Clin Radiol 2007;62(3):233–237

[7] de Perrot M, Chaparro C, McRae K, et al. Twenty-year experience of lung transplantation at a single center: Influence of recipient diagnosis on long-term survival. J Thorac Cardiovasc Surg 2004;127(5):1493–1501

[8] Krishnam MS, Suh RD, Tomasian A, et al. Postoperative complications of lung transplantation: radiologic findings along a time continuum. Radiographics 2007;27(4):957–974

[9] Frost AE, Jammal CT, Cagle PT. Hyperacute rejection following lung transplantation. Chest 1996;110(2):559–562

[10] King-Biggs MB. Acute pulmonary allograft rejection. Mechanisms, diagnosis, and management. Clin Chest Med 1997;18(2):301–310

[11] Loubeyre P, Revel D, Delignette A, Loire R, Mornex JF. High-resolution computed tomographic findings associated with histologically diagnosed acute lung rejection in heart-lung transplant recipients. Chest 1995;107(1):132–138

[12] Collins J. Imaging of the chest after lung transplantation. J Thorac Imaging 2002;17(2):102–112

[13] Sharples LD, McNeil K, Stewart S, Wallwork J. Risk factors for bronchiolitis obliterans: a systematic review of recent publications. J Heart Lung Transplant 2002;21(2):271–281

[14] Collins J, Hartman MJ, Warner TF, et al. Frequency and CT findings of recurrent disease after lung transplantation. Radiology 2001;219(2):503–509

[15] Knisely BL, Mastey LA, Collins J, Kuhlman JE. Imaging of cardiac transplantation complications. Radiographics 1999;19(2):321–339, discussion 340–341

[16] Fletcher C, Ostergaard C, Menzies R. Dressler syndrome after minimally invasive coronary artery bypass surgery. J Am Board Fam Pract 2004;17(3):230–232

[17] Kabukcu M, Demircioglu F, Yanik E, Basarici I, Ersel F. Pericardial tamponade and large pericardial effusions: causal factors and efficacy of percutaneous catheter drainage in 50 patients. Tex Heart Inst J 2004;31(4):398–403

[18] Kim TJ, Lee KH, Kim YH, et al. Postoperative imaging of esophageal cancer: what chest radiologists need to know. Radiographics 2007;27(2):409–429

[19] Kim EA, Lee KS, Shim YM, et al. Radiographic and CT findings in complications following pulmonary resection. Radiographics 2002;22(1):67–86

[20] Gompelmann D, Eberhardt R, Herth F. Endoscopic volume reduction in COPD- a critical review. Dtsch Arztebl Int 2014;111(49):827–833

[21] Choi MH, Jung JI, Chung WD, et al. Acute pulmonary complications in patients with hematologic malignancies. Radiographics 2014;34(6):1755–1768

[22] Panoskaltsis-Mortari A, Griese M, Madtes DK, et al; American Thoracic Society Committee on Idiopathic Pneumonia. An official American Thoracic Society research statement: noninfectious lung injury after hematopoietic stem cell transplantation: idiopathic pneumonia syndrome. Am J Respir Crit Care Med 2011;183(9):1262–1279

[23] Franquet T, Müller NL, Lee KS, Giménez A, Flint JD. High-resolution CT and pathologic findings of noninfectious pulmonary complications after hematopoietic stem cell transplantation. AJR Am J Roentgenol 2005;184(2):629–637

Chapter 18

Occupational Lung Diseases

18

18 Occupational Lung Diseases

Beate Rehbock

18.1 Introduction

Occupational or work-related disease is the term used to describe health disorders fully or partially attributable to work activity. These are usually caused by multiple factors, exhibit nonspecific symptoms, and very often have a chronic course. Lung diseases account for almost half of all occupational diseases and, at 87%, are statistically the leading cause of related deaths.

The most common pulmonary occupational disease is pneumoconiosis (black lung) which is caused by inorganic dust—in particular the clinical disease entities of silicosis and mixed-dust pneumoconiosis as well as asbestosis and asbestos-related pleural disease. A specific feature of most occupational lung diseases is the long latency period (years to decades) between exposure to the hazardous substance and the appearance of radiographic findings or clinical symptoms. Imaging plays a key role in diagnosis and monitoring of asbestosis, asbestos-related pleural disease, and silicosis.

18.2 Imaging Modalities

18.2.1 Chest Radiography

Chest radiography is the first imaging modality used for all occupational lung diseases (posteroanterior and optional left lateral radiograph); the International Labour Organization (ILO) classification system (▶Fig. 18.1) is commonly used to report radiographic findings of pneumoconioses, especially in preventive medical checkups and medical opinions.[1,2] This standardized diagnostic schema is an epidemiological instrument for internationally uniform description of radiographic changes following exposure to hazardous substances. It is not designed to provide a definitive diagnosis or information to establish compensation; instead, it is aimed at assignment of opacity types to pulmonary and pleural inhalation damage. Furthermore, the schema can be used for quantification of the disease extent and as a prognostic predictor as well as for detection of other diseases causing respiratory symptoms.[3] The findings are evaluated by comparison with reference films available as hard copies and in digital format.

The ILO classification system can be used for any occupational lung or pleural disease. No image pattern is pathognomonic for dust exposure. An occupational disease can only be diagnosed by taking a detailed occupational history and through ascertainment of an occupational exposure to hazardous substances linked to a specific image pattern.

18.2.2 Computed Tomography

Since sensitivity and specificity of CT are superior to those of chest radiography, it is increasingly used for diagnostic imaging of occupational lung diseases.

In view of the fact that the majority of occupational lung diseases manifest interstitially, CT should be primarily used as a high-resolution (HR), weight-adapted, low-dose, unenhanced multidetector CT technique. Sequential thin slices should only be obtained if needed additionally on expiration (suspected air trapping) or in the prone position (for differentiation between fibrosis and dependent opacities).

Semi-quantitative classification of the CT findings is performed in accordance with the International Classification of HRCT for Occupational and Environmental Respiratory Diseases (ICOERD),[4] which is similar to the ILO classification system (▶Fig. 18.2), and for which digital reference films are also available.[5] Likewise, in this purely descriptive diagnostic schema, the letters and symbols merely serve as descriptors with no claim to conferring etiologic or pathogenetic insights. However, (in the "Remarks" column) a conclusive assignment should be made to a disease entity or suspected diagnosis, with reference to differential diagnosis if applicable.

IV contrast is needed for diagnosis of suspected tumors (pulmonary nodule, lung cancer, mesothelioma, pleural effusion).

18.2.3 Other Imaging Modalities

MRI has presently no established role in primary diagnosis of occupational lung diseases but can be superior to CT in resolving certain tumor-related diagnostic issues in lung cancer and pleural mesothelioma (e.g., local invasion of adjacent structures).[6] MRI is reported to be advantageous in differentiating between progressive massive fibrosis and a malignant tumor (see ▶Fig. 18.11)[7] as well as between rounded atelectasis and lung cancer.[8] Likewise, PET-CT and ultrasonography are reserved for particular individual cases.

18.3 Disease Entities

18.3.1 Inorganic Dust-Induced Lung Diseases (Pneumoconiosis)

Pneumoconiosis presents as a result of a lung tissue reaction to inhaled dust particles that reach the alveoli. There is no clear-cut definition of pneumoconiosis or of how occupational lung diseases are classified as such. While the term coined in 1867 by Zenker also included organic dust, "pneumoconiosis" is currently generally understood to mean lung diseases caused by inorganic dust (▶Table 18.1). Pneumoconiosis may be fibrogenic or nonfibrogenic (▶Table 18.2). While berylliosis is also classified as pneumoconiosis, it occupies a special place because of its immunologic pathogenesis.[3] Beryllium is a metal used, for example, in the automobile and aircraft construction industries as well as in aerospace technology but may also be found as traces in dental alloys.

II

READING SHEET FOR

Complete ILO (2000) International Classification of Radiographs of Pneumoconioses

Reader code ☐☐☐ Radiograph identifier ☐☐☐☐☐☐☐☐☐

Date of reading ☐☐–☐☐–☐☐☐☐ Date of radiograph ☐☐–☐☐–☐☐☐☐

Technical quality

GRADE 1, 2, 3, or 4 (Mark appropriate box) 1 2 3 4

If grade not 1, Comment required here

Comment on technical quality :

Parenchymal abnormalities

Small opacities

Profusion (12-pooint scale)

0/- 0/0 0/1 1/0 1/0 1/1 1/2 2/1 2/2 2/3 3/2 3/3 3/+

(Consult standard radiographs – mark profusion subcategory.)

0/- 0/0 0/1
1/0 1/1 1/2
2/1 2/2 2/3
3/2 3/3 3/+

Affected zones

(Mark ALL affected zones)

	R	L
Upper	☐	☐
Middle	☐	☐
Lower	☐	☐

Shape and size : p, q, r, s, t, or u
(Consult standard radiographs. Two symbols required ;

mark one primary and one secondary.)

Primary		Secondary	
p	s	p	s
q	t	q	t
r	u	r	u

Large opacities Mark 0 for none or mark A, B, or C O A B C

Pleural abnormalities Yes ☐ No ☐

If "No" go to ***SYMBOLS**

(0=None R=Right L=Left)

Pleural plaques

Site
(Mark appropriate boxes)

Calcification
(Mark)

Extent (chest wall ; combined for in-profile and face-on)
up to ¼ of lateral chest wall = 1
¼ to ½ of lateral chest wall = 2
>½ of lateral chest wall = 3

Width (optional)
(3 mm minimum width required)
3 to 5 mm = a
5 to 10 mm = b
> 10 mm = c

	Site	Calcification	Extent		Width	
Chest wall in profile	O R L	O R L	O R	O L	R	L
			1 2 3	1 2 3	a b c	a b c
face–on	O R L	O R L				
Diaphragm	O R L	O R L				
Other site(s)	O R L	O R L				

Costophrenic angle obliteration O R L

Diffuse pleural thickening

(Mark appropriate boxes)

Calcification
(Mark)

Extent (chest wall ; combined for in-profile and face-on)
up to ¼ of lateral chest wall = 1
¼ to ½ of lateral chest wall = 2
>½ of lateral chest wall = 3

Width (optional)
(3 mm minimum width required)
3 to 5 mm = a
5 to 10 mm = b
> 10 mm = c

	Site	Calcification	Extent		Width	
Chest wall in profile	O R L	O R L	O R	O L	R	L
			1 2 3	1 2 3	a b c	a b c
face-on	O R L	O R L				

***Symbols** Yes ☐ No ☐

aa at ax bu ca cg cn co cp cv di ef em es

fr hi ho id ih kl me pa pb pi px ra rp tb od

(Circle as appropriate ; if **od** *circled,* **COMMENT** *must be made below)*

Comments Yes ☐ No ☐

Fig. 18.1 ILO classifications form—several variants of this form are available. Instructions for use and a key to the symbols are given in International Labour Office.[9] (Reproduced with permission from © International Labour Organization, 2002.)

CT- Classification

Name/No.	CT-No. / Date				Quality	Position
	No. slices		Sequential	KV	1	Prone
	Slice thickness		Single slice spir.	mA	2	Supine
	Window setting		Multi slice spiral	sec	3	
					4	

CT-FINDING 2001

Is the film completely negative? No Yes

Symbols: Ø, AX, BE, BR, BU, CA, CG, CV, DI, DO, EF, ES, FP, FR, HI, ME, MP, OD, PB, RA, SC, TB, TD

Lung

Well defined rounded opacities — No Yes

	No	Yes
P = <1.5 mm		
Q = 1.5 -3 mm		
R = >3-10 mm		

Predominant Size

Zones Profusion

	R				L			
U	0	1	2	3	0	1	2	3
M	0	1	2	3	0	1	2	3
L	0	1	2	3	0	1	2	3

Sum Grade

Irregular and /or linear opacities — No Yes

	No	Yes
Intralobular		
Interlobular		

Predominant Size

Grade

	R				L			
U	0	1	2	3	0	1	2	3
M	0	1	2	3	0	1	2	3
L	0	1	2	3	0	1	2	3

Sum Grade

Inhomogeneous attenuation — No Yes

Ground glass opacity grade — No Yes

	R				L			
U	0	1	2	3	0	1	2	3
M	0	1	2	3	0	1	2	3
L	0	1	2	3	0	1	2	3

Sum Grade

Honeycombing grade — No Yes

	R				L			
U	0	1	2	3	0	1	2	3
M	0	1	2	3	0	1	2	3
L	0	1	2	3	0	1	2	3

Sum Grade

Emphysema grade — No Yes

	R				L			
U	0	1	2	3	0	1	2	3
M	0	1	2	3	0	1	2	3
L	0	1	2	3	0	1	2	3

Sum Grade

Large opacities — No Yes

A / B / C

	R	L
U		
M		
L		

Predominant Parenchymal: RO IR GGO HC EM LO

Pleura

Pleural calcifications — No Yes

		No	Yes
W	panetal type		
	visceral type		
M			
D			

Predominant

	R	L
U		
M		
L		

Extent /Width

R				L			
0	1	2	3	0	1	2	3
0	a	b	c	0	a	b	c

Pleural calcifications — No Yes

Localisation: W M D

Comments /Summary

Date /signature

Date	Signature

Fig. 18.2 CT classification form according to ICOERD. (Reproduced with permission from Kusaka et al.[4])

In terms of pathogenesis of pneumoconioses, it is thought that larger dust particles are eliminated by the ciliated epithelia of the tracheobronchial system or are deposited in the nasopharyngeal region. Dust particles measuring less than 5 µm in diameter and fibrogenic particles may be retained depending on the amount of dust and exposure time,

Table 18.1 Principal types of inorganic dust-induced pneumoconiosis

Pneumoconiosis	Occupations
Silicosis/coal workers' pneumoconiosis	Stone quarry, stonemason, glass and ceramics industry, coal mining, foundry
Silicotuberculosis	
Asbestosis/asbestos-related pleural disease	Roofer, fitter, insulator, etc. Currently, (generally little) exposure especially in demolition work
Aluminum-induced lung disease	Aluminum powder production (pyro grinding), aluminum welding, production of corundum for grinding wheels
Hard metal lung disease	Production of hard metal tools, e.g., drill heads
Siderofibrosis	Welding processes: with extreme and prolonged exposure to welding smoke and gases
Dental technician lung disease	With prolonged (18-year) exposure to mixed dusts; prevalence 10% (chromium, cobalt, molybdenum, beryllium, etc.)

Table 18.2 Common fibrogenic and nonfibrogenic dusts and resulting pneumoconiosis

Fibrogenic dust	Nonfibrogenic dust
Quartz, sand, and other silicic acid-containing minerals → silicosis	Iron oxide ("inert") → siderosis
Asbestos (white and blue asbestos) → asbestosis and asbestos-related pleural disease	Carbon (soot, graphite) → anthracosis (coal workers' lung disease)
	Tin dust → stannosis
Talc soapstone (usually with quartz and/or asbestos content) → talcosis	Barium sulfate → baritosis
Aluminum dust → alumininosis	
Hard metals (including titanium, tungsten carbide, cobalt) → hard metal lung disease	

Table 18.3 Principal occupational causes of hypersensitivity pneumonitis

Disease entity	Antigens	Occupational risks
Farmer lung	Thermophilic actinomycetes	Agriculture, gardeners
Bird fancier lung	Animal-based antigens	Bird handlers, veterinarians
Air humidifier lung	Molds	Air-conditioning systems, air humidifiers
Baker lung	Moldy flour	Bakers, millers
Isocyanate alveolitis	Isocyanate compounds	Chemical workers

individual disposition and the integrity of the mucociliary clearance function (phagocytosis by alveolar macrophages). The mucociliary clearance function is adversely affected by cigarette smoking and toxic gases. After alveolar deposition the dust particles can trigger a chronic inflammatory reaction in the lung interstitium or be transported in the lymphatic and blood systems. Asbestos fibers can alter the pleura through pleural drift. All fibrogenic substances have the potential to cause irreversible damage to the lung parenchyma. The associated radiologic features will range from reticular (e.g., asbestosis) through reticulonodular to predominantly nodular pattern (e.g., silicosis) depending on the dust composition and severity of damage. Short-term exposure identified at an early stage often exhibits a nodular pattern with ground-glass opacity on HRCT (which applies also to rare types of pneumoconiosis). The more chronic the exposure and disease process, the more widespread the fibrosing pattern.

Clinically, inorganic—including fibrosing—pneumoconiosis can remain silent for a very long time. This is usually followed by onset of symptoms of restrictive lung function. In particular, in silicosis obstructive ventilation disorders are also observed.

18.3.2 Organic Dust-Induced Lung Diseases

Organic dust of animal and plant origin can trigger an allergic reaction of the airways. Hypersensitivity pneumonitis is a collective term that includes a number of disease entities with similar symptoms that may be triggered by various allergens (▸Table 18.3); for more details, please consult Section 7.1.3.

Byssinosis is a disease caused by the toxic potential of inhaled uncleaned cotton which may manifest clinically as chronic bronchitis and emphysema but is not associated with any specific radiographic features.

Pathophysiologically, hypersensitivity pneumonitis is caused by a type III and IV immunologic response. Its pathohistology is characterized by bronchocentric lymphocytic alveolitis with granulomatous inflammation that may evolve to fibrosis.[10]

Clinically, acute hypersensitivity pneumonitis may manifest with flu-like symptoms, including dyspnea and cough 6 to 8 hours after exposure. The acute variant is often self-limiting and reversible if allergen exposure is avoided early on. Persistent exposure can lead to interstitial fibrosis.

Table 18.4 Most common exposures that can cause a malignant tumor

Noxae	Malignant tumors
Asbestos	Asbestos-induced lung cancer
	Asbestos-induced pleural mesothelioma
	Lung cancer due to interaction between asbestos dust and polycyclic aromatic hydrocarbons
Ionizing radiation	Lung cancer
Silicium dioxide	Lung cancer in quartz dust–related lung disease (silicosis or silicotuberculosis)

18.3.3 Acute Inhalation Toxicity

The place and extent of damage are determined by the physical state, water solubility, dose, and pH value of the noxae. The following disease entities may result:

- *Acute toxic tracheitis and bronchitis*: Water-soluble substances (e.g., ammonia, chlorine gas, hydrochloric acid, and formaldehyde) cause damage especially to the upper respiratory tract.
- *Chemical irritation or toxic asthma* (reactive airways dysfunction syndrome): sulfur dioxide, sulfuric acid, isocyanate, and formaldehyde can trigger acute reflex bronchoconstriction with or without reversible obstruction.
- *Organizing pneumonia*: Following inhalational injury with high doses of, e.g., nitrogen dioxide, sulfur dioxide, ammonia, or chlorine gas, organizing pneumonia can manifest after a latency period of only up to 3 weeks.
- *Pulmonary edema*: Substances with poor water solubility (e.g., phosgene and ozone) as well as lipophilic substances, such as nitrogen dioxide, can cause intra-alveolar edema that manifests clinically only after a dose-related latency period. Bacterial pneumonia is common because of the damage to the immune function of the alveolar macrophages.

Note

The role of imaging in relation to inhalation toxicity is to exclude acute complications (pulmonary edema). Because of the latency period, the possibility of delayed complications must be considered (pneumonia, cryptogenic organizing pneumonia). CT should be used early on if there is any discrepancy between the radiographic and clinical findings.

18.3.4 Chronic Bronchitis and Asthma

There are myriad workplace-related hazardous substances that can cause chronic as well as acute irritation disorders of the airways not amenable to primary diagnostic imaging. Exceptions to that rule are chronic obstructive pulmonary diseases like chronic bronchitis and emphysema; imaging plays an important role in these disease entities when they present in the following circumstances:

- As a complication of silicosis and silicotuberculosis.
- In underground coalminers exposed to a cumulative dose of more than 100 fine dust years ([mg/m^3] × years).

In addition to the pathognomonic changes following quartz dust exposure, special attention should be paid on chest radiography, and possibly HRCT, and to emphysema criteria since this can present as a complication of occupational chronic bronchitis.

18.3.5 Malignant Occupational Diseases of the Lung and Pleura

Malignant tumors of the lung and pleura quantitatively account for the majority of occupational cancer diseases (▸Table 18.4). In particular, these are asbestos- and quartz dust–related lung cancers as well as asbestos-related pleural mesotheliomas. While imaging is unable to directly impute the tumor to an occupational pathogenesis, through indirect radiologic signs it can often establish a probable link to asbestosis, asbestos-induced pleural disease, or silicosis.

18.4 Diagnostic Imaging of Special Disease Entities

18.4.1 Asbestosis and Asbestos Dust–Related Pleural Disease

As per its definition, asbestosis consists of diffuse, bilateral interstitial fibrosis caused by inhalation of asbestos fibers. Asbestos-induced fibrosis can affect the pulmonary interstitium (asbestosis) as well as the parietal and/or visceral pleura.[11] Histologic evidence of asbestos bodies in the lung parenchyma is only a marker of exposure and in itself does not constitute disease.

High asbestos exposure levels are generally responsible for parenchymal fibrosis with a latency of more than 20 years.[3] Compared to lung fibrosis, pleural changes already appear at lower levels of asbestos exposure. Therefore, they are today more common findings than lung fibrosis because of the ban on the use of asbestos in numerous countries from its historical peak in 1980 and the introduction of extensive occupational safety measures. During the first decade of asbestos exposure, the pleura often reacts with exudation (asbestos pleuritis), only later followed by areas of discrete pleural thickening (pleural plaques) as well as pleural fibrosis (visceral pleural thickening).[3]

Note

The imaging findings associated with asbestos may have a pleural and a pulmonary component. The term "asbestosis" (better: asbestos-related lung disease) refers only to the asbestos-induced lung fibrosis.[12] The term "pleural asbestosis" is incorrect.

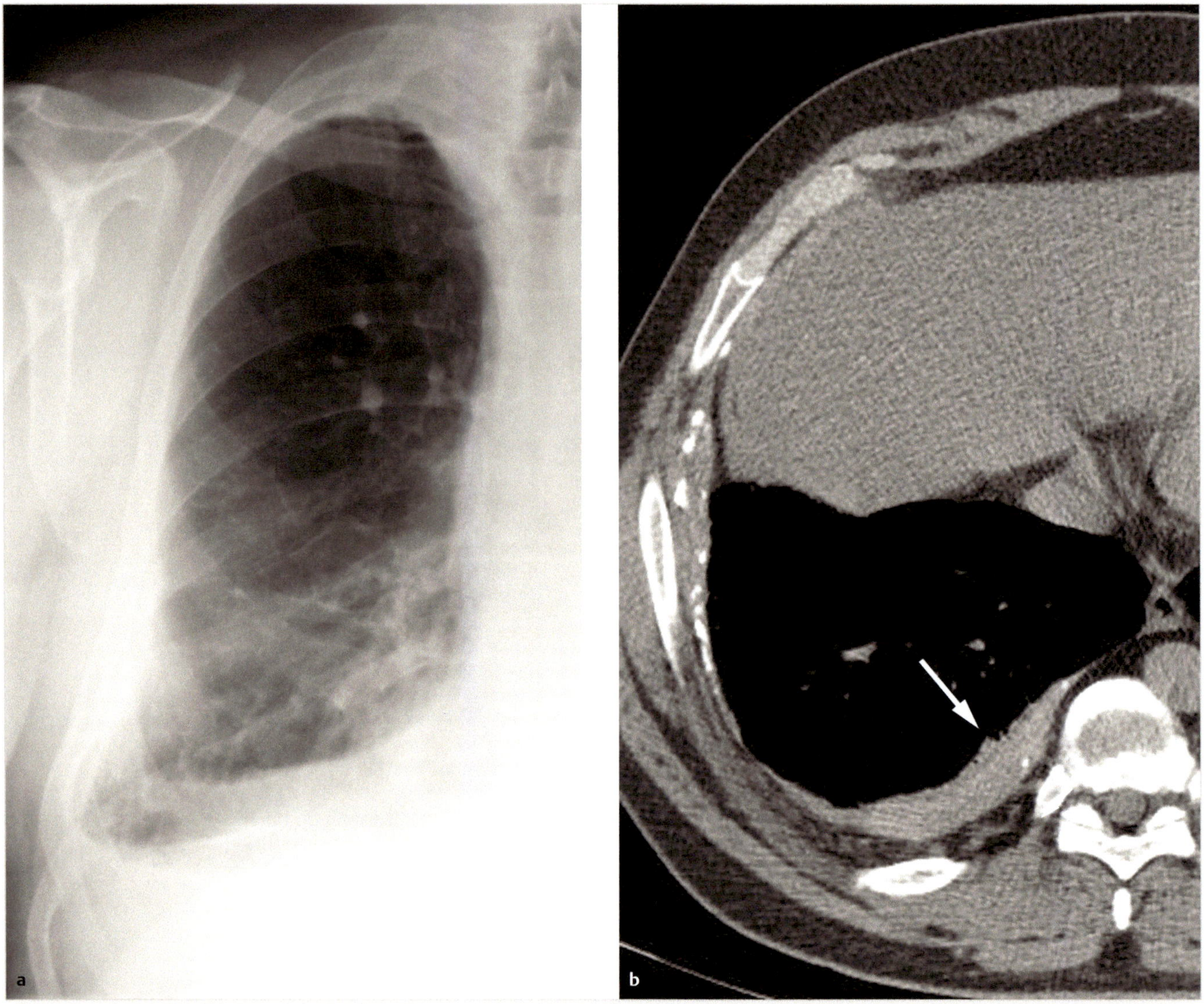

Fig. 18.3 Diffuse pleural thickening (ILO 2b) with involvement of the right recess consistent with hyalinosis complicata. (a) Magnified section of a radiograph. **(b)** On CT, virtually circumferential, partially calcified thickening of the costal pleura (ICOERD w [=wall] of visceral type) with subpleural parenchymal reaction and fibrosis. Ill-defined, lung-sided delineation of the area of pleural thickening, with parenchymal involvement (*arrow*).

Pleural Asbestos-Related Changes

Pleural plaques are areas of discrete hyaline or calcified fibrosis of predominantly the parietal pleura (costal, diaphragmatic, and mediastinal pleura).[7] The following variations in attenuation are observed:

- Noncalcified (hyaline): probably primary.
- Calcified: partial or complete.
- Location of calcifications: at the center or base of the plaque or isolated pleural calcification.

A distinction must be made between the following morphologic types:

- Table mountain–shaped (deemed pathognomonic for asbestos exposure and usually smoothly marginated [parietal type]; predominantly located in the costal pleura).
- Hill- and spindle-shaped pleural thickening.
- Thickening at the level of the pleura.
- Visceral pleural thickening (with ill-defined, lung-sided margin, consistent with subpleural parenchymal changes like local subpleural fibrosis; ▶Fig. 18.3).

The following locations are characteristic:

- *Costal pleura*: Usually bilateral and often symmetrical.
  - *Plaques in the upper and middle zones*: Predominantly anterior and anterolateral, in the lower zones paravertebral and posterior.
  - *Pleural dome and recesses*: Generally spared.
- *Diaphragmatic pleura*: Predominantly at the central tendon with confluent tendency along its course.
- *Mediastinal pleura*: Differentiation versus pericardial calcification often not possible.
- *Unilateral pleural thickening*: Prevalence of up to 35% and no dominant side.
- *Parietal pleura*: The most common; less common interlobar plaques confined to the visceral pleura.

Diffuse pleural thickening is defined as fibrosis of the visceral pleura or the visceral and parietal pleura and the subpleural lung parenchyma. It generally develops secondary to asbestos pleuritis (*pleural effusion*) with effusion-induced pleural thickening and may present with or without involvement of the phrenocostal recess as well as with or without calcification.

Asbestos-Related Lung Disease (Asbestosis)

In asbestosis *interstitial pulmonary fibrosis* is usually classified as a pattern of usual interstitial pneumonia with variable severity. Less commonly, a pattern of nonspecific interstitial pneumonia is also seen.[3]

Rounded atelectasis is caused by retractile fibrosis of the visceral pleura due to pleural invagination into the parenchyma.[3]

Imaging Findings

In addition to a verbal description, ILO coding (see ▶Fig. 18.1) and CT classification according to ICOERD (see ▶Fig. 18.2) with a semi-quantitative diagnostic schema can be undertaken.

Discrete Pleural Thickening

Discrete pleural thickening is associated with the following findings on imaging:

- Chest radiography (▶Fig. 18.4):
  - Tangential as circumscribed hump in the region of the lateral chest wall.
  - In en face views seen as cord-like or nodular opacity if there is involvement of the anterior and/or posterior pleura.
  - Diaphragmatic waviness.
  - Calcification facilitates plaque detection, in particular along the pericardium or mediastinal pleura and on the diaphragm.
- *HRCT* (▶Fig. 18.5):
  - Evaluation of aforementioned criteria (density, morphology, location, and distribution).
  - Accurate differentiation between parietal and visceral type.

Diffuse Pleural Thickening

Diffuse pleural thickening (see ▶Fig. 18.3) may exhibit the following features on imaging:

- *Chest radiography:* Hyalinosis complicata (pleural thickening) with or without curved parenchymal bands (so-called "crow's feet"); transition to rounded atelectasis is possible
- *CT:*
  - Diffuse pleural thickening identified on chest radiography according to the ILO classification is not necessarily indicative of visceral pleural thickening as per the CT classification since visceral pleural thickening may also be discrete.
  - Confluent, extensive pleural thickening, usually with a consecutive changes in lung parenchyma.

Interstitial Fibrosis and Rounded Atelectasis

Asbestosis manifests as follows on imaging:

- Chest radiography:
  - Basal and peripheral predominance, usually symmetrical linear and reticular opacities, small irregular opacities according to the ILO classification (s, t, and u; see ▶Fig. 18.4).

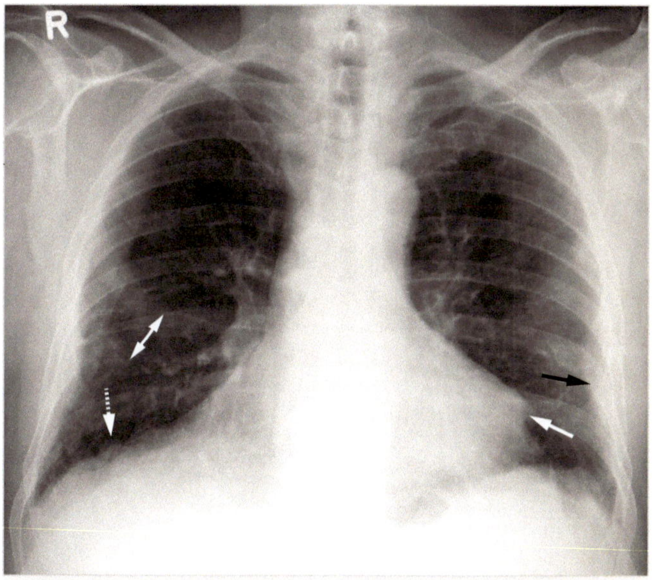

Fig. 18.4 Asbestos-related discrete pleural thickening. Chest radiography. *Black arrow* = tangential area of pleural thickening at the lateral left chest wall. *White arrow* = calcified pleural thickening at the mediastinal pleura. *Double arrow* = calcified pleural thickening of the costal pleura in en face view. *Dashed arrow* = diaphragmatic waviness pointing to noncalcified pleural thickening of the right diaphragmatic pleura.

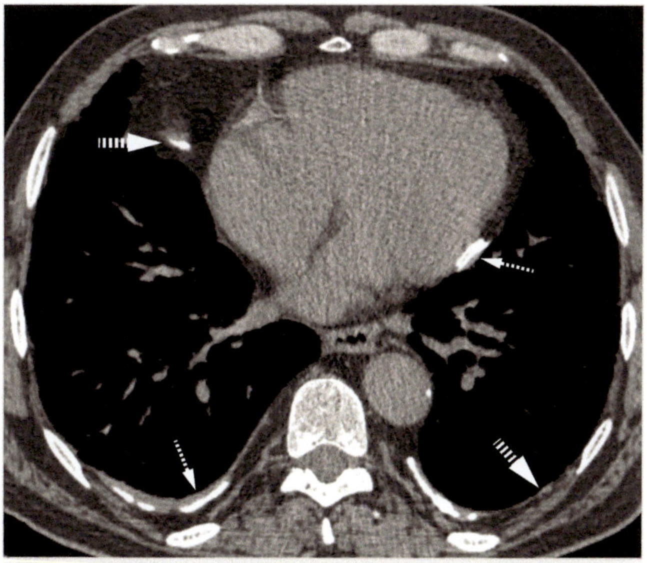

Fig. 18.5 Asbestos-related pleural thickening. CT of the chest, lower zone. *Right thick dashed arrow* = calcification of the right diaphragmatic pleura. *Right thin dashed arrow* = right paravertebral costal pleura with partially calcified pleural thickening—basal to central calcification. *Left thin dashed arrow* = calcification of the left mediastinal pleura. *Left thick dashed arrow* = costal pleura with partially portions of subtotally calcified and noncalcified ("hyaline") thickening.

- Rounded atelectasis, often tumor-like (always in contact with the pleura). CT:
- Early fibrosis: Subpleural dots and subtle branched intralobular opacities as a correlate of peribronchiolar fibrosis (▶ Fig. 18.6).[13]
- Interlobular septal thickening and intralobular lines with subpleural and basal predominance.
- Honeycombing with or without traction bronchiectasis (optional).
- Subpleural curvilinear lines.
- Parenchymal bands (always in contact with the pleura).
- Rounded atelectasis: always in contact with the pleura, distorted bronchovascular bundles in a curvilinear disposition particularly recognizable in multiplanar reformations.

Specific Aspects of Differential Diagnosis

Specific aspects of differential diagnosis *pleural findings*:

- At chest radiography, differential diagnosis of "pleural thickening versus extrapleural fat" and "nodule versus plaque in en face views (lateral plane!)" should be considered.
- Caution: Plaque-shaped pleural thickening is also seen in around 3% of the normal population due to a natural background occurrence of asbestos minerals in the environment.
- Asbestos-related pleural calcification is not usually found in the pleural dome or recesses. Coarsely calcified pleural thickening due to tuberculosis is a relevant differential diagnosis.
- In settings of pleural thickening and rounded atelectasis, differential diagnosis should include all postinflammatory, posttraumatic, or postoperative states; these findings have the lowest specificity for asbestos.
- In talcosis, characteristic asbestos-related pleural findings may also be seen if the talc has a high asbestos content.

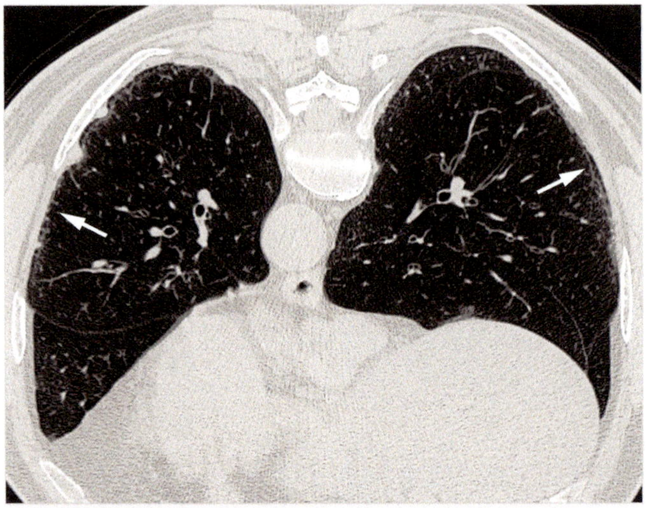

Fig. 18.6 Asbestosis. HRCT of chest in prone position. Subtle bilateral subpleural, intralobular lines in the peripheral interstitium—consistent with early fibrosis with concomitant plaque-shaped pleural thickening. Right arrow lower zone = subpleural dots and fine branched parenchymal opacities (ICOERD: IR [= irregular] – intralobular – U [=lower zone] – grade /profusion: 1). Left arrow lower zone = curvilinear line (ICOERD: symbol SC).

The following findings are significant for differential diagnosis of *lung fibrosis*:

- Idiopathic pulmonary fibrosis also exhibits the pattern of usual interstitial pneumonia. Asbestosis can only be reliably diagnosed in conjunction with the aforementioned pleural findings and a history of asbestos exposure. Curvilinear lines and parenchymal bands are more common in asbestosis than in idiopathic pulmonary fibrosis.[14]
- In siderofibrosis, the fibrosis does not necessarily exhibit the CT pattern of usual interstitial pneumonia.
- In hard metal fibrosis, both the CT pattern of the usual interstitial pneumonia and nonspecific interstitial pneumonia fibrosis are seen.
- In alumininosis, the pattern of usual interstitial pneumonia or of nonspecific interstitial pneumonia may be present.

Note

- A clear conceptual distinction must be made on CT between early fibrosis and the histologically defined minimal asbestosis which cannot be visualized on imaging.[15]
- Fibrosis of the lung parenchyma with no pleural findings has the lowest specificity and can thus, even in settings of asbestos exposure, be a coexisting lung fibrosis of different etiology.
- Pleural plaques which occur most commonly after asbestos exposure have an indicator function.

18.4.2 Silicosis

Silicosis is caused by inhalation of fibrogenic, quartz-containing dust. In the workplace, especially in underground mines, this is usually a mixed dust whose variable quartz percentage can have pathogenetic implications in different work settings. The quartz content can be as high as 80% in coalmines and in the stone industry. Since the dust to which the coalminers are exposed is coal- and quartz-containing mixed dust rather than pure quartz dust, the resulting anthracosilicosis is classified as a separate disease entity known as "coal workers' pneumoconiosis" (CWP); its imaging features are similar to those of silicosis.

The latency for the classical silicosis at low exposure doses is between 10 and 30 years. Shorter exposure to high concentrations of fine-particle silicates gives rise to acute disease courses.[16]

The characteristic pathologic correlate is the nodular granuloma encapsulated by fibrosis that can progress even on termination of exposure, depending on the fibrogenic potential of the silicate. In the course of disease, it may cause characteristic perifocal emphysema. Lymph nodes are affected only if silicate-laden macrophages migrate to the hili and mediastinum.[17]

Types

The following types of silicosis are distinguished:

- Acute silicosis[16]:
  - Rare, e.g., in sandblasters and tunnel workers.
  - Onset within months to a few years with fulminant dyspnea.

- Manifests as silicoproteinosis with intra-alveolar proteinaceous material, histologically similar to pulmonary alveolar proteinosis.
- Accelerated and chronic silicosis:
  - Accelerated silicosis: within 4 to 10 years after high exposure; pathologic and radiologic signs identical to those of the chronic type occur.
  - Chronic silicosis: synonym: classical silicosis.
    - Simple type.
      - No symptoms in early stages and no restricted lung function.
      - In advanced stages, chronic bronchitis and a combination of restrictive and obstructive lung function disorder and impaired gas exchange.
    - Complicated type:
      - Development of bilateral perihilar masslike lesions, the so-called progressive massive fibrosis (defined as fibrotic mass with anthracotic pigmentation).[18]
      - CWP on exposure to coalmine dust and generally smaller quartz content.
- Emphysema and bronchitis:
  - Chronic bronchitis and emphysema in cases with anthracofibrosis.
- *Silicotuberculosis* (including atypical mycobacteriosis):
  - Nowadays, rare complication.
  - Probably due to the toxic effect of quartz dust on the alveolar macrophages.[19]
  - Either exacerbation of existing tuberculosis or new tuberculous colonization with predilection for necrotic consolidations.
- Caplan syndrome:
  - Rare coincidence of rheumatoid arthritis and pneumoconiosis.
  - Probably no causal relationship between the two dise.ases.

Imaging Findings

Acute Silicosis/Silicoproteinosis

The following imaging findings are seen in acute silicosis:

- *Chest radiography*:
  - Bilateral consolidations.
  - Perihilar predominance.
- *HRCT*:
  - Bilateral consolidations and ground-glass opacities.
  - Posterior predominance.
  - Centrilobular, ill-defined nodules with confluence (differential diagnosis versus pulmonary alveolar proteinosis the latter has no nodules).

Chronic, Accelerated, and Coalminer Silicosis

These silicosis types manifest as follows on chest radiography and CT:

- Chest radiography:
  - Simple type:
    - Largely well-defined rounded and oval opacities (according to the ILO classification, small rounded opacities of categories p, q, and r).
    - Partial and complete calcification possible.
    - Predominantly in the posterior portions of the upper and middle zones.
    - Possibly, signs of emphysema.
    - Possibly, calcified hilar and/or mediastinal lymph nodes
  - Complicated type:
    - Perihilar, usually symmetrical consolidations with diameter measuring more than 1 cm (according to the ILO classification, large opacities) due to coalescence of the silicotic nodules.
    - Consolidations may undergo liquefaction due to necrobiosis (differential diagnosis to include silicotuberculosis and lung carcinoma).
    - Consolidations migrate over time toward both the hilum and the periphery.
    - Usually bilateral, rarely unilateral.[19]
- HRCT:
  - Simple form (▶Fig. 18.7):
    - Largely well-defined nodules (less than 1.5 up to 10.0 mm).
    - With little fibrogenic dust (CWP) peribronchiolar, ill-defined small ground-glass nodules (according to ICOERD, $P < 1.5$ mm).[20]
    - Centrilobular location and perilymphatic distribution.
    - Tendency to coalescence (CT classification: symbol ax).
    - Pleural pseudoplaques due to subpleural coalescence.[21]
    - Perifocal emphysema and traction bronchiectasis, in particular in confluent consolidations.
    - Possibly peripherally calcified lymph nodes (eggshell calcification); this is not pathognomonic since it may also be seen in sarcoidosis and berylliosis).[19,20]
    - Lymph node involvement may precede changes to the lung parenchyma, hence this may be the only finding identified.
  - Complicated type:
    - Perihilar, often dumbbell-shaped mass of soft-tissue density (fibrosis) measuring more than 1 cm (see ▶Fig. 18.7).
    - Hilar retraction with emphysema between the hilum and pleura.
    - Usually symmetrical but asymmetrical and unilateral appearance is also possible.
    - Possibly cavity due to ischemic necrosis (see above for differential diagnosis).
    - Calcified or noncalcified lymphadenopathy.

Silicotuberculosis

Tuberculosis must be considered in silicosis if rapidly changing findings and sudden onset cavitation[19] are observed on chest radiography and CT and if additionally nodular, possibly ill-defined opacities are seen on CT, especially in the upper and middle zones.

Specific Aspects of Differential Diagnosis

The following disease entities should be included in differential diagnosis:

- In silicoproteinosis:
  - Subacute hypersensitivity pneumonitis.
  - Siderosis, aluminninosis, hard metal lung disease.
- In silicosis:
  - Sarcoidosis: On CT it may not be possible to reliably differentiate between sarcoidosis and silicosis without an

II

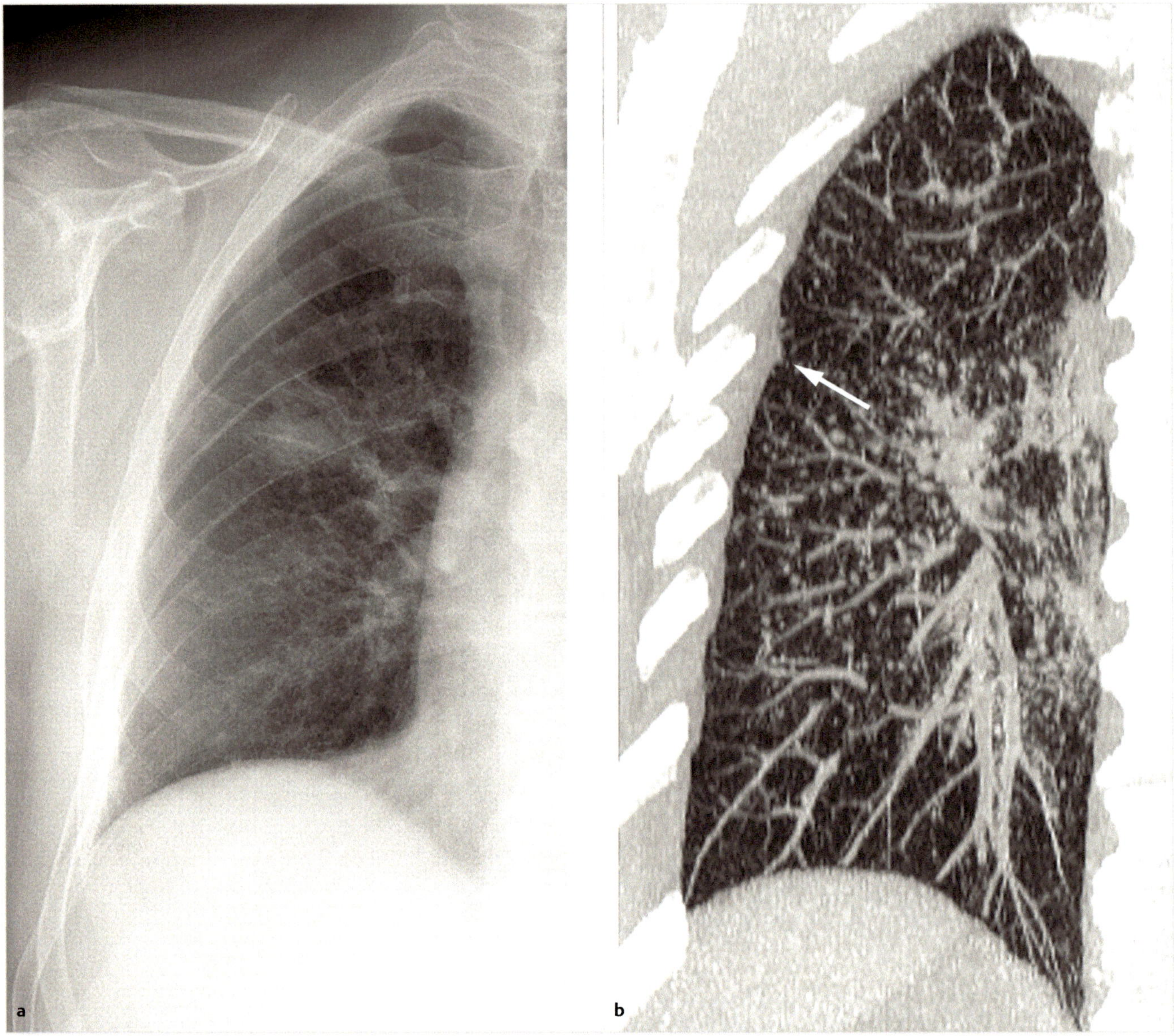

Fig. 18.7 **Silicosis in a stonemason.** In the upper and middle zones, small rounded opacities (ILO: q and ICOERD: Q each predominant) consistent with silicotic granulomas. Additionally, in the perihilar middle zone a large opacity secondary to coalescence with agglomeration and fibrosis (incipient progressive massive fibrosis). Note the perilymphatic distribution of the nodules on CT. Isolated subpleural granulomas—pleural plaques (**b**, *arrow*). **(a)** Magnified section of radiograph. **(b)** CT of right chest, coronal MIP.

exposure history. Calcifications of identical morphology may be seen in association with lymphadenopathy.

- Berylliosis: This cannot be distinguished from sarcoidosis through imaging (caution: including eggshell calcified lymphadenopathy) or histopathology.[3] Unlike silicosis, the nodules are arranged along the bronchovascular bundle (as in sarcoidosis but not also in centrilobular regions like in silicosis) and there is more evidence of interlobular septal thickening, ground-glass opacities but rarely of consolidations.[17]
- Talcosis[22]: The nodules are located in the centrilobular and subpleural regions. Consolidations (if symmetrical and perihilar, differential diagnosis should include progressive massive fibrosis) of high density and lymphadenopathy (correlate of talc deposition). Emphysema tends to exhibit basal predominance.[20]

N!

Note

Nodules predominantly in the upper fields are a characteristic diagnostic imaging pointer in silicosis. MIP reconstructions can help detect these diagnostic indicators at high-resolution CT.

The morphology of the *coal workers' pneumoconiosis* usually seen is not consistent and depends on the dust composition:

- The higher the content of fibrogenic quartz dust, the higher the proportion of classical well-defined silicotic nodules.
- The higher the content of nonfibrogenic dust (e.g., coal), the greater the presence of imaging findings of bronchiolitis.

Diagnosis of silicosis is based on clinical and radiologic criteria in conjunction with a relevant exposure history.

18.4.3 Hypersensitivity Pneumonitis

As per its definition, hypersensitivity pneumonitis is an immune-mediated diffuse, granulomatous diffuse parenchymal lung disease affecting the lung parenchyma and terminal airways. It is triggered by inhalation of organic antigens and of low-molecular-weight chemicals (e.g., isocyanates). Occupational and nonoccupational exposure is often difficult to differentiate.

A distinction is made both clinically and on imaging between overlapping types of acute or subacute and chronic hypersensitivity pneumonitis.

Diagnosis is based on a combination of exposure and occupational history, and possibly restrictive ventilation disorders and/or impaired gas exchange, lymphocytosis in bronchoalveolar lavage, positive allergen tests, and compatible radiographic and CT findings as well as optional lung biopsy.[10]

Acute or Subacute Hypersensitivity Pneumonitis

Imaging Findings

The *acute type* exhibits the following findings on imaging:

- *Chest radiography*: often normal; bilateral consolidations and small rounded opacities.[23]
- *HRCT*: the main findings are diffuse ground-glass opacities and, less commonly, consolidations and ground-glass nodules with basal predominance.[23]

The *subacute type* can be differentiated on imaging from the acute type by means of the following:

- *Chest radiography*: noncharacteristic; subtle nodular to reticulonodular opacities
- *HRCT*: characteristic, with the following findings:
  - Ill-defined small centrilobular ground-glass nodules.
  - Geographic or diffuse ground-glass opacities (▶Fig. 18.8).
  - Sparing of the subpleural space, including at the fissures.
  - Mosaic attenuation pattern (in particular on expiratory scans verifiable air trapping as a sign of concomitant bronchiolitis[20]).
  - Rarely, cysts (of unknown etiology).[24]
  - Reactive lymphadenopathy possible.

18

Specific Aspects of Differential Diagnosis

For subacute hypersensitivity pneumonitis, the following disease entities should be included in differential diagnosis, in particular in terms of occupational diseases:

- *Alumininosis* (early): centrilobular nodules of higher density and predominantly in the upper lobes.[25]

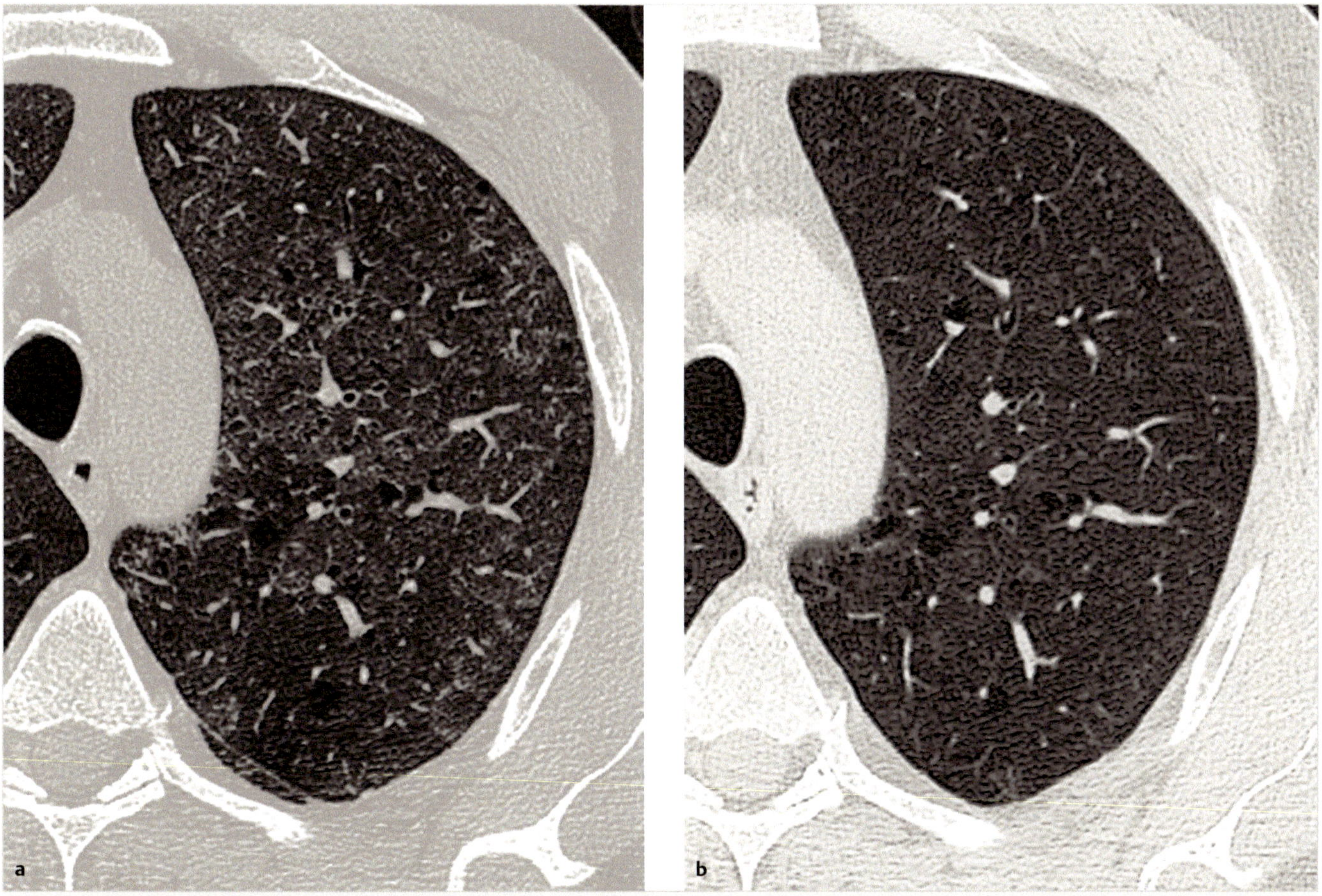

Fig. 18.8 Subacute hypersensitivity pneumonitis in pigeon breeder. HRCT of chest. **(a)** Baseline findings: partially diffuse, partially patchy ground-glass opacities (ICOERD: GGO – grade/profusion 2) and mild centrilobular emphysema. **(b)** Course after 6 months with no allergen exposure: resolution of ground-glass opacities confirms the diagnosis of hypersensitivity pneumonitis.

II

- *Siderosis*: reversible centrilobular ground-glass nodules,[20] branching seen in some cases.
- *Hard metal lung disease* (early stages): ground-glass nodules with basal predominance.
- *Gas intoxication*: chemical pneumonitis due to toxic vapors from chlorine gas and other gases (centrilobular ground-glass nodules, exposure serves as diagnostic pointer[20]).
- *Respiratory bronchiolitis with diffuse parenchymal lung disease*: frequently, co-exposure to cigarette smoke and occupational dust.

Chronic Hypersensitivity Pneumonitis

Imaging Findings

Chronic hypersensitivity pneumonitis manifests as follows on imaging:

- *Chest radiography*: patchy and variable reticular pattern.
- *HRCT*: All signs of fibrosis.
- Peripheral and peribronchial, often fine intralobular lines of no clear predominance, but often less pronounced in basal regions.[26]
- Ground-glass opacities (GGO according to CT classification).
- Traction bronchiectasis.
- Mosaic attenuation pattern and other findings of subacute hypersensitivity pneumonitis such as centrilobular ground-glass nodules.[26]
- Honeycombing in advanced cases.

Specific Aspects of Differential Diagnosis

Differential diagnosis of *chronic hypersensitivity pneumonitis* comprises the following disease entities:

- *Asbestosis*: pleural findings are pathognomonic; basal predominance of fibrosis.
- *Alumininosis* (chronic): fibrosis with peripheral (patterns of usual interstitial pneumonia or nonspecific interstitial pneumonia) or axial distribution (like sarcoidosis).[20]
- *Siderofibrosis*: uncharacteristic signs of fibrosis.[27]
- *Hard metal lung disease* (chronic): all signs of fibrosis as well as consolidations (correlate of intra-alveolar desquamation of giant cells).[20]

> **Note**
>
> Onset of *acute hypersensitivity pneumonitis* is seen around 4 to 6 hours after exposure of sensitized individuals to high antigen levels. Hence, this is rarely seen on imaging.
>
> For the more common *subacute hypersensitivity pneumonitis* triggered by chronic exposure to lower levels of organic antigens, centrilobular ground-glass nodules and geographic or diffuse ground-glass opacities on HRCT are virtually pathognomonic. Less common, predominantly early or acute manifestations of other, including inorganic, dusts may exhibit identical findings on HRCT.
>
> Chronic hypersensitivity pneumonitis presents a diagnostic challenge because of overlapping patterns of usual interstitial pneumonia and nonspecific interstitial pneumonia. Differential diagnosis should include all forms of pneumoconiosis associated with fibrosis.

18.4.4 Occupational Malignant Thoracic Tumors

Asbestos-Related Lung Cancer and Pleural Mesothelioma

Persons exposed to asbestos are at higher risk for development of lung cancer and pleural mesothelioma because of the carcinogenic potential of asbestos fibers (in particular crocidolite, the so-called blue asbestos). Due to the long latency period, a rising incidence is still expected until 2020.

Lung Cancer

Asbestos exposure and concomitant nicotine abuse multiply the risk of lung cancer. Asbestos-related lung cancer does not differ from lung cancers of other etiology on imaging.[28]

The role of diagnostic imaging is to ascertain whether there is any causative link between the lung cancer and the asbestos exposure by identifying asbestosis or asbestos-induced pleural disease on chest radiography or CT. The following findings are suggestive of a probable asbestos-induced etiology of the tumor:

- *Asbestos-related pleural disease*: Table mountain–like, parietal pleural thickening (pleural plaque) has the highest specificity.
- *Asbestosis*: Without concomitant pleural findings, these radiologic images are not specific. Lung fibrosis of different etiology also presents a risk of lung cancer.

Pleural Mesothelioma

At least 80% of all pleural mesotheliomas are attributable to asbestos exposure. Therefore, pleural mesothelioma (▶ Fig. 18.9) is considered a signal tumor of asbestos exposure and is thought to be linked to short-term exposure to high levels. Less commonly, mesotheliomas can also have their origin in the pericardium or peritoneum.

A unilateral pleural effusion is the first disease symptom identified on imaging in 80% of cases. In advanced stages the most salient finding is volume loss on the affected side despite the space-occupying effect of the tumor lining the pleura. This contrasts with pleural carcinosis which usually has a space-occupying effect.

> **Note**
>
> Pleural plaques are not a precancerosis of pleural mesothelioma.

Lung Cancer in Silicosis and/or Silicotuberculosis

Diagnostic imaging of lung cancer in silicosis is challenging because of the preexisting nodular pattern. The implicated tumor may be a mass some distance away from the silicotic changes or a scar carcinoma within the silicotic changes. The pathogenetic link is the carcinogenic potential of quartz dust.

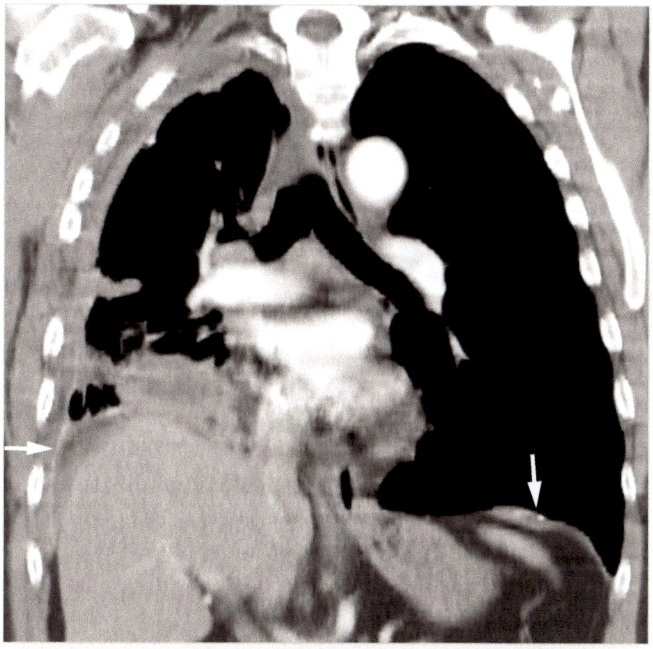

Fig. 18.9 Right pleural mesothelioma. CT, coronal MPR of contrast enhanced tumor. Combination of solid tumor portions with invasion of the minor (horizontal) fissure and mild residual effusion secondary to talc pleurodesis (*right arrow:* talc residues in the right recess → no asbestos-related changes!). On the left, pathognomonic for asbestos exposure, partially calcified thickening of the diaphragmatic pleura (*left arrow*) in the region of the central tendon of diaphragm.

Imaging Indicators of Lung Cancer

In cases of *known underlying disease*, the following findings are suggestive of lung cancer:

- Any sudden new onset nodule, in particular outside the predilection sites for silicosis, for example, in the lower zones (▶ Fig. 18.10).
- Sudden progressive growth of existing nodules and consolidations as well as increasingly blurred margins.
- Newly detected cavities (differential diagnosis versus silicotuberculosis).
- Newly detected, clinically unexplained pleural effusion and on CT an increase in the proportion of noncalcified, enlarged lymph nodes.

In cases of *unknown underlying disease*, the possibility of an occupational disease should be considered when the specific constellation of findings of nodular parenchymal changes and suspected tumor are seen on chest radiography or CT.

Aspects of Differential Diagnosis

Differentiation between (in particular unilateral) progressive massive fibrosis and carcinoma is challenging:

- *Chest radiography*: The lateral border delineating areas of progressive massive fibrosis typically runs parallel to the chest wall, while that of a tumor tends to be more convex arch shaped.
- *CT*: Progressive massive fibrosis has more a retraction than a space-occupying effect.
- *MRI*: Progressive massive fibrosis appears hypointense on T2-weighted images (▶ Fig. 18.11); a high signal on T2-weighted images is suggestive of a lung cancer.[7]

18

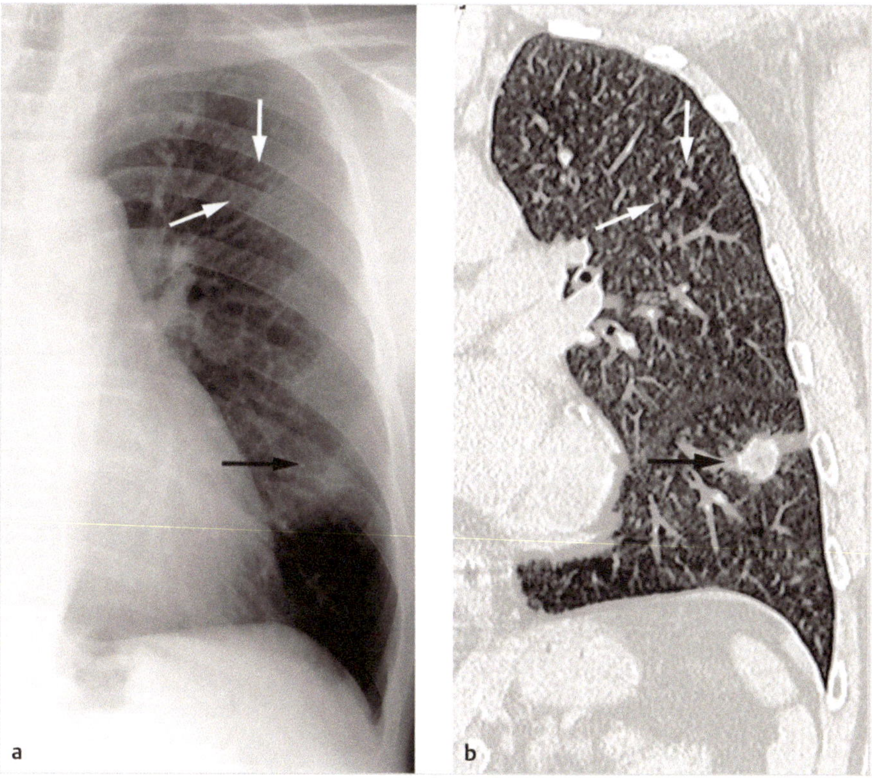

Fig. 18.10 Lung cancer in silicosis. Occupational; quartz-dust exposure from long-term employment in a foundry, 30-year latency of lung cancer. **(a)** Magnified section of radiograph of the left chest. On the radiograph in the upper zone, small rounded opacities of categories q and r with profusion/ grade 1/1 according to the ILO classification (*white arrows*). **(b)** CT according to ICOERD. Small rounded opacities of categories Q and R (*white arrows*). Different nodular opacity in the left lower zone (a, b, *black arrows*), histologically, adenocarcinoma.

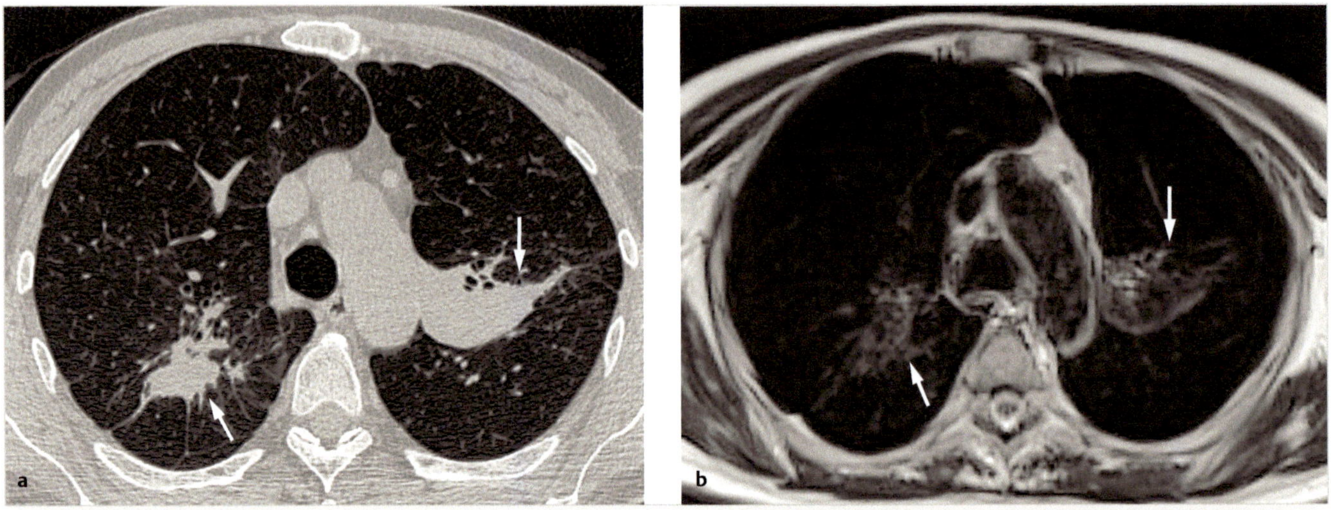

Fig. 18.11 **Silicosis.** Fibrotic consolidations in both upper lobes with retraction and perifocal emphysema. **(a)** CT image. Consolidation, consistent with progressive massive fibrosis (*arrows*), furthermore, small rounded opacities of categories P and Q. **(b)** MRI image. Hypointensity of fibrosis on T2-weighted images (*arrows*).

Note

Rapidly changing imaging findings are signal signs of lung cancer in silicosis. Silicotuberculosis must always be excluded as an alternative diagnosis.

18.5 Summary

Almost half of occupational diseases involve the lung. It is therefore important that radiologists should be conversant with the typical imaging patterns encountered in the lung.

A standardized semi-quantitative schema should be used for reporting of pulmonary occupational diseases. To that effect, the severity of pathologic changes is compared with reference images. The ILO classification form is available for assessment of chest radiographs (see ▸Fig. 18.1).

The term "pneumoconiosis" is used to describe lung diseases caused by inorganic dust, especially asbestos, quartz dust, and quartz-containing mixed dust.

Asbestos-containing dust leads to characteristic pleural changes:

- Bilateral parietal pleural plaques that may become calcified
- Fibrosis and thickening of the visceral pleura
- Lung fibrosis (asbestos-related lung disease or asbestosis; asbestos-induced lung fibrosis without concomitant pleural findings is rare; therefore, imaging cannot prove asbestosis in such cases).

Unilateral pleural findings should also raise the possibility of a cause other than asbestos exposure, e.g., historic tuberculosis or residual findings of pleura empyema or hemothorax.

Silicosis and anthracosilicosis (CWP) present in different forms. Characteristic radiologic findings are as follows:

- Nodular pattern with perilymphatic distribution showing upper and middle zone predominance.
- Bilateral perihilar consolidations or conglomerate tumors (progressive massive fibrosis).

At times it can be almost impossible to differentiate between silicosis and sarcoidosis on imaging.

Hypersensitivity pneumonitisis caused by myriad antigens, often in the occupational setting. The associated disease manifestations are described in detail in Chapter 7.

Acknowledgments

My thanks to Prof. Dr. Thomas Kraus, Faculty of Occupational and Social Medicine at University Hospital, RWTH Aachen, for his cooperation and advice on aspects of occupational medicine. I thank Dr. K.G. Hering for kindly checking the manuscript.

References

[1] International Labour Office. Guidelines for the use of the ILO international classification of radiographs of pneumoconioses. 2000 Aufl. Geneva: International Labour Office; 2002. Available at: http://www.ilo.org/wcmsp5/groups/public/-ed_protect/-protrav/-safework/documents/publication/wcms_108 568.pdf

[2] International Labour Office. Guidelines for the use of the ILO International Classification of Radiographs of Pneumoconioses (OSH 22). 2011 Aufl. Geneva: International Labour Office; 2011. Available at: http://www.ilo.org/wcmsp5/groups/public/-ed_protect/-protrav/-safework/documents/publication/wcms_168260.pdf

[3] Gevenois PA, de Vuyst P, Akira M. Imaging of Occupational and Environmental Disorders of the Chest. Berlin: Springer; 2006

[4] Kusaka Y, Hering KG, Parker JE. International Classification of HRCT for Occupational and Environmental Respiratory Diseases. Tokyo: Springer; 2005

[5] Suganuma N, Kusaka Y, Hering KG, et al. Selection of reference films based on reliability assessment of a classification of high-resolution computed tomography for pneumoconioses. Int Arch Occup Environ Health 2006;79:472–476

[6] Biederer J, Beer M. Hirsch Wet al. MRI of the lung (2/3). Why... when... how? Insights Imaging 2012;3:355–371

[7] Matsumoto S, Mori H, Miyake H, et al. MRI signal characteristics of progressive massive fibrosis in silicosis. Clin Radiol 1998;53:510–514

[8] Horn M, Oechsner M, Gardarsdottir M, et al. Dynamic contrast-enhanced MR imaging for differentiation of rounded atelectasis from neoplasm. J Magn Reson Imaging 2010;31:1364–1370

[9] International Labour Office. Guidelines for the use of the ILO International Classification of Radiographs of Pneumoconioses (OSH 22). 1st ed. International Labour Office, Geneva; 2011

[10] Selman M, Buendía-Roldán I. Immunopathology, diagnosis, and management of hypersensitivity pneumonitis. Semin Respir Crit Care Med 2012;33:543–554
[11] American Thoracic Society. Medical section of the American Lung Association: the diagnosis of nonmalignant diseases related to asbestos. Am Rev Respir Dis 1986;134:363–368
[12] American Thoracic Society. Diagnosis and initial management of nonmalignant diseases related to asbestos. Am J Respir Crit Care Med 2004;170:691–715
[13] Akira M, Yokoyama K, Yamamoto S, et al. Early asbestosis: evaluation with high-resolution CT. Radiology 1991;178:409–416
[14] Akira M, Yamamoto S, Inoue Y, et al. High-resolution CT of asbestosis and idiopathic pulmonary fibrosis. AJR Am J Roentgenol 2003;181:163–169
[15] Craighead JE, Abraham JL, Churg A, et al. The pathology of asbestos-associated diseases of the lungs and pleural cavities: diagnostic criteria and proposed grading schema. Report of the Pneumoconiosis Committee of the College of American Pathologists and the National Institute for Occupational Safety and Health. Arch Pathol Lab Med 1982;106:544–596
[16] Marchiori E, Souza CA, Barbassa TG, et al. Silicoproteinosis: high-resolution CT findings in 13 patients. AJR Am J Roentgenol 2007;189:1402–1406
[17] Sirajuddin A, Kanne JP. Occupational lung disease. J Thorac Imaging 2009;24:310–320
[18] Chong S, Lee KS, Chung MJ, et al. Pneumoconiosis: comparison of imaging and pathologic findings. Radiographics 2006;26:59–77
[19] Kim JS, Lynch DA. Imaging of nonmalignant occupational lung disease. J Thorac Imaging 2002;17:238–260
[20] Akira M. Imaging of occupational and environmental lung diseases. Clin Chest Med 2008;29:117–131
[21] Arakawa H, Honma K, Saito Y, et al. Pleural disease in silicosis: pleural thickening, effusion, and invagination. Radiology 2005;236:685–693
[22] Flors L, Domingo ML, Leiva-Salinas C, et al. Uncommon occupational lung diseases: high-resolution CT findings. AJR Am J Roentgenol 2010;194:W20–W26
[23] Silver SF, Müller NL, Miller RR, et al. Hypersensitivity pneumonitis: evaluation with CT. Radiology 1989;173:441–445
[23] Franquet T, Hansell DM, Senbanjo T, et al. Lung cysts in subacute hypersensitivity pneumonitis. J Comput Assist Tomogr 2003;27:475–478
[24] Kraus T, Schaller KH, Angerer J, et al. Aluminosis – detection of an almost forgotten disease with HRCT. J Occup Med Toxicol 2006;1:b5–b13
[25] Silva CIS, Müller NL, Lynch DA, et al. Chronic hypersensitivity pneumonitis: differentiation from idiopathic pulmonary fibrosis and nonspecific interstitial pneumonia by using thin-section CT. Radiology 2008;246:288–297
[26] Buerke U, Schneider J, Rösler J, et al. Interstitial pulmonary fibrosis after severe exposure to welding fumes. Am J Ind Med 2002;41:259–268
[27] Roberts HC, Patsios DA, Paul NS, et al. Screening for malignant pleural mesothelioma and lung cancer in individuals with a history of asbestos exposure. J Thorac Oncol 2009;4:620–628

Chapter 19

Congenital Thoracic Diseases and Malformations

19 Congenital Thoracic Diseases and Malformations

The lungs, airways, and pulmonary vessels are involved in several developmental anomalies. There is no uniform system for classification of such developmental anomalies. A breakdown into malformations affecting the airways, vascular architecture, or a combination of both has been proposed.[1] The disease entities presented in ▶Table 19.1 are classified according to that system.

19.1 Congenital Lobar Emphysema

Congenital overinflation of a lung lobe is known as congenital lobar emphysema or, more pathogenetically accurate, as congenital lobar overinflation. Frequent causes include abnormal softening of the bronchial cartilage, its complete absence, or external compression of the lobe bronchus (e.g., because of a bronchogenic cyst or pulmonary artery).[2] In almost half of all cases, the disease involves the left upper lobe, followed by the middle lobe.

Three clinical types of congenital lobar emphysema are distinguished[3,4]:

- *Type I*: in infants, the most severe form, causes early respiratory distress.
- *Type II*: in older children, with milder symptoms.
- *Type III*: in adults or older children, asymptomatic incidental finding.

Types II and III are rare.

On imaging, the diseased lobe appears enlarged and hyperlucent (▶Fig. 19.1). If diagnosis is not made during the first month after birth, it may be difficult to distinguish congenital lobar emphysema from Swyer–James syndrome but the latter is not always strictly confined to a single lobe.

19.2 Bronchial Atresia

Bronchial atresia is a rare malformation where the bronchus of a lobe, segment, or subsegment is not fully formed. That implies discrete occlusion of the bronchial lumen.[5] Distal to the atresia, the bronchus may be filled with mucus and dilated. Overinflation of the affected lung regions is markedly less pronounced than in congenital lobar emphysema and is caused by air admitted via collateral ventilation from adjacent lung areas. Bronchial atresia is often asymptomatic and identified only as an incidental finding on imaging. Surgical resection of the diseased lung regions is indicated if it causes recurrent pulmonary infections.

On CT, the occluded bronchus and resultant distal bronchoceles (mucoid impacted, dilated bronchial lumen) can usually be identified[2] (▶Fig. 19.2). These bronchoceles are predominantly found in the upper lobes, in particular in segment 1/2 of the left upper lobe.

19

19.3 Congenital Pulmonary Airway Malformation

Congenital pulmonary airway malformation (CPAM) was previously known as congenital cystic adenomatoid malformation of the lung. The current term is more accurate since only three of the five histologic types of CPAM are of a cystic nature and only one contains adenomatoid components.[6] Depending on the histologic type, it involves developmental anomalies at different levels of the tracheobronchial system ranging from the trachea to major bronchi to the alveolar ducts or distal acini.[2]

Imaging is unable to differentiate the histologic types. Instead, these are classified into three categories based on the cyst size (Table 19.2). The cystic structure of types I and II is routinely identified on CT, but the type III microcystic structure is not. The latter is included in the differential diagnosis of solitary pulmonary nodules and has no pathognomonic radiologic features. The types I and II cysts associated with CPAM can be connected with the bronchial system, in which case they may be purely air filled or contain air–fluid levels (▶Fig. 19.3). They become completely filled with fluid in the absence of bronchial drainage (▶Fig. 19.4). The small-cystic type II, in particular, may occasionally have

Table 19.1 Classification of congenital disease according to affected structures[1,2]

Airways	Vessels	
	Not affected	**Affected**
Not affected	–	• Pulmonary arteriovenous malformation • Pulmonary arterial anomalies • Anomalous pulmonary venous drainage
Affected	• Congenital lobar emphysema • Bronchial atresia • Congenital pulmonary airway malformation (formerly: congenital cystic adenomatoid malformation)	• Pulmonary agenesis, aplasia and hypoplasia • Bronchopulmonary sequestration (intralobar and extralobar) • Scimitar syndrome

abnormal systemic blood supply. In that respect, it is similar to sequestration. These hybrid lesions exhibit radiologic features of both entities (▶ Fig. 19.5).[5]

Often, CPAM constitutes an incidental imaging finding. At times, it becomes symptomatic because of recurrent pulmonary infections or because of its size and space-occupying effect.[2] Elective resection should be considered due to the potential susceptibility to malignant transformation.[7]

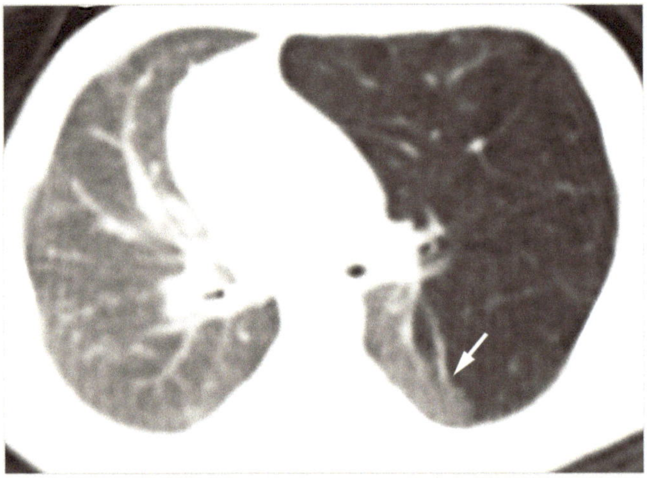

Fig. 19.1 **Congenital lobar emphysema in the left upper lobe of infant.** CT image. Hypodensity and overinflation of the left upper lobe causing mediastinal shift to the right. Normal density of the left lower lobe apex (*arrow*).

19.4 Bronchogenic Cysts

Bronchogenic cysts are caused by an embryonic developmental anomaly of the tracheobronchial tree branching.[2] These are found most commonly in the mediastinal region close to the tracheal bifurcation and are less frequently seen in the lung parenchyma, in the vicinity of the pleura or diaphragm.[8]

Table 19.2 Radiologic types of congenital pulmonary airway malformation[1]

Types	Cyst size	Radiologic features
I	2–10 cm	Large thin-walled cysts
II	0.5–2 cm	Conglomerate of small thin-walled cysts
III	Microcystic	Nodule or mass, of soft-tissue density and smoothly marginated

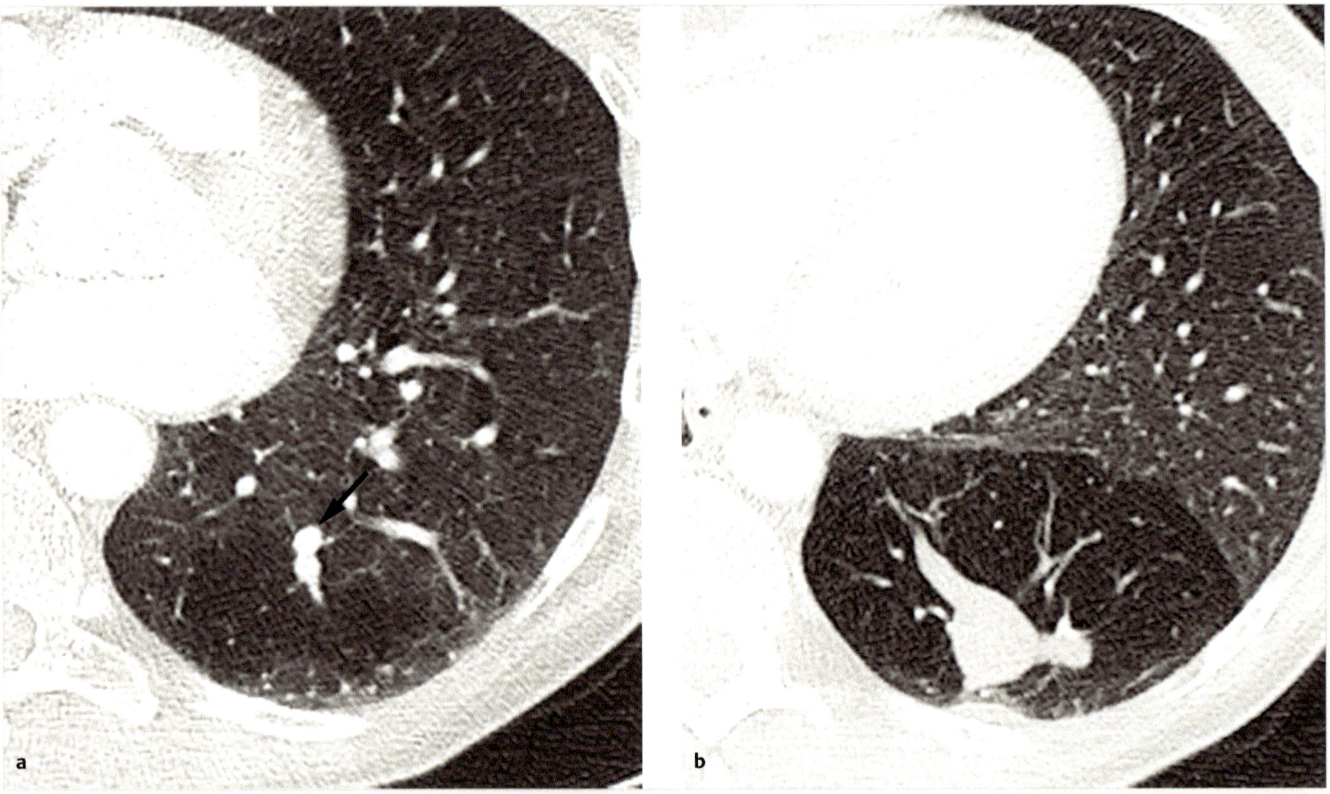

Fig. 19.2 **Bronchial atresia in segment 10, on the left. (a)** CT image at level of bronchial atresia. Absent lumen of left segmental bronchus 10 (*arrow*). **(b)** CT image somewhat more caudal. Mucocele in left segment 10 and overinflation of the affected segment.

Occasionally, the cysts cause recurrent infections; then their resection is indicated.[2] Otherwise, asymptomatic bronchogenic cysts are incidental findings.

On imaging, intrapulmonary bronchogenic cysts manifest as smoothly marginated nodules or masses. Mediastinal cysts appear as smoothly marginated masses in the middle or posterior mediastinum. Because of their protein or lime milk content, the cysts have a density above 0 HU on CT. Likewise on MRI, cysts often exhibit a signal pattern different from that of water (▶Fig. 19.6). On T2-weighted sequences, bronchogenic cysts are hyperintense, while on T1-weighted sequences the signal intensity is determined by the cyst content. On rare occasions, they contain an air–fluid level or are purely air filled.[3,8] The cyst content exhibits no contrast enhancement but infected cysts may have a thick, somewhat irregular, wall showing intense contrast enhancement and an inflammatory reaction of surrounding structures.

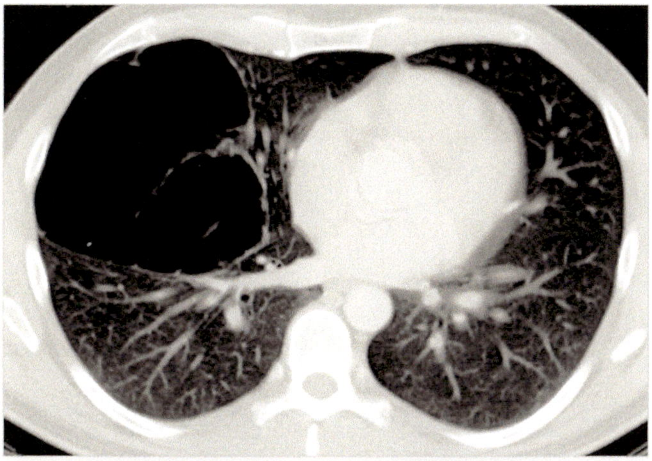

Fig. 19.3 Congenital pulmonary airway malformation, type I. CT image. Large thin-walled cyst in the middle lobe.

Differential diagnosis should include duplication cysts of different genesis (esophageal cysts, neurenteric cysts) as well as CPAMs, in particular types I and II cysts (see above). Infected cysts can grow and develop ill-defined margins, with the risk of confusion with a malignant tumor. The latter has a solid component within the cyst wall.[3]

19.5 Vascular Anomalies

19

19.5.1 Anomalies of the Pulmonary Arteries

Agenesis of a pulmonary artery affects more commonly the right than the left lung. This results in hypoplasia of the respective lung which receives its blood supply exclusively from systemic arteries.[9] There is also increased lung hyperlucency but, unlike in Swyer–James syndrome, no air trapping.[1] The uncommon agenesis of the left pulmonary artery is usually associated with other cardiovascular malformations.

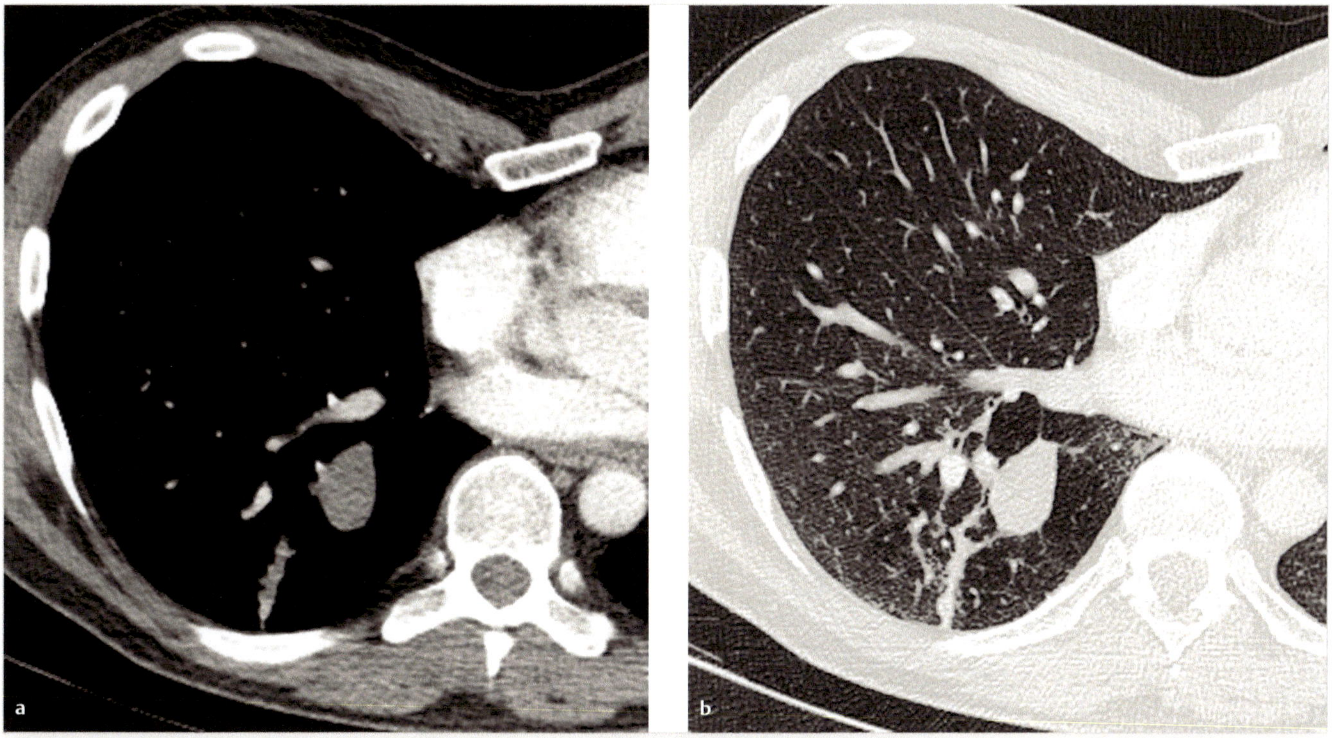

Fig. 19.4 Congenital pulmonary airway malformation type I, in the right lower lobe. CT image. Thin-walled cyst completely filled with fluid. Besides, funnel chest. **(a)** Soft-tissue window. **(b)** Lung window.

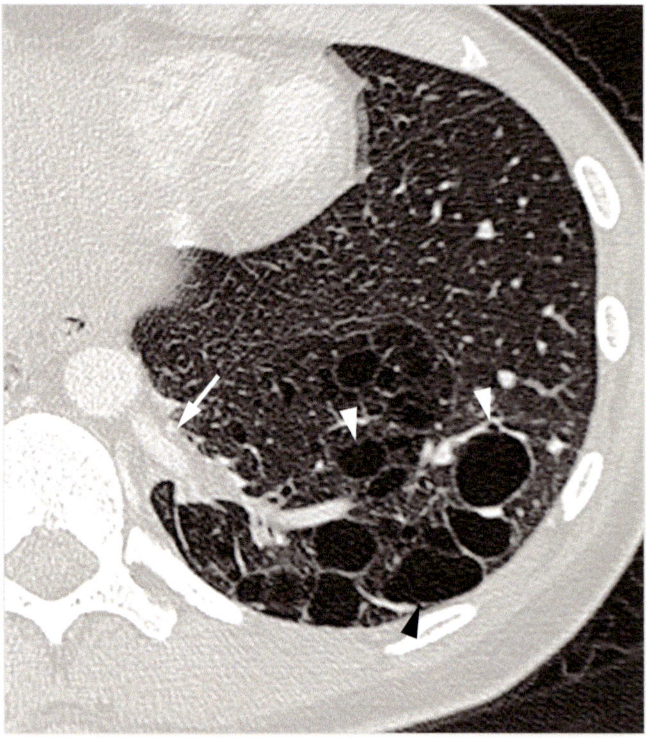

Fig. 19.5 **Hybrid lesion consisting of congenital pulmonary airway malformation type II and sequestration.** CT image. The arterial blood supply is obtained directly from the aorta (*arrow*). Multiple pulmonary cysts in type II congenital pulmonary airway malformation (*arrowheads*).

Often, the *anomalous origin of the left pulmonary artery from the right* becomes symptomatic already during infancy because the aberrant left pulmonary artery runs posteriorly through the retrotracheal space causing external compression of the trachea, major bronchi, or esophagus. Occasionally, it constitutes an incidental finding in asymptomatic adults.

19.5.2 Anomalous Pulmonary Venous Drainage

In anomalous pulmonary venous drainage, the pulmonary venous blood is returned to the systemic veins. *Total anomalous pulmonary venous drainage* requires a right-to-left shunt, for example, via a patent ductus arteriosus or septal defect[1]; otherwise, this malformation is not consistent with life.

Partial anomalous pulmonary venous drainage, which is much more common, predominantly involves the left upper lobe (▶Fig. 19.7). Anomalous drainage is either into the right atrium, superior vena cava, brachiocephalic veins, or infradiaphragmatic veins.[1] The existing left-to-right shunt may continue to be asymptomatic or lead to reduced physical stamina.

19.6 Pulmonary Arteriovenous Malformation

Pulmonary arteriovenous malformation (PAVM) occurs sporadically or, in around half of cases, in association with a syndrome (hereditary hemorrhagic telangiectasias, also known

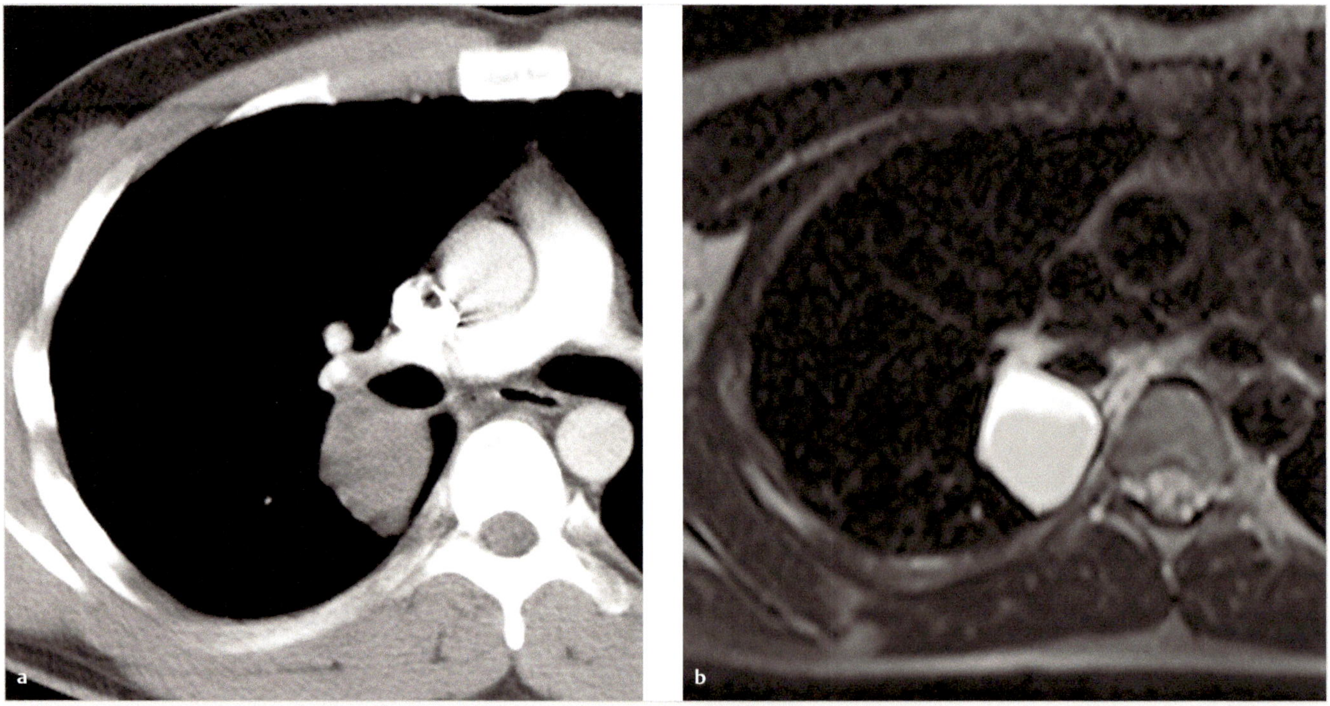

Fig. 19.6 **Bronchogenic cyst posterior to the right mainstem bronchus. (a)** Axial CT image. Smoothly marginated, fluid-isodense nodule. **(b)** Axial T2w MRI image with fat saturation. Smoothly marginated, hyperintense nodule with internal structures.

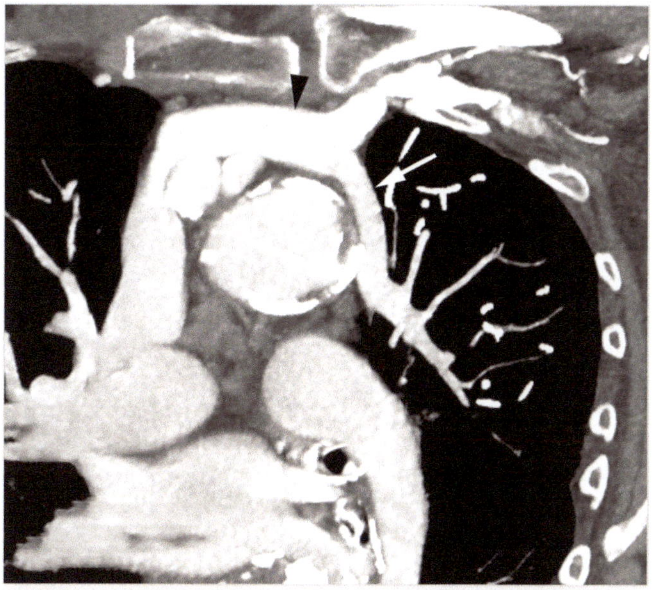

Fig. 19.7 **Partial anomalous pulmonary venous drainage.** CT, paracoronal MIP. Left upper pulmonary vein (*arrow*) draining into left brachiocephalic vein (*arrowhead*). Furthermore, aortic arch aneurysm.

as *Osler–Rendu–Weber*).[1] Multiple PAVM lesions may be seen, especially in Osler–Rendu–Weber disease, and tend to increase in size and number over time.[10]

Chest radiography and CT visualize PAVMs as smoothly marginated, often polycyclic, nodules. They are predominantly found in the middle lobe and lingula. At times, the characteristically dilated supplying and draining vessels can be identified already on radiography. CT reliably demonstrates the findings and allows for definite diagnosis of PAVM (▶ Fig. 19.8).

Treatment is required for a large right-to-left shunt or because of the risk of neurologic complications of paradoxical emboli. The usual treatment procedure is interventional embolization of the PAVM.[10]

19.7 Underdevelopment of the Lung

Complete absence of one lung is termed *agenesis*. In most cases, this is associated with other malformations (patent foramen ovale, patent ductus arteriosus, esophagotracheal fistula, anus imperforatus, spinal segmentation anomalies, extremity malformations). On one side of the thorax, there is no lung tissue, bronchial system, or pulmonary vascular architecture.

As opposed to agenesis, in *aplasia* a short, blind ending mainstem bronchus exists but no lung parenchyma or pulmonary vasculature on the aplastic side.

While in lung *hypoplasia*, the lung parenchyma, associated bronchial system, and pulmonary vasculature are present, they are diminutive (▶ Fig. 19.9). Often, pulmonary hypoplasia occurs secondarily to an extrapulmonary mass (e.g., a large congenital diaphragmatic hernia).

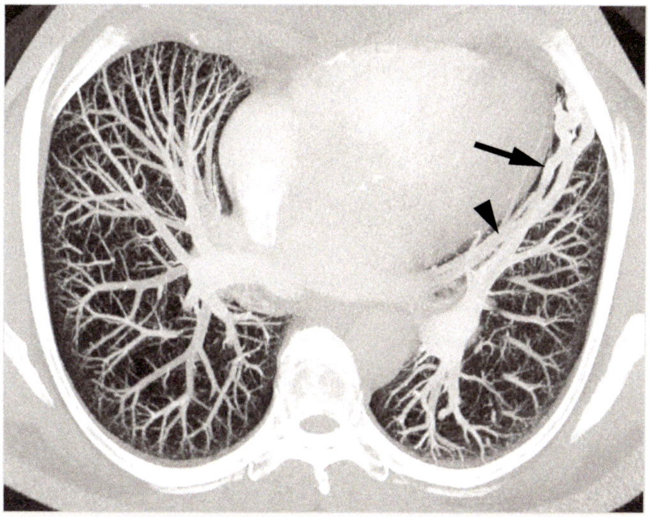

Fig. 19.8 **Pulmonary arteriovenous malformation in the lower lingula segment.** CT, axial MIP. Dilated supplying pulmonary artery (*arrow*) and dilated draining pulmonary vein (*arrowhead*).

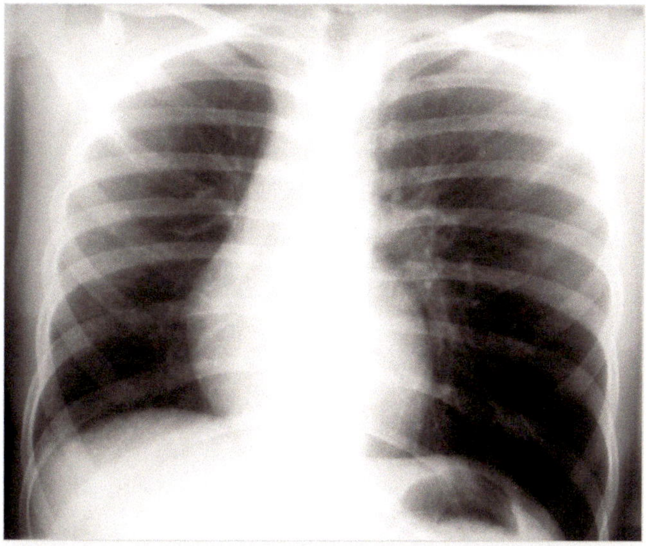

Fig. 19.9 **Hypoplasia of the right lung.** Radiograph. Mediastinal shift to the right and high-riding diaphragm due to right lung volume loss. Rarefaction of the right lung vascular architecture.

19.8 Bronchopulmonary Sequestration

The term "sequestration" refers to lung tissue that is not connected to the bronchial system or the pulmonary artery. The blood supply to the sequestration comes from systemic arteries, usually directly from the thoracic or abdominal aorta. It frequently becomes clinically manifest through recurrent infections. Sequestrations are thought to arise during embryonic development from a supernumerary lung bud.[2,3] Two types are distinguished:

- *Extralobar sequestration*: The sequestration has its own visceral pleural covering and is thus separated from the

19

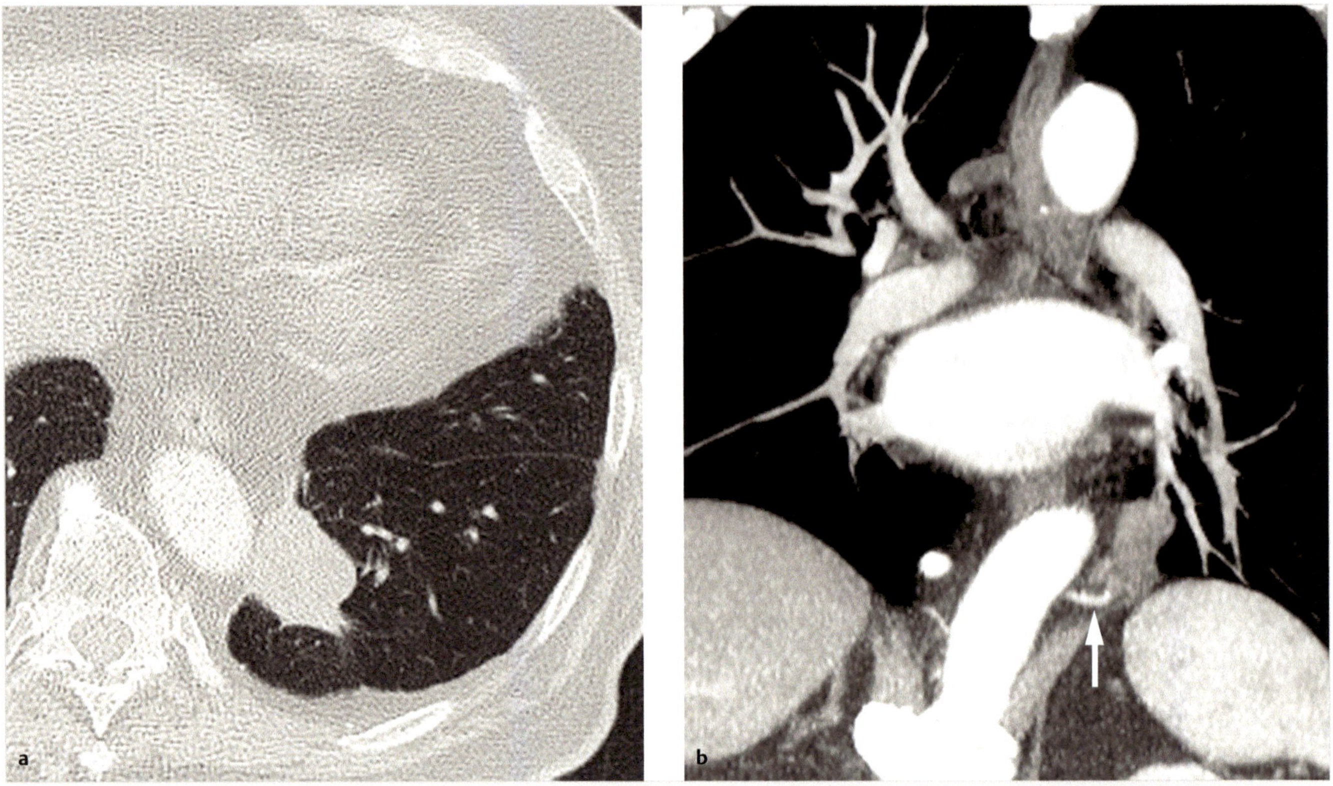

Fig. 19.10 Intralobar bronchopulmonary sequestration in the left lower lobe. CT images. **(a)** Axial lung window: smoothly marginated paramediastinal consolidation in left segment 10. **(b)** Soft-tissue window, coronal MPR: vascular supply to sequester from the aorta (*arrow*).

normal lung tissue. It is usually drained via the systemic veins. Occasionally, this condition is associated with other malformations, e.g., congenital diaphragmatic hernias, cardiac lesions, or pulmonary hypoplasia.[11] Rarely, infradiaphragmatic sequestrations are seen and risk being confused with retroperitoneal masses.[12]

- *Intralobar sequestration*: The sequestration together with the surrounding normal lung tissue is covered by the same visceral pleura. Venous drainage is usually via the pulmonary veins, less commonly via systemic veins.

Imaging demonstrates sequestrations as multiple cysts, soft-tissue density structures (see ▶Fig. 19.5) or overinflated lung tissue, predominantly found in the paramediastinal left lower lobe, especially in segment 10. The supplying artery (often arising directly from the aorta) is often evident on CT (▶Fig. 19.10); in sequestrations of soft-tissue density, this serves as a criterion for differential diagnosis versus type III microcystic CPAM.

19.9 Scimitar Syndrome

Scimitar syndrome is a rare condition that has several synonyms: venolobar syndrome or hypogenetic lung syndrome. In its fully developed form, the following findings are seen[3,13]:

- Venous drainage of part of, or the entire, right lung into a systemic vein, usually the inferior vena cava or the right atrium.
- Hypoplasia of the right lung.
- Right displacement of the heart.
- Hypoplasia or another anomaly of the right pulmonary artery.
- Blood supply to the right lower lobe via systemic arteries, usually from the abdominal aorta.

It almost always occurs on the right side.

The resultant left-to-right shunt may be massive and in such cases the diagnosis is made already in infancy because of the symptoms exhibited. By contrast, a small shunt volume continues to be symptomless for a long time, hence its detection as an incidental imaging finding in adults is not uncommon.[2]

The draining pulmonary vein manifests on chest radiography as a thick right paramediastinal curvilinear structure; it is shaped like an oriental sabre (scimitar). Right lung hypoplasia can also be identified on radiographs. The anomalous vascular supply to the right lung is well visualized on CT.

19.10 Summary

Congenital thoracic diseases are classified as bronchopulmonary anomalies, vascular anomalies, or a combination of both.

Bronchopulmonary Anomalies

The term *congenital lobar emphysema* is used to describe overinflation of a lung lobe because of congenital bronchial stenosis. It most commonly affects the left upper lobe. Imaging shows a hyperlucent lung of increased volume.

In *bronchial atresia*, one—usually segmental or subsegmental—short portion of the bronchus has no lumen. Distal to that occlusion, the usually dilated bronchi are mucus impacted (bronchoceles). The lung parenchyma distal to the bronchial atresia receives air via collateral ventilation; air trapping is often visible. Bronchial atresia occurs predominantly in the upper lobes, in particular in left segment 1/2.

CPAM was formerly known as congenital cystic adenomatoid malformation. It is a malformation originating from the airways. Three different types are distinguished based on the cyst size:

- *Type I*: > 2 cm cysts.
- *Type II*: 0.5–2.0 cm cysts.
- *Type III*: microcysts.

In CPAM, imaging demonstrates cystic structures (filled with air or containing fluid) (type I and II) or a smoothly marginated nodule of soft-tissue density (type III).

Vascular Anomalies

PAVMs occur spontaneously or in association with Osler–Rendu–Weber disease, with the latter often involving multiple lesions. The diagnosis can be made on imaging if one or more well-defined nodules are seen to have a dilated supplying pulmonary artery as well as a likewise dilated draining pulmonary vein.

Agenesis of a pulmonary artery affects more commonly the right than the left lung. Systemic arteries supply the affected hypoplastic lung. If the aberrant left pulmonary artery originates from the right pulmonary artery, it courses retrotracheally and can cause stenosis of the central airways and esophagus.

In order to survive, patients with *total anomalous pulmonary venous drainage* into the venous system require a right-to-left shunt via a septal defect or a patent ductus arteriosus. The left upper lobe is most commonly affected by *partial anomalous pulmonary venous drainage*. Pulmonary venous drainage is either into the systemic veins or right atrium.

Bronchopulmonary sequestration refers to parts of the lung tissue not connected to the bronchial system and pulmonary arterial blood supply. These receive their arterial blood supply via systemic arteries, usually directly from the aorta. An extralobar sequestration has its own visceral pleural covering and is thus anatomically separated from the rest of the lung. Venous drainage is usually via systemic veins. By contrast, the intralobar sequestration is located within the lung, does not have its own pleural covering, and venous drainage is usually via the pulmonary veins. The majority of sequestrations are found in the left posterobasal lower lobe segment. Imaging demonstrates the sequestration as a smoothly marginated consolidation, multiple cysts, or as overinflation of the affected lung parenchyma. The detection of arterial blood supply on CT arising directly from the aorta serves as a diagnostic pointer.

Combined Anomalies

Underdevelopment of the lung is classified as:

- *Agenesis*: The bronchial system is not formed; there are no vessels or lung tissue. Other anomalies are often coexisting.
- *Aplasia*: A rudimentary bronchus with blind ending is present but there are no vessels or lung tissue.
- *Hypoplasia*: The bronchial system, vessels, and lung tissue are present but only in a rudimentary form.

Scimitar syndrome (synonyms: venolobar syndrome, hypogenetic lung syndrome) is a complex vascular and pulmonary malformation. Its name derives from the shape of the aberrant right lower pulmonary vein seen on radiography which typically drains into the inferior vena cava. Aspects of scimitar syndrome include:

- Venous drainage of parts of the right lung into a systemic vein.
- Hypoplasia of the right lung.
- Right displacement of the heart.
- Hypoplasia of the right pulmonary artery.
- Systemic arterial blood supply.

References

[1] Zylak CJ, Eyler WR, Spizarny DL, Stone CH. Developmental lung anomalies in the adult: radiologic-pathologic correlation. Radiographics 2002;22(Spec No):S25–S43

[2] Biyyam DR, Chapman T, Ferguson MR, Deutsch G, Dighe MK. Congenital lung abnormalities: embryologic features, prenatal diagnosis, and postnatal radiologic-pathologic correlation. Radiographics 2010;30(6):1721–1738

[3] Berrocal T, Madrid C, Novo S, Gutiérrez J, Arjonilla A, Gómez-León N. Congenital anomalies of the tracheobronchial tree, lung, and mediastinum: embryology, radiology, and pathology. Radiographics 2004;24(1):e17

[4] Myers NA. Congenital lobar emphysema. Aust N Z J Surg 1960;30:32–35

[5] Langston C. New concepts in the pathology of congenital lung malformations. Semin Pediatr Surg 2003;12(1):17–37

[6] Stocker JT. Congenital pulmonary airway malformation: a new name for and an expanded classification of congenital cystic adenomatoid malformation of the lung. Histopathology 2002;41:424–431

[7] Azizkhan RG, Crombleholme TM. Congenital cystic lung disease: contemporary antenatal and postnatal management. Pediatr Surg Int 2008;24(6):643–657

[8] McAdams HP, Kirejczyk WM, Rosado-de-Christenson ML, Matsumoto S. Bronchogenic cyst: imaging features with clinical and histopathologic correlation. Radiology 2000;217(2):441–446

[9] Castañer E, Gallardo X, Rimola J, et al. Congenital and acquired pulmonary artery anomalies in the adult: radiologic overview. Radiographics 2006;26(2):349–371

[10] Swanson KL, Prakash UB, Stanson AW. Pulmonary arteriovenous fistulas: Mayo Clinic experience, 1982–1997. Mayo Clin Proc 1999;74(7):671–680

[11] Newman B. Congenital bronchopulmonary foregut malformations: concepts and controversies. Pediatr Radiol 2006;36(8):773–791

[12] Lager DJ, Kuper KA, Haake GK. Subdiaphragmatic extralobar pulmonary sequestration. Arch Pathol Lab Med 1991;115(5):536–538

[13] Husain AN, Hessel RG. Neonatal pulmonary hypoplasia: an autopsy study of 25 cases. Pediatr Pathol 1993;13(4):475–484

Chapter 20

Nonvascular Interventions

20 Nonvascular Interventions

Conduct of percutaneous diagnostic and therapeutic interventions in the thorax is long established. These are carried out under the guidance of different imaging modalities (fluoroscopy, ultrasound, CT, including fluoro-CT, and MRI). The choice of modality is determined by the available equipment, location and size of the suspicious lesion, and the radiologist's experience and preferences. These imaging techniques differ considerably in terms of costs, availability, ease of handling and control, and radiation dose (▶Table 20.1).

As for all interventions, three preconditions must be met for interventions in the chest:

- *Indication*: The following sections give a detailed account of the indications for the various techniques.
- *Patient information*: While severe or life-threatening complications are rare in thoracic interventions, they do occur. Therefore, on the day before the intervention by the latest a physician with experience of the proposed intervention should inform the patient about the risks involved and obtain the patient's written informed consent.
- *Appropriate coagulation*: Except for chest wall interventions, hemostasis through manual compression is generally not possible for the chest organs. Functional blood coagulation is therefore paramount. To ensure that this is the case, an in-depth history of blood coagulation must be taken (bleeding events and anticoagulant medication). Interventions should only be carried out if there is no clinical or paraclinical evidence of coagulation disorders or when any such existing disorder has been effectively treated.

20.1 Biopsy

Transthoracic biopsies are performed to harvest tissue samples for histologic or cytologic analysis. There are two techniques available: fine needle aspiration and core biopsy. The first lends itself only to cytological and microbiological analysis, while histologic analysis can only be performed after core biopsy. Accordingly, core biopsy should be conducted for differential diagnosis in cases of suspected lung cancer. Furthermore, novel treatment approaches to lung cancer require molecular genetic analysis of the biopsy specimen; hence, enough tissue must be available.

20.1.1 Indications

Note

Important indications for obtaining tissue specimens (transthoracic biopsy) from a pulmonary or mediastinal pathologic process[1,2]:

- Pulmonary nodule or mass of unclear etiology.
- Suspected malignant pulmonary nodule if no primary surgical treatment is prescribed or minimally invasive surgery is planned (intraoperative confirmation based on frozen section is not possible).
- Nodule in patient with history of malignant tumor, tumor in clinical remission, or multiple primary tumors.
- Residual nodule following radiotherapy or chemotherapy.
- Tissue harvesting for molecular biology tests.
- For pathogen isolation in suspected inflammatory process in immunoincompetent patients.

Other indications may apply in an individual case. Indications should always be based on multidisciplinary consultation.

While tissue sampling of centrally located lesions is a domain of bronchoscopy, lesions in the lung periphery can better be approached with transthoracic biopsy.[3]

20.1.2 Preprocedure Assessment

A safe venous approach is needed to treat any complications arising during the intervention. Provision should be made for pulse oximetry and a control monitor. In principle, sedation compromises the patient's cooperation capability and should therefore be reserved for unavoidable exceptional cases.

Patient positioning will depend on the chosen access route (see below). In general, the prone position confers greatest stability since chest wall breathing movements are minimal. The supine position assures good conditions, too. However, the lateral position is the least stable because even shallow breathing causes maximum chest movements and minimal changes to the patient positioning have major effects.

Table 20.1 Comparison of imaging techniques for guidance of thoracic interventions[1]

Modality	Cost	Availability	Radiation (patient/ physician)	Length of procedure	Access to central lesions	Real-time control	Mobilization of the patient
Ultrasound	+	+++	0	+ +	0	+++	+ + +
Fluoroscopy	+	+++	+ / +	+	+	+++	+ + +
CT	+ +	++	+ + /0	+ + +	+ +	0	+
Fluoro-CT	+ +	++	++/+	+ +	+ + +	++	+ +
MRI	+ + +	+	0	+ + +	+ + +	+	+

II

20.1.3 Technique

A local anesthetic is administered before beginning the intervention, while avoiding puncture of vessels or the pleura; this is assured by means of aspiration while advancing the needle. In addition to the skin, the parietal pleura, which is very sensitive to pain, must be anesthetized.

Biopsy cannulas with a diameter of more than 18 G are more likely to cause bleeding complications than are thinner cannulas. This is particularly true for interventions in the vicinity of major vessels or highly vascularized lesions. To avoid multiple pleural passes with the biopsy needle, a coaxial system is used in principle for pulmonary core biopsies. But caution is advised for lesions with air bronchogram since the use of a coaxial system increases the risk of air embolism.[4]

The risk of vascular injury is the chief determinant of the access route chosen. In particular, the internal thoracic vessels and intercostal arteries must be protected. The number of pleural passes should be kept to a minimum; in particular, needle pass of pulmonary fissures should be avoided. Emphysematous lung areas, especially emphysematous bullae, present a high risk of pneumothorax and should be evaded. For biopsy of mediastinal masses, preference is given to an extrapleural over a transpulmonary access approach.[5] Widening of the mediastinum by injection of several 10 mL of saline solution in the mediastinal fat may establish an extrapleural access in some cases.

The biopsy cannula is inserted into the suspicious lesion under imaging guidance. Due to the risk of false-negative results, the biopsies should be taken from a peripheral region, especially in the case of large nodules with central necrosis. Several core biopsies are obtained from different parts of the lesion by using different angulations during needle insertion.

Imaging is conducted again after removal of the biopsy cannula to rule out complications. If there is evidence of pneumothorax this can be aspirated immediately after the intervention. Postinterventional radiography after a few hours is also indicated for transpleural punctures.

20.1.4 Complications

The complication incidence of fine needle aspiration is similar to that of core biopsy. There is only a loose correlation between onset of pneumothorax and the biopsy cannula gauge. Only the bleeding risk is somewhat higher when using large-gauge cannulas.[4] The typical complications associated with biopsy of chest organs are summarized in ▶Table 20.2.

Table 20.2 Typical complications of transthoracic biopsies[1]

Incidence	Complications
Common	• Pneumothorax (8–60%, requiring chest tube insertion around 5%) • Bleeding (<10%)
Rare	• Infection • Tumor cell seeding along needle track • Air embolism • Death (0.02%)

Pneumothorax is by far the most common complication. But the majority of pneumothoraces do not require any specific treatment. However, placement of a chest tube is indicated in certain cases:

- Large pneumothorax.
- Clinical symptoms related to the pneumothorax, especially new onset dyspnea.
- Persistence or recurrence of pneumothorax after attempted aspiration.

Hemorrhage may be accompanied by hemoptysis and is usually self-limiting.

20.2 Drainage Therapy

Imaging-guided placement of drains is an alternative to their surgical placement and helps enhance effectiveness and safety compared with a blind approach.[1] Aspiration or drainage of pleural, pericardial, intrapulmonary, or mediastinal fluid collections can also be effected under imaging guidance.

20.2.1 Indications

Potential indications are summarized in Table 20.3. An imaging-guided drainage technique is essentially advisable for all intrathoracic fluid collections requiring drainage. However, in many uncomplicated cases, surgical, non-imaging-guided techniques are safe to perform and have few complications. Therefore, the indication should be based on multidisciplinary decision-making, while taking account of the available resources.

20.2.2 Preprocedure Assessment

The preprocedure assessment is similar to that described in Section 20.1. But sedation and analgesia are needed additionally.

Table 20.3 Potential indications for drainage of thoracic fluid collections[1]

Location of fluid collection	Indications
Pleura	• Pleural empyema • Malignant pleural effusion • Hematothorax • Pneumothorax
Lung	• Lung abscess • Pneumatocele
Mediastinum	• Mediastinal abscess • Pericardial effusion • Tension pneumomediastinum • Ectopic pancreatic pseudocysts • Other mediastinal cysts

20.2.3 Technique

The access route is planned while taking into consideration the details outlined in Section 20.1. A sufficiently large puncture incision is required after local anesthesia to permit pass of the drainage catheter through the skin.

Conventional percutaneous drainage catheters consist of a three-component coaxial system:

- External soft pigtail drainage catheter with additional side holes.
- Rigid hollow, metallic obturator for catheter stretching on insertion.
- A sharply polished mandrin that is inserted into the obturator.

There are two alternative procedures for placement of the drainage catheter:

- *Trocar technique*: All three components of the catheter are used. Under imaging guidance, the rigid catheter containing the mandrin is advanced directly into the fluid collection. Next the obturator together with the mandrin is withdrawn and the catheter now assumes its original pigtail shape within the fluid collection.
- *Seldinger technique*: The drainage system comprises only the drainage catheter and obturator; the mandrin is not used. First the fluid collection is punctured with a thin puncture cannula under imaging guidance. Next a rigid guidewire is advanced through the puncture cannula and placed in the fluid collection and then the cannula is withdrawn. If necessary, dilators of increasing diameter are advanced via the in situ guidewire as far as the fluid collection. Now the drainage catheter that has been stretched with the obturator is placed over the guidewire and advanced by means of the obturator far into the fluid collection. Once in the fluid collection, the obturator is withdrawn, and the drainage catheter assumes its original pigtail shape. Finally, obturator and guidewire are completely removed.

The Seldinger technique is suitable for deep lesions of difficult access. By contrast, the trocar technique is quicker and easier to use, and consumes fewer materials.

To finish off, the drainage catheter is secured to the skin with sutures or a suitable adhesive material.

20.2.4 Complications

Compared with the complications discussed in Section 20.1, pneumothorax is less prevalent when placing chest drains since the visceral pleura is usually not breached. Apart from a bleeding risk, there is a higher risk of injury to adjacent organs since relatively large-bore drains are used and the instruments used for drain insertion are rigid. If inflammatory processes, in particular abscesses, are drained, there is a risk of bacteria entering the blood stream and causing sepsis. Patients requiring drainage are usually in a worse general condition than patients undergoing biopsy. Accordingly, drain-related morbidity and mortality are generally higher than for diagnostic punctures.[6,7]

20.3 Thermal Ablation of Lung Tumor

Thermal ablation of lung tumors is a minimally invasive procedure used in oncology to treat lung tumors. Heat or cold is thought to destroy lung tumors. Several different techniques are available (▶Table 20.4).

A common feature of all procedures is CT-controlled percutaneous insertion of an applicator that releases the energy or cold in the region of the tissue to be destroyed. The aim is to trigger necrosis of the tumor and adjacent healthy tissue.

The longest and most extensive experience is available for radiofrequency ablation. Proximity to major vessels or impedance problems may result in delivery of inadequate amounts of energy to the tumor tissue.[10] Local recurrences may present because of incomplete tumor ablation. The experiences hitherto with microwave ablation suggest that the latter might be associated with better local tumor control rates.[10,11] So far, only limited data are available on other tumor ablation procedures such as laser-induced thermal therapy[12,13] and cryoablation.[14]

20

20.3.1 Indications

Note

Indications for thermal ablation of lung tumors should always be based on multidisciplinary consultation. This gives a picture of the patient's overall cancer status and potential treatment alternatives can be considered.

Thermal ablation is performed for small primary lung cancers in functionally inoperable patients; this procedure competes with the well-established radiotherapy with curative intent. Thermal ablation may be indicated, in particular, for postradiotherapy local recurrence or in settings of restricted lung function and limited tolerance of any radiation pneumonitis, e.g., following contralateral pneumonectomy (▶Fig. 20.1).

Table 20.4 Technical procedures and their principle of action for local ablation of lung tumors[8,9]

Procedure	Principle of action
Radiofrequency ablation	High-frequency alternating current (375–500 kHz)
Microwave ablation	Electromagnetic radiation (0.9–2.5 GHz)
Laser-induced thermal therapy	Nd:YAG laser (1,064 nm) or diode laser (820 nm)
Cryoablation	Cooling agent: argon or helium, –40°C

In certain oncology settings, local treatment of lung metastases from extrapulmonary primary tumors may appear advisable. Here, thermal ablation is seen as an adjunct to surgical resection. Clinical influence factors that favor thermal ablation over surgery are as follows[8]:

- Surgery refusal by the patient.
- Restricted lung function (FEV1 below 40%, diffusion capacity below 40%).
- Cardiac comorbidity (NYHA III, restricted cardiac function).
- Multiple comorbidities.
- Status post partial lung resection.
- Status post contralateral pneumonectomy.
- Status post pleurodesis.
- Status post thoracic radiotherapy.

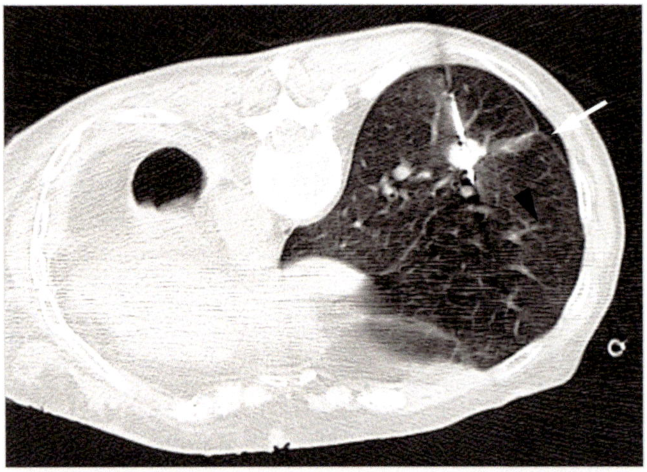

Fig. 20.1 **Microwave ablation of a lung carcinoma following contralateral pneumonectomy.** CT image. Microwave antenna placed within tumor. Small lateral pneumothorax (*arrow*) following prophylactic insertion of chest drain for risk minimization.

20.3.2 Technique

This intervention is conducted under general anesthesia or under conscious sedation.[15,16] The main advantage of general anesthesia is that in principle it allows better control of any arising complications. Peri-interventional antibiotic prophylaxis has been recommended[17,18] but is not always used.[9]

The principles described in Section 20.1 apply with regard to the choice of access approach for the ablation probe. The extent of the necrotic zone expected must be taken into account when planning the intervention. Injury to important structures must be avoided, e.g., the phrenic nerve, during ablation of paramediastinal tumors. To minimize the risk of local recurrence, the necrotic zone should extend by at least several millimeters beyond the tumor. Access route ablation can also be performed when removing the ablation probe to prevent tumor cell seeding in the probe access tract.

Immediate postinterventional CT usually visualizes only subtle ground-glass opacities surrounding the tumor and reflecting the necrotic zone. Demarcation of the necrotic zone bounded by an area of linear opacity is seen within a few days (▶Fig. 20.2). This is later usually followed by a consolidation covering the entire necrotic zone, persisting and then gradually shrinking over the course of months. Any increase noted in this consolidation after weeks or months is suggestive of local recurrence.

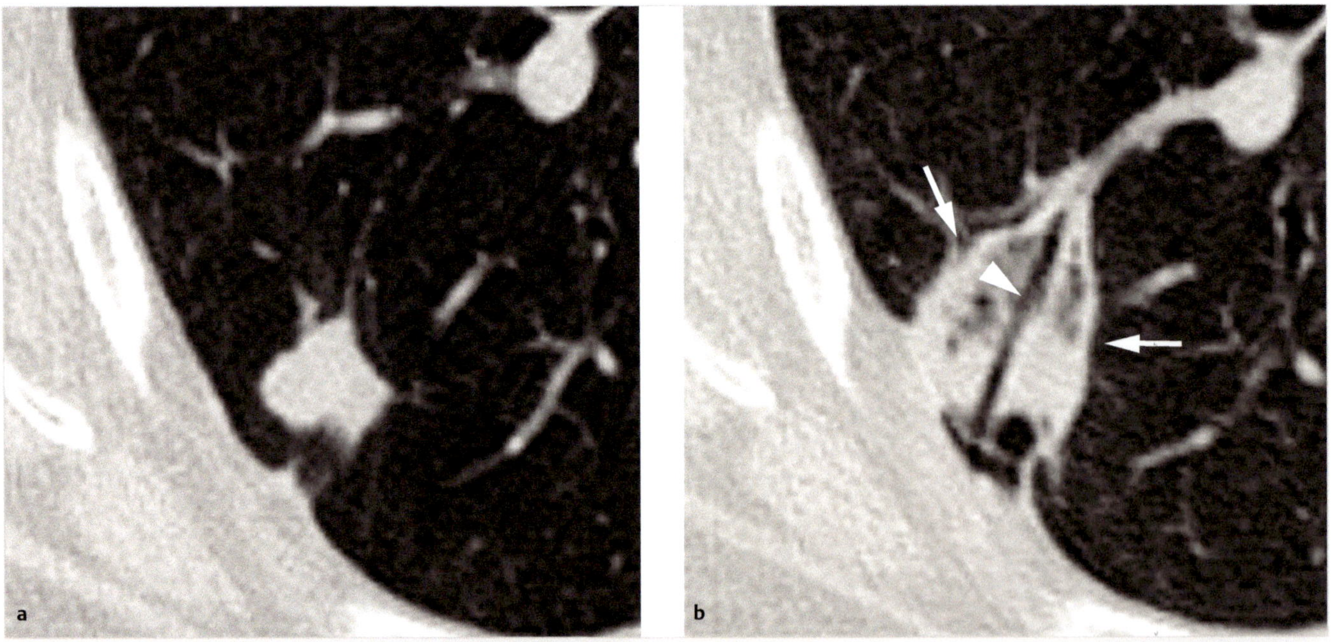

Fig. 20.2 **Postablation course following microwave ablation of lung metastasis.** CT images. **(a)** Preinterventional. **(b)** Postinterventional week 6: the metastasis is surrounded on all sides by a sharply demarcated necrotic zone (*arrows*). The microwave antenna needle track can still be identified within the coagulation necrosis (*arrowhead*).

20.3.3 Complications

Note

Complications of lung tumor thermal ablation of[9]:

- Pneumothorax (40% of cases, requiring chest tube in 10% of cases).
- Hemorrhage (8% of cases, of these 4% with hemoptysis).
- Pleural effusion (2–7%).
- Pleuritic pain.
- Fever.
- Infection (abscess, pneumonia).
- Tumor cavitation.
- Pneumatocele.
- Chest wall or mediastinal emphysema.
- Tumor cell propagation.
- Skin burns (in radiofrequency ablation).
- Neurological deficits (intercostal nerves, phrenic nerve, recurrent laryngeal nerve).
- Air embolism.

Pneumothorax is the most common complication of lung tumor thermal ablation. Despite the large gauge ablation probes (around 13–15 G), it hardly occurs more often than in transthoracic lung biopsies. The same applies for the pneumothorax requiring chest tube insertion.

Hemorrhage is usually self-limiting but bronchoscopic removal of the endobronchial coagula may be required to prevent atelectasis. Cavitation of the ablated tumor is not, strictly speaking, a complication; rather, it is a treatment effect but can develop into a pneumatocele. Slight to moderate postinterventional pain may persist for a few days, in particular after ablation of tumors close to the parietal pleura. This pain can be well controlled with nonsteroidal anti-inflammatories.

References

[1] Ghaye B, Dondelinger RF. Imaging guided thoracic interventions. Eur Respir J 2001;17(3):507–528

[2] Klein JS, Zarka MA. Transthoracic needle biopsy: an overview. J Thorac Imaging 1997;12(4):232–249

[3] National Institute for Health and Care Excellence (NICE) Guideline. Lung Cancer: Diagnosis and Management. Clinical guideline [NG122]. March 2019

[4] Lal H, Neyaz Z, Nath A, Borah S. CT-guided percutaneous biopsy of intrathoracic lesions. Korean J Radiol 2012;13(2):210–226

[5] Gupta S, Seaberg K, Wallace MJ, et al. Imaging-guided percutaneous biopsy of mediastinal lesions: different approaches and anatomic considerations. Radiographics 2005;25(3):763–786, discussion 786–788

[6] Kabukcu M, Demircioglu F, Yanik E, Basarici I, Ersel F. Pericardial tamponade and large pericardial effusions: causal factors and efficacy of percutaneous catheter drainage in 50 patients. Tex Heart Inst J 2004;31(4):398–403

[7] vanSonnenberg E, D'Agostino HB, Casola G, Wittich GR, Varney RR, Harker C. Lung abscess: CT-guided drainage. Radiology 1991;178(2):347–351

[8] Schneider T, Heussel CP, Herth FJF, Dienemann H. Thermal ablation of malignant lung tumors. Dtsch Arztebl Int 2013;110(22):394–400

[9] Steinke K. Radiofrequency ablation of pulmonary tumours: current status. Cancer Imaging 2008;8:27–35

[10] de Baere T, Farouil G, Deschamps F. Lung cancer ablation: what is the evidence? Semin Intervent Radiol 2013;30(2):151–156

[11] Smith SL, Jennings PE. Lung radiofrequency and microwave ablation: a review of indications, techniques and post-procedural imaging appearances. Br J Radiol 2015;88(1046):20140598

[12] Hosten N, Stier A, Weigel C, et al. Laser-induced thermotherapy (LITT) of lung metastases: description of a miniaturized applicator, optimization, and initial treatment of patients [in German]. RoFo Fortschr Geb Rontgenstr Nuklearmed 2003;175(3):393–400

[13] Vogl TJ, Straub R, Lehnert T, et al. Percutaneous thermoablation of pulmonary metastases. Experience with the application of laser-induced thermotherapy (LITT) and radiofrequency ablation (RFA), and a literature review [in German]. RoFo Fortschr Geb Rontgenstr Nuklearmed 2004;176(11):1658–1666

[14] Hinshaw JL, Lee FT Jr, Laeseke PF, Sampson LA, Brace C. Temperature isotherms during pulmonary cryoablation and their correlation with the zone of ablation. J Vasc Interv Radiol 2010;21(9):1424–1428

[15] Bargellini I, Bozzi E, Cioni R, Parentini B, Bartolozzi C. Radiofrequency ablation of lung tumours. Insights Imaging 2011;2(5):567–576

[16] Hoffmann RT, Jakobs TF, Lubienski A, et al. Percutaneous radiofrequency ablation of pulmonary tumors--is there a difference between treatment under general anaesthesia and under conscious sedation? Eur J Radiol 2006;59(2):168–174

[17] Gadaleta C, Mattioli V, Colucci G, et al. Radiofrequency ablation of 40 lung neoplasms: preliminary results. AJR Am J Roentgenol 2004;183(2):361–368

[18] Lee JM, Jin GY, Goldberg SN, et al. Percutaneous radiofrequency ablation for inoperable non-small cell lung cancer and metastases: preliminary report. Radiology 2004;230(1):125–134

Part III

Differential Diagnostic Considerations and Incidental Findings

III

Chapter 21

Pulmonary Nodules

21 Pulmonary Nodules

21.1 Solitary Nodule

By definition, a pulmonary nodule is a rounded opacity in the lung parenchyma measuring up to 3 cm. It is surrounded by aerated lung parenchyma and is smoothly marginated, with no adjacent atelectasis or associated lymphadenopathy.[1] This presents a common diagnostic dilemma in the clinical setting.

A large variety of benign and malignant diseases cause pulmonary nodules. ▶Table 21.1 gives an overview of the histologic entities that can manifest as a pulmonary nodule.

21.1.1 Differential Diagnosis

In the vast majority of cases, the radiographic or CT morphology of nodules is not pathognomonic for a particular histologic entity. There are only a few imaging findings that permit a definitive diagnosis of a nodule. For example, detection of fat inside the nodule on CT or of characteristic popcorn-like calcification in a sharply marginated nodule is pathognomonic for a hamartoma (▶Fig. 21.1).

The main focus of differential diagnosis is on distinguishing between the benignity and malignancy of a nodule.

N!

Note

Radiologic criteria of benignity of solid pulmonary nodules:

- At least 2-year stability.
- Fat detection.
- Detection of a benign calcification pattern:
  - Homogeneous calcification.
  - Central calcification.
  - Lamellar calcification.
  - Popcorn-like calcification.

Evidence of at least 2-year *stability* is deemed proof of the benignity of a solid nodule. This is often demonstrated on the basis of previous images in which the finding (possibly only retrospectively) appears identical.

On CT, fat and popcorn-like *calcification* are found in hamartomas, while the other benign calcification patterns are seen, in particular, in inflammatory residual findings (see ▶Fig. 21.1). All other calcification types, especially eccentric and amorphous types, are also found in malignant tumors (▶Fig. 21.2).

Growth detection is the best noninvasive predictor of malignancy. Volumetry with special software lends itself better than manual determination of the nodule diameter[3,4,5] for detection of pulmonary nodule growth. Thin-slice CT datasets are needed to that effect. Based on the tumor volume, the nodule doubling time can be determined using the modified Schwartz formula.[6,7] The following doubling time is calculated from the baseline volume and the volume on follow-up:

$$VDT = \frac{t \cdot \log 2}{\log\left(\frac{V_t}{V_0}\right)}$$

Table 21.1 Disease entities that can manifest as solitary pulmonary nodule[2]

Disease entities	Examples
Tumors:	
• Malignant tumors	• Lung cancer • Carcinoid • Metastasis • Lung sarcoma • Kaposi sarcoma • Hodgkin disease • Non-Hodgkin lymphoma • Malignant fibrous histiocytoma
• Benign tumors	• Hamartochondroma • Bronchial adenoma • Cylindroma • Papilloma • Fibroma • Leiomyoma • Lipoma • Neurogenic tumors • Inflammatory pseudotumor
Inflammatory processes	• Tuberculoma • Chronic pneumonia • Abscess • Septic embolism • Lipoid pneumonia • Echinococcus cyst • Aspergillosis (invasive or aspergilloma) • Histoplasmosis • Other mycoses • Rheumatoid nodules • Progressive massive fibrosis
Other	• Endometriosis • Sequestration • Pulmonary arterial aneurysm • Arteriovenous malformation • Type III congenital pulmonary airway malformation (formerly congenital cystic adenomatoid malformation) • Pulmonary varicose veins • Pulmonary infarction • Pulmonary hematoma • Rounded atelectasis • Interlobar effusion • Bronchogenic cyst • Bronchial atresia (mucocele) • Amyloidosis • Eosinophilic granuloma

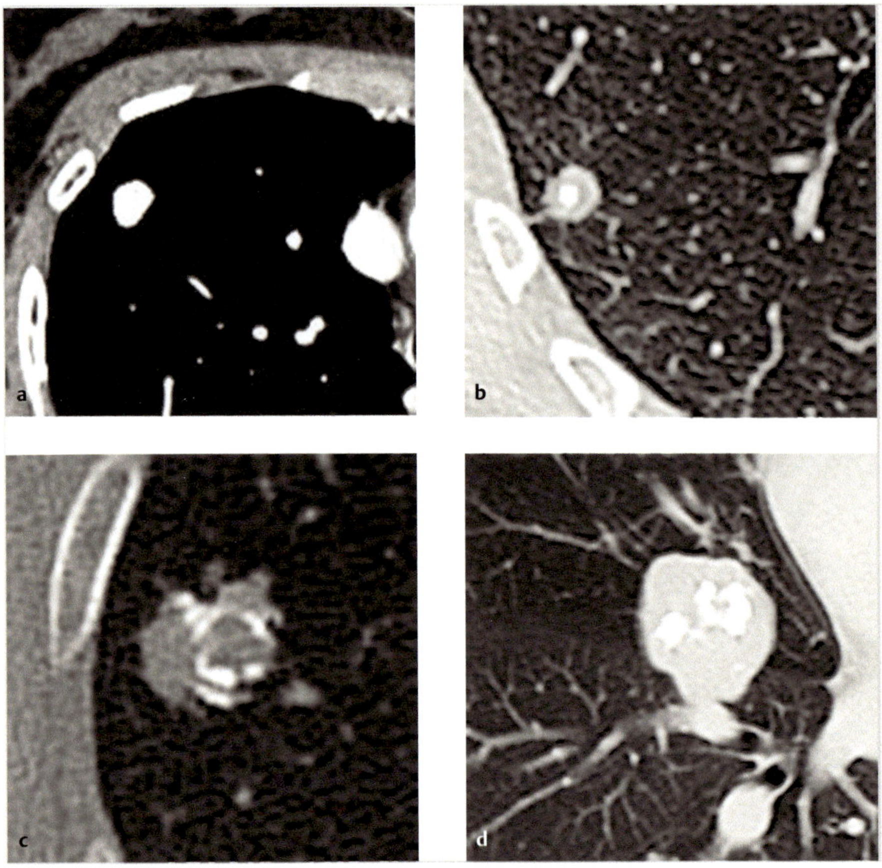

Fig. 21.1 Benign calcification patterns in nodules. (a) Homogeneous calcification. **(b)** Central calcification. **(c)** Lamellar calcification. **(d)** Popcorn-like calcification.

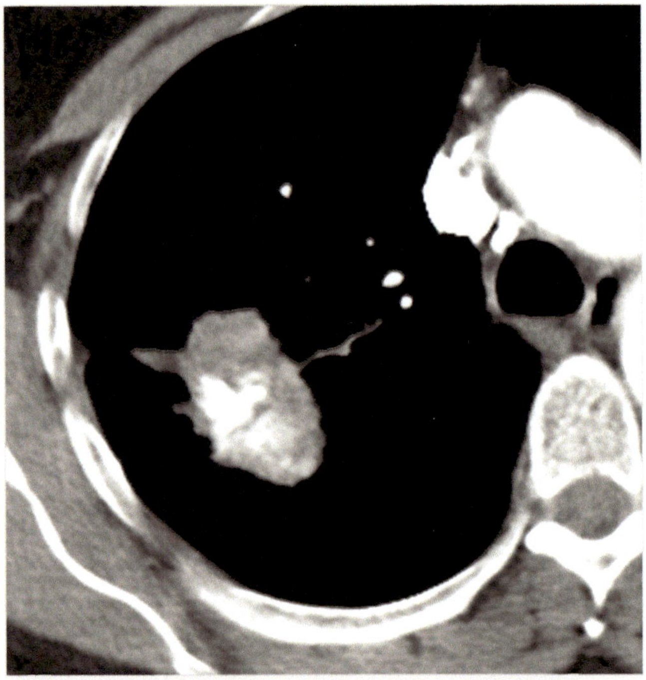

Fig. 21.2 Amorphous calcification in a small cell lung cancer.

where

VDT	= volume doubling time of tumor
t	= time between baseline volume determination and follow-up
V_0	= baseline tumor volume
V_t	= tumor volume on follow-up

Many volumetry systems automatically calculate the tumor doubling time from the nodule volumes measured. In general, volume doubling times of between 20 and 400 days are considered to be suspicious for malignancy. There have also been reports of rare cases of lung cancers with extremely short (7 days) but likewise very long doubling time (4.5 years).[8,9,10,11]

Dynamic contrast CT and PET-CT are two other imaging modalities used in this field, with both able to visualize *functional parameters* (vascularization and glucose uptake) of the nodule. The advantage of contrast dynamic CT is its high negative predictive value (96%). Absence of contrast enhancement of the nodule—or analogously absence or only minimal glucose uptake (SUV [standard uptake value] of less than 2.5) on PET—means that malignancy is very unlikely. Both modalities are suitable for nodules measuring more than 8 mm.

21.1.2 Management

Nodules identified as incidental findings on chest radiography often measure more than 1 cm and should be further investigated since they are viewed as potentially malignant until proven otherwise.[12] In general, CT is the next diagnostic modality indicated, with two exceptions that need no further investigation:

- If previous images show at least 2-year nodule stability.
- If an extrapulmonary location of the nodule is suspected (e.g., mammillary shadows or rib osteoma; this can be further explored on chest radiography using mammilla markings or rotational fluoroscopy, thus with markedly lower radiation exposure than on CT). CT is often able to visualize small, incidentally detected, nodules not found

on chest radiography or only identifiable retrospectively in relation to the CT findings. Several lung cancer screening studies with low-dose CT have already produced extensive data on the potential malignancy of incidentally detected nodules. At least one nodule was identified on CT in up to two-thirds of all study participants at high risk for lung carcinoma. The majority of these nodules were very small. In all studies, more than 95% of these pulmonary nodules proved to be benign.

N!

Note

The diagnostic dilemma posed by a small nodule derives from the fact that, while it is the most common presentation of early lung cancer, it is also an extremely widespread but only rarely malignant incidental finding.

Growth exclusion is a good predictor of nodule benignity. Two-year stability of solid pulmonary nodules (of soft-tissue density) is generally accepted as a benignity criterion. Subsolid nodules can prove to be a slowly growing adenocarcinoma even after 2-year stability and therefore must be followed up beyond that period up to 5 years.[13]

Management of pulmonary nodules depends on their likelihood of malignancy and the expected growth pattern. Because the latter differs between solid and subsolid nodules, recommendations vary dependent on nodule attenuation as described below.

Several recommendations for management of incidental pulmonary nodules have been published, starting with the first recommendation for management of solid nodules of the Fleischner Society in 2005,[14] followed by a recommendation for management of subsolid nodules in 2013.[15] The newest recommendation from 2017 includes recommendations for solid and subsolid nodules and will be presented in more detail below.[13]

Solid Nodules

If the benignity of a nodule can be demonstrated on the basis of the listed criteria, there is no need for further measures. In all other cases, the choice of further procedure will depend on the nodule size and presence of risk factors.

N!

Note

Risk factors for malignancy of a pulmonary nodule[14,16]:

- History of smoking (smoker, current or during the previous 10 years, passive smoker).
- History of known malignant tumor.
- Family history of lung cancer.
- Chronic obstructive pulmonary disease.
- Lung fibrosis.
- Inhalation exposure to:
  - Asbestos.
  - Quartz.
  - Cadmium.
  - Arsenic.
  - Beryllium.
  - Nickel.
  - Chromium.
  - Polycyclic aromatic hydrocarbons.
  - Radioactive substances such as uranium or radon.

▸Table 21.2 lists the recommended procedure for nodules measuring less than 8 mm in relation to diameter size and risk of malignancy[13]:

- Nodules with a mean diameter (average of longest diameter and diameter perpendicular to the longest diameter, rounded to the nearest full millimeter) of less than 6 mm in patients with no risk factors have such a low risk of malignancy that no further investigation or follow-up is recommended. In persons with known risk factors or if the nodule looks morphologically suspicious, a 12-month follow-up CT scan can be performed.
- If a decrease in the size of a nodule has been observed during follow-up or the nodule disappears completely, follow-up is no longer required. Nodule benignity is just about proven.
- If there is evidence of nodule stability, follow-up is advisable at variable intervals tailored to the individual risk.
- Progressive growth of a nodule during follow-up is suggestive of malignancy and normally needs further investigation (histologic confirmation).

Nodules measuring more than 8 mm have a markedly higher risk of malignancy than smaller pulmonary. Hence, further

21

Table 21.2 Recommendations for CT follow-up intervals and management of solid pulmonary nodules that do not meet benignity criteria depending on mean nodule diameter (average of long and short axis, rounded to the nearest millimeter) or nodule volume[13]

Nodule type	Risk	<6 mm (<100 mm³)	6–8 mm (100–250 mm³)	>8 mm (>250 mm³)
Single	Low	No routine follow-up	6–12 months, consider 18–24 months	3 months or PET or tissue sampling
	High	Optional 12 months	6–2 months, 18–24 months	3 months or PET or tissue sampling
Multiple	Low	No routine follow-up	3–6 months, consider 18–24 months	
	High	Optional 12 months	3–6 months, 18–24 months	

Note: High risk: at least one risk factor (see above); low risk: no such known risk factor.

diagnostic work-up should be considered. A multidisciplinary decision on necessary diagnostic measures is recommended, with pneumonologists and thoracic surgeons taking into consideration the aspects listed in ▶Table 21.3. There is no need for further invasive investigation if malignancy appears unlikely in the context of the described morphology criteria. This may also apply in the individual case if PET or contrast dynamic CT yield a negative result.

In principle, patients with equivocal or suspicious nodules measuring more than 8 mm should be referred to a specialist center where radiologists, pneumologists, thoracic surgeons, and radiotherapists can take a multidisciplinary decision on the choice of procedure. That decision is based on several aspects:

- *Medical risk and general condition*: If an invasive procedure presents an increased medical risk, caution is exercised when indicating biopsy, especially for nodules with low probability of malignancy. Instead, follow-up is generally recommended and invasive diagnostic exploration is advisable only if there is nodule growth.
- *Operability*: The technical and functional operability are estimated. The latter can be decisive for the choice of ensuing procedure if, as in the case of a central pulmonary nodule, surgery is expected to result in major lung volume loss.
- *Probability of nodule malignancy*: Statistical models are available to estimate the probability of malignancy of the nodule, e.g., the formula for calculation of the probability of malignancy nodule given in Gould et al[18]:

$$\text{Probability of malignancy} = \frac{e^x}{1+e^x}$$

where $x = -6.8272$

$+ 0.0391 \times$ age (in years)

$+ 0.7917 \times$ smoker (1 = yes; 0 = no)

$+ 1.3388 \times$ carcinoma in the previous 5 years (1 = yes; 0 = no)

$+ 0.1274 \times$ nodule diameter (in mm)

$+ 1.0407 \times$ spiculated margin (1 = yes; 0 = no)

$+ 0.7838 \times$ located in upper lobe (1 = yes; 0 = no)

Here, a probability of malignancy of less than 5% is interpreted as low risk and of over 60% as high risk.[18] Thus, the quantitatively estimated probability correlates well with the qualitative estimate of clinical experts[18]; hence, with appropriate experience there is no need to calculate the probability of malignancy. Based on the estimated likelihood of malignancy, diagnostic options as presented in ▶Table 21.3 are to be decided in a multidisciplinary discussion.

- *Patient preference*: The patient should be given information on the potential dangers associated with the nodule as well as on the risks of the proposed diagnostic procedures. Consideration will be given to patient preference when planning the choice of procedure. Occasionally, a nodule with only a low probability of malignancy, or even when radiologic benignity criteria are met, must be resected since the existence of the nodule causes considerable anxiety to the patient.

Subsolid Nodules

Ground-glass nodules as well as part-solid nodules are collectively classified as subsolid nodules. They are common manifestations of adenocarcinomas or their precursors. That is particularly true for part-solid nodules which in addition to ground-glass components also have a solid component. Many of these tumors grow very slowly and must be followed up for at least 5 years to exclude any growth suspicious for malignancy. ▶Table 21.4 lists the recommended intervals for CT follow-up based on the nodule size.[15] PET examination is not recommended for pure ground-glass nodules since false-negative results are very common.

Interpretation of the follow-up findings for subsolid pulmonary nodules is more complicated than for solid

Table 21.3 Case-by-case decision for management of solid pulmonary nodules measuring more than 8 mm that do not meet benignity criteria: considerations and available diagnostic options[17,18]

Influence factor	Diagnostic options[a]

• General status
• Surgical risk
• Technical operability
• Functional operability
• Probability of malignancy:
  – Clinical data
  – CT morphology
  – Possibly, PET and dynamic contrast findings
• Patient preference
	• CT follow-up
	• PET-CT and/or dynamic contrast
	• Biopsy:
	  – Bronchoscopic
	  – Transthoracic (CT-guided)
	• Video-assisted thoracoscopy (VATS)
	• Thoracotomy

[a]The invasiveness of the diagnostic methods increases in descending order.

Table 21.4 Recommended CT follow-up intervals and management for part-solid nodules and ground-glass nodules depending on mean nodule diameter (average of long and short axis, rounded to the nearest millimeter) or nodule volume[13]

Nodule type	Density	<6 mm (<100 mm³)	≥6 mm (≥100 mm³)
Single	Ground-glass	No routine follow-up (consider 2 and 4 years in suspicious nodule)	6–12 months, then every 2 years until 5 years
	Part-solid	No routine follow-up	3–6 months. If persistent: • Solid part <6 mm: annual until 5 years • Solid part ≥6 mm: should be considered highly suspicious
Multiple		3–6 months, if stable consider 2 and 4 years	3–6 months. If persistent management based on most suspicious nodule

Table 21.5 Malignancy criteria for solid and subsolid nodules at CT follow-up

Solid nodule	Subsolid nodule	
	Part-solid pulmonary nodule	**Ground-glass nodule**
Progressive growth	Progressive growth	Progressive growth
	Increased density[a]	Increased density[a]
	Progressive growth of solid component[a]	New-onset solid component[a]

[a]Continues to be a malignancy criterion even if there is simultaneous reduction in overall size.

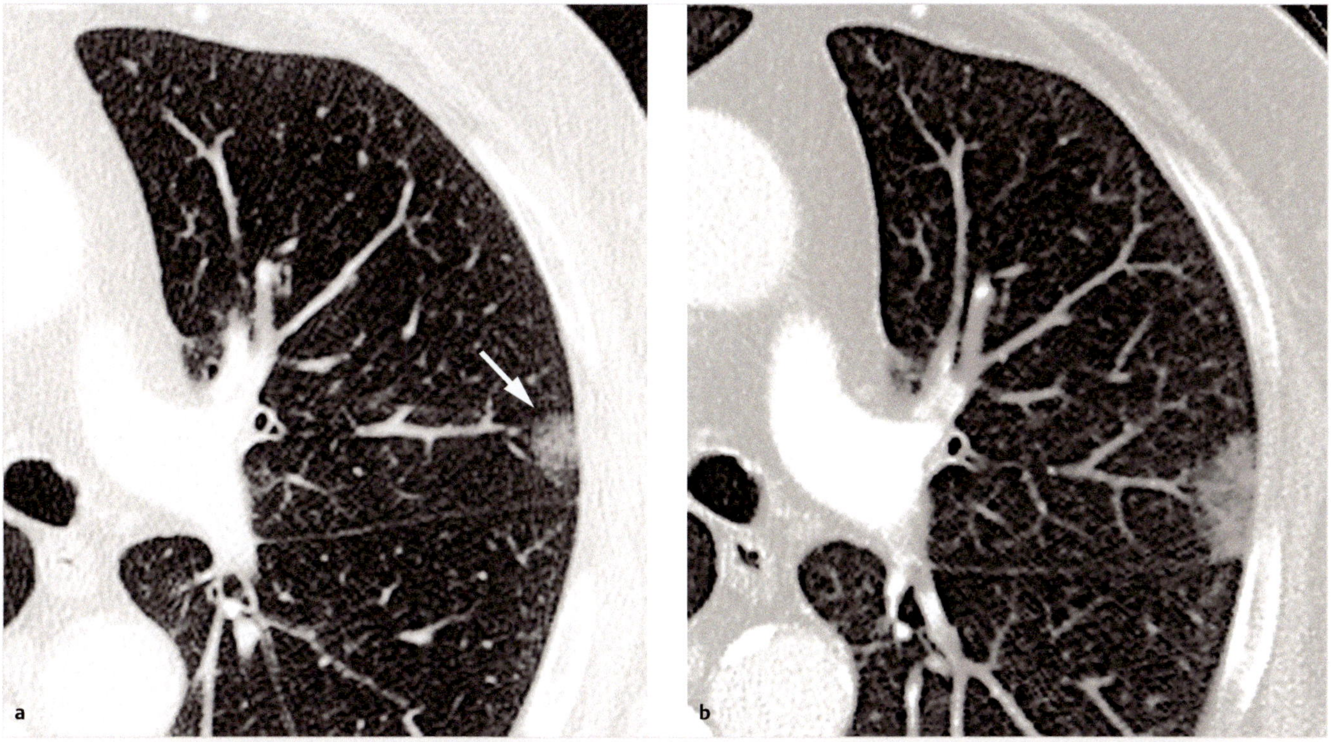

Fig. 21.3 Criteria for malignancy of subsolid nodules. Progressive growth of a ground-glass nodule (**a**, *arrow*) over 4 years; histologically, adenocarcinoma. **(a)** Baseline examination. **(b)** Follow-up examination at 4 years.

pulmonary nodules. The malignancy criteria are presented in Table 21.5. As for solid nodules, an increase in size is deemed a malignancy criterion (▶Fig. 21.3 and ▶Fig. 21.4). Likewise, an increase in density is suggestive of malignancy (▶Fig. 21.5). This often derives from increasing alveolar collapse which can result in a simultaneous decrease in nodule size. Therefore, the latter should not be interpreted as evidence of benignity, unlike in the case of solid nodules. The same applies for an increase in the size of the solid nodule component but no change in the overall diameter of a part-solid nodule (▶Fig. 21.6).

> **Note**
>
> Part-solid nodules with a solid component measuring more than 5 mm in diameter which persist or progress over 3 months are viewed as potentially malignant. They must be further investigated through biopsy since such nodules are often adenocarcinomas.

Solitary Nodules in Tumor Patients

Solitary nodules in patients with known extrapulmonary malignant tumor should not automatically be viewed as metastases. Several studies have demonstrated that the vast majority of small nodules in tumor patients are benign.[3,19,20,21,22] The size of solid nodules determines the probability of malignancy: nodules measuring less than 5 mm are probably benign, while conversely those measuring more than 10 mm are suspected metastases. Subsolid nodules very rarely prove to be pulmonary metastases from extrapulmonary tumors and should not be reported as such. The diagnostic procedure is subject to the aforementioned criteria. If malignant, these nodules are much more likely to be a primary lung cancer (second tumor) than lung metastasis from an extrapulmonary malignant tumor.

21.2 Multiple Nodules

Multiple pulmonary nodules are common, with studies detecting them in 7 to 23% of healthy older smokers.[23,24] The vast majority of these nodules were small and benign. As outlined

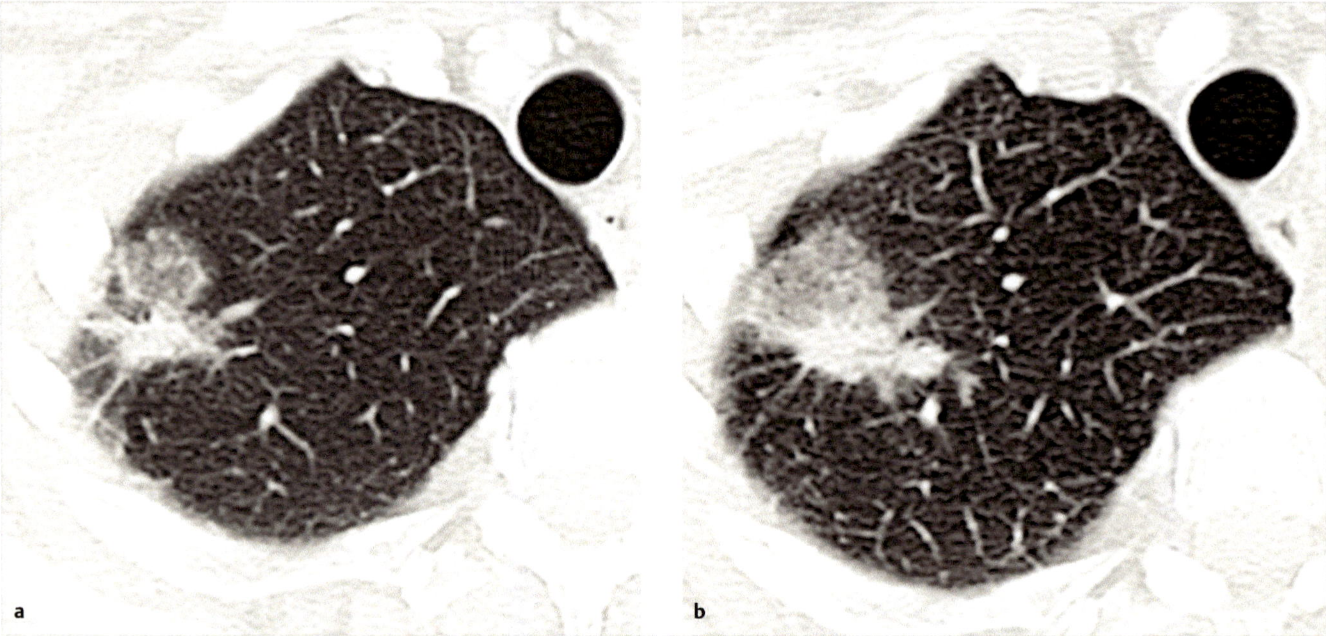

Fig. 21.4 Criteria for malignancy of subsolid nodules. Progressive growth of part-solid nodule over 6 months; histologically, adenocarcinoma. **(a)** Baseline examination. **(b)** Follow-up examination at 6 months.

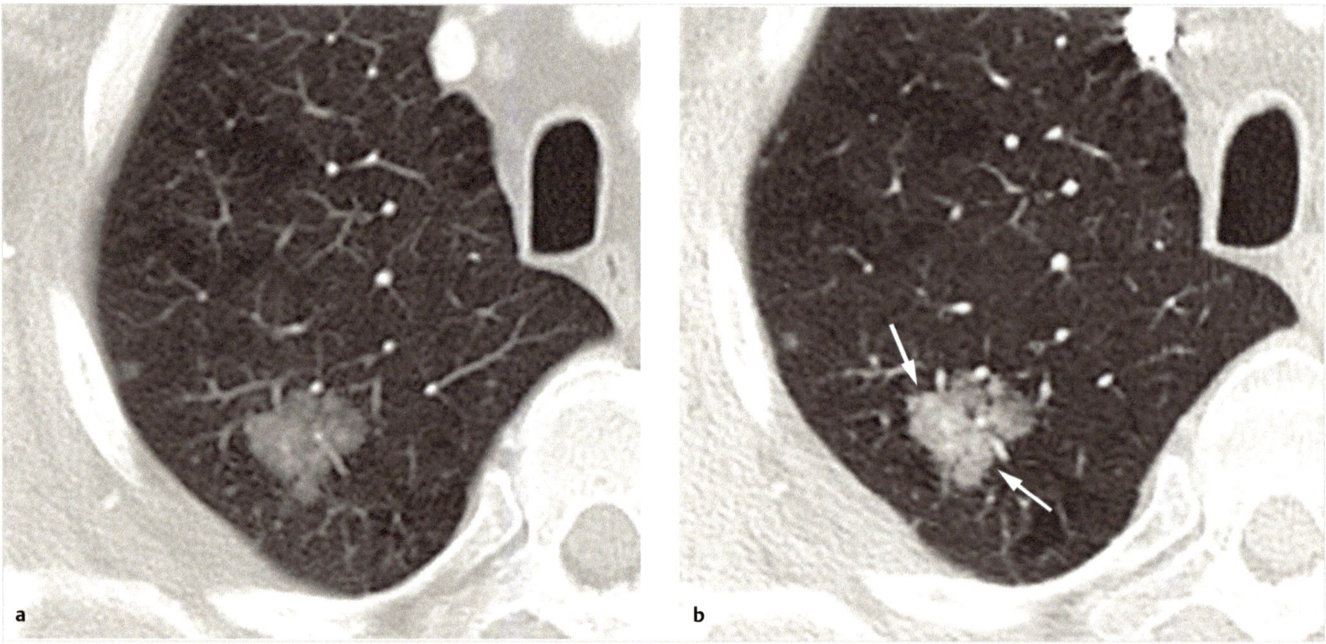

Fig. 21.5 Criteria for malignancy of subsolid nodules. Increase in nodule density (**b**, *arrows*) over 4 months and size stability of ground-glass nodule; histologically, adenocarcinoma. **(a)** Baseline examination. **(b)** Follow-up examination at 4 months.

in the concepts presented in Section 21.1 for solitary nodules, the small, usually less than 5 mm, multiple pulmonary nodules incidentally detected on CT are viewed as being highly probably benign. Multiple nodules detected on chest radiography usually measure more than 1 cm and are often malignant, quite probably metastases. Differential diagnosis and management are largely determined by the clinical context and are explained in greater detail below.

21.2.1 Differential Diagnosis

The broad spectrum of possible differential diagnoses is essentially based on the following parameters:

- Nodule size.
- Number of nodules.
- History of malignant tumor.

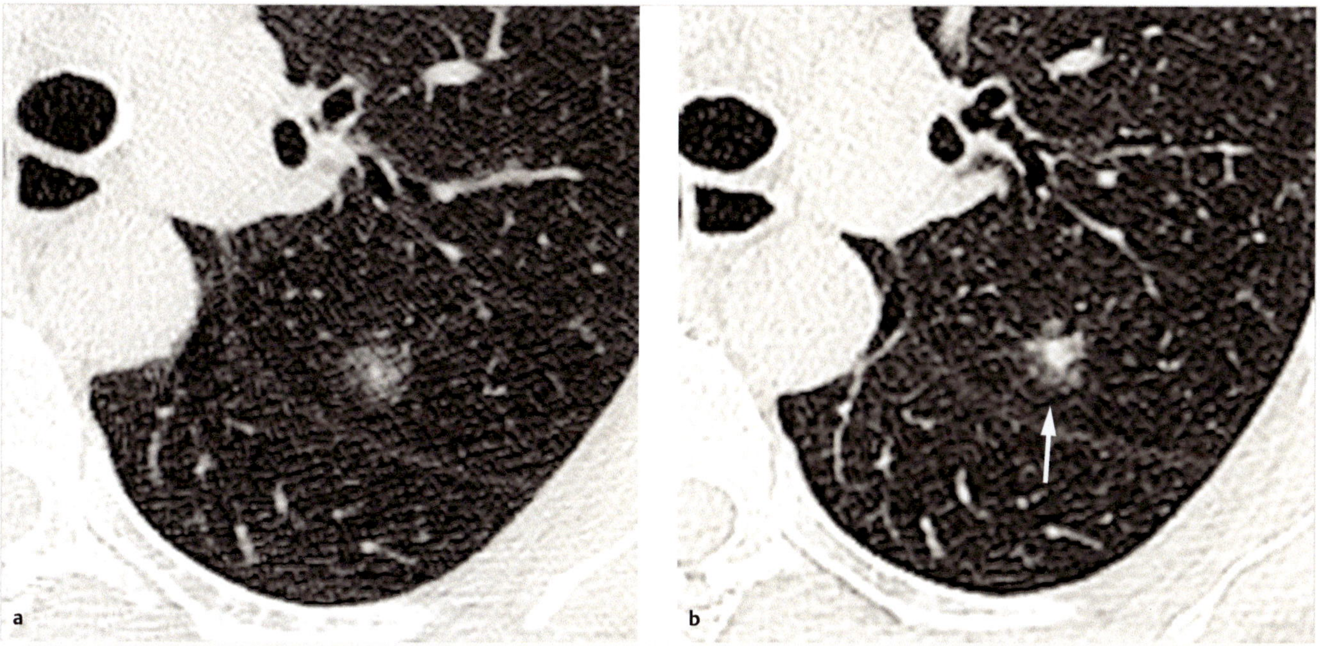

Fig. 21.6 Criteria for malignancy of subsolid nodules. Progressive growth of solid component (b, *arrow*) over 12 months and no change in overall nodule size; histologically, adenocarcinoma. **(a)** Baseline examination. **(b)** Follow-up at 12 months.

A Few Small Nodules in Nononcology Patients

These are usually nodules incidentally detected on CT. From lung cancer screening studies, it is known that a considerable percentage of smokers are found to have several benign, small nodules on CT. These predominantly prove to be benign granulomas or intrapulmonary lymph nodes. The latter often have a characteristic longitudinal-oval shape and are generally located in the subpleural region or at the periphery of the lung parenchyma at a maximum distance of 1 cm from the pleura (▶Fig. 21.7).

By contrast, metastases from a hitherto unknown primary tumor are much less likely and should therefore only be included in differential diagnosis if the criteria listed in ▶Table 21.6 apply. CT morphology confers few insights in this setting: depending on the primary tumor, metastases can be either well defined or spiculated, and central cavities are found in both metastases and inflammatory lesions.

The aforementioned guidelines for management of incidental pulmonary nodules[13] also cover the topic of multiple nodules. The recommended CT follow-up intervals to exclude growth that is highly suspicious for malignancy are summarized in ▶Table 21.2 for solid and in ▶Table 21.4 for subsolid nodules.

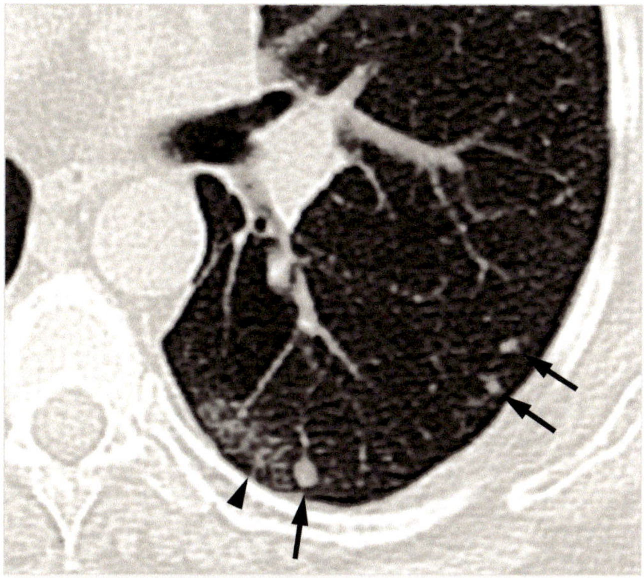

Fig. 21.7 Intrapulmonary lymph nodes. Few subpleural, oval, well-defined nodules in the left lower lobe (*arrows*). Additionally, dependent opacity in the posterior left lower lobe (*arrowhead*).

Multiple Small Nodules in Nononcology Patients (Nodular Pattern)

In general, patients have an underlying disease that needs further, even invasive, diagnostic exploration (bronchoscopy, biopsy). A differential diagnosis is illustrated in Fig. 24.5 and Fig. 24.6.

Large Nodules in Nononcology Patients

▶Table 21.7 gives a summary of common differential diagnoses for multiple, large pulmonary nodules.

Conversancy with the patient's clinical and paraclinical history is required to limit the myriad differential diagnoses that are possible. In certain cases, a review of the patient history and the suggestive imaging findings suffice for diagnosis, but in most cases further invasive diagnostic measures are needed to reach a diagnosis (bronchoscopy, biopsy). CT follow-up alone is advisable only in exceptional cases, e.g., for patients with rheumatoid arthritis found to have typical rheumatoid nodules on CT or for nodules with dilated supplying and draining vessels and family history of Osler–Rendu–Weber disease.

Table 21.6 Criteria for suspected lung metastases from unknown primary tumor

Feature	Suspected metastasis if
Size	• Variable • >10 mm
Location	• Not exclusively peripheral • Basal predominance
Additional findings	• Interlobular septal thickening • Pleural effusion

Nodules in Oncology Patients

The probability that multiple nodules in patients with a history of malignant tumor are lung metastases is markedly higher than in nononcology patients. Although several studies[3,19,20,21,22] have revealed that the majority of small nodules proved to be benign even in these patients, the probability of metastases rises sharply in line with nodule size. Furthermore, metastases of certain primary tumors may have specific imaging features as presented in Table 21.8; detection of these criteria supports the assumption that nodules are metastases. The rather challenging assessment of whether nodules are metastatic is illustrated in ▸Fig. 21.8. The following aspects should be considered:

- *Pretest probability*: How likely do lung metastases occur at a given time point in a patient with a specific tumor? An important aspect here is the time lag between primary tumor diagnosis and onset of pulmonary nodules (synchronous vs.

Table 21.7 Differential diagnoses of multiple large nodules in patients with no known malignant tumor[2]

Etiology	Disease entities	Special features
Tumor (initial diagnosis)	Lung metastasis	Rarely cavitary, very rarely ground-glass nodules, at times interlobular septal thickening (lymphangitic carcinomatosis)
	Multifocal pulmonary adenocarcinoma	Often with large consolidations or ground-glass nodules and ground-glass opacities, at times cavitary
	Multiple carcinoids	Often associated with bronchus
	Lymphoma	Usually secondary lung involvement with known extrapulmonary lymphoma, very rarely primary pulmonary lymphoma
	Kaposi sarcoma	Very rarely, in AIDS patients
Infection	Lung abscess	Hypodense or cavitary center
	Septic embolism	Often cavitary
	Mycobacteriosis	Often calcified, often other findings (consolidations, ground-glass opacities)
	Fungal pneumonia	In immunoincompetent patients, often halo sign, air-crescent sign (late sign)
Noninfectious inflammation	Sarcoidosis	Apical predominance, perilymphatic distribution, usually with lymphadenopathy
	Silicosis/coal workers' pneumoconiosis	Apical predominance, perilymphatic distribution, often with subpleural nodules and pleural pseudoplaques
	Granulomatous polyangiitis	Often cavitary, possibly also ground-glass opacities consistent with alveolar hemorrhage, positive c-ANCA in blood
	Organizing pneumonia	Usually irregular nodules and consolidations
	Eosinophilic granulomatosis with polyangiitis (Churg–Strauss syndrome)	Usually with multiple ground-glass opacities, positive p-ANCA in blood
	Pulmonary Langerhans cell histiocytosis	Often cavitary nodules and cysts, apical predominance sparing the costophrenic angles
	Eosinophilic pneumonia	Often with surrounding, relatively sharply marginated ground-glass opacities, usually blood eosinophilia
	Necrotizing sarcoid granulomatosis	Rarely, consolidations, apical predominance
	Bronchocentric granulomatosis	Rarely, often cavitary, consolidations
Other	Rheumatoid nodules	In known rheumatoid arthritis, necrotic center, at times coexistent with diffuse parenchymal lung disease (generally of usual interstitial pneumonia pattern)
	Amyloidosis	Often predisposing underlying disease
	Mucoceles	Predisposing airway disease, almost fluid-isodense density values, at times stag-antler-like branching
	Arteriovenous malformations	In Osler–Rendu–Weber disease dilated supplying and draining vessels

Abbreviations: c-ANCA, cytoplasmic antineutrophil cytoplasmic antibodies; p-ANCA, perinuclear antineutrophil cytoplasmic antibodies.

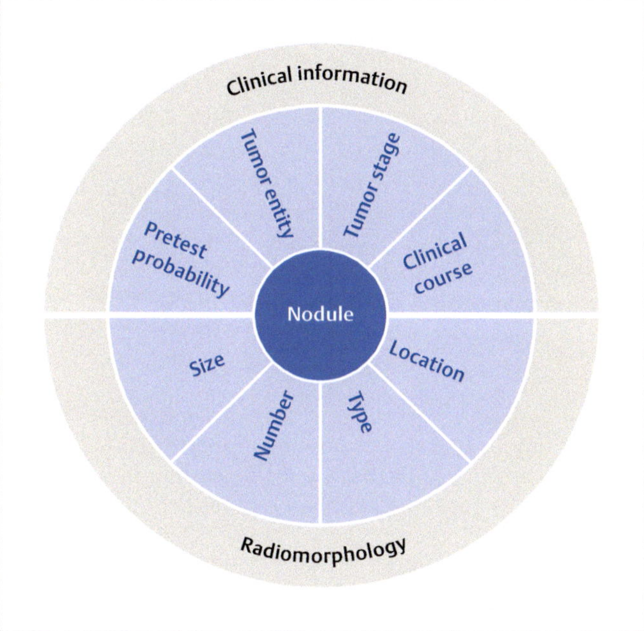

Fig. 21.8 Aspects to be considered in the assessment of the likelihood of metastatic etiology of nodules in oncology patients.

metachronous occurrence). For example, synchronous lung metastases are rare at the time when a breast cancer is first diagnosed. The probability increases over several years and then decreases—late metastases after decades are increasingly less likely.

- *Tumor entity*: How commonly does the known primary tumor metastasize to the lung? Are the typical metastasis pathways and timelines followed?
- *Tumor stage*: Is lung metastasis occurrence probable in the current tumor stage? If an early-stage primary tumor was completely resected, metastasis are unlikely.
- *Clinical course*: Does the clinical course suggest alternative diagnoses? If new-onset nodules appear during or after chemotherapy that led to a decrease in the primary tumor size, inflammatory lesions or reactive intrapulmonary lymph nodes should be considered.
- *Location*: Lung metastases reach the lung through hematogenous dissemination. Accordingly, they exhibit basal predominance and a random distribution pattern in respect of the lobule structures. Other distribution patterns suggest alternative diagnoses.
- *Shape*: An oval shape of well-defined subpleural nodules is suggestive of intrapulmonary lymph nodes and reduces the likelihood of metastasis. A summary of other characteristic morphologic features of specific tumor entities is given in ▶Table 21.8.
- *Number*: Different tumor entities tend to have specific lung metastasis patterns. Whereas thyroid gland carcinomas, for example, are commonly associated with diffuse small nodular metastases, colorectal carcinomas usually have few but larger nodules.
- *Size*: The bigger the nodules, the higher the probability of metastasis. Likewise, nodules of variable size are probably metastases. Specific to renal cell carcinoma is the occurrence of spontaneous remission of lung metastases after resection

Table 21.8 Special CT morphology features of lung metastasis of different tumor entities

Imaging feature	Typical primary tumor
Spiculated margin	• Colorectal cancer (largish nodules) • Breast cancer • Pancreatic cancer
Subpleural/pleural location	Renal cell carcinoma
Intensive contrast enhancement (strong vascularization)	Renal cell carcinoma
Cystic lung metastases	• Bladder cancer • Pulmonary adenocarcinoma or squamous cell carcinoma • Sarcoma (often with pneumothorax)
Ground-glass nodules	Rarely, pulmonary adenocarcinoma
Calcification	• Osteosarcoma • Rarely, thyroid cancer
Fat-equivalent density values	• Liposarcoma • Rarely, renal cell carcinoma
Necrosis	Nonsmall cell lung cancer
Interlobular septal thickening (additional lymphangitic carcinomatosis)	• Gastrointestinal adenocarcinomas • Breast cancer • Pulmonary adenocarcinoma

of the primary tumor; hence, decrease of nodule size without specific therapy does not rule out lung metastasis in renal cell carcinoma.

21.2.2 Management

Management of multiple nodules is essentially determined by the clinical context and varies greatly from one setting to another. For incidental multiple nodules, guidelines have been recently published[13] and are summarized in ▶Table 21.2 and ▶Table 21.4. These recommendations are not applicable to patients in an oncological setting or with immunosuppression. To date, no clinical guidelines are available for multiple nodules in these patients, thus reflecting the multiple factors influencing the likelihood of various differential diagnosis as discussed above. Nonetheless, general considerations are given below for certain characteristic clinical situations.

Incidental Imaging Finding, No History of Malignant Tumor

Management depends on the size of the nodules and potential risk factors as discussed in Section 21.1.2. The Fleischner Society recommendations for management are presented in ▶Table 21.2 for solid nodules and in ▶Table 21.4 for subsolid nodules.

Remarkably, no routine follow-up is recommended for multiple solid nodules with a mean diameter of less than 6 mm and a nodule volume of less than 100 mm³ in the absence of risk factors because in these patients malignancy of the lesions is exceedingly rare.

Incidental Imaging Finding, History of Known Malignant Tumor

In patients with a known history of a malignant tumor, metastases must, in general, be considered as a relevant differential diagnosis. Aspects that influence the probability of metastases in the specific case are discussed in Section 21.2. In patients with a known malignant tumor, previous images might be available, e.g., dating back to the time of earlier tumor treatment. An attempt to demonstrate long-term stability of these findings and obtain confirmation of their benignity could be undertaken. New-onset—or only retrospectively identified—nodules exhibiting progressive growth, regardless of their size, are suggestive of metastatic etiology.

Nodule morphology can be of great differential diagnostic value as described in the previous section.

If diagnostic exploration is unsuccessful, the choice of further diagnostic and therapeutic procedures should be discussed with a clinician well versed in oncology. Histologic confirmation is often necessary if the morphology is not very suggestive of benignity. Otherwise, short-term follow-up for at least 2 years can help differentiate between metastases and benign findings.

Primary Staging of a Malignant Tumor

In this setting, the availably of suitable previous imaging is less likely than in the aforementioned case. The issue of metastasis can be easily clarified if previous images are available. Otherwise, the ensuing procedure should be discussed in a multidisciplinary tumor consultation. Tissue sampling and PET or CT follow-up are commonly the most relevant options. If previous imaging is available, the general rule is that nodules exhibiting progressive growth and already identifiable on previous examinations are most likely metastases. Likewise, new-onset nodules with no plausible alternative diagnosis must be viewed as metastases. Conversely, nodules showing long-term stability are most probably benign.

Immunoincompetent Patient on Systemic Oncological Treatment

This represents a special situation compared with the settings described above. Inflammatory changes are more common than in the normal population or in immunocompetent tumor patients.

If fever of unknown origin presents in an immunoincompetent patient (especially patient with bone marrow suppression), any concurrent, new-onset multiple nodules will be chiefly attributable to pneumonia, most likely fungal pneumonia.

Small, pre-existing nodules showing progressive growth may be inflammatory reactive *intrapulmonary lymph nodes* or *lung metastases*. Differential diagnosis should take into account the response of other known tumor manifestations to systemic therapy.

Note

Some rules for differential diagnosis of multiple nodules in tumor patients:

- Not all multiple nodules are metastases!
- Plausible alternative diagnoses must be actively sought.
- Knowledge of tumor biology is essential:
  - Synchronous or metachronous metastasis?
  - Customary metastasis pathways and timelines?
  - Probability of hematogenous metastasis in current tumor stage?
  - Tumor response to treatment hitherto?
- Discussion of differential diagnoses with referring clinicians is crucial.

References

[1] Tuddenham WJ. Glossary of terms for thoracic radiology: recommendations of the Nomenclature Committee of the Fleischner Society. AJR Am J Roentgenol 1984;143(3):509–517

[2] Webb WR, Müller NL, Naidich DP. High-Resolution CT of the Lung. 4th ed Philadelphia, PA: Wolters Kluwer/Lippincott Williams & Wilkins; 2009

[3] Benjamin MS, Drucker EA, McLoud TC, Shepard JA. Small pulmonary nodules: detection at chest CT and outcome. Radiology 2003;226(2):489–493

[4] Takashima S, Sone S, Li F, et al. Small solitary pulmonary nodules (< or =1 cm) detected at population-based CT screening for lung cancer: Reliable high-resolution CT features of benign lesions. AJR Am J Roentgenol 2003;180(4):955–964

[5] Yankelevitz DF, Henschke CI. Does 2-year stability imply that pulmonary nodules are benign? AJR Am J Roentgenol 1997;168(2):325–328

[6] Schwartz M. A biomathematical approach to clinical tumor growth. Cancer 1961;14:1272–1294

[7] Usuda K, Saito Y, Sagawa M, et al. Tumor doubling time and prognostic assessment of patients with primary lung cancer. Cancer 1994;74(8):2239–2244

[8] Aoki T, Nakata H, Watanabe H, et al. Evolution of peripheral lung adenocarcinomas: CT findings correlated with histology and tumor doubling time. AJR Am J Roentgenol 2000;174(3):763–768

[9] Hasegawa M, Sone S, Takashima S, et al. Growth rate of small lung cancers detected on mass CT screening. Br J Radiol 2000;73(876):1252–1259

[10] Shyu CL, Lee YC, Perng RP. Fast-growing squamous cell lung cancer. Lung Cancer 2002;36(2):199–202

[11] Winer-Muram HT, Jennings SG, Tarver RD, et al. Volumetric growth rate of stage I lung cancer prior to treatment: serial CT scanning. Radiology 2002;223(3):798–805

[12] Tan BB, Flaherty KR, Kazerooni EA, Iannettoni MD; American College of Chest Physicians. The solitary pulmonary nodule. Chest 2003;123(1, Suppl):89S–96S

[13] MacMahon H, Naidich DP, Goo JM, et al. Guidelines for management of incidental pulmonary nodules detected on CT images: From the Fleischner Society 2017. Radiology 2017;284(1):228–243

[14] MacMahon H, Austin JHM, Gamsu G, et al; Fleischner Society. Guidelines for management of small pulmonary nodules detected on CT scans: a statement from the Fleischner Society. Radiology 2005;237(2):395–400

[15] Naidich DP, Bankier AA, MacMahon H, et al. Recommendations for the management of subsolid pulmonary nodules detected at CT: a statement from the Fleischner Society. Radiology 2013;266(1):304–317

[16] National Comprehensive Cancer Network. NCCN Clinical Practice Guidelines in Oncology (NCCN Guidelines®) Lung Cancer Screening (26.10.2011). Available at: http://www.nccn.org/professionals/physician_gls/pdf/lung_screening.pdf

[17] Gould MK, Donington J, Lynch WR, et al. Evaluation of individuals with pulmonary nodules: when is it lung cancer? Diagnosis and management of lung cancer, 3rd ed: American College of Chest Physicians evidence-based clinical practice guidelines. Chest 2013;143(5 Suppl):e93S–e120S

[18] Gould MK, Fletcher J, Iannettoni MD, et al; American College of Chest Physicians. Evaluation of patients with pulmonary nodules: when is it lung cancer?: ACCP evidence-based clinical practice guidelines (2nd edition). Chest 2007;132(3 Suppl):108S–130S

[19] Grampp S, Bankier AA, Zoubek A, et al. Spiral CT of the lung in children with malignant extra-thoracic tumors: distribution of benign vs malignant pulmonary nodules. Eur Radiol 2000;10(8):1318–1322

[20] Keogan MT, Tung KT, Kaplan DK, Goldstraw PJ, Hansell DM. The significance of pulmonary nodules detected on CT staging for lung cancer. Clin Radiol 1993;48(2):94–96

[21] Kim YH, Lee KS, Primack SL, et al. Small pulmonary nodules on CT accompanying surgically resectable lung cancer: likelihood of malignancy. J Thorac Imaging 2002;17(1):40–46

[22] Yuan Y, Matsumoto T, Hiyama A, et al. The probability of malignancy in small pulmonary nodules coexisting with potentially operable lung cancer detected by CT. Eur Radiol 2003;13(11):2447–2453

[23] Diederich S, Wormanns D, Semik M, et al. Screening for early lung cancer with low-dose spiral CT: prevalence in 817 asymptomatic smokers. Radiology 2002;222(3):773–781

[24] Henschke CI, McCauley DI, Yankelevitz DF, et al. Early Lung Cancer Action Project: overall design and findings from baseline screening. Lancet 1999;354(9173):99–105

Chapter 22

Cavities

22 Cavities

The term "cavity" is used to describe nodules, masses, or consolidations with an air-filled central space (synonyms: cavern, cavitary nodule). They are formed following bronchial drainage of necrotic material from the center of a lesion, resulting in the necrotic cavity manifesting as an air-filled hollow space on imaging.

Differential diagnosis varies in accordance with the number of nodules (solitary or multiple) and the nodule size (▶Table 22.1).

The probability of malignancy of large cavities increases in line with the thickness and irregularity of the cavity wall. But there are also adenocarcinomas that present as very thin-walled, smoothly marginated cavities, with a virtually cyst-like appearance.

The diagnostic and therapeutic procedure is largely determined by the clinical context. For example, if there is evidence of an inflammatory process and a visible cavity suggestive of an abscess on imaging, antibiotics are prescribed as first-line treatment. Lesion regression in response to treatment is considered ex juvantibus confirmation of the diagnosis. Further diagnostic measures, with more extensive laboratory diagnosis, CT, and bronchoscopy, are taken only if the lesion persists or even enlarges. One aim of bronchoscopy is to isolate the implicated pathogen in the case of infection. Furthermore, bronchoscopic biopsy is useful for differential diagnosis. If there is no evidence of an inflammatory process, invasive diagnostic tests are performed without resorting to prior antibiotic treatment.

Table 22.1 Differential diagnosis of solitary and multiple cavitary lesions

Diagnoses	Solitary	Multiple	Remarks
Lung cancer	+ +	(+)	• Squamous cell carcinoma: solitary, thick-walled • Adenocarcinoma: thin-walled, occasionally multifocal
Metastasis	(+)	++	Thin-walled, usually small nodules; common primary tumors: bladder cancer, pulmonary adeno- and squamous cell carcinomas, sarcomas
Abscess	+ +	+	Generally clinical and paraclinical inflammatory symptoms
Septic embolism	–	+ +	Generally severe inflammatory symptoms
Tuberculosis	++	++	Postprimary tuberculosis. Concomitant findings: consolidations, bronchial wall thickening, tree-in-bud pattern
Rheumatoid nodules	(+)	++	In known rheumatoid arthritis: cavitary and solid nodules, usually smoothly marginated
Granulomatous polyangiitis	–	++	Positive c-ANCA, furthermore, diffuse alveolar hemorrhage (ground-glass opacities and consolidations)
Langerhans cell histiocytosis	–	++	Small nodules, of which some solid with apical predominance, sparing the costophrenic angles
Necrotizing sarcoid granulomatosis	–	++	Rare; multiple nodules or largish masses, some cavitary
Bronchocentric granulomatosis	–	+ +	Rare; consolidations and liquefying nodules

Abbreviation: c-ANCA, cytoplasmic antineutrophil cytoplasmic antibodies.

Chapter 23

Persistent or Migratory Pulmonary Infiltrates

23 Persistent or Migratory Pulmonary Infiltrates

Pulmonary infiltrates are very commonly detected in clinical practice. On chest radiography, they are usually interpreted as pneumonia, when this is consistent with the clinical symptoms, and treated with antibiotics. The initial working diagnosis must be critically reviewed if timely follow-up reveals:

- Absence of adequate regression, or even progression, of the infiltrates.
- New-onset infiltrates at hitherto unaffected locations (even in settings of infiltrate regression at the initial locations).

The myriad relevant differential diagnoses cannot be reliably excluded on imaging alone. Discussion of the further diagnostic and therapeutic procedures with clinicians is helpful in this situation. In addition to further clinical work-up, a chest CT scan should definitely be obtained. A summary of relevant differential diagnoses is given in ▶Table 23.1.

Bronchoscopy is generally needed as part of the further clinical work-up. The radiologic differential diagnoses impact the bronchoscopic procedure, e.g., conduct of transbronchial biopsy or of bronchoalveolar lavage.

Inflammatory markers identified in routine laboratory tests provide the first diagnostic insights.

23.1 Raised Inflammatory Markers

23.1.1 Infection

Calculated antibiotic therapy will not be able to achieve adequate resolution of pneumonia (▶Fig. 23.1) if the chosen antibiotic is not effective against the causative pathogen. Bronchoscopy is aimed at identifying the causative pathogen; therefore, antibiotic treatment must be stopped prior to bronchoscopy to avoid suppression of bacterial growth in the obtained samples. Furthermore, pneumonia types against which conventional antibiotics are not effective must be considered:

- *In immunocompetent patients*:
  - Viral pneumonia: extensive, often bilateral ground-glass opacities and consolidations (▶Fig. 23.2).
  - Primary tuberculosis: solitary consolidation, often with surrounding ground-glass opacities and hilar lymphadenopathy (▶Fig. 23.3).

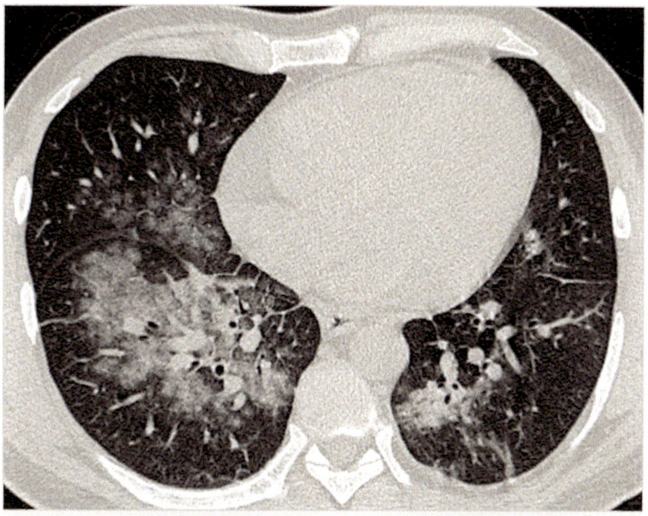

Fig. 23.1 Bacterial bronchopneumonia in both lower lobes. CT image.

Table 23.1 Differential diagnoses of persistent or migratory pulmonary infiltrates

Disease entity	Bilateral	Migration	Disease course on steroid therapy	Consolidation	Ground-glass opacities	Inflammatory markers	Other
Cryptogenic organizing pneumonia	(+)	+	↓	+	(+)	↑	Bronchoalveolar lavage: lymphocytosis
Infectious pneumonia	(+)	–	↑	+	+	↑	
Eosinophilic pneumonia	(+)	+	↓	+	+	↑	Bronchoalveolar lavage and blood: eosinophilia
Eosinophilic granulomatosis with polyangiitis (Churg–Strauss syndrome)	+	+	↓	(+)	+	↑	p-ANCA +
Allergic bronchopulmonary aspergillosis	+	+	↓	+	(+)	↑	Central bronchiectasis
Diffuse alveolar hemorrhage	+	+	↓	(+)	+	–(↑)	• c-ANCA+: Granulomatous polyangiitis • Glomerular basement membrane antibodies: Goodpasture syndrome
Pulmonary alveolar proteinosis	+	+	=	(+)	+	–	Crazy-paving pattern
Adenocarcinoma	– or +	–	↑	+	+	–	

Abbreviations: c-ANCA, cytoplasmic antineutrophil cytoplasmic antibodies; p-ANCA, perinuclear antineutrophil cytoplasmic antibodies.

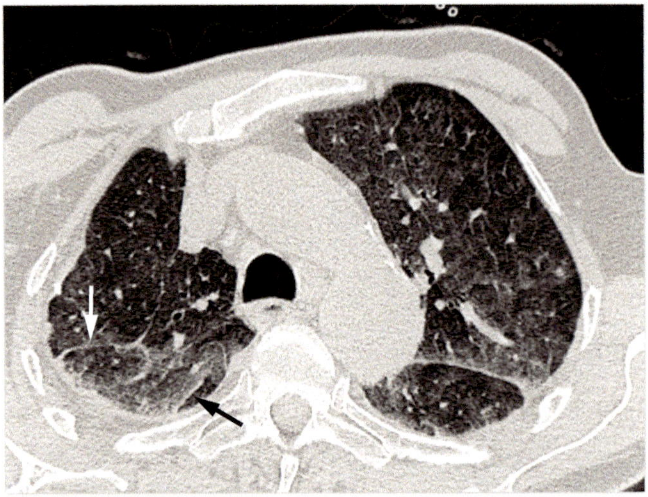

Fig. 23.2 Herpes simplex pneumonia. CT image. Bilateral ground-glass opacities; furthermore, historic inflammatory changes in the right upper lobe (*arrows*).

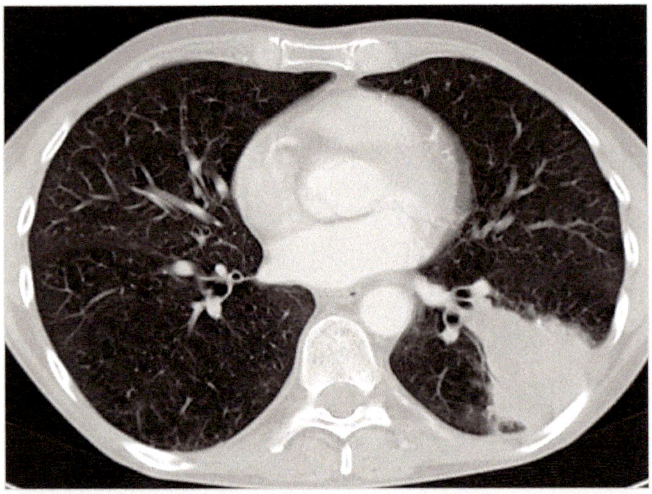

Fig. 23.3 Primary tuberculosis. CT image. Solitary consolidation in the left lower lobe.

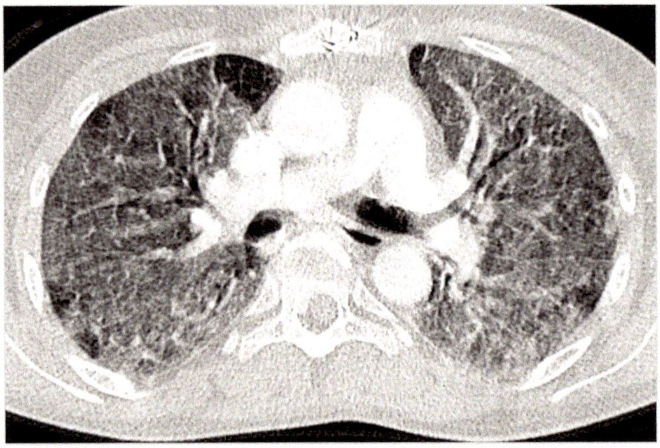

Fig. 23.4 *Pneumocystis jirovecii* pneumonia. CT image. Extensive bilateral ground-glass opacities.

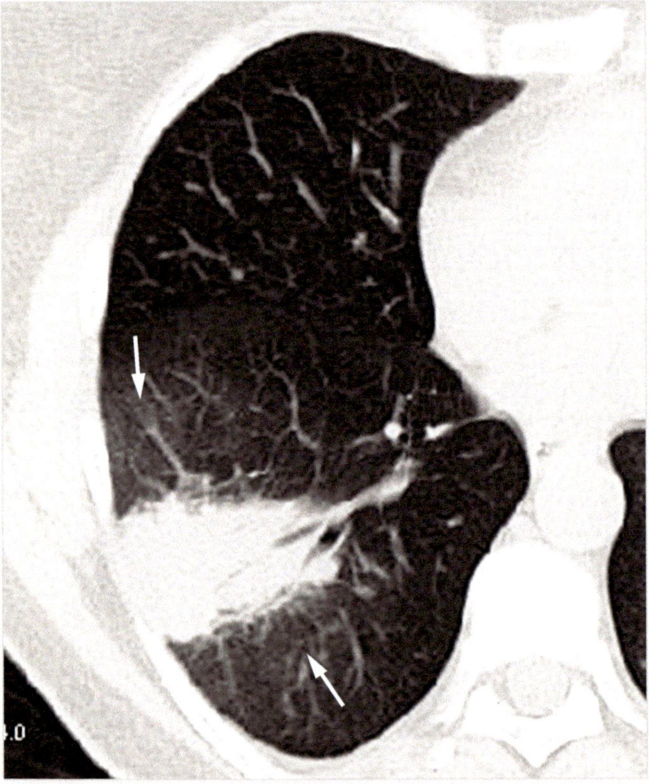

Fig. 23.5 Fungal pneumonia. CT image. Invasive pulmonary aspergillosis in the right lower lobe. Triangular pleural-based consolidation with intralesional open bronchi and perifocal ground-glass opacities, "halo sign" (*arrows*).

- *Additionally, in immunoincompetent patients*:
  - *Pneumocystis jirovecii* pneumonia: extensive, usually bilateral ground-glass opacities, often with relative sparing of the subpleural space (▶Fig. 23.4).
  - Fungal pneumonia: depending on the causative fungus, multiple nodules, or consolidations, often with surrounding ground-glass opacities (▶Fig. 23.5).

Bronchoscopy is aimed at identification of the causative pathogen; only then can antibiotic therapy that takes account of specific resistances of the organisms be prescribed. Furthermore, bronchoscopy is aimed at excluding an underlying cause of pneumonia, e.g., bronchial obstruction.

23.1.2 Cryptogenic Organizing Pneumonia

Antibiotic-resistant, bilateral, rather sharply marginated consolidations and inflammatory clinical manifestations are suggestive of cryptogenic organizing pneumonia (▶Fig. 23.6). This can often be confirmed on transbronchial biopsy. Lymphocytosis is a conspicuous finding on bronchoalveolar lavage. Once organizing pneumonia has been confirmed on histology, known causes must be ruled out clinically to reach a diagnosis of cryptogenic organizing pneumonia.

23.1.3 Eosinophilic Pneumonia

Solitary or multiple consolidations with surrounding, relatively sharply marginated ground-glass opacities are suggestive of Löffler syndrome (eosinophilic pulmonary infiltrates; ▶Fig. 23.7). Acute eosinophilic pneumonia is characterized by

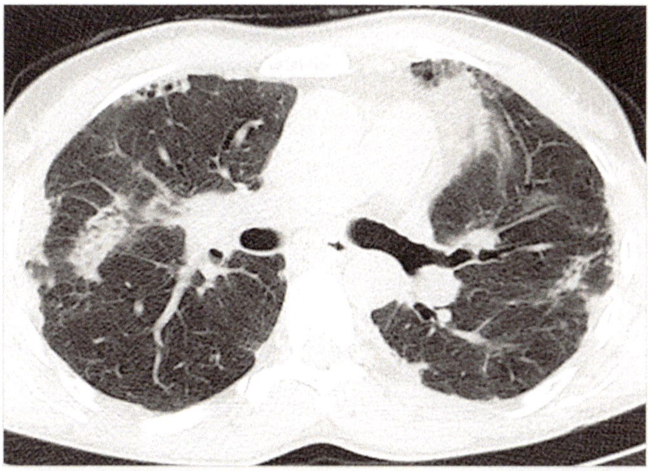

Fig. 23.6 **Cryptogenic organizing pneumonia.** CT image. Bilateral well-defined consolidations.

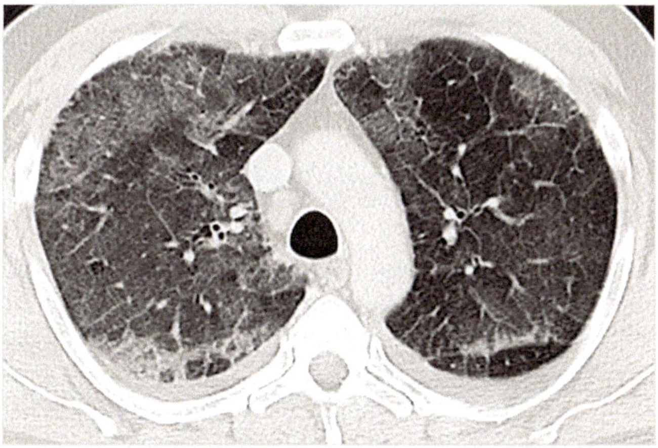

Fig. 23.8 **Acute eosinophilic pneumonia.** CT image. Bilateral, extensive ground-glass opacities; besides, slight bilateral pleural effusion.

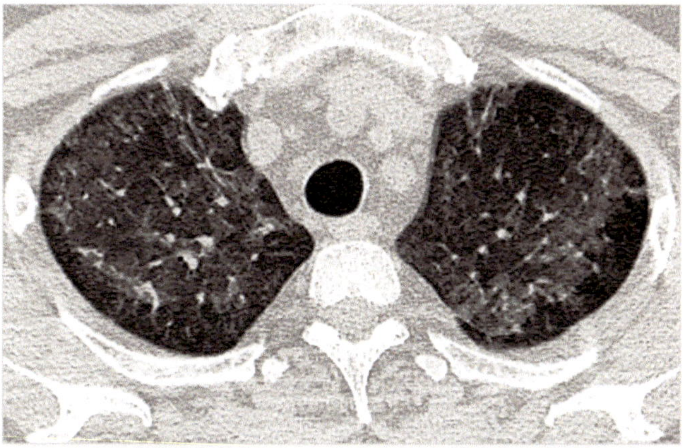

Fig. 23.10 **Eosinophilic granulomatosis with polyangiitis (Churg–Strauss syndrome).** CT image. Bilateral ground-glass opacities and intralobular lines.

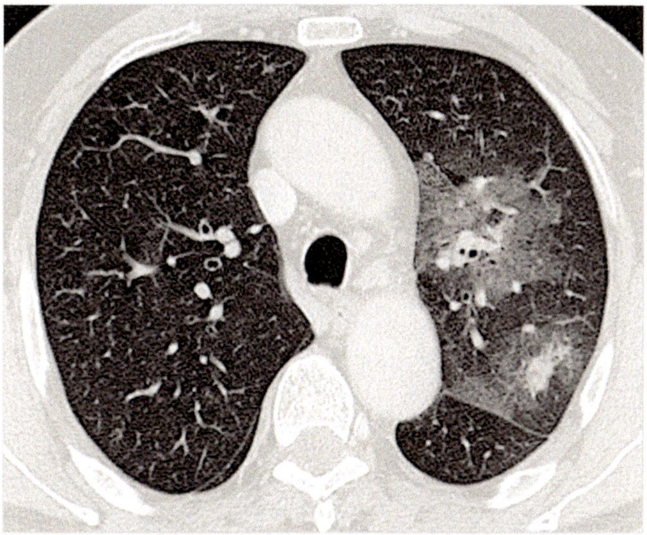

Fig. 23.7 **Löffler syndrome and eosinophilic pulmonary infiltrates.** CT image. Consolidations and surrounding ground-glass opacities in the left upper lobe.

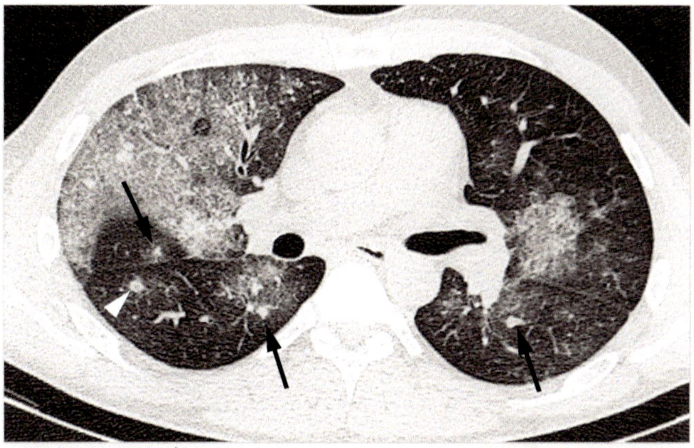

Fig. 23.9 **Granulomatous polyangiitis** CT image. Bilateral ground-glass opacities; furthermore, several nodules (*arrows*), some with incipient cavitation (*arrowhead*).

extensive bilateral ground-glass opacities (▶Fig. 23.8), while conversely chronic eosinophilic pneumonia is associated with peripheral bilateral consolidations. Peripheral blood eosinophilia is seen in both Löffler syndrome and in chronic, but not acute, eosinophilic pneumonia. Bronchoscopic confirmation is made through bronchoalveolar lavage showing elevated eosinophil counts (over 25%).

23.1.4 Vasculitis

Elevated serum levels of certain autoantibodies serve as diagnostic pointers:

- *c-ANCA*: Granulomatous polyangiitis, often with involvement of the nasal sinuses or kidneys. Characteristic features are cavitary nodules as well as bilateral infiltrates, consistent with hemorrhage (▶Fig. 23.9).
- *p-ANCA*: Eosinophilic granulomatosis with polyangiitis (Churg–Strauss syndrome), characterized by peripheral blood and bronchoalveolar lavage eosinophilia (▶Fig. 23.10).

23.1.5 Radiation Pneumonitis

Radiation pneumonitis manifests a few weeks to months after radiotherapy administered at nodule dose of at least 20 to 30 Gy. The opacities do not respect anatomic boundaries and extend beyond, e.g., lobar fissures, generally in the vicinity of the irradiated tumor (▶Fig. 23.11).

III

23.2 Normal Inflammatory Markers

23.2.1 Lung Cancer

A lung cancer manifests as either a solitary lesion or—in the case of pulmonary adenocarcinoma—at times as multifocal solid nodules, consolidations, or ground-glass nodules as well as diffuse ground-glass opacities that can also present bilaterally (▶Fig. 23.12). A typical hallmark is gradual progression of opacities despite administration of antibiotics and corticoids; regression cannot be expected without cytostatic treatment. The diagnosis is confirmed on bronchoscopic biopsy.

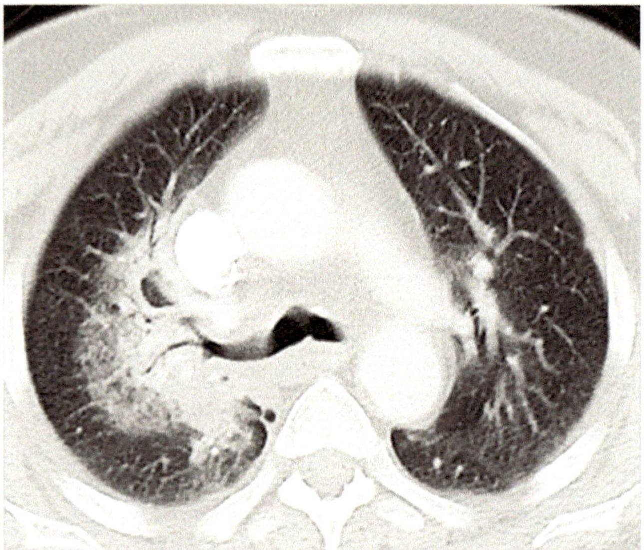

Fig. 23.11 **Radiation pneumonitis.** CT image. Right central lung cancer, surrounded by consolidations and ground-glass opacities.

23.2.2 Diffuse Alveolar Hemorrhage

There are several known causes[1,2] but only those of relevance in the clinical context of persistent or migratory pulmonary infiltrates are addressed below:

- Impaired coagulation.
- Autoimmune disease, e.g., in association with antiphospholipid syndrome (▶Fig. 23.13), Goodpasture syndrome with antibodies against glomerular basement membranes, or in vasculitis, but with elevated inflammatory markers in the latter case.
- Cardiovascular diseases such as left-sided congestive heart failure, mitral valve disease, pulmonary veno-occlusive disease, endocarditis, malignant hypertension.
- Drug-induced lung disease (there are around 100 drugs known to trigger hemorrhage).
- Illicit drugs, in particular crack cocaine.

23.2.3 Allergic Bronchopulmonary Aspergillosis

There is generally underlying asthma, in addition to blood eosinophilia and antibodies against *Aspergillus* antigens. The diagnosis is supported by other findings on CT: central bronchiectasis, mucoid impaction, and atelectasis (▶Fig. 23.14).

23.2.4 Pulmonary Alveolar Proteinosis

Pulmonary alveolar proteinosis is a rare disease entity characterized by ground-glass opacities with overlying interlobular septal thickening and intralobular lines (crazy-paving pattern; ▶Fig. 23.15). The diagnosis is confirmed on bronchoscopy.

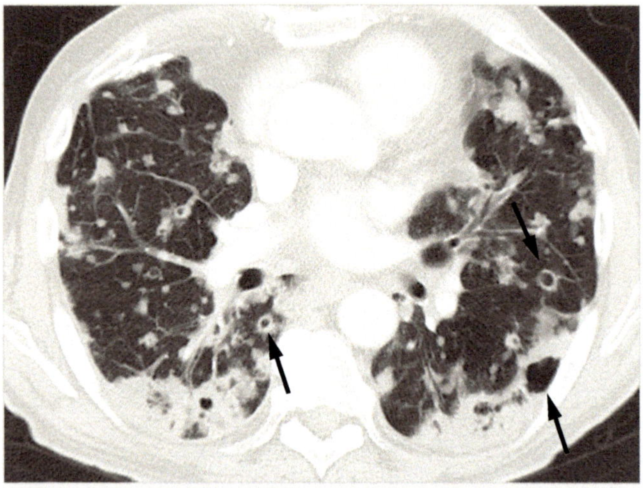

Fig. 23.12 **Multifocal pulmonary adenocarcinoma.** CT image. Bilateral lesions and central cavitation of several nodules (*arrows*).

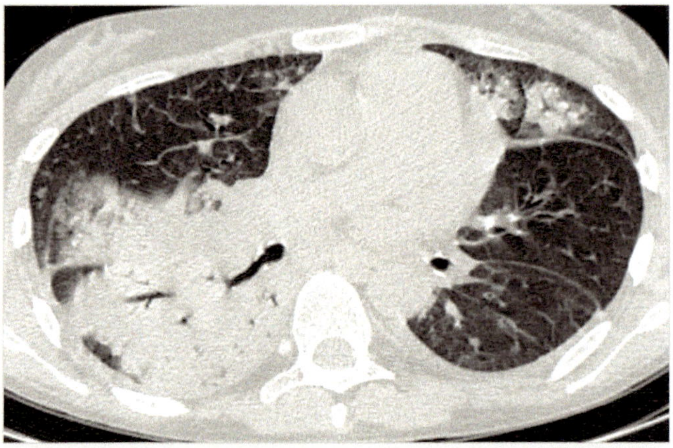

Fig. 23.13 **Diffuse alveolar hemorrhage.** CT image. Antiphospholipid syndrome in association with systemic lupus erythematosus: bilateral consolidations largely sparing the subpleural space.

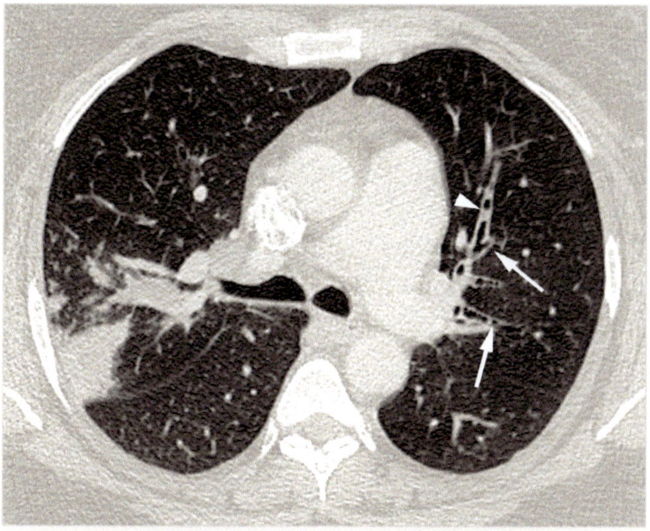

Fig. 23.14 Allergic bronchopulmonary aspergillosis. CT image. Consolidations in the right upper lobe as well as central bronchiectasis in the left upper lobe (*arrows*) with mucoid impaction (*arrowhead*).

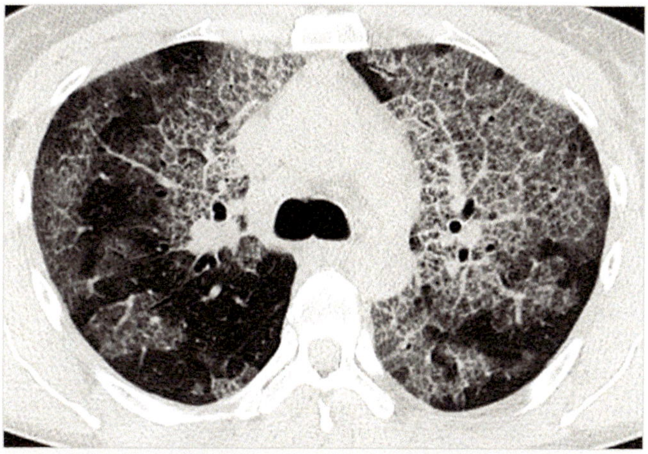

Fig. 23.15 Pulmonary alveolar proteinosis. CT image. Bilateral geographic ground-glass opacities with overlying interlobular septal thickening and intralobular lines (crazy-paving muster).

References

[1] Schreiber J, Knolle J, Kachel R, Schück R. Differential diagnosis of diffuse pulmonary haemorrhage [in German] Pneumologie 2006;60(6):347–354

[2] Krause ML, Cartin-Ceba R, Specks U, Peikert T. Update on diffuse alveolar hemorrhage and pulmonary vasculitis. Immunol Allergy Clin North Am 2012;32(4):587–600

Chapter 24

Diagnostic Schema for Typical Computed Tomography Findings of Diffuse Pulmonary Diseases

24 Diagnostic Schema for Typical Computed Tomography Findings of Diffuse Pulmonary Diseases

As in an identification guide, differential diagnosis of diffuse parenchymal lung diseases is presented on the basis of typical patterns of findings. This enables rapid orientation and quickly leads to the first suspected diagnosis. However, this overview is not a substitute for complete differential diagnosis tables on the various image patterns.

The differential diagnoses are presented in relation to a main finding. Further differentiation is made via an additionally present second image pattern that is less dominant than the main finding.

First, the main finding must be identified, as illustrated with different color backgrounds in ▸Fig. 24.1. The respective color leads the way to another table that queries the existence of an additional image pattern. This thus often narrows differential diagnosis down to a few diseases; some findings are even pathognomonic.

For nodules, a further differentiation into interstitial and airspace nodules is needed. Deviating from the normal procedure (i.e., an additional image pattern), differential diagnosis of interstitial nodules is based on their predominant distribution pattern.

To narrow the differential diagnosis sufficiently, inclusion of an additional image pattern is not enough for highly ambiguous main findings, such as ground-glass opacities. Other characteristic constellations of findings may in this case additionally point to potential diagnoses.

Main findings		Other differential diagnosis
Interlobular septal thickening	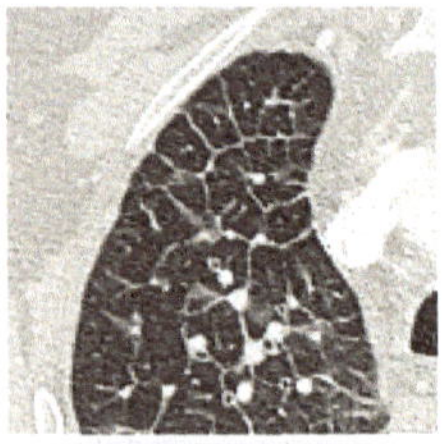	See Fig. 24.2
Intralobular lines	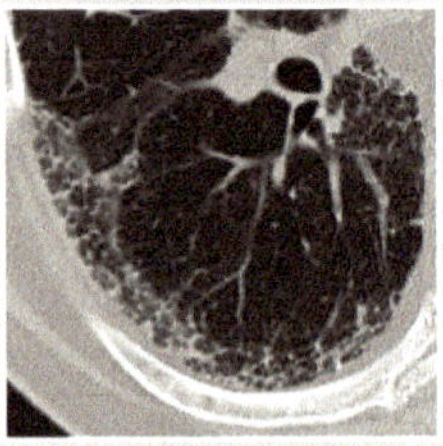	See Fig. 24.3
Nodules	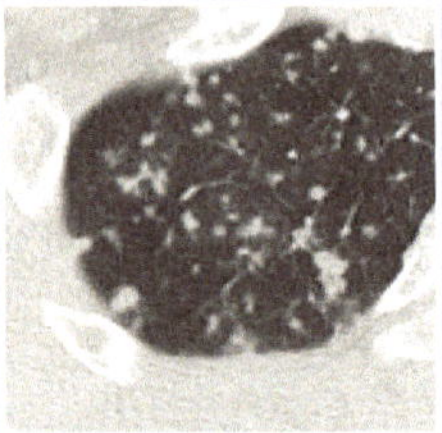	See Fig. 24.4
Ground-glass opacities	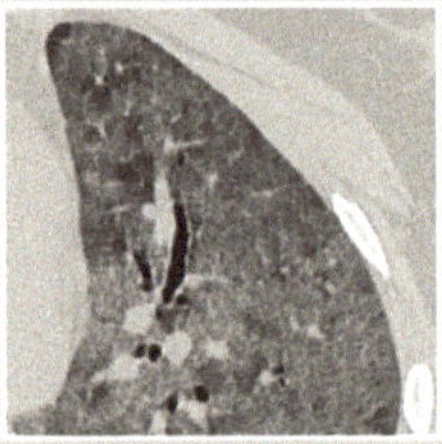	See Fig. 24.7
Consolidations	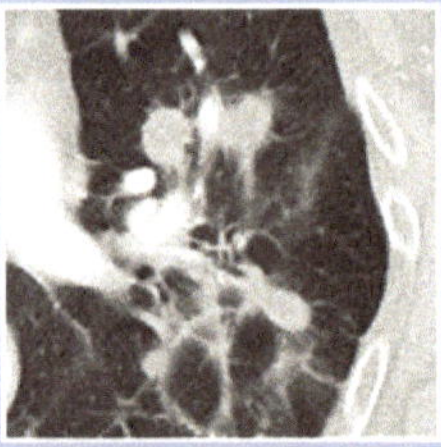	See Fig. 24.9
Cysts	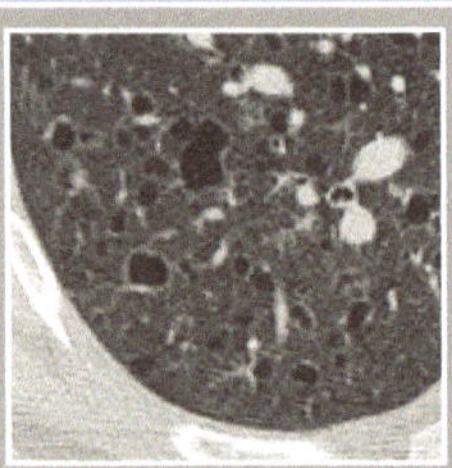	See Fig. 24.10
Tree-in-bud pattern	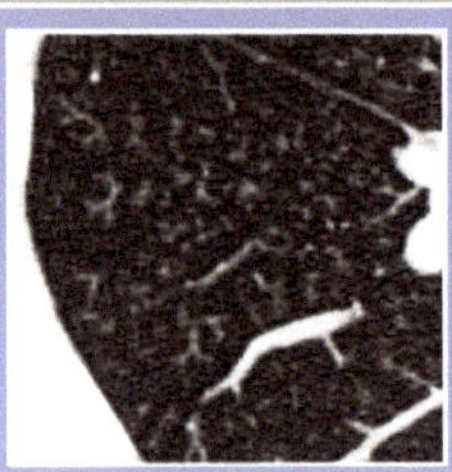	Bronchiolitis (see Section 10.2)

Fig. 24.1 Main finding on CT for diffuse pulmonary diseases.

24.1 Main Finding: Interlobular Septal Thickening

► Fig. 24.2 illustrates the differential diagnoses for the main finding: interlobular septal thickening.

Findings		Differential diagnoses	
No other image patterns	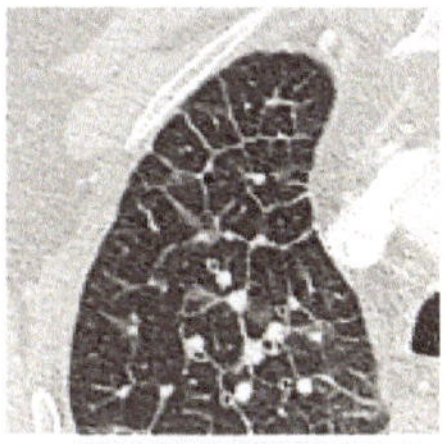	• *Bilateral symmetrical:* – Hydrostatic pulmonary edema – Lymphangitic carcinomatosis	• *Unilateral:* – Often, lymphangitic carcinomatosis – Rarely, unilateral hydrostatic pulmonary edema • *Nodular interlobular septal thickening:* – Lymphangitic carcinomatosis (beaded septum sign)
+Ground-glass opacities	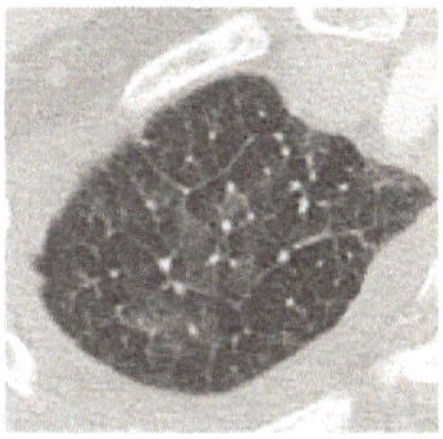	• *Diffuse or basal predominance:* – Often, hydrostatic pulmonary edema	• *Mosaic attenuation pattern:* – Hydrostatic pulmonary edema – Rarely, pulmonary alveolar proteinosis
+Nodules	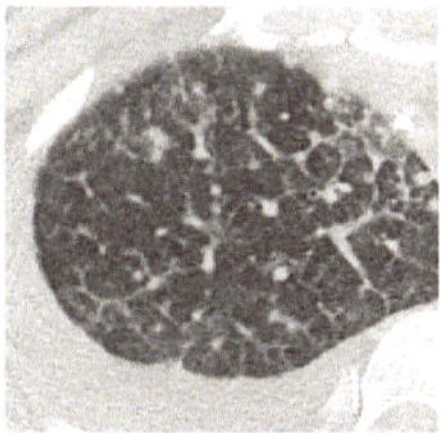	• *Nodules in interlobular septal thickening:* – Lymphangitic carcinomatosis	• *Nodules in random distribution:* – Lymphangitic carcinomatosis and additional nodular metastasis

Fig. 24.2 **Main finding: interlobular septal thickening.**

24.2 Main Finding: Intralobular Lines

▶Fig. 24.3 illustrates the differential diagnoses for the main finding: intralobular lines.

Findings		Differential diagnoses	
No other image patterns	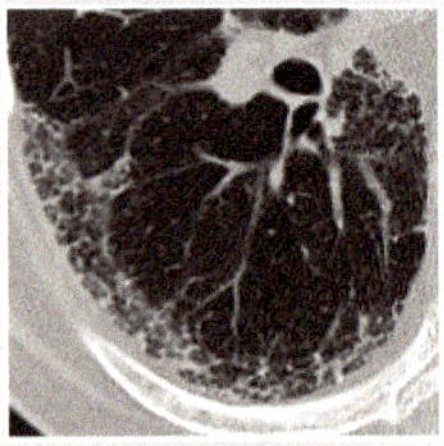	• *Basal and peripheral predominance:* – Usual interstitial pneumonia – Nonspecific interstitial pneumonia – Asbestosis	• *Other predominance:* – Lung involvement in collagen vascular diseases – Chronic hypersensitivity pneumonitis
+Honeycombing	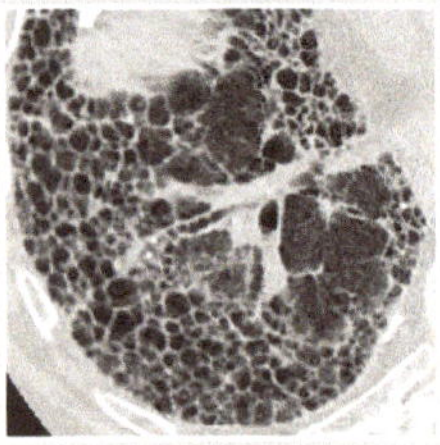	• *Basal and peripheral predominance:* – Usual interstitial pneumonia	• *Other predominance:* – Nonspecific interstitial pneumonia – Chronic hypersensitivity pneumonitis
+Traction bronchiectasis	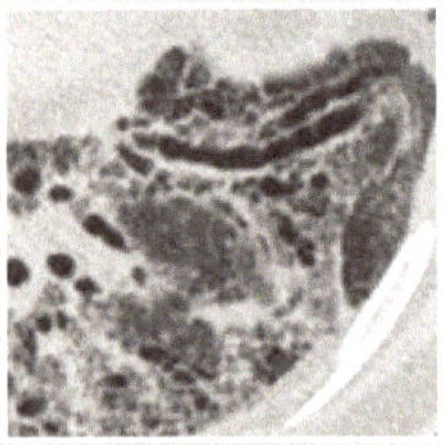	• *Basal and peripheral predominance:* – Usual interstitial pneumonia	• *Other predominance:* – Chronic hypersensitivity pneumonitis – Nonspecific interstitial pneumonia
+Ground-glass opacities	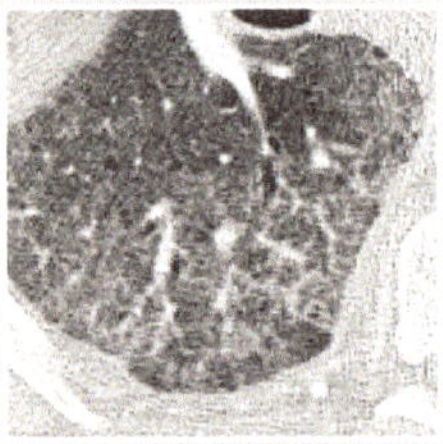	• *Ground-glass opacity predominance:* – Nonspecific interstitial pneumonia	• *Mild ground-glass opacities:* – Usual interstitial pneumonia
+Nodules	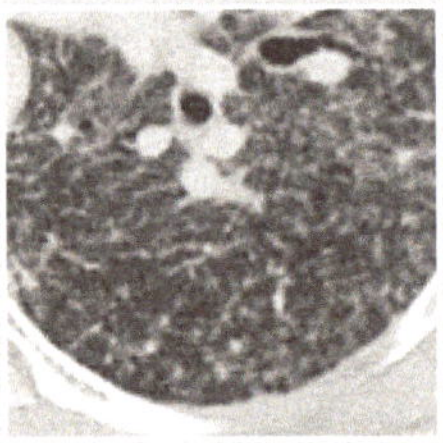	• *Nodules in perilymphatic distribution:* – Sarcoidosis	

Fig. 24.3 **Main finding: intralobular lines.**

24.3 Main Finding: Nodules

The following overviews present the differential diagnosis for image patterns with multiple small nodules with an average size of less than 10 mm. Differential diagnosis of large nodules is very different and is discussed in Section 21.2.

▶Fig. 24.4 differentiates the CT morphology into interstitial (▶Fig. 24.5) and airspace nodules (▶Fig. 24.6).

Findings		Differential diagnoses
• **Interstitial nodules:** – Measuring only a few millimeters – Sharply marginated – Soft-tissue-like density	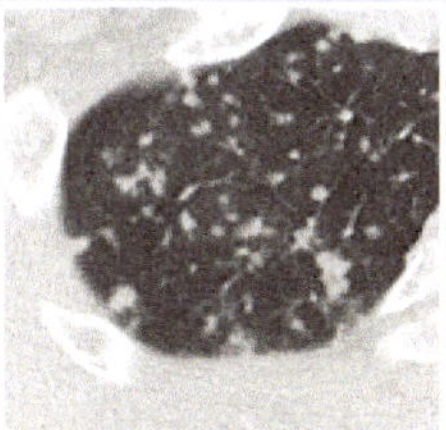	*Differential diagnosis based on lobule distribution predominance:* See Fig. 24.5
• **Airspace nodules:** – Approx. 5–10 mm in size – Ill-defined margins – Ground-glass-like density	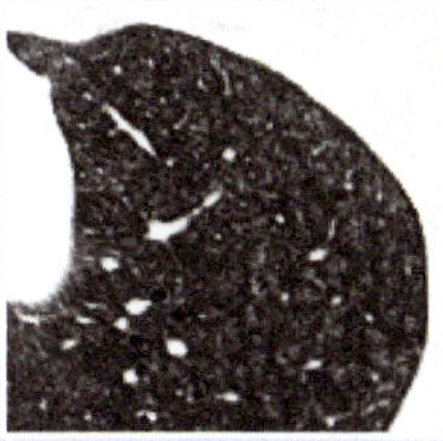	*Differential diagnosis based on 2nd image pattern:* See Fig. 24.6

Fig. 24.4 **CT morphology of multiple small nodules.**

Distribution pattern		Differential diagnoses
Random distribution (not oriented to lobule structures)	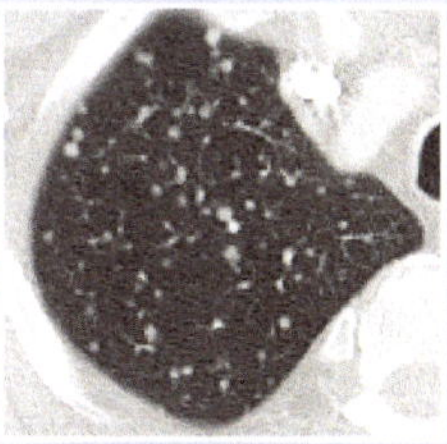	• *Hematogenous origin* – Nodular metastasis – Miliary tuberculosis – *Candida pneumonia*
Perilymphatic distribution (peribronchovascular, subpleural, in interlobular septa)	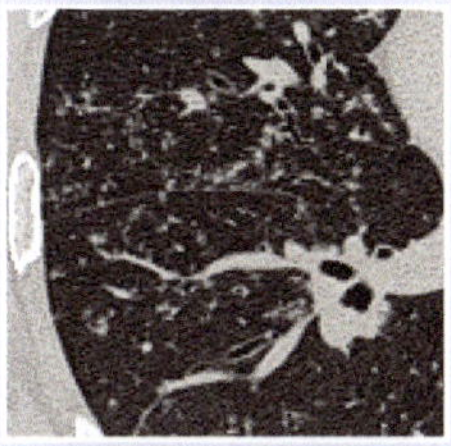	– Sarcoidosis – Silicosis (with subpleural pseudoplaques) – Lymphangitic carcinomatosis (usually with interlobular septal thickening, nodules predominantly in interlobular septa)
Centrilobular distribution (somewhat equidistant distribution of nodules, approx. 5–10 mm)	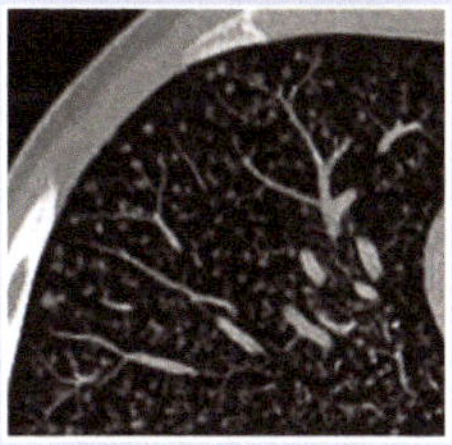	• *Terminal/respiratory bronchiole disease:* – Infectious bronchiolitis (often with tree-in-bud pattern) – Respiratory bronchiolitis – Rarely, bronchiolitis obliterans – Rarely, lymphocytic interstitial pneumonia

Fig. 24.5 **Main finding: interstitial nodules.**

III

Findings		Differential diagnoses
No other image patterns	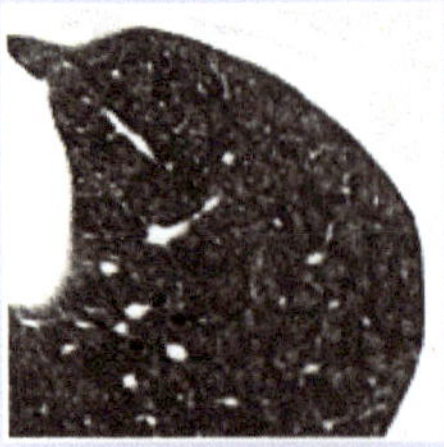	• *Focal:* – Bronchopneumonia • *Diffuse:* – Bronchopneumonia – Bronchiolitis – Rarely, lung metastasis from adenocarcinomas with lepidic growth pattern
+Tree-in-bud pattern	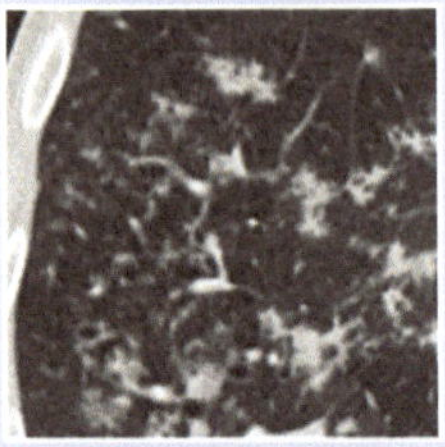	• *Focal or multifocal:* – Bronchopneumonia – Infectious bronchiolitis – Tuberculosis • *Diffuse:* – Rarely, panbronchiolitis
+Ground-glass opacities	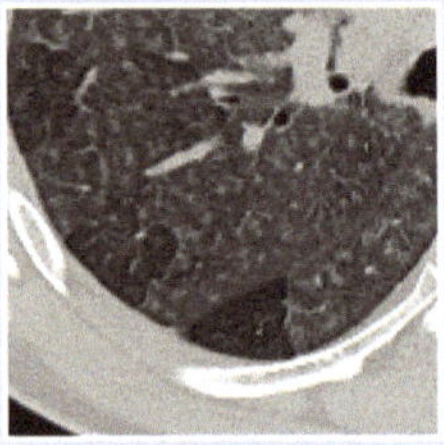	• *Focal:* – Bronchopneumonia • *Diffuse: mosaic attenuation pattern:* – Subacute hypersensitivity pneumonitis – Respiratory bronchiolitis – Sarcoidosis – Capillary leak edema – Rarely, lymphocytic interstitial pneumonia
+Consolidations	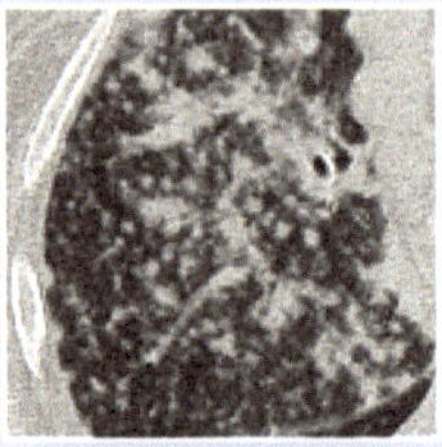	• *Focal:* – Bronchopneumonia • *Diffuse:* – Cryptogenic organizing pneumonia – Sarcoidosis – Rarely, lymphocytic interstitial pneumonia
+Hyperinflation	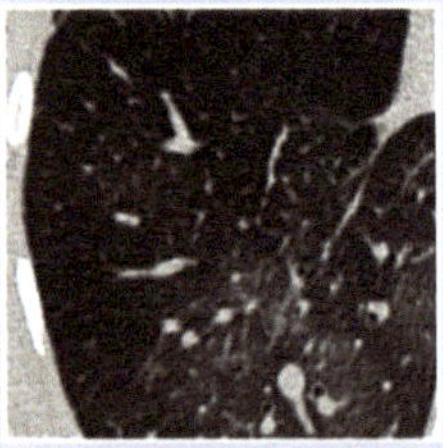	• *Diffuse:* – Bronchiolitis obliterans
+Cysts	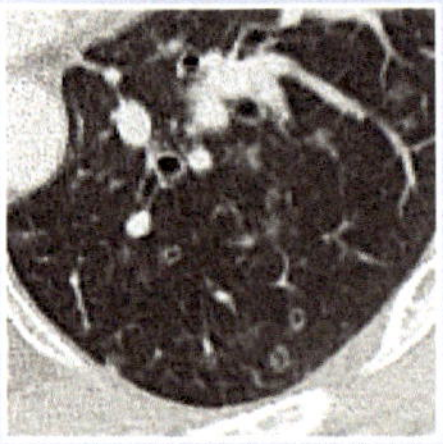	• *Isolated or diffuse* – Rarely, pulmonary Langerhans cell histiocytosis – Rarely, lymphocytic interstitial pneumonia

Fig. 24.6 **Main finding: airspace nodules.**

24.4 Main Finding: Ground-Glass Opacities

▶Fig. 24.7 illustrates the differential diagnoses for the main finding: ground-glass opacities. ▶Fig. 24.8 presents additional information on differential diagnosis for specific findings associated with ground-glass opacities.

24

Findings		Differential diagnoses	
No other image patterns	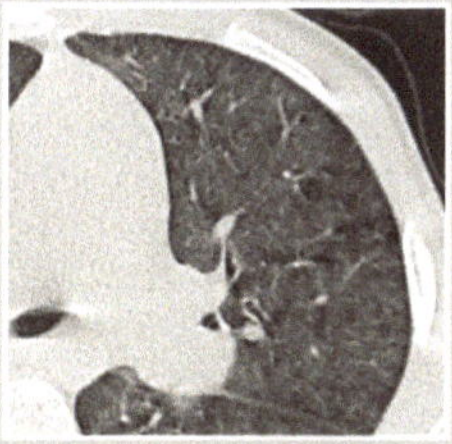	• *Focal: pneumonia* • *Multifocal:* – Vasculitis – Alveolar hemorrhage – Viral pneumonia	• *Diffuse, mosaic attenuation pattern:* – Pulmonary edema – Pneumocystis pneumonia – Subacute hypersensitivity pneumonitis – Acute eosinophilic pneumonia – Respiratory bronchiolitis – Desquamative interstitial pneumonia
+Consolidations	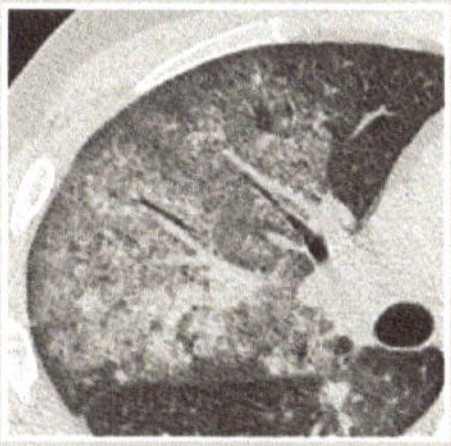	• *Focal, multifocal:* – Pneumonia – Alveolar hemorrhage – Adenocarcinoma	• *Diffuse:* – Pneumonia – Adult respiratory distress syndrome – Acute interstitial pneumonia – Capillary leak edema – Vasculitis
+Nodules	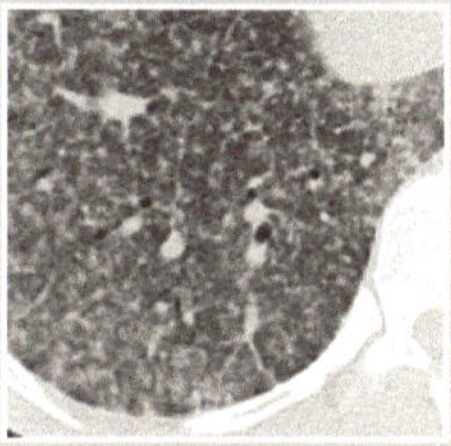	• *Interstitial nodules:* – Interstitial nodules:	• *Airspace nodules:* – Subacute hypersensitivity pneumonitis – Infection, pneumocystis pneumonia
+Intralobular lines	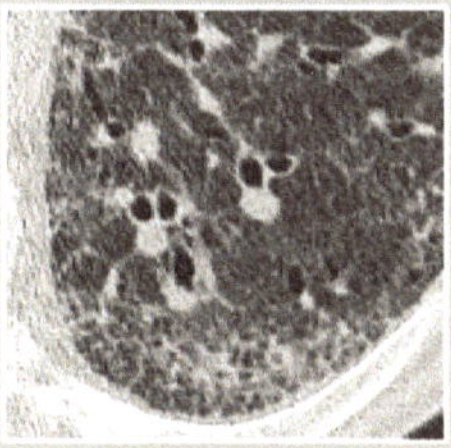	• *Focal or multifocal:* – Viral pneumonia	• *Diffuse:* – Pneumocystis pneumonia – Nonspecific interstitial pneumonia
+Interlobular septal thickening	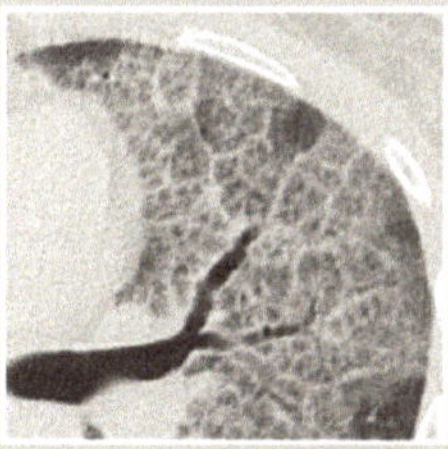	• *Diffuse or multifocal:* – Hydrostatic pulmonary edema	• *Mosaic attenuation pattern:* – Alveolar hemorrhage – Rarely, pulmonary alveolar proteinosis
+Cysts	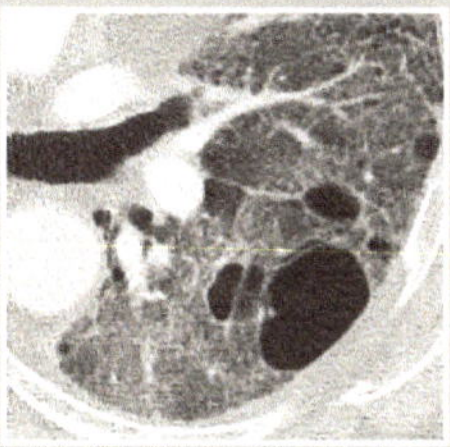	• Subacute hypersensitivity pneumonitis • Rarely, pneumocystis pneumonia • Rarely, lymphocytic interstitial pneumonia	

Fig. 24.7 **Main finding: ground-glass opacities.**

Findings		Differential diagnoses
Sharply marginated	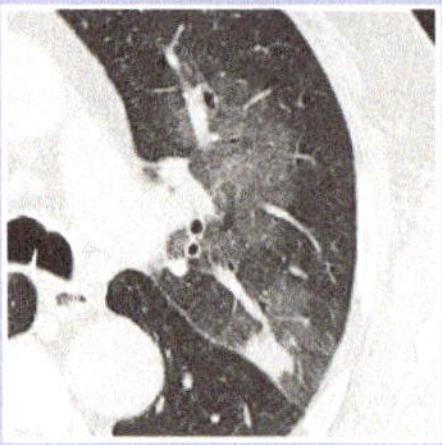	• *Focal or multifocal:* – Adenocarcinoma – Löffler syndrome (eosinophilic pulmonary infiltrate)
Ill-defined margins	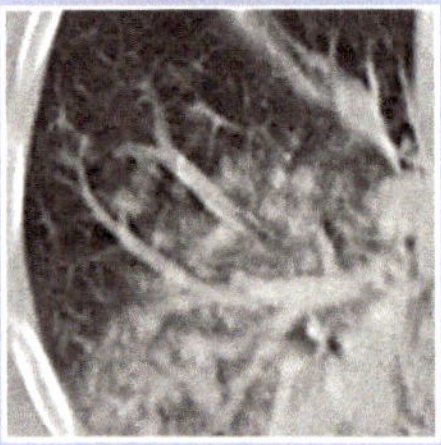	• *Focal, or multifocal:* – Pneumonia – Hemorrhage
Sparing of subpleural space	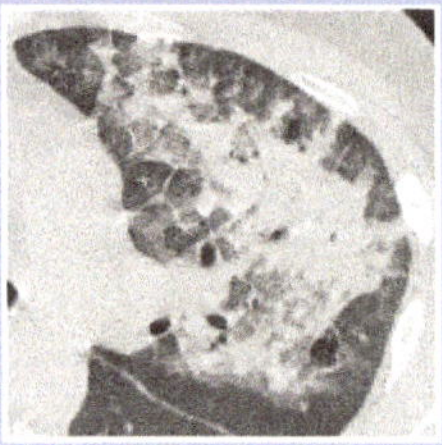	• *Focal or multifocal:* – Alveolar hemorrhage • *Diffuse, mosaic attenuation pattern:* – Pneumocystis pneumonia

Fig. 24.8 **Differential diagnosis: ground-glass opacities with or without consolidations and other specific findings.**

24.5 Main Finding: Consolidations

▶Fig. 24.9 illustrates the differential diagnoses for the main finding: consolidations.

Findings		Differential diagnoses	
No other image patterns	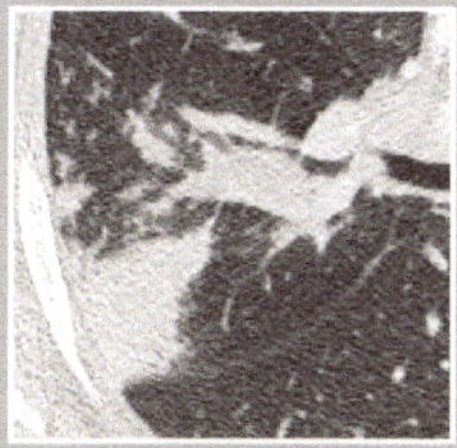	• Pneumonia • Sarcoidosis • Silicosis • Septic embolism • Granulomatous polyangiitis	• Cryptogenic organizing pneumonia • Chronic eosinophilic pneumonia • Lung metastasis • Amyloidosis
+Ground-glass opacities	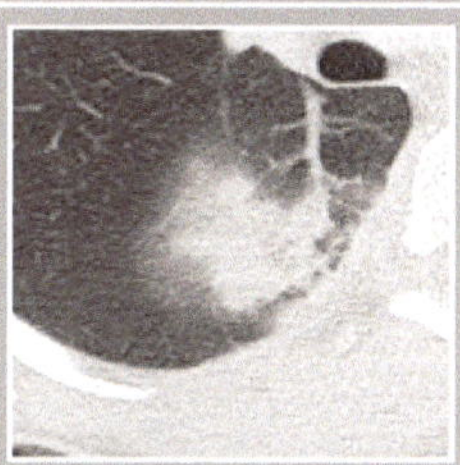	• *Ill-defined margins:* – Pneumonia – Hemorrhage – Cryptogenic organizing pneumonia	• *Sharply marginated* – Löffler syndrome (eosinophilic pulmonary infiltrate) – Adenocarcinoma
+Calcifications	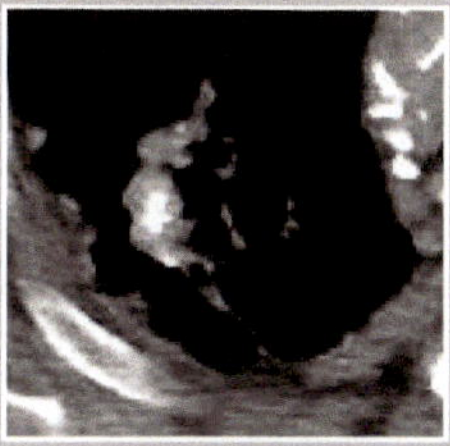	• Sarcoidosis • Tuberculosis • Silicosis	
+Cavities	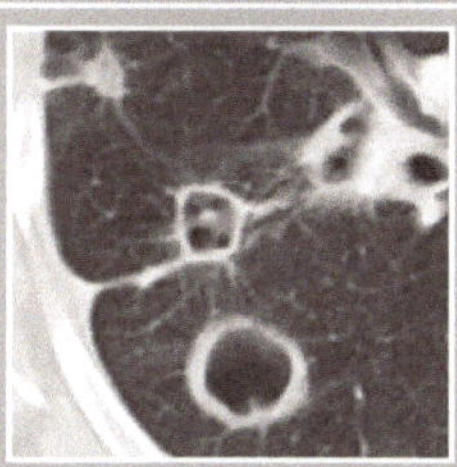	• Septic embolism • Granulomatous polyangiitis • Tuberculosis • Rarely, lung metastasis • For other rare differential diagnoses see Chapter 22	
+Nodules	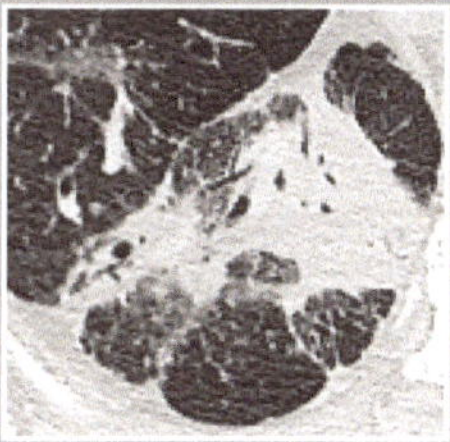	• *In perilymphatic distribution:* – Sarcoidosis – Silicosis	

Fig. 24.9 **Main finding: consolidations.**

24.6 Main Finding: Cysts

▶Fig. 24.10 illustrates the differential diagnoses for the main finding: cysts.

Findings		Differential diagnoses	
No other image patterns	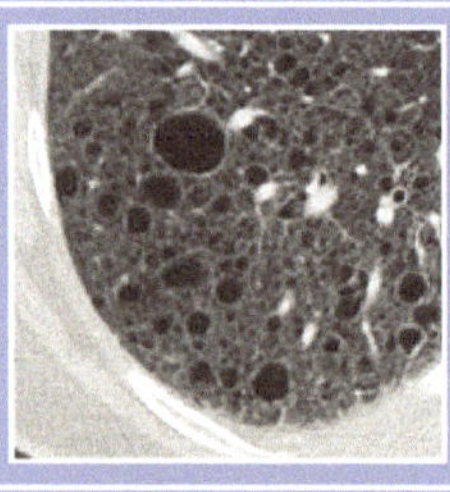	• Cystic bronchiectasis • Cystic lung metastasis • *Only in middle-aged women:* Lymphangioleiomyomatosis • *In adolescents:* Pulmonary Langerhans cell histiocytosis	• *In older smokers* – Centrilobular pulmonary emphysema (caution: no actual cysts) – Pulmonary Langerhans cell histiocytosis
+Nodules	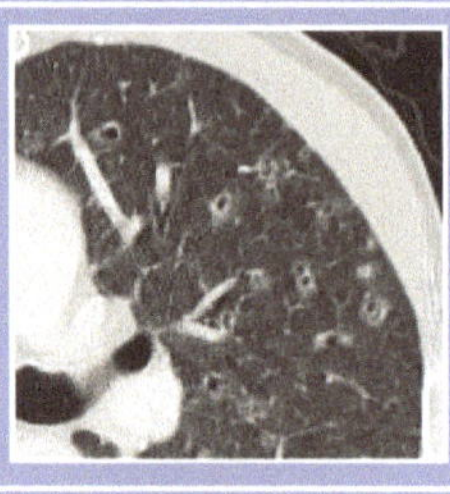	• Cystic lung metastasis • *In older smokers or adolescents:* Pulmonary Langerhans cell histiocytosis	
+Ground-glass opacities	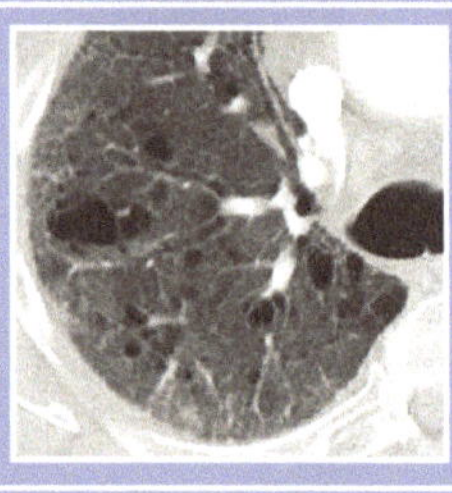	• Pneumocystis pneumonia • Cystic bronchiectasis with florid inflammation • Lymphocytic interstitial pneumonia	
+Calcifications	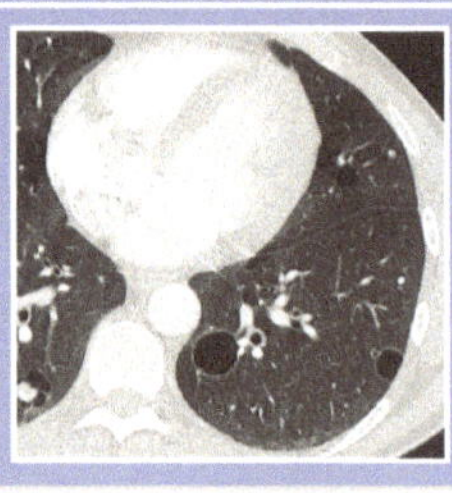	• Amyloidosis • Mycobacteriosis	

Fig. 24.10 **Main finding: cysts.**

Part IV

Glossary

IV

Chapter 25

Fleischner Society Glossary of Terms for Thoracic Imaging

25 Fleischner Society Glossary of Terms for Thoracic Imaging

25.1 Preliminary Remarks

The Fleischner Society is an international society for thoracic radiology, founded in 1969 to provide a forum for the presentation and discussion of scientific matters.[1] It has for decades been active in defining and standardizing terms to describe findings in thoracic imaging. As a consequence, the Society published the first glossary of terms for thoracic imaging in 1984.[2] Updates to that glossary were issued in 1996[3] and 2008.[4] The glossary presented here is the 2008 version and newest one available. Since then, the Fleischner Society has published further recommendations on specific topics—in particular, on subsolid pulmonary nodules[5] and emphysema.[6] Relevant terms not contained in the 2008 glossary but defined in these more recent publications have been incorporated in this chapter in a separate section (Section 25.3). Moreover, a few terms not contained in the glossary, but thought to be useful for understanding the definitions, have been added to that section (e.g., mucoid impaction and random distribution).

25.2 Glossary[a]

Acinus

Anatomy—The acinus is a structural unit of the lung distal to a terminal bronchiole and is supplied by first-order respiratory bronchioles; it contains alveolar ducts and alveoli. It is the largest unit in which all airways participate in gas exchange and is approximately 6 to 10 mm in diameter. One secondary pulmonary lobule contains between 3 and 25 acini.[7]

Radiographs and CT scans—Individual normal acini are not visible, but acinar arteries can occasionally be identified on thin-section CT scans. Accumulation of pathologic material in acini may be seen as poorly defined nodular opacities on chest radiographs and thin-section CT images. (See also *nodules*.)

[a]Reprinted with permission from RSNA. Original publication: Hansell DM, Bankier AA, MacMahon H, et al. Fleischner Society: Glossary of terms for thoracic imaging. Radiology 2008;246:697–722. Radiology is owned and published by the Radiological Society of North America, Inc. (RSNA).

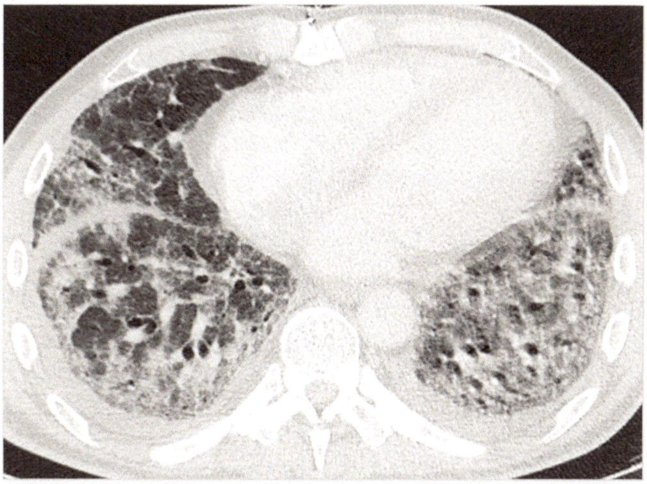

Fig. 25.1 Transverse CT scan in a patient with acute interstitial pneumonia.

Acute interstitial pneumonia, or AIP

Pathology—The term *acute interstitial pneumonia* is reserved for diffuse alveolar damage of unknown cause. The acute phase is characterized by edema and hyaline membrane formation. The later phase is characterized by airspace and/or interstitial organization.[8] The histologic pattern is indistinguishable from that of acute respiratory distress syndrome.

Radiographs and CT scans—In the acute phase, patchy bilateral ground-glass opacities are seen,[9] often with some sparing of individual lobules, producing a geographic appearance; dense opacification is seen in the dependent lung (▸Fig. 25.1). In the organizing phase, architectural distortion, traction bronchiectasis, cysts, and reticular opacities are seen.[10]

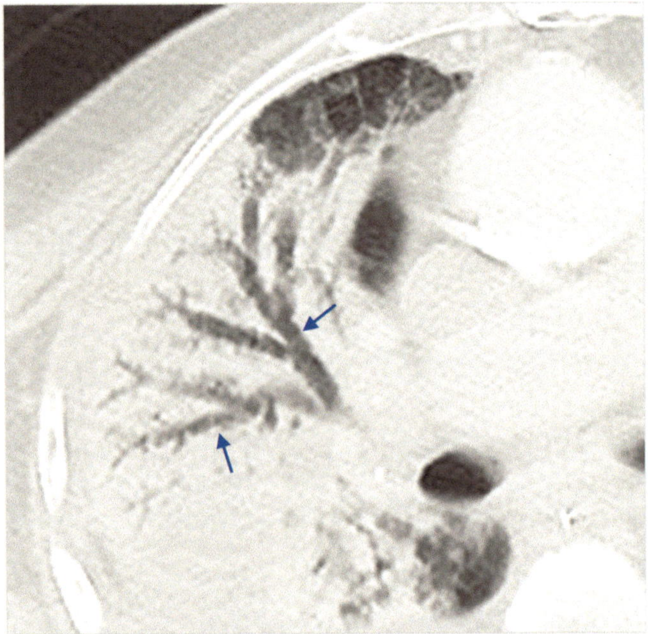

Fig. 25.2 Transverse CT scan shows air bronchogram as air-filled bronchi (*arrows*) against background of high-attenuation lung.

Air bronchogram

Radiographs and CT scans—An air bronchogram is a pattern of air-filled (low-attenuation) bronchi on a background of opaque (high-attenuation) airless lung (▶Fig. 25.2). The sign implies (1) patency of proximal airways and (2) evacuation of alveolar air by means of absorption (atelectasis) or replacement (e.g., pneumonia) or a combination of these processes. In rare cases, the displacement of air is the result of marked interstitial expansion (e.g., lymphoma).[11]

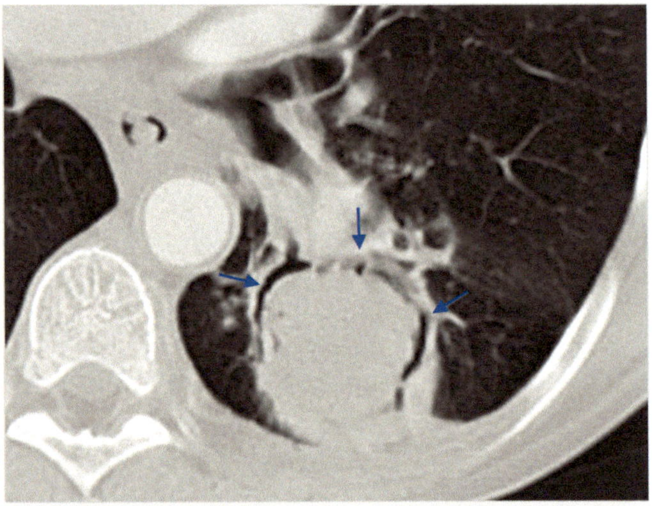

Fig. 25.3 Transverse CT scan shows air crescent (*arrows*) adjacent to mycetoma.

Air crescent

Radiographs and CT scans—An air crescent is a collection of air in a crescentic shape that separates the wall of a cavity from an inner mass (▶Fig. 25.3). The air crescent sign is often considered characteristic of either *Aspergillus* colonization of preexisting cavities or retraction of infarcted lung in angioinvasive aspergillosis.[12,13] However, the air crescent sign has also been reported in other conditions, including tuberculosis, Wegener granulomatosis, intracavitary hemorrhage, and lung cancer. (See also *mycetoma*.)

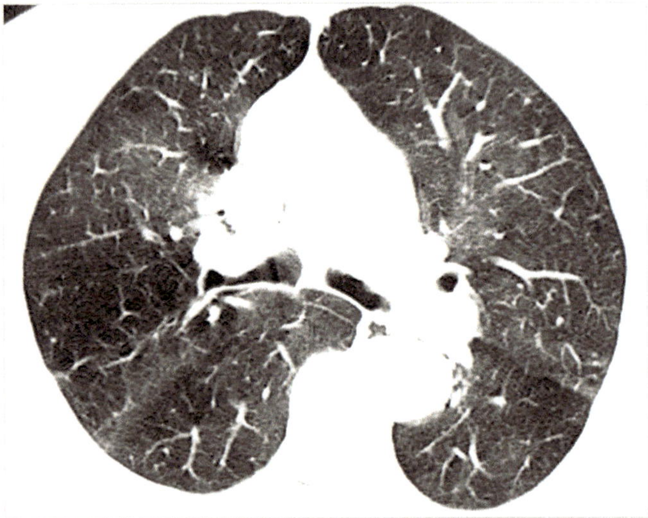

Fig. 25.4 Transverse CT scans at end expiration shows air trapping.

Air trapping

Pathophysiology—Air trapping is retention of air in the lung distal to an obstruction (usually partial).

CT scans—Air trapping is seen on end-expiration CT scans as parenchymal areas with less than normal increase in attenuation and lack of volume reduction. Comparison between inspiratory and expiratory CT scans can be helpful when air trapping is subtle or diffuse[14,15] (▶Fig. 25.4). Differentiation from areas of decreased attenuation resulting from hypoperfusion as a consequence of an occlusive vascular disorder (e.g., chronic thromboembolism) may be problematic,[16] but other findings of airways versus vascular disease are usually present. (See also *mosaic attenuation pattern.*)

Airspace

Anatomy—An airspace is the gas-containing part of the lung, including the respiratory bronchioles but excluding purely conducting airways, such as terminal bronchioles.

Radiographs and CT scans—This term is used in conjunction with consolidation, opacity, and nodules to designate the filling of airspaces with the products of disease.[17]

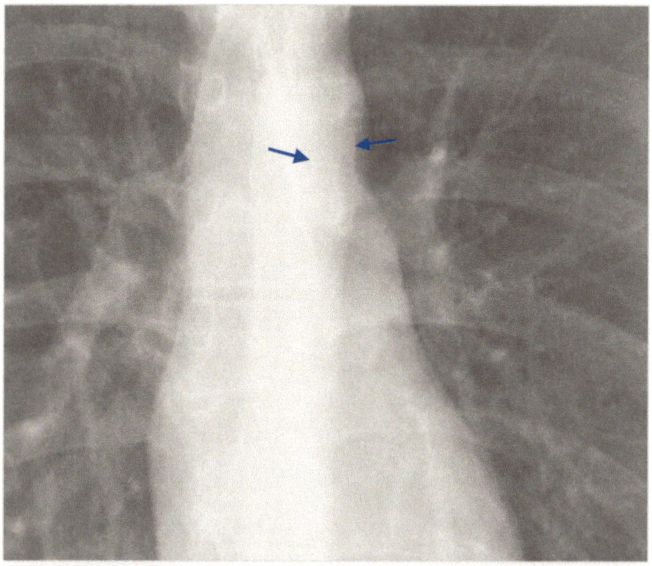

Fig. 25.5 Magnified chest radiograph shows aortopulmonary window (*arrows*).

Aortopulmonary window

Anatomy—The aortopulmonary window is the mediastinal region bounded anteriorly by the ascending aorta, posteriorly by the descending aorta, cranially by the aortic arch, inferiorly by the left pulmonary artery, medially by the ligamentum arteriosum, and laterally by the pleura and left lung.[18,19]

Radiographs and CT scans—Focal concavity in the left mediastinal border below the aorta and above the left pulmonary artery can be seen on a frontal radiograph (▶Fig. 25.5). Its appearance may be modified by tortuosity of the aorta. The aortopulmonary window is a common site of lymphadenopathy in a variety of inflammatory and neoplastic diseases.

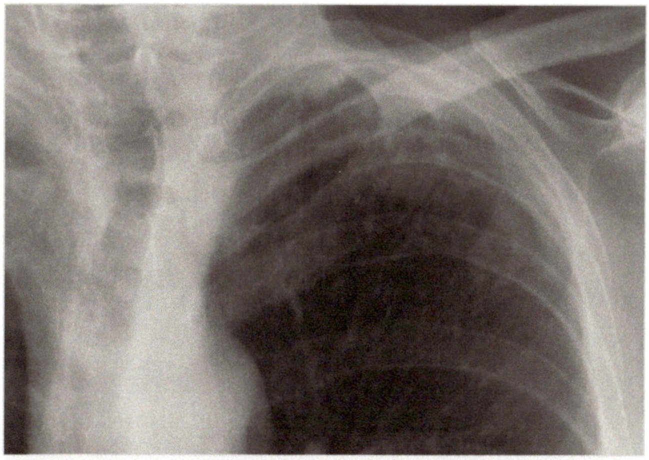

Fig. 25.6 Magnified chest radiograph shows apical cap.

Apical cap

Pathology—An apical cap is a caplike lesion at the lung apex, usually caused by intrapulmonary and pleural fibrosis pulling down extrapleural fat[20] or possibly by chronic ischemia resulting in hyaline plaque formation on the visceral pleura.[21] The prevalence increases with age. It can also be seen in hematoma resulting from aortic rupture or in other fluid collection associated with infection or tumor, either outside the parietal pleura or loculated within the pleural space.[22]

Radiographs and CT scans—The usual appearance is of homogeneous soft-tissue attenuation capping the extreme lung apex (uni- or bilaterally), with a sharp or irregular lower border (▶Fig. 25.6). Thickness is variable, ranging up to about 30 mm.[20] An apical cap occasionally mimics apical consolidation on transverse CT scans.

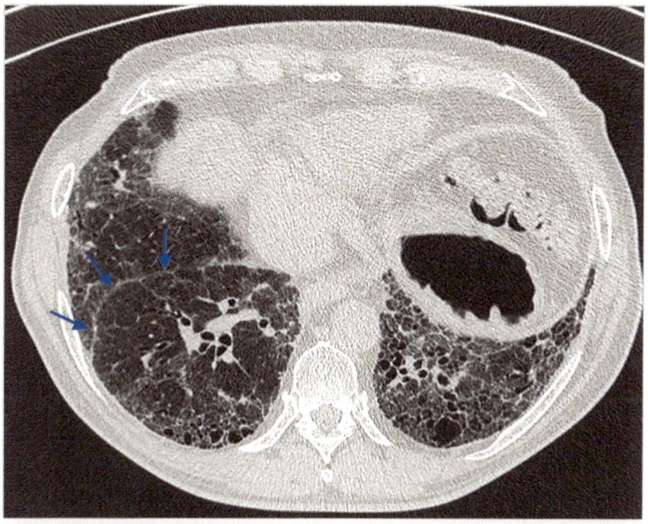

Fig. 25.7 Transverse CT scan shows architectural distortion caused by pulmonary fibrosis (*arrows*).

Architectural distortion

Pathology—Architectural distortion is characterized by abnormal displacement of bronchi, vessels, fissures, or septa caused by diffuse or localized lung disease, particularly interstitial fibrosis.

CT scans—Lung anatomy has a distorted appearance and is usually associated with pulmonary fibrosis (▶Fig. 25.7) and accompanied by volume loss.

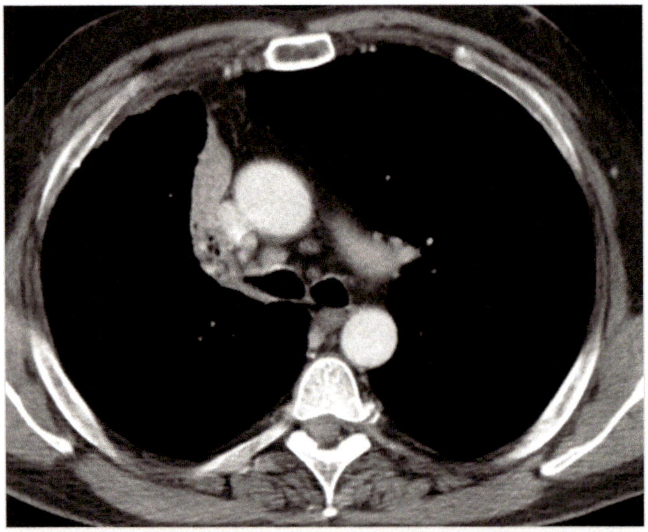

Fig. 25.8 Transverse CT scan shows atelectasis of right upper lobe as increased attenuation adjacent to the mediastinum.

Atelectasis

Pathophysiology—Atelectasis is reduced inflation of all or part of the lung.[23] One of the commonest mechanisms is resorption of air distal to airway obstruction (e.g., an endobronchial neoplasm).[24] The synonym collapse is often used interchangeably with atelectasis, particularly when it is severe or accompanied by obvious increase in lung opacity.

Radiographs and CT scans—Reduced volume is seen, accompanied by increased opacity (chest radiograph) or attenuation (CT scan) in the affected part of the lung (▶Fig. 25.8). Atelectasis is often associated with abnormal displacement of fissures, bronchi, vessels, diaphragm, heart, or mediastinum.[25] The distribution can be lobar, segmental, or subsegmental. Atelectasis is often qualified by descriptors such as linear, discoid, or platelike. (See also *linear atelectasis, rounded atelectasis.*)

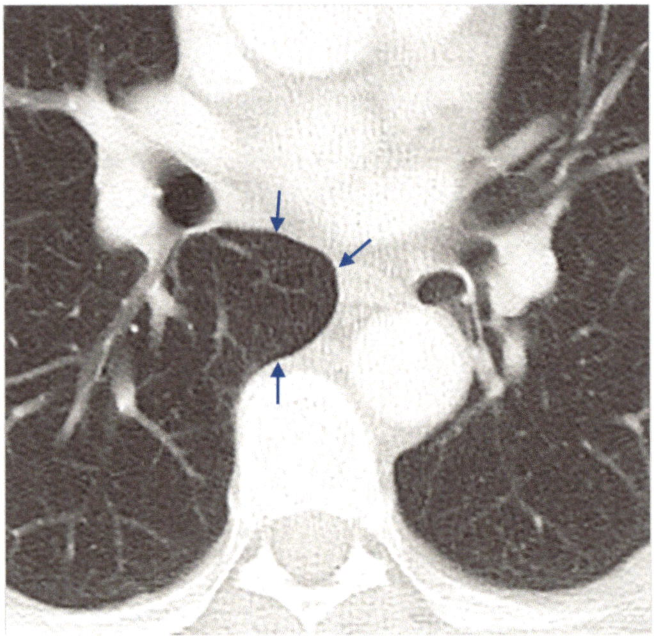

Fig. 25.9 Transverse CT scan shows azygoesophageal recess (*arrows*).

Azygoesophageal recess

Anatomy—The azygoesophageal recess is a right posterior mediastinal recess into which the edge of the right lower lobe extends. It is limited superiorly by the azygos arch, posteriorly by the azygos vein and pleura anterior to the vertebral column, and medially by the esophagus and adjacent structures.

Radiographs and CT scans—On a frontal chest radiograph, the recess is seen as a vertically oriented interface between the right lower lobe and the adjacent mediastinum (the medial limit of the recess). Superiorly, the interface is seen as a smooth arc with convexity to the left. Disappearance or distortion of part of the interface suggests disease (e.g., subcarinal lymphadenopathy). On CT scans, the recess (▶Fig. 25.9) merits attention because small lesions located in the recess will often be invisible on chest radiographs.[26]

Azygos fissure

See fissure.

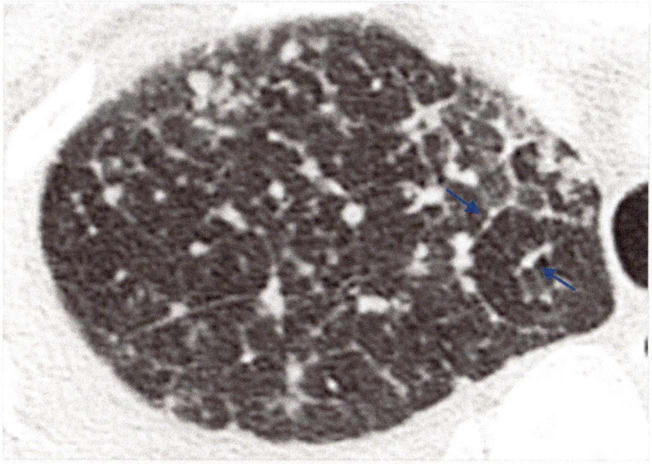

Fig. 25.10 Transverse CT scan shows beaded septum sign (*arrows*).

Beaded septum sign

CT scans—This sign consists of irregular and nodular thickening of interlobular septa reminiscent of a row of beads (▶ Fig. 25.10). It is frequently seen in lymphangitic spread of cancer and less often in sarcoidosis.[27]

Bleb

Anatomy—A bleb is a small gas-containing space within the visceral pleura or in the subpleural lung, not larger than 1 cm in diameter.[28]

CT scans—A bleb appears as a thin-walled cystic air space contiguous with the pleura. Because the arbitrary (size)-distinction between a bleb and bulla is of little clinical importance, the use of this term by radiologists is discouraged.

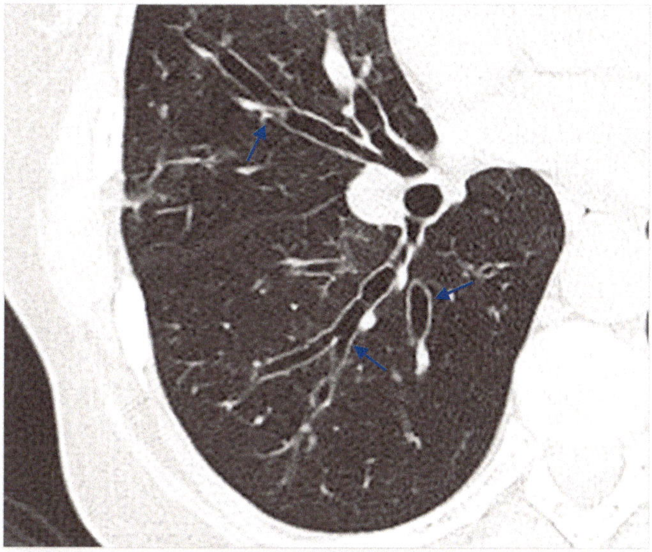

Fig. 25.11 Transverse CT scan shows varicose bronchiectasis (*arrows*).

Bronchiectasis

Pathology—Bronchiectasis is irreversible localized or diffuse bronchial dilatation, usually resulting from chronic infection, proximal airway obstruction, or congenital bronchial abnormality.[29] (See also *traction bronchiectasis*.)

Radiographs and CT scans—Morphologic criteria on thin-section CT scans include bronchial dilatation with respect to the accompanying pulmonary artery (signet ring sign), lack of tapering of bronchi, and identification of bronchi within 1 cm of the pleural surface[30] (▶ Fig. 25.11). Bronchiectasis may be classified as cylindric, varicose, or cystic, depending on the appearance of the affected bronchi. It is often accompanied by bronchial wall thickening, mucoid impaction, and small-airways abnormalities.[30,31,32] (See also *signet ring sign*.)

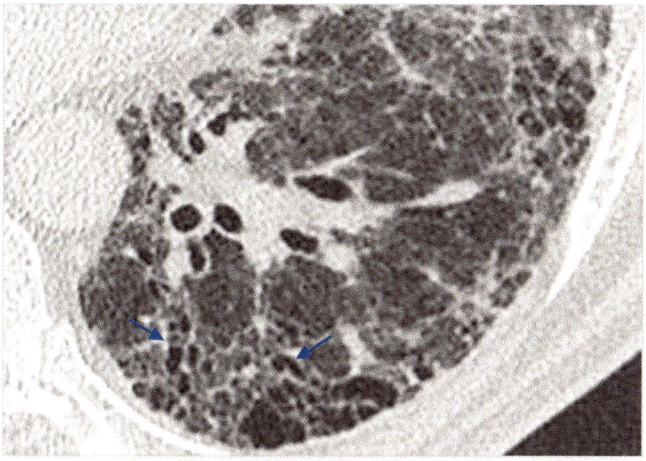

Fig. 25.12 Transverse CT scan shows bronchiolectasis within fibrotic lung (*arrows*).

Bronchiole

Anatomy—Bronchioles are non–cartilage-containing airways. Terminal bronchioles are the most distal of the purely conducting airways; they give rise to respiratory bronchioles, from which the alveoli arise and permit gas exchange. Respiratory bronchioles branch into multiple alveolar ducts.[33]

Radiographs and CT scans—Bronchioles are not identifiable in healthy individuals, because the bronchiolar walls are too thin.[7] In inflammatory small-airways disease, however, thickened or plugged bronchioles may be seen as a nodular pattern on a chest radiograph or as a tree-in-bud pattern on CT scans.

Bronchiolectasis

Pathology—Bronchiolectasis is defined as dilatation of bronchioles. It is caused by inflammatory airways disease (potentially reversible) or, more frequently, fibrosis.

CT scans—When dilated bronchioles are filled with exudate and are thick walled, they are visible as a tree-in-bud pattern or as centrilobular nodules.[34,35] In traction bronchiolectasis, the dilated bronchioles are seen as small, cystic, tubular airspaces, associated with CT findings of fibrosis (▶ Fig. 25.12). (See also *traction bronchiectasis and traction bronchiolectasis, tree-in-bud pattern*.)

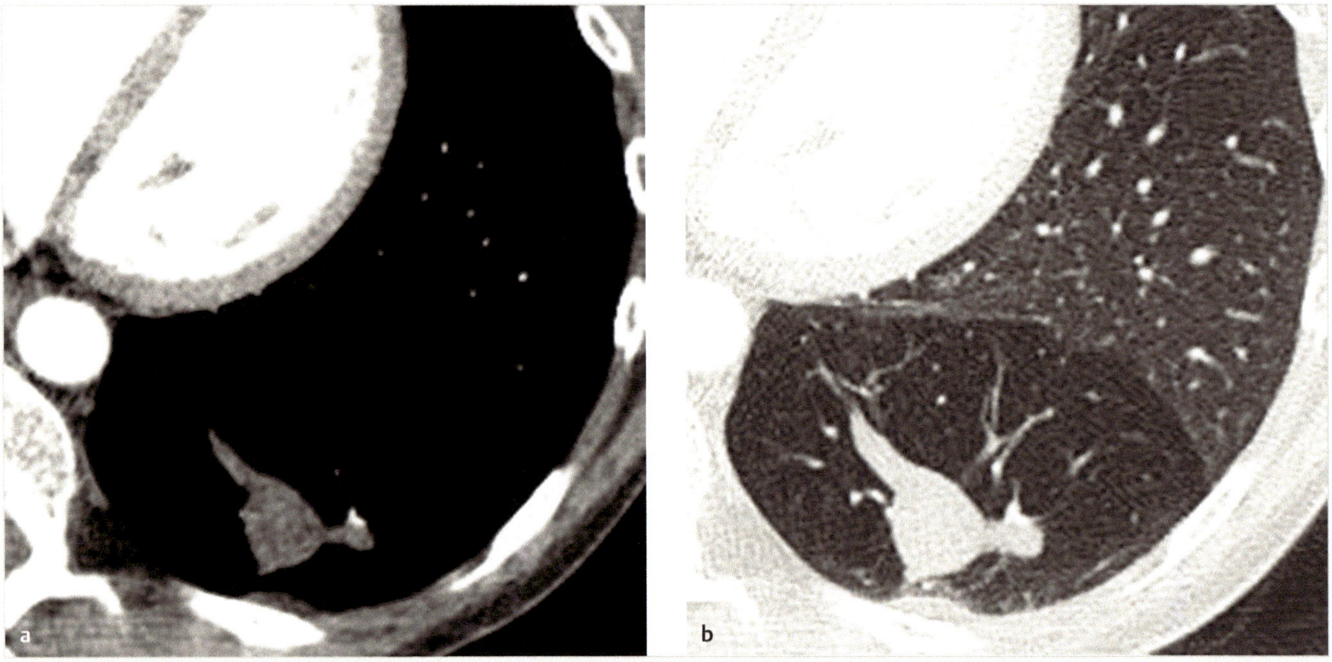

Fig. 25.13 Transverse CT scan shows bronchocele. **(a)** Soft-tissue window. **(b)** Lung window.

Bronchiolitis

Pathology—Bronchiolitis is bronchiolar inflammation of various causes.[36]

CT scans—This direct sign of bronchiolar inflammation (e.g., infectious cause) is most often seen as the tree-in-bud pattern, centrilobular nodules, and bronchiolar wall thickening on CT scans. (See also *small-airways disease, tree-in-bud pattern.*)

Bronchocele

Pathology—A bronchocele is bronchial dilatation due to retained secretions (mucoid impaction) usually caused by proximal obstruction, either congenital (e.g., bronchial atresia) or acquired (e.g., obstructing cancer).[37]

Radiographs and CT scans—A bronchocele is a tubular or branching Y or V-shaped structure that may resemble a gloved finger (▸Fig. 25.13). The CT attenuation of the mucus is generally that of soft tissue but may be modified by its composition (e.g., high-attenuation material in allergic bronchopulmonary aspergillosis). In the case of bronchial atresia, the surrounding lung may be of decreased attenuation because of reduced ventilation and, thus, perfusion.

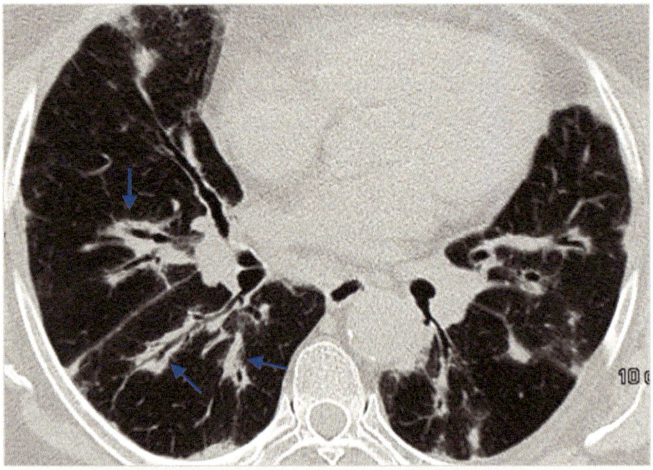

Fig. 25.14 Transverse CT scan shows consolidation with bronchocentric distribution (*arrows*).

Bronchocentric

CT scans—This descriptor is applied to disease that is conspicuously centered on macroscopic bronchovascular bundles (▸Fig. 25.14). Examples of diseases with a bronchocentric distribution include sarcoidosis,[38] Kaposi sarcoma,[39] and organizing pneumonia.[40]

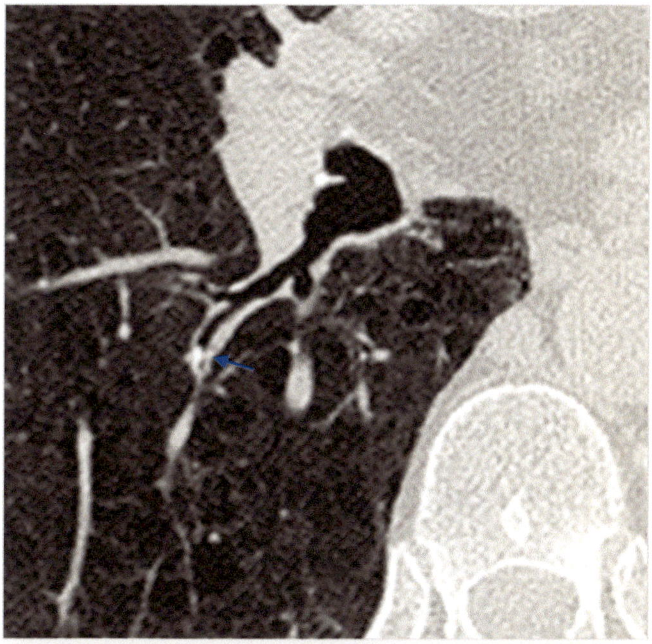

Fig. 25.15 Transverse CT scan shows a broncholith (*arrow*). (With kind permission of B. Rehbock, Berlin, Germany.)

Broncholith

Pathology—A broncholith, a calcified peribronchial lymph node that erodes into an adjacent bronchus, is most often the consequence of *Histoplasma* or tuberculous infection.

Radiographs and CT scans—The imaging appearance is of a small calcific focus in or immediately adjacent to an airway (▶ Fig. 25.15), most frequently the right middle lobe bronchus. Broncholiths are readily identified on CT scans.[41] Distal obstructive changes may include atelectasis, mucoid impaction, and bronchiectasis.

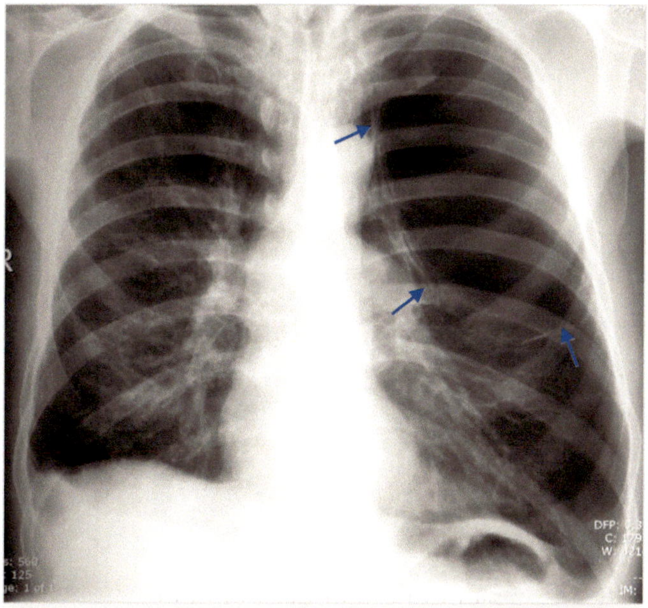

Fig. 25.16 Chest radiograph shows large bulla in left upper lung zone.

Bulla

Pathology—An airspace measuring more than 1 cm—usually several centimeters—in diameter, sharply demarcated by a thin wall that is no greater than 1 mm in thickness. A bulla is usually accompanied by emphysematous changes in the adjacent lung. (See also *bullous emphysema.*)

Radiographs and CT scans—A bulla appears as a rounded focal lucency or area of decreased attenuation, 1 cm or more in diameter, bounded by a thin wall (▶ Fig. 25.16). Multiple bullae are often present and are associated with other signs of pulmonary emphysema (centrilobular and paraseptal).

Bullous emphysema

Pathology—Bullous emphysema is bullous destruction of the lung parenchyma, usually on a background of paraseptal or panacinar emphysema. (See also *emphysema, bulla.*)

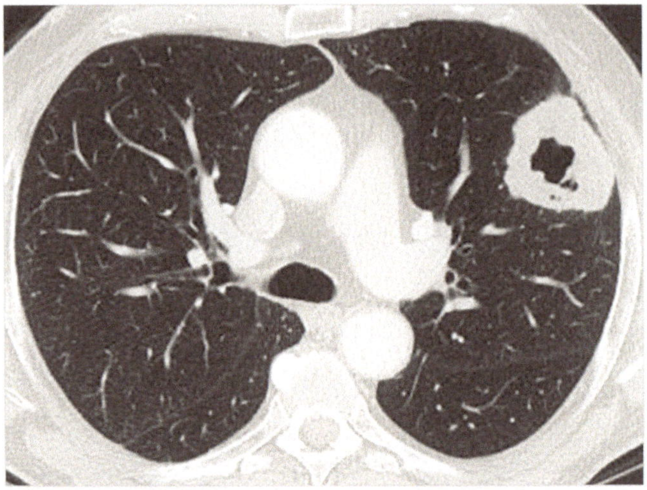

Fig. 25.17 Transverse CT scan shows cavitating mass in left upper lobe.

Cavity

Radiographs and CT scans—A cavity is a gas-filled space, seen as a lucency or low-attenuation area, within pulmonary consolidation, a mass, or a nodule (▶ Fig. 25.17). In the case of cavitating consolidation, the original consolidation may resolve and leave only a thin wall. A cavity is usually produced by the expulsion or drainage of a necrotic part of the lesion via the bronchial tree. It sometimes contains a fluid level. Cavity is not a synonym for abscess.

Centrilobular

Anatomy—Centrilobular describes the region of the bronchiolovascular core of a secondary pulmonary lobule.[7,42,43] This term is also used by pathologists to describe the location of lesions beyond the terminal bronchiole that center on respiratory bronchioles or even alveolar ducts.

CT scans.–A small dotlike or linear opacity in the center of a normal secondary pulmonary lobule, most obvious within 1 cm of a pleural surface, represents the intralobular artery (approximately 1 mm in diameter).[44] Centrilobular abnormalities include (1) nodules, (2) a tree-in-bud pattern indicating small-airways disease, (3) increased visibility of centrilobular structures due to thickening or infiltration of the adjacent interstitium, or (4) abnormal areas of low attenuation caused by centrilobular emphysema.[7] (See also *lobular core structures*.)

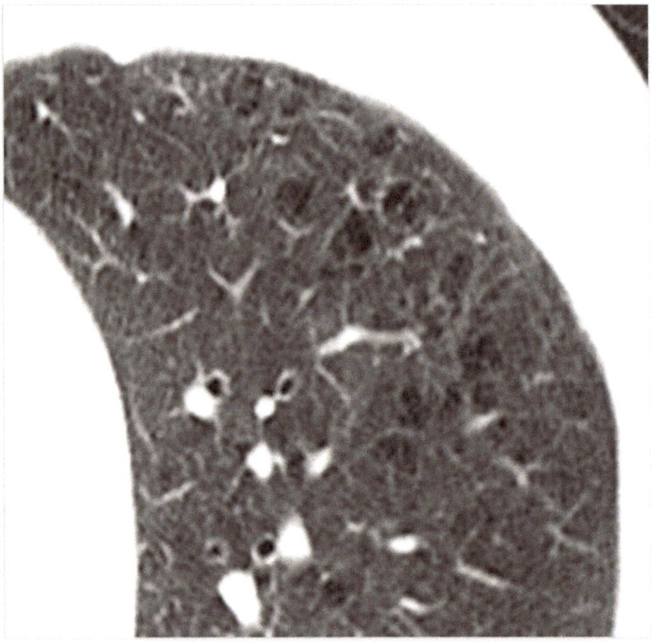

Fig. 25.18 Transverse CT scan shows centrilobular emphysema.

Centrilobular emphysema

Pathology—Centrilobular emphysema is characterized by destroyed centrilobular alveolar walls and enlargement of respiratory bronchioles and associated alveoli.[45,46] This is the commonest form of emphysema in cigarette smokers.

CT scans—CT findings are centrilobular areas of decreased attenuation, usually without visible walls, of nonuniform distribution and predominantly located in upper lung zones[47] (▶ Fig. 25.18). The term centriacinar emphysema is synonymous. (See also *emphysema*.)

Collapse

See atelectasis.

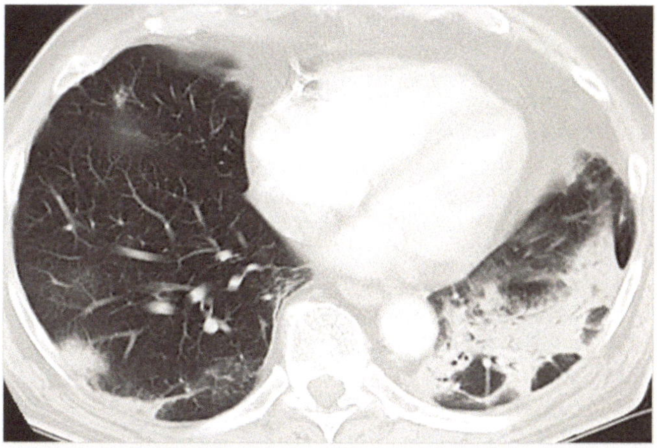

Fig. 25.19 Transverse CT scan shows multifocal consolidation.

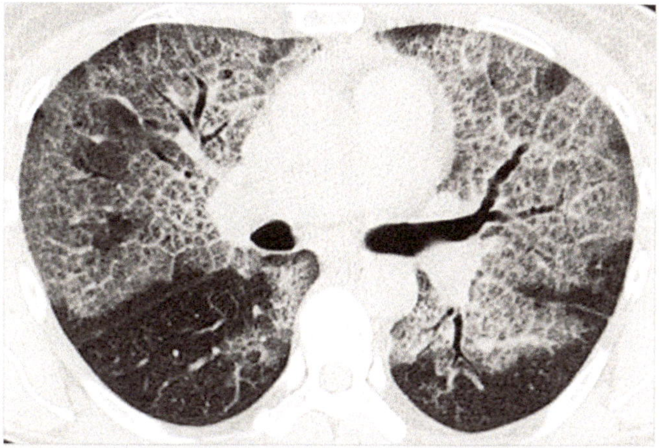

Fig. 25.20 Transverse CT scan shows crazy-paving pattern.

Consolidation

Pathology—Consolidation refers to an exudate or other product of disease that replaces alveolar air, rendering the lung solid (as in infective pneumonia).

Radiographs and CT scans—Consolidation appears as a homogeneous increase in pulmonary parenchymal attenuation that obscures the margins of vessels and airway walls[48] (▶Fig. 25.19). An air bronchogram may be present. The attenuation characteristics of consolidated lung are only rarely helpful in differential diagnosis (e.g., decreased attenuation in lipoid pneumonia[49] and increased in amiodarone toxicity[50]).

Crazy-paving pattern

CT scans—This pattern appears as thickened interlobular septa and intralobular lines superimposed on a background of ground-glass opacity (▶Fig. 25.20), resembling irregularly *shaped paving stones. The crazy-paving* pattern is often sharply demarcated from more normal lung and may have a geographic outline. It was originally reported in patients with pulmonary alveolar proteinosis[51] and is also encountered in other diffuse lung diseases[52] that affect both the interstitial and airspace compartments, such as lipoid pneumonia.[53]

Cryptogenic organizing pneumonia, or COP

See organizing pneumonia.

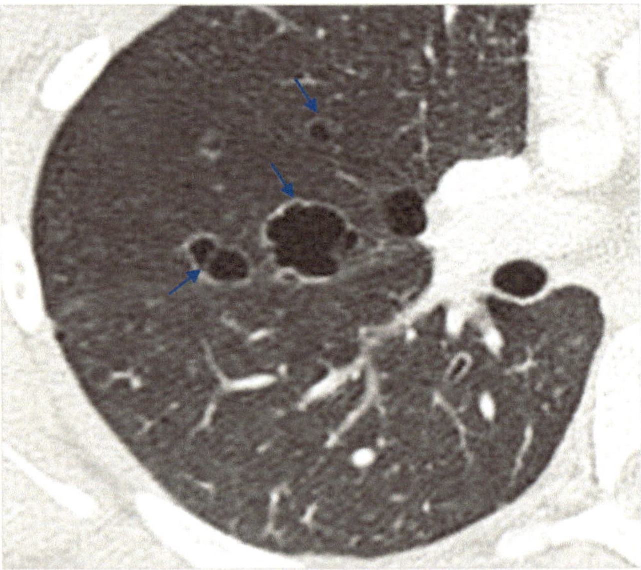

Fig. 25.21 Transverse CT scan shows cysts (*arrows*).

Cyst

Pathology—A cyst is any round circumscribed space that is surrounded by an epithelial or fibrous wall of variable thickness.[54]

Radiographs and CT scans—A cyst appears as a round parenchymal lucency or low-attenuating area with a well-defined interface with normal lung. Cysts have variable wall thickness but are usually thin-walled (<2 mm) and occur without associated pulmonary emphysema (▶ Fig. 25.21). Cysts in the lung usually contain air but occasionally contain fluid or solid material. The term is often used to describe enlarged thin-walled airspaces in patients with lymphangioleiomyomatosis[55] or Langerhans cell histiocytosis[56]; thicker walled honeycomb cysts are seen in patients with end-stage fibrosis.[57] (See also *bleb, bulla, honeycombing, pneumatocele.*)

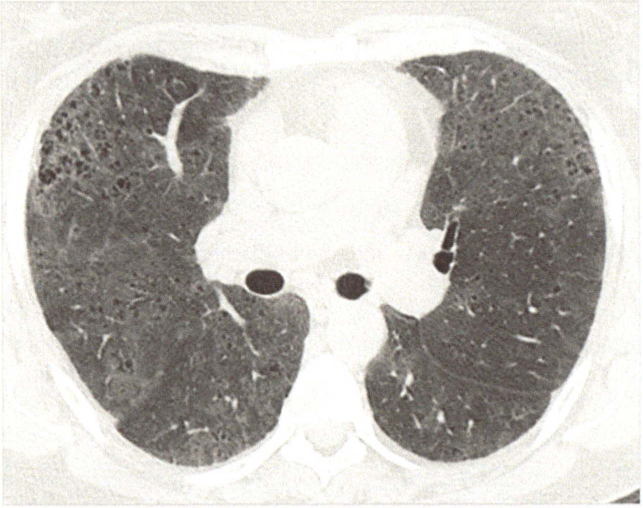

Fig. 25.22 Transverse CT scan in a patient with desquamative interstitial pneumonia.

Desquamative interstitial pneumonia, or DIP

Pathology—Histologically, DIP is characterized by the widespread accumulation of an excess of macrophages in the distal airspaces. The macrophages are uniformly distributed, unlike in respiratory bronchiolitis–interstitial lung disease, in which the disease is conspicuously bronchiolocentric. Interstitial involvement is minimal. Most cases of DIP are related to cigarette smoking, but a few are idiopathic or associated with rare inborn errors of metabolism.[8]

Radiographs and CT scans—Ground-glass opacity is the dominant abnormality and tends to have a basal and peripheral distribution (▶ Fig. 25.22). Microcystic or honeycomb changes in the area of ground-glass opacity are seen in some cases.[58]

Diffuse alveolar damage, or DAD

See acute interstitial pneumonia.

Emphysema

Pathology—Emphysema is characterized by permanently enlarged airspaces distal to the terminal bronchiole with destruction of alveolar walls.[45,46] Absence of “obvious fibrosis” was historically regarded as an additional criterion,[45] but the validity of that criterion has been questioned because some interstitial fibrosis may be present in emphysema secondary to cigarette smoking.[59,60] Emphysema is usually classified in terms of the part of the acinus predominantly affected: proximal (centriacinar, more commonly termed centrilobular, emphysema), distal (paraseptal emphysema), or whole acinus (panacinar or, less commonly, panlobular emphysema).

CT scans—The CT appearance of emphysema consists of focal areas or regions of low attenuation, usually without visible walls.[61] In the case of panacinar emphysema, decreased attenuation is more diffuse. (See also *bullous emphysema, centrilobular emphysema, panacinar emphysema, paraseptal emphysema.*)

Fissure

Anatomy—A fissure is the infolding of visceral pleura that separates one lobe or part of a lobe from another; thus, the interlobar fissures are produced by two layers of visceral pleura. Supernumerary fissures usually separate segments rather than lobes. The azygos fissure, unlike the other fissures, is formed by two layers each of visceral and parietal pleura. All fissures (apart from the azygos fissure) may be incomplete.

Radiographs and CT scans—Fissures appear as linear opacities, normally 1 mm or less in thickness, that correspond in position and extent to the anatomic fissural separation of pulmonary lobes or segments. Qualifiers include minor, major, horizontal, oblique, accessory, anomalous, azygos, and inferior accessory.

Folded lung

See *rounded atelectasis.*

Fungus ball

See *mycetoma.*

Gas trapping

See *air trapping.*

Ground-glass nodule

See *nodule.*

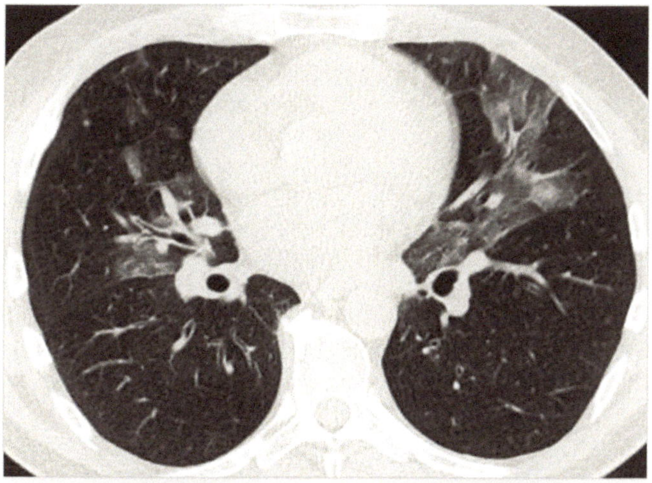

Fig. 25.23 Transverse CT scan shows ground-glass opacity.

Ground-glass opacity

Radiographs and CT scans—On chest radiographs, ground-glass opacity appears as an area of hazy increased lung opacity, usually extensive, within which margins of pulmonary vessels may be indistinct. On CT scans, it appears as hazy increased opacity of lung, with preservation of bronchial and vascular margins (▶Fig. 25.23). It is caused by partial filling of airspaces, interstitial thickening (due to fluid, cells, and/or fibrosis), partial collapse of alveoli, increased capillary blood volume, or a combination of these, the common factor being the partial displacement of air.[62,63] Ground-glass opacity is less opaque than consolidation, in which bronchovascular margins are obscured. (See also *consolidation*.)

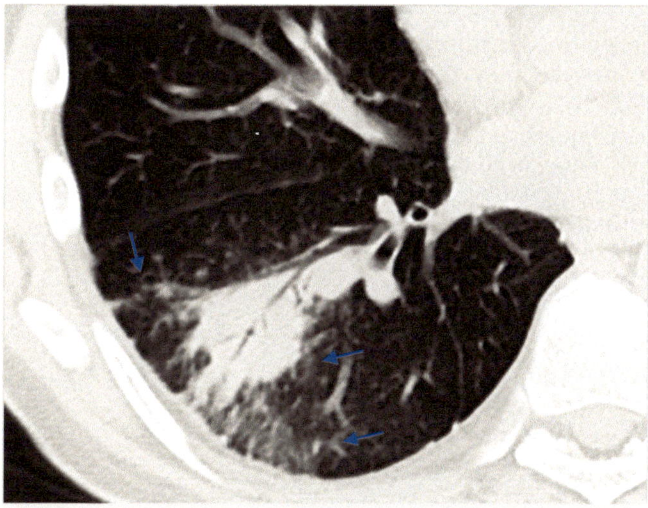

Fig. 25.24 Transverse CT scan shows nodule exhibiting the halo sign (*arrows*).

Halo sign

CT scans—The halo sign is a CT finding of ground-glass opacity surrounding a nodule or mass (▶Fig. 25.24). It was first described as a sign of hemorrhage around foci of invasive aspergillosis.[64] The halo sign is nonspecific and may also be caused by hemorrhage associated with other types of nodules[65] or by local pulmonary infiltration by neoplasm (e.g., adenocarcinoma). (See also *reversed halo sign*.)

Hilum

Anatomy—Hilum is a generic term that describes the indentation in the surface of an organ, where vessels and nerves connect with the organ. It is the site on the medial aspect of the lung where the vessels and bronchi enter and leave the lung.

Radiographs and CT scans—A hilum appears as a composite opacity at the root of each lung produced by bronchi, arteries, veins, lymph nodes, nerves, and other tissue. The terms hilum (singular) and hila (plural) are preferred to hilus and hili, respectively; the adjectival form is hilar.

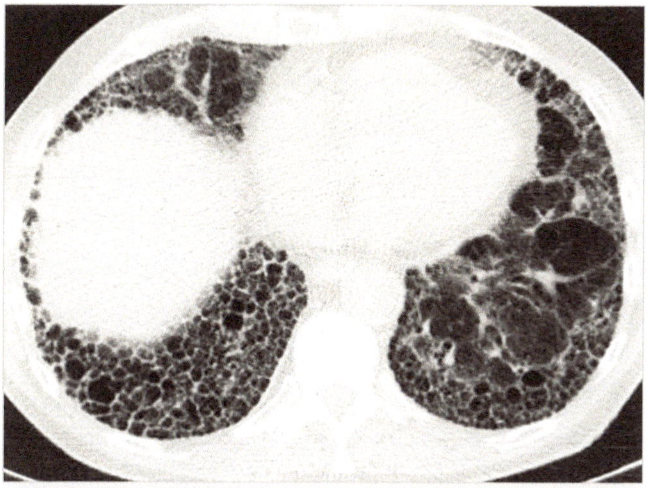

Fig. 25.25 Transverse CT scan shows honeycombing.

Honeycombing

Pathology—Honeycombing represents destroyed and fibrotic lung tissue containing numerous cystic airspaces with thick fibrous walls, representing the late stage of various lung diseases, with complete loss of acinar architecture. The cysts range in size from a few millimeters to several centimeters in diameter, have variable wall thickness, and are lined by metaplastic bronchiolar epithelium.[54]

Radiographs and CT scans—On chest radiographs, honeycombing appears as closely approximated ring shadows, typically 3 to 10 mm in diameter with walls 1 to 3 mm in thickness, that resemble a honeycomb; the finding implies end-stage lung disease. On CT scans, the appearance is of clustered cystic air spaces, typically of comparable diameters on the order of 3 to 10 mm but occasionally as large as 2.5 cm (▶Fig. 25.25). Honeycombing is usually subpleural and is characterized by well-defined walls.[57] It is a CT feature of established pulmonary fibrosis.[8] Because honeycombing is often considered specific for pulmonary fibrosis and is an important criterion in the diagnosis of usual interstitial pneumonia,[66] the term should be used with care, as it may directly impact patient care.

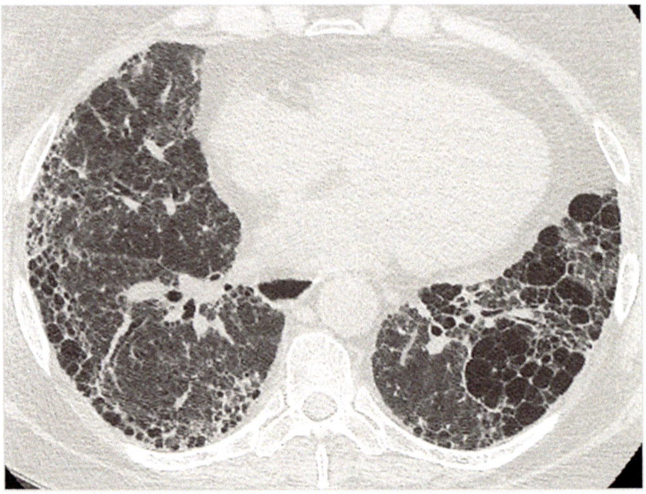

Fig. 25.26 Transverse CT scan shows reticular opacities and honeycombing in the lower zones, typical of idiopathic pulmonary fibrosis.

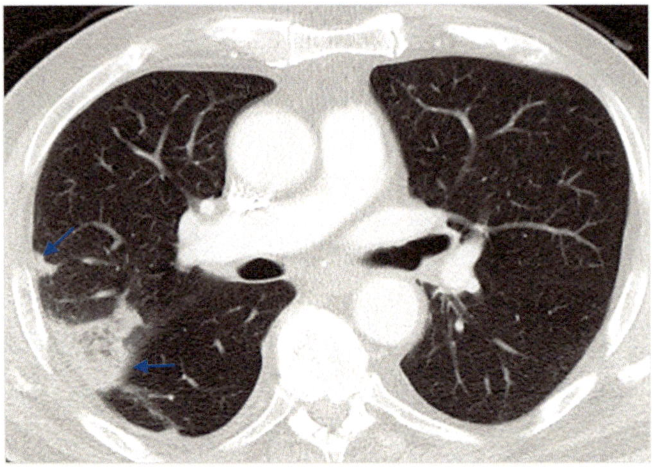

Fig. 25.27 Transverse CT scan shows pulmonary infarction (*arrows*).

Idiopathic pulmonary fibrosis

Pathology—Idiopathic pulmonary fibrosis is a specific form of chronic fibrosing interstitial pneumonia of unknown cause and is characterized by a histologic pattern of usual interstitial pneumonia.[8,67]

Radiographs and CT scans—The typical imaging findings are reticular opacities and honeycombing, with a predominantly peripheral and basal distribution (▶Fig. 25.26). Ground-glass opacity, if present, is less extensive than reticular and honeycombing patterns. The typical radiologic findings[68,69] are also encountered in usual interstitial pneumonia secondary to specific causes, such as asbestos-induced pulmonary fibrosis (asbestosis), and the diagnosis is usually one of exclusion. (See also *usual interstitial pneumonia.*)

Infarction

Pathology—Infarction is a process that may result in ischemic necrosis, usually the consequence of vascular compromise such as occlusion of a feeding pulmonary artery by an embolus (venous infarction is rare but recognized). Necrosis is relatively uncommon because tissue viability is maintained by the bronchial arterial blood supply. Pulmonary infarction may be secondary to a vasculitis (e.g., Wegener granulomatosis).

Radiographs and CT scans—A pulmonary infarct is typically triangular or dome-shaped, with the base abutting the pleura and the apex directed toward the hilum (▶Fig. 25.27). The opacity represents local hemorrhage with or without central tissue necrosis.[70,71]

Infiltrate

Radiographs and CT scans—Formerly used as a term to describe a region of pulmonary opacification caused by airspace or interstitial disease seen on radiographs and CT scans. Infiltrate remains controversial because it means different things to different people.[72] The term is no longer recommended, and has been largely replaced by other descriptors. The term opacity, with relevant qualifiers, is preferred.

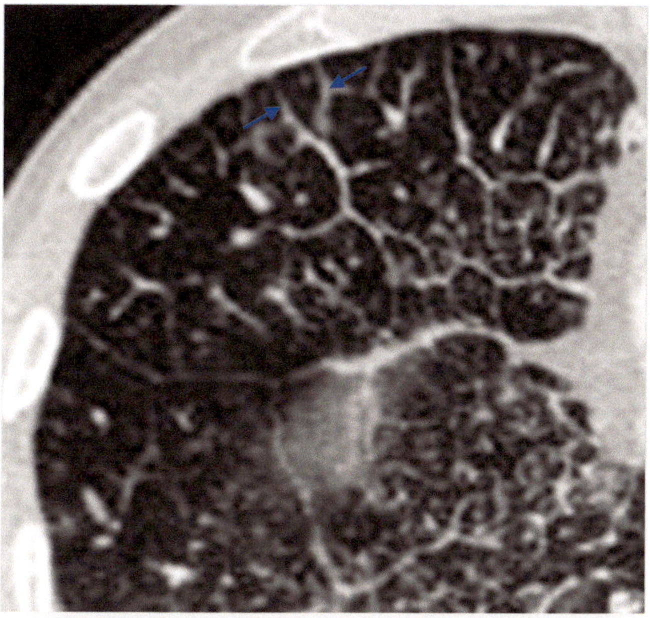

Fig. 25.28 Transverse CT scan shows interlobular septal thickening (*arrows*).

Interlobular septal thickening

Radiographs and CT scans—This finding is seen on chest radiographs as thin linear opacities at right angles to and in contact with the lateral pleural surfaces near the lung bases (Kerley B lines); it is seen most frequently in lymphangitic spread of cancer or pulmonary edema. Kerley A lines are predominantly situated in the upper lobes, are 2 to 6 cm long, and can be seen as fine lines radially oriented toward the hila. In recent years, the anatomically descriptive terms septal lines and septal thickening have gained favor over Kerley lines. On CT scans, disease affecting one of the components of the septa (see interlobular septum) may be responsible for thickening and so render septa visible. On thin-section CT scans, septal thickening may be smooth or nodular[73] (▸Fig. 25.28), which may help refine the differential diagnosis. (See also *interlobular septum, beaded septum.*)

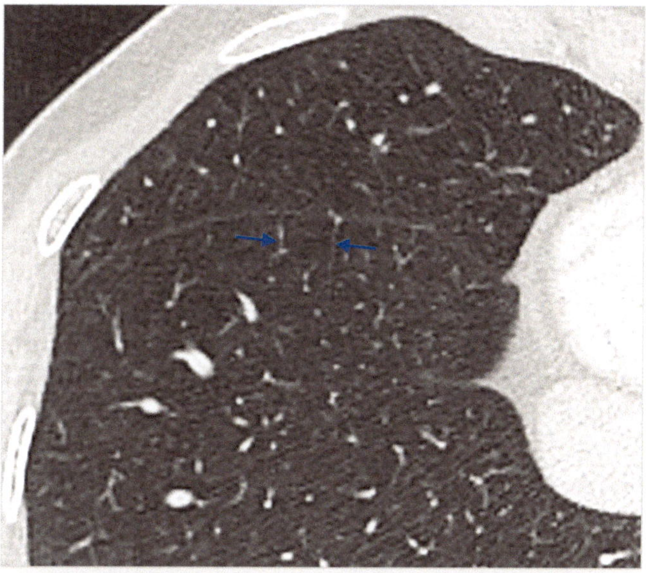

Fig. 25.29 Transverse CT scan shows interlobular septa (*arrows*) in a healthy individual.

Interlobular septum

Anatomy—Interlobular septa are sheetlike structures 10- to 20-mm long that form the borders of lobules; they are more or less perpendicular to the pleura in the periphery. Interlobular septa are composed of connective tissue and contain lymphatic vessels and pulmonary venules.

Radiographs and CT scans—Interlobular septa appear as thin linear opacities between lobules (▸Fig. 25.29); these septa are to be distinguished from centrilobular structures. They are not usually seen in the healthy lung (normal septa are approximately 0.1 mm thick) but are clearly visible when thickened (e.g., by pulmonary edema). (See also *interlobular septal thickening, lobule.*)

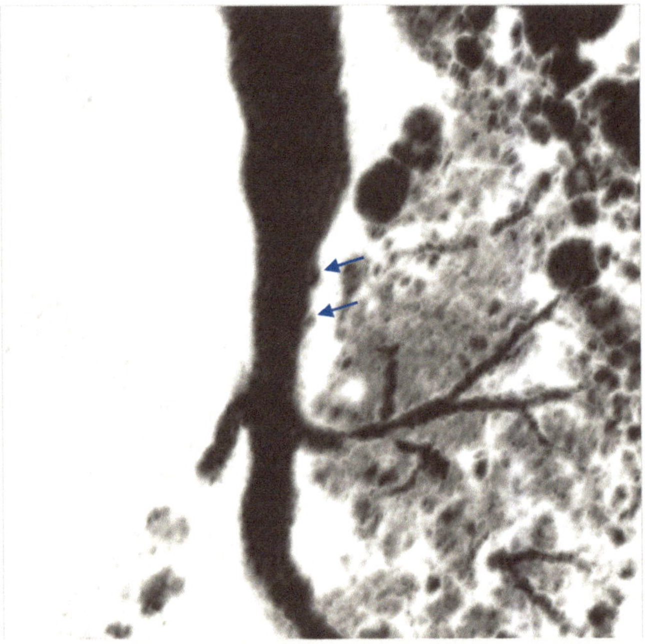

Fig. 25.30 Paracoronal CT scan shows interstitial emphysema (*arrow*).

Interstitial emphysema

Pathology—Interstitial emphysema is characterized by air dissecting within the interstitium of the lung, typically in the peribronchovascular sheaths, interlobular septa, and visceral pleura. It is most commonly seen in neonates receiving mechanical ventilation.

Radiographs and CT scans—Interstitial emphysema is rarely recognized radiographically in adults and is infrequently seen on CT scans (▶Fig. 25.30). It appears as perivascular lucent or low-attenuating halos and small cysts.[74,75]

Interstitium

Anatomy—The interstitium consists of a continuum of connective tissue throughout the lung comprising three subdivisions: (1) the bronchovascular (axial) interstitium, surrounding and supporting the bronchi, arteries, and veins from the hilum to the level of the respiratory bronchiole; (2) the parenchymal (acinar) interstitium, situated between alveolar and capillary basement membranes; and (3) the subpleural connective tissue contiguous with the interlobular septa.[76]

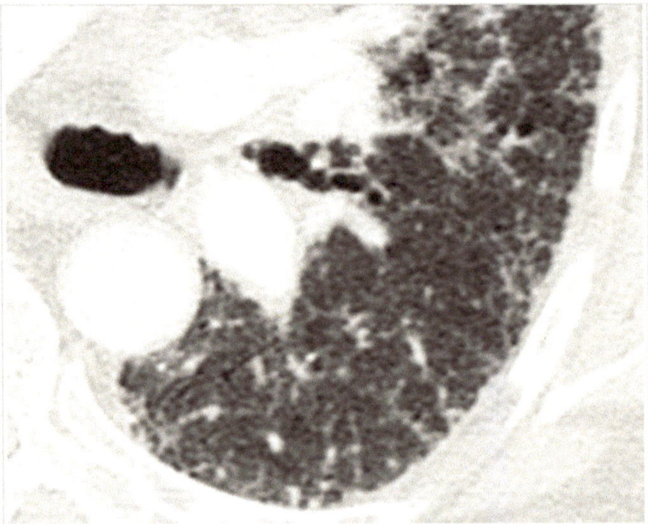

Fig. 25.31 Transverse CT scan shows intralobular lines.

Intralobular lines

CT scans—Intralobular lines are visible as fine linear opacities in a lobule when the intralobular interstitial tissue is abnormally thickened (▶Fig. 25.31). When numerous, they may appear as a fine reticular pattern. Intralobular lines may be seen in various conditions, including interstitial fibrosis and pulmonary alveolar proteinosis.[44]

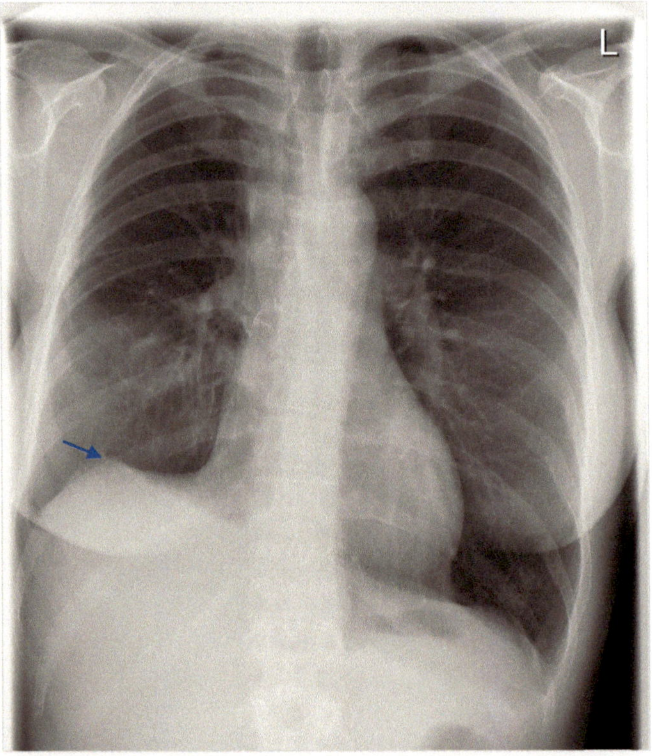

Fig. 25.32 Chest radiograph shows juxtaphrenic peak of the right hemidiaphragm (*arrow*).

Juxtaphrenic peak

Radiographs and CT scans—A juxtaphrenic peak is a small triangular opacity based at the apex of the dome of a hemidiaphragm, associated with upper lobe volume loss of any cause (e.g., postirradiation fibrosis or upper lobectomy).[77] It is most readily appreciated on a frontal chest radiograph (▶Fig. 25.32). The peak is caused by upward retraction of the inferior accessory fissure[78] or an intrapulmonary septum associated with the pulmonary ligament.[79]

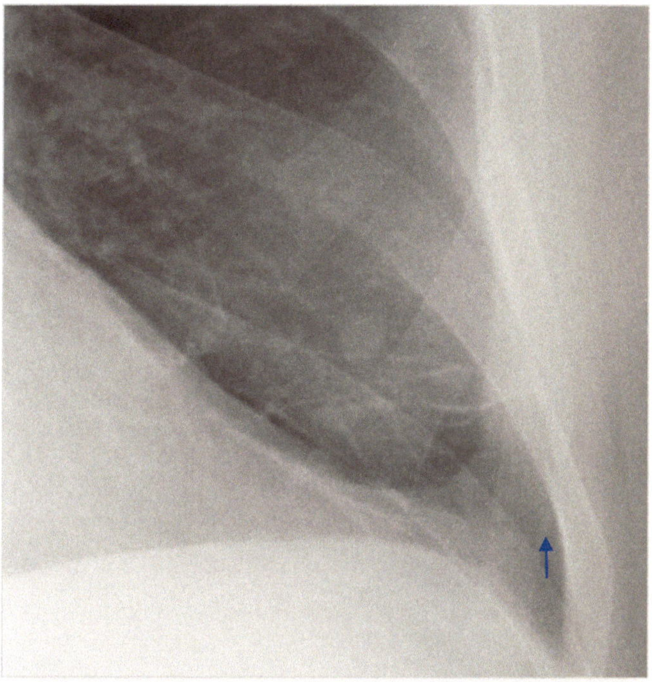

Fig. 25.33 Magnified chest radiograph shows basal linear atelectasis (*arrow*).

Linear atelectasis

Radiographs and CT scans—Linear atelectasis is a focal area of subsegmental atelectasis with a linear configuration, almost always extending to the pleura.[b,80] It is commonly horizontal but sometimes oblique or vertical. The thickness of the atelectasis may range from a few millimeters to more than 1 cm (▶Fig. 25.33). Linear atelectasis is also referred to as discoid or platelike atelectasis. (See also *atelectasis*.)

Lobe

Anatomy—The lobe is the principal division of the lungs (normally, three lobes on the right and two on the left); each lobe is enveloped by visceral pleura, except at the lung root (hilum) and when an interlobar fissure is incomplete.

[b]Dag Wormanns' note: In original publication,[4] erroneously referenced as Kattan et al.[66]

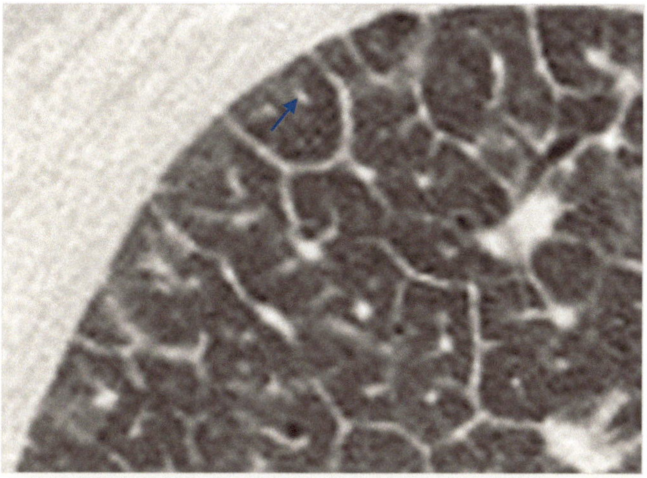

Fig. 25.34 Transverse CT scan shows lobular core structure (*arrow*).

Lobular core structures

Anatomy—Lobular core structures are the central structures in secondary pulmonary lobules and consist of a centrilobular artery and bronchiole.[42]

CT scans—The pulmonary artery and its immediate branches are visible in the center of a secondary lobule on thin-section CT scans, particularly if thickened (e.g., by pulmonary edema) (▶Fig. 25.34). These arteries measure approximately 0.5 to 1.0 mm in diameter. However, the normal bronchiole in the center of the secondary pulmonary lobule cannot be seen on thin-section CT scans because of the thinness of its wall (approximately 0.15 mm).[7,44] (See also *centrilobular, lobule*.)

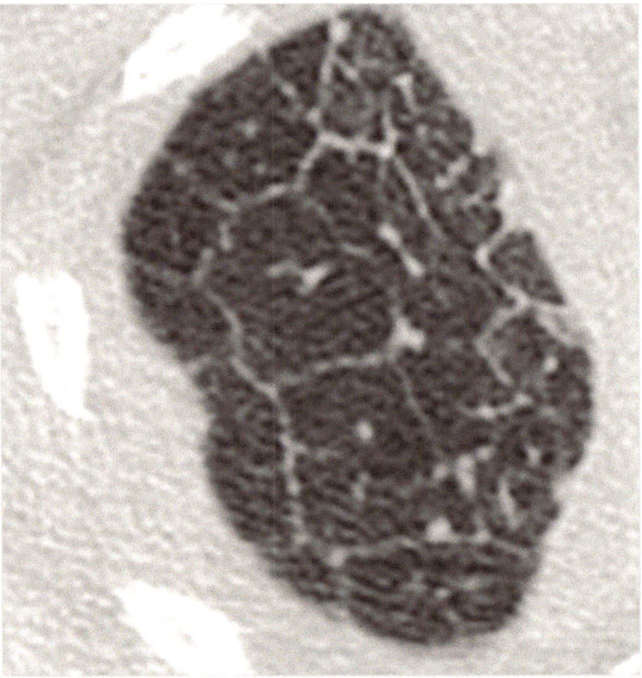

Fig. 25.35 Transverse CT scan shows lobules.

Lobule

Anatomy—The lobule is the smallest unit of lung surrounded by connective tissue septa, as defined by Miller[81] and Heitzman et al.[42] The lobule is also referred to as the secondary pulmonary lobule; it contains a variable number of acini, is irregularly polyhedral in shape, and varies in size from 1.0 to 2.5 cm in diameter. The centrilobular structures, or core structures, include bronchioles and their accompanying pulmonary arterioles and lymphatic vessels. The connective-tissue septa surrounding the pulmonary lobule—the interlobular septa, which contain veins and lymphatic vessels—are best developed in the periphery in the anterior, lateral, and juxtamediastinal regions of the upper and middle lobes.

CT scans—On thin-section CT scans, the three basic components of the lobule—the interlobular septa and septal structures, the central lobular region (centrilobular structures), and the lobular parenchyma—can be identified, particularly in disease states. Peripheral lobules are more uniform in appearance and pyramidal in shape than are central lobules[7] (▶Fig. 25.35). (See also *interlobular septa, lobular core structures.*)

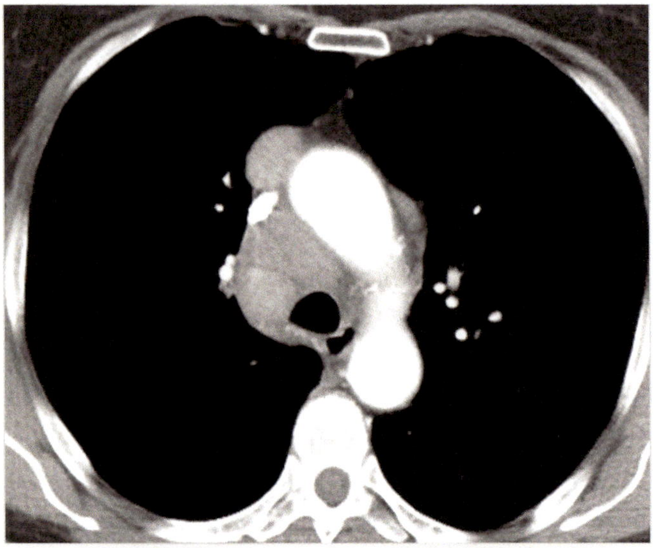

Fig. 25.36 Transverse CT scan shows lymphadenopathy (enlarged mediastinal lymph nodes).

Lymphadenopathy

Pathology—By common usage, the term lymphadenopathy is usually restricted to enlargement, due to any cause, of the lymph nodes. Synonyms include lymph node enlargement (preferred) and adenopathy.

CT scans—There is a wide range in the size of normal lymph nodes. Mediastinal and hilar lymph nodes range in size from sub-CT resolution to 12 mm. Somewhat arbitrary thresholds for the upper limit of normal of 1 cm in short-axis diameter for mediastinal nodes[82] and 3 mm for most hilar nodes[83] have been reported, but size criteria do not allow reliable differentiation between healthy and diseased lymph nodes (▶Fig. 25.36).

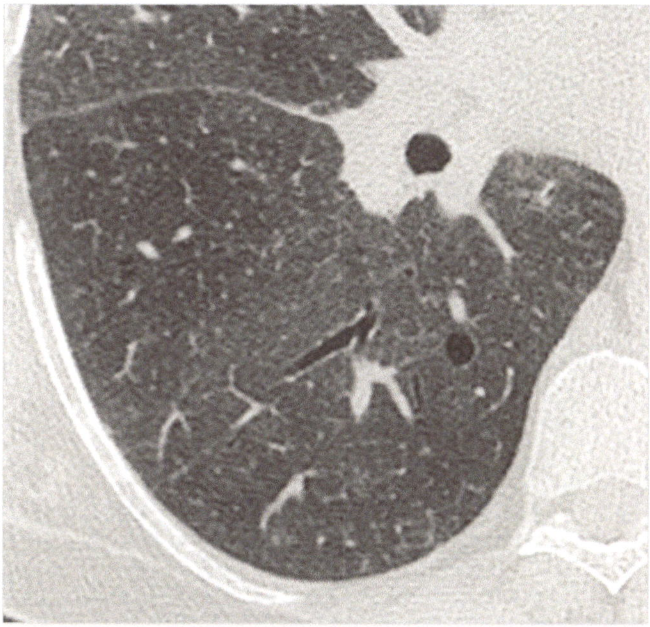

Fig. 25.37 Transverse CT scan shows ground-glass opacities and a perivascular cyst in a patient with lymphoid interstitial pneumonia.

Lymphoid interstitial pneumonia, or LIP

Pathology—LIP is a rare disease characterized by diffuse pulmonary lymphoid proliferation with predominant interstitial involvement. It is included in the spectrum of interstitial pneumonias and is distinct from diffuse lymphomas of the lung. Features include diffuse hyperplasia of bronchus-associated lymphoid tissue and diffuse polyclonal lymphoid cell infiltrates surrounding the airways and expanding the lung interstitium. LIP is usually associated with autoimmune diseases or human immunodeficiency virus infection.[8,84]

CT scans—Ground-glass opacity is the dominant abnormality, and thin-walled perivascular cysts may be present (▶Fig. 25.37). Lung nodules, a reticular pattern, interlobular septal and bronchovascular thickening, and widespread consolidation may also occur.[85,86]

Mass

Radiographs and CT scans—A mass is any pulmonary, pleural, or mediastinal lesion seen on chest radiographs as an opacity greater than 3 cm in diameter (without regard to contour, border, or density characteristics). Mass usually implies a solid or partly solid opacity. CT allows more exact evaluation of size, location, attenuation, and other features. (See also *nodule*.)

Mediastinal compartments

Anatomy—Nominal anatomic compartments of the mediastinum include the anterior, middle, posterior, and (in some schemes) superior compartments. The anterior compartment is bounded anteriorly by the sternum and posteriorly by the anterior surface of the pericardium, the ascending aorta, and the brachiocephalic vessels. The middle compartment is bounded by the posterior margin of the anterior division and the anterior margin of the posterior division. The posterior compartment is bounded anteriorly by the posterior margins of the pericardium and great vessels and posteriorly by the thoracic vertebral bodies. In the four-compartment model, the superior compartment is defined as the compartment above the plane between the sternal angle to the T4–T5 intervertebral disk or, more simply, above the aortic arch.[87,88] Exact anatomic boundaries between the compartments do not exist, and there are no barriers (other than the pericardium) to prevent the spread of disease between compartments. Other classifications exist, but the three- and four-compartment models are the most commonly used.

Micronodule

CT scans—A micronodule is a discrete, small, round, focal opacity. A variety of diameters have been used in the past to define a micronodule; for example, a diameter of no greater than 7 mm.[89] Use of the term is most often limited to nodules with a diameter of less than 5 mm[90] or less than 3 mm.[91] It is recommended that the term be reserved for opacities less than 3 mm in diameter. (See also *nodule, miliary pattern.*)

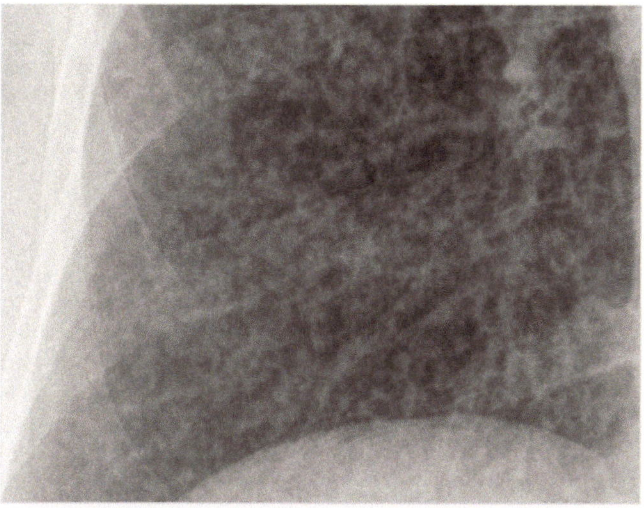

Fig. 25.38 Magnified chest radiograph shows miliary pattern.

Miliary pattern

Radiographs and CT scans—On chest radiographs, the miliary pattern consists of profuse tiny, discrete, rounded pulmonary opacities (≤3 mm in diameter) that are generally uniform in size and diffusely distributed throughout the lungs (▶Fig. 25.38). This pattern is a manifestation of hematogenous spread of tuberculosis and metastatic disease. Thin-section CT scans show widespread, randomly distributed micronodules.

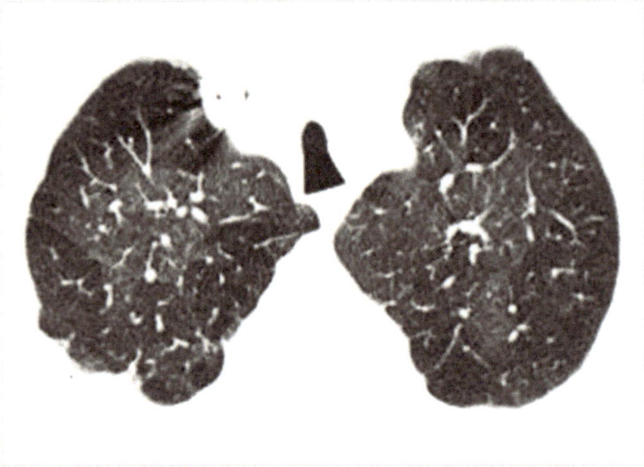

Fig. 25.39 Transverse CT scan shows mosaic attenuation pattern.

Mosaic attenuation pattern

CT scans—This pattern appears as patchwork of regions of differing attenuation that may represent (1) patchy interstitial disease, (2) obliterative small-airways disease (▶Fig. 25.39), or (3) occlusive vascular disease.[92] Mosaic attenuation pattern is a more inclusive term than the original terms mosaic oligemia and perfusion.[93] Air trapping secondary to bronchial or bronchiolar obstruction may produce focal zones of decreased attenuation, an appearance that can be enhanced by using expiratory CT.[94,95] The mosaic attenuation pattern can also be produced by interstitial lung disease characterized by ground-glass opacity; in this situation, areas of higher attenuation represent the interstitial process and areas of lower attenuation represent the normal lung.

Mosaic oligemia, perfusion

See *mosaic attenuation pattern*.

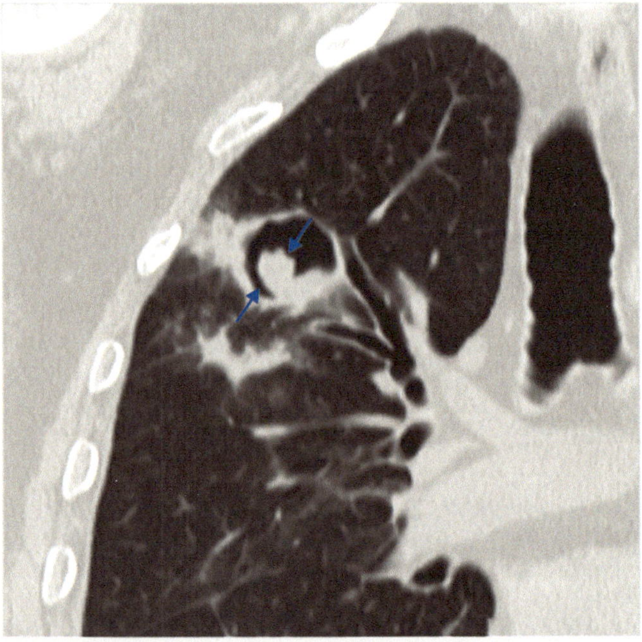

Fig. 25.40 Coronal CT scan shows mycetoma (*arrows*).

Mycetoma

Pathology—A mycetoma is a discrete mass of intertwined hyphae, usually of an *Aspergillus* species, matted together by mucus, fibrin, and cellular debris colonizing a cavity, usually from prior fibrocavitary disease (e.g., tuberculosis or sarcoidosis).

Radiographs and CT scans—A mycetoma may move to a dependent location when the patient changes position and may show an air crescent sign (▶Fig. 25.40). CT scans may show a spongelike pattern and foci of calcification in the mycetoma.[96] A synonym is fungus ball. (See also *air crescent*.)

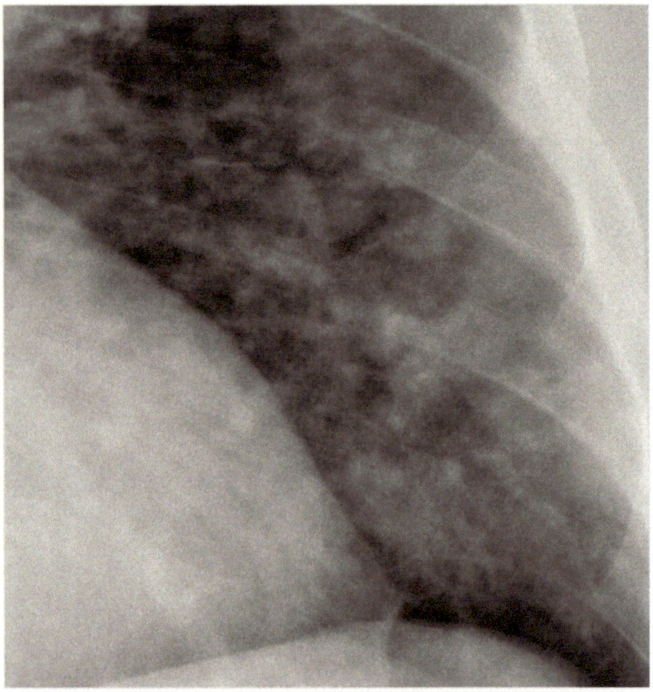

Fig. 25.41 Magnified chest radiograph shows a nodular pattern.

Nodular pattern

Radiographs and CT scans—A nodular pattern is characterized on chest radiographs by the presence of innumerable small rounded opacities that are discrete and range in diameter from 2 to 10 mm (▶Fig. 25.41). The distribution is widespread but not necessarily uniform. On CT scans, the pattern may be classified as one of three anatomic distributions: centrilobular, perilymphatic,[c] or random. (See also *nodule*.)

[c]Dag Wormanns' note: In original publication,[4] erroneously: lymphatic.

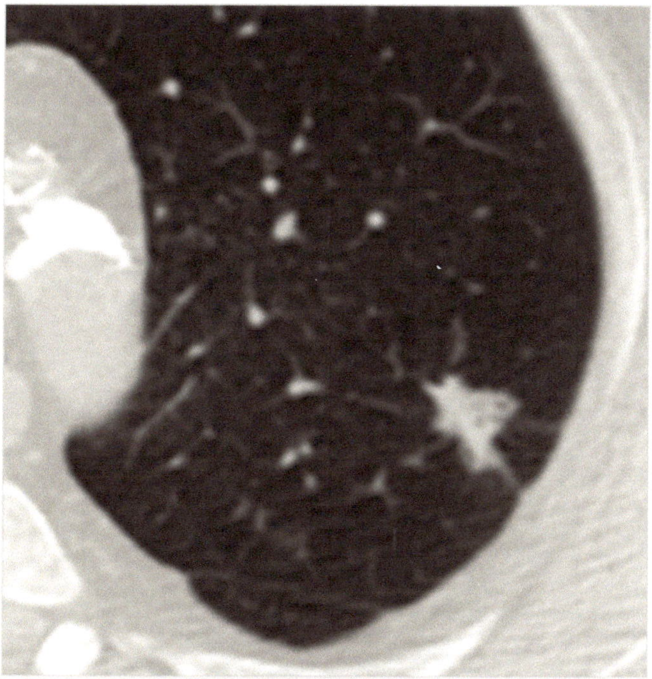

Fig. 25.42 Transverse CT scan shows irregular nodule in left upper lobe.

Nodule

Radiographs and CT scans—The chest radiographic appearance of a nodule is a rounded opacity, well or poorly defined, measuring up to 3 cm in diameter. (1) Acinar nodules are round or ovoid poorly defined pulmonary opacities approximately 5 to 8 mm in diameter, presumed to represent an anatomic acinus rendered opaque by consolidation. This classification is used only in the presence of numerous such opacities. (2) A pseudonodule mimics a pulmonary nodule; it represents, for example, a rib fracture, a skin lesion, a device on the surface of the patient, anatomic variants, or composite areas of increased opacity.[97] On CT scans, a nodule appears as a rounded or irregular opacity, well or poorly defined, measuring up to 3 cm in diameter (▶Fig. 25.42). (1) Centrilobular nodules appear separated by several millimeters from the pleural surfaces, fissures, and interlobular septa. They may be of soft-tissue or ground-glass attenuation. Ranging in size from a few millimeters to a centimeter, centrilobular nodules are usually ill-defined.[7] (2) A micronodule is less than 3 mm in diameter (see also *micronodule*). (3) A ground-glass nodule (synonym, nonsolid nodule) manifests as hazy increased attenuation in the lung that does not obliterate the bronchial and vascular margins. (4) A solid nodule has homogenous soft-tissue attenuation. (5) A part-solid nodule (synonym, semisolid nodule) consists of both ground-glass and solid soft-tissue attenuation components. (See also *mass*.)

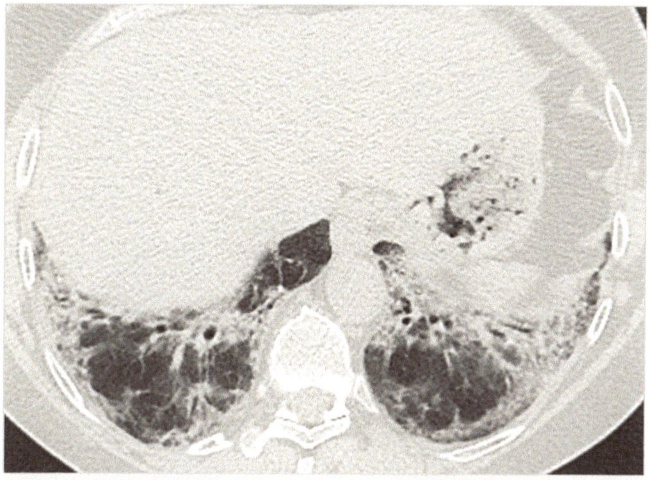

Fig. 25.43 Transverse CT scan shows nonspecific interstitial pneumonia.

Nonspecific interstitial pneumonia, or NSIP

Pathology—NSIP is characterized by a histologic pattern of uniform interstitial involvement by varying degrees of chronic inflammation or fibrosis. NSIP may be idiopathic or seen in other settings, including collagen vascular disease, hypersensitivity pneumonitis, drug-induced lung disease, infection, and immunodeficiency (including human immunodeficiency virus infection).[8]

CT scans—NSIP has variable thin-section CT appearances: the most frequent is ground-glass opacities with reticulation, traction bronchiectasis or bronchiolectasis, and little or no honeycombing (▶Fig. 25.43). The distribution is usually basal and subpleural.[98]

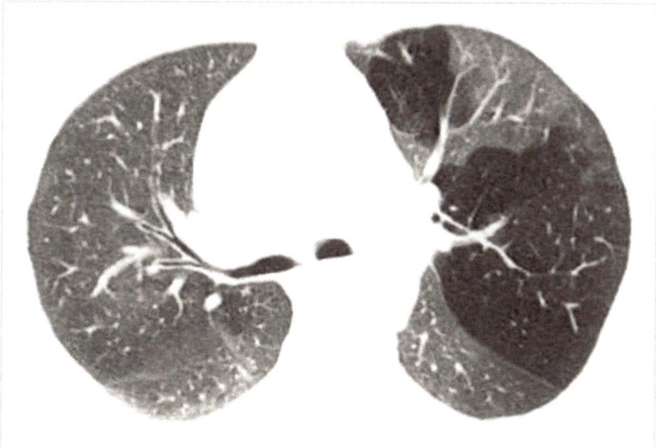

Fig. 25.44 Transverse CT scan shows oligemia (*arrows*) in left lung.

Oligemia

Pathophysiology—Oligemia is a reduction in pulmonary blood volume. Most frequently, this reduction is regional, but occasionally it is generalized. Regional oligemia is usually associated with reduced blood flow in the oligemic area.

Radiographs and CT scans—Oligemia appears as a regional or widespread decrease in the size and number of identifiable pulmonary vessels (▶Fig. 25.44), which is indicative of less than normal blood flow. (See also *mosaic attenuation pattern, pulmonary blood flow redistribution.*)

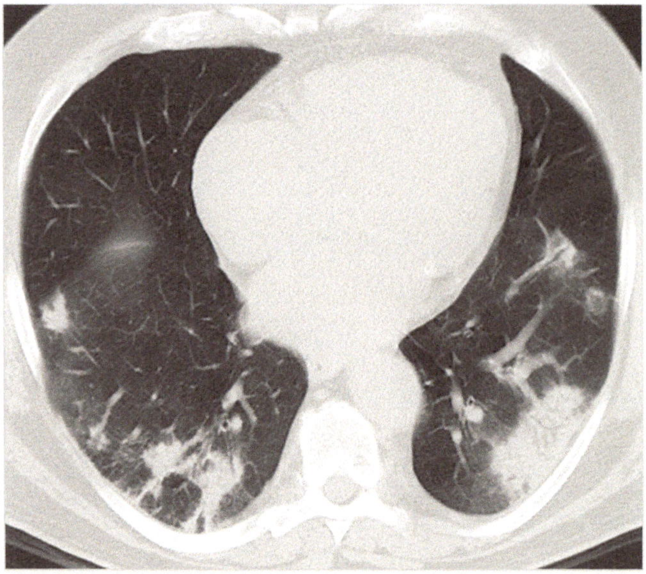

Fig. 25.45 Transverse CT scan shows cryptogenic organizing pneumonia with subpleural and basal distribution.

Organizing pneumonia

Pathology—Organizing pneumonia manifests as a histologic pattern characterized by loose plugs of connective tissue in the airspaces and distal airways. Interstitial inflammation and fibrosis are minimal or absent. Cryptogenic organizing pneumonia, or COP, is a distinctive clinical disorder among the idiopathic interstitial pneumonias,[8] but the histologic pattern of organizing pneumonia is encountered in many different situations, including pulmonary infection, hypersensitivity pneumonitis, and collagen vascular diseases.

Radiographs and CT scans—Airspace consolidation is the cardinal feature of organizing pneumonia on chest radiographs and CT scans. In COP, the distribution is typically subpleural and basal (▶Fig. 25.45) and sometimes bronchocentric.[99] Other manifestations of organizing pneumonia include ground-glass opacity, tree-in-bud pattern, and nodular opacities.[40]

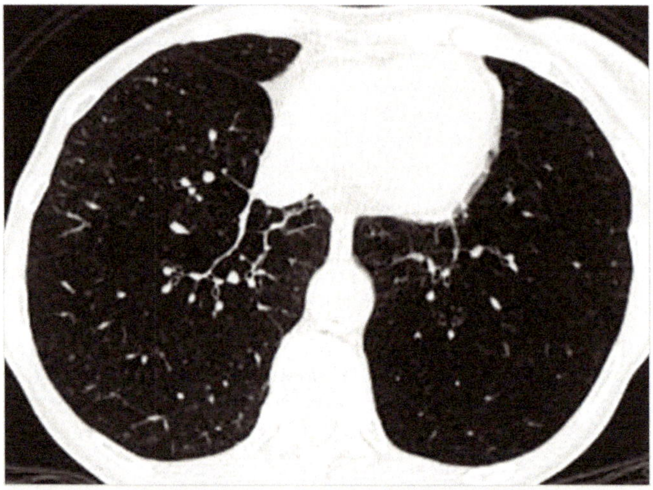

Fig. 25.46 Transverse CT scan shows panacinar emphysema.

Panacinar emphysema

Pathology—Panacinar emphysema involves all portions of the acinus and secondary pulmonary lobule more or less uniformly.[45] It predominates in the lower lobes and is the form of emphysema associated with α1-antitrypsin deficiency.

CT scans—Panacinar emphysema manifests as a generalized decrease of the lung parenchyma with a decrease in the caliber of blood vessels in the affected lung[100,101] (▶Fig. 25.46). Severe panacinar emphysema may coexist and merge with severe centrilobular emphysema. The appearance of featureless decreased attenuation may be indistinguishable from severe constrictive obliterative bronchiolitis.[102] The term panlobular emphysema is synonymous. (See also *emphysema*.)

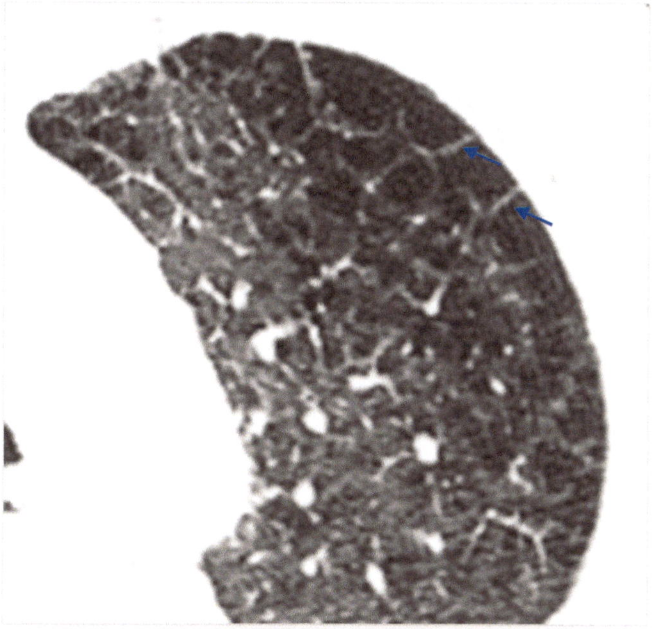

Fig. 25.47 Transverse CT scan shows paraseptal emphysema (*arrows*).

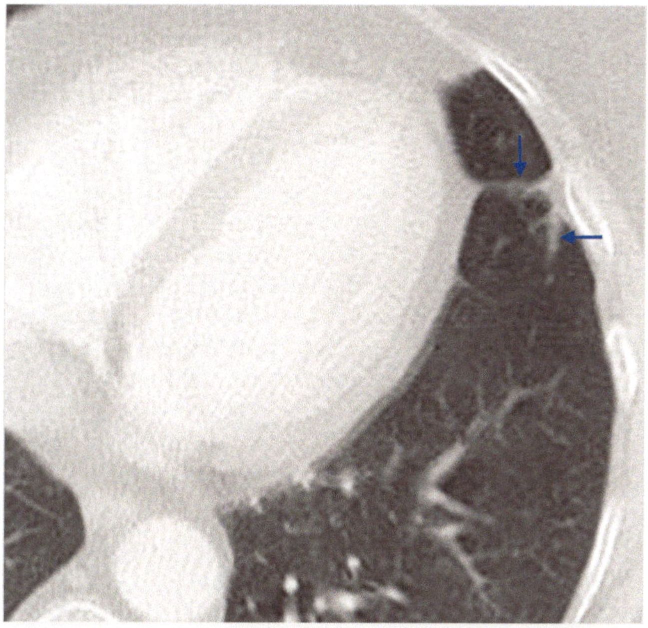

Fig. 25.48 Transverse CT scan shows parenchymal bands (*arrows*).

Paraseptal emphysema

Pathology—Paraseptal emphysema is characterized by predominant involvement of the distal alveoli and their ducts and sacs. It is characteristically bounded by any pleural surface and the interlobular septa.[45,46]

CT scans—This emphysema is characterized by subpleural and peribronchovascular regions of low attenuation separated by intact interlobular septa (▶Fig. 25.47), sometimes associated with bullae. The term distal acinar emphysema is synonymous. (See also *emphysema*.)

Parenchyma

Anatomy—Parenchyma refers to the gas-exchanging part of the lung, consisting of the alveoli and their capillaries.

Radiographs and CT scans—The portion of the lung exclusive of visible pulmonary vessels and airways.

Parenchymal band

Radiographs and CT scans—A parenchymal band is a linear opacity, usually 1 to 3 mm thick and up to 5 cm long that usually extends to the visceral pleura (which is often thickened and may be retracted at the site of contact) (▶Fig. 25.48). It reflects pleuroparenchymal fibrosis and is usually associated with distortion of the lung architecture. Parenchymal bands are most frequently encountered in individuals who have been exposed to asbestos.[103,104]

Parenchymal opacification

Radiographs and CT scans—Parenchymal opacification of the lungs may or may not obscure the margins of vessels and airway walls.[48] Consolidation indicates that definition of these margins (excepting air bronchograms) is lost within the dense opacification, whereas ground-glass opacity indicates a smaller increase in attenuation, in which the definition of underlying structures is preserved.[63] The more specific terms consolidation and ground-glass opacity are preferred. (See also *consolidation*, ground-glass opacity.)

Peribronchovascular interstitium

Anatomy—The peribronchovascular interstitium is a connective-tissue sheath that encloses the bronchi, pulmonary arteries, and lymphatic vessels. It extends from the hila to the lung periphery.

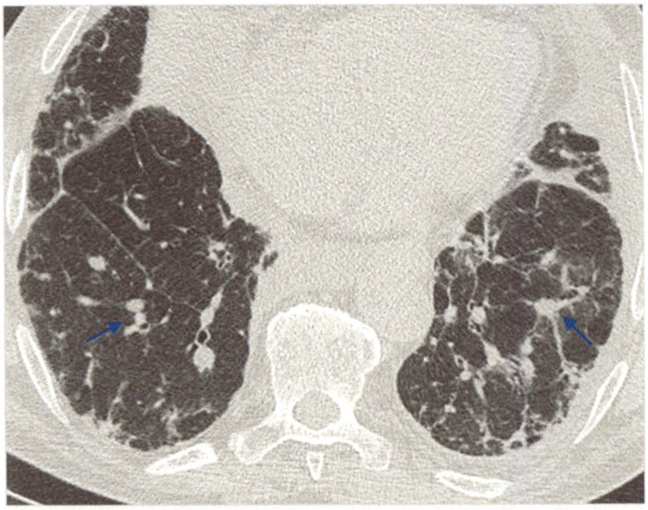

Fig. 25.49 Transverse CT scan shows organizing pneumonia in a perilobular distribution (*arrows*).

Perilobular distribution

Anatomy—The perilobular region comprises the structures bordering the periphery of the secondary pulmonary lobule.

CT scans—This pattern is characterized by distribution along the structures that border the pulmonary lobules (i.e., interlobular septa, visceral pleura, and vessels).[105] The term is most frequently used in the context of diseases (e.g., perilobular organizing pneumonia) that are distributed mainly around the inner surface of the secondary pulmonary lobule[106] (▸Fig. 25.49). This may resemble indistinct thickening of the interlobular septa.

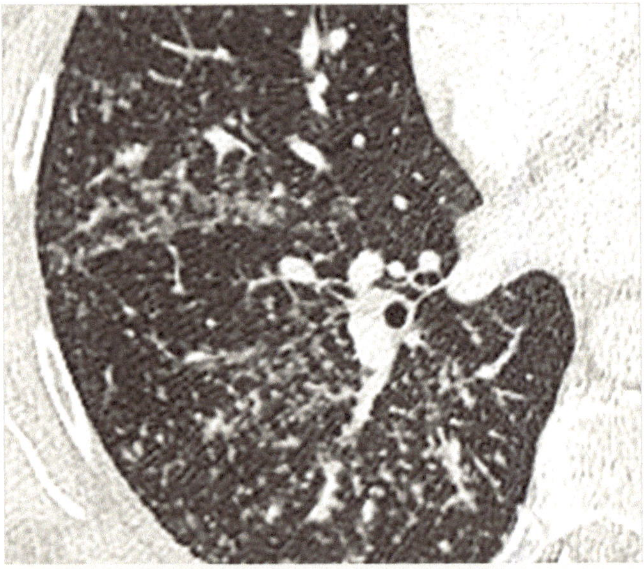

Fig. 25.50 Transverse CT scan shows sarcoidosis with a perilymphatic distribution.

Perilymphatic distribution

Anatomy—This pattern is characterized by distribution along or adjacent to the lymphatic vessels in the lung. The routes of lymphatics are found along bronchovascular bundles, in the interlobular septa, around larger pulmonary veins, and in the pleura; alveoli do not have lymphatics.

CT scans—Abnormalities along the pathway of the pulmonary lymphatics— that is, in the perihilar, peribronchovascular, and centrilobular interstitium, as well as in the interlobular septa and subpleural locations—have a perilymphatic distribution.[107] A perilymphatic distribution typically seen in sarcoidosis (▸Fig. 25.50) and lymphangitic spread of cancer.

Platelike atelectasis

See linear atelectasis.

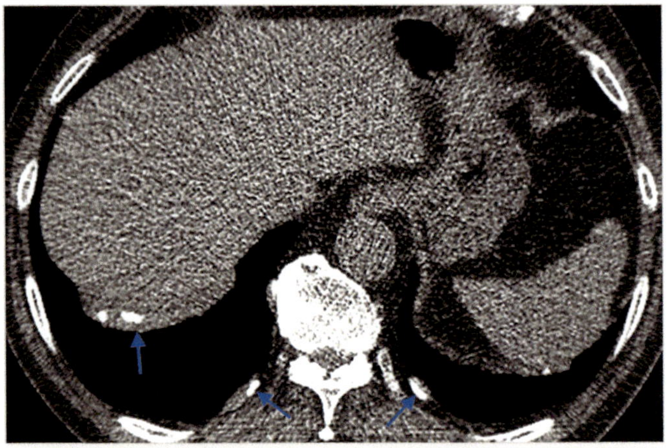

Fig. 25.51 Transverse CT scan shows bilateral pleural plaques (*arrows*).

Pleural plaque

Pathology—A pleural plaque is a fibrohyaline, relatively acellular lesion arising predominantly on the parietal pleural surface, particularly on the diaphragm and underneath ribs.[108] Pleural plaques are almost invariably the consequence of previous (at least 15 years earlier) asbestos exposure.

Radiographs and CT scans—Pleural plaques are well-demarcated areas of pleural thickening, seen as elevated flat or nodular lesions that often contain calcification (▸Fig. 25.51). Plaques are of variable thickness, range from less than 1 to approximately 5 cm in diameter, and are more easily identified on CT scans than on chest radiographs.[109] An en face plaque may simulate a pulmonary nodule on chest radiographs. (See also *pseudoplaque*.)

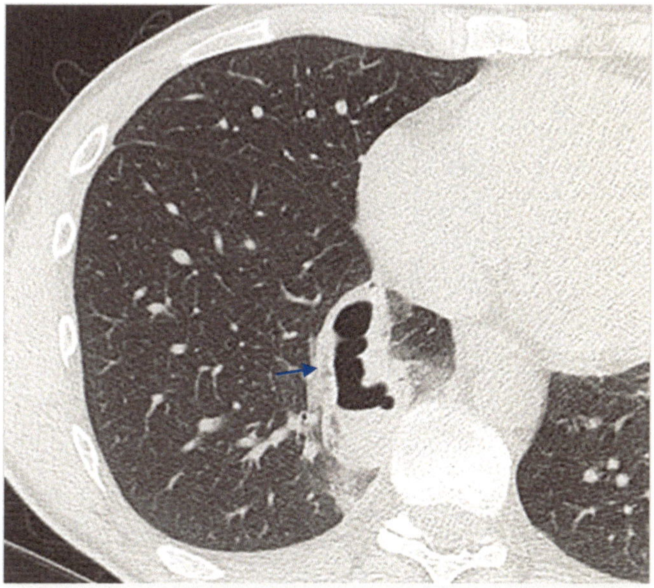

Fig. 25.52 Transverse CT scan shows a pneumatocele (*arrows*).

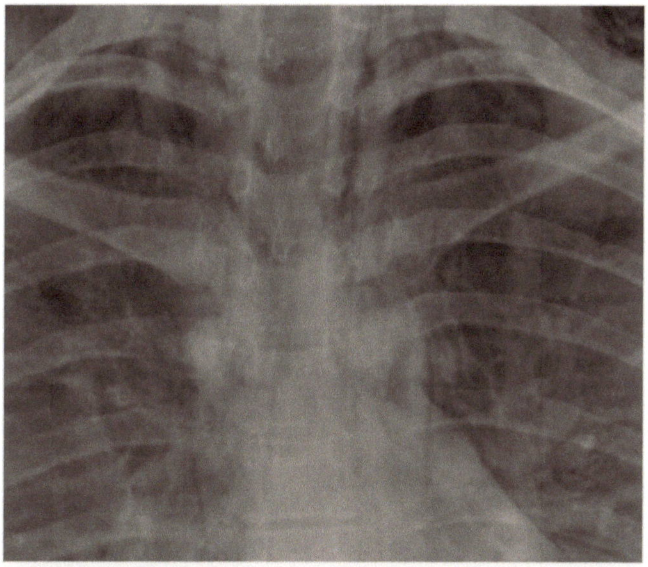

Fig. 25.53 Magnified chest radiograph shows pneumomediastinum.

Pneumatocele

Pathology—A pneumatocele is a thin-walled, gas-filled space in the lung. It is most frequently caused by acute pneumonia, trauma, or aspiration of hydrocarbon fluid and is usually transient. The mechanism is believed to be a combination of parenchymal necrosis and check-valve airway obstruction.[110]

Radiographs and CT scans—A pneumatocele appears as an approximately round, thin-walled airspace in the lung (▶Fig. 25.52).

Pneumomediastinum

Pathology—Pneumomediastinum is the presence of gas in mediastinal tissue outside the esophagus and tracheobronchial tree. It may be caused by spontaneous alveolar rupture, with subsequent tracking of air along the bronchovascular interstitium into the mediastinum. Pneumomediastinum is particularly associated with a history of asthma, severe coughing, or assisted ventilation.

Radiographs and CT scans—Pneumomediastinum appears as lucent streaks on chest radiographs, mostly vertically oriented (▶Fig. 25.53). Some of these streaks may outline vessels and main bronchi. (See also *pneumopericardium*.)

Pneumonia

Pathology—Pneumonia is inflammation of the airspaces and/or interstitium (e.g., due to infection, as in bacterial pneumonia). Infective pneumonia is characterized by exudate resulting in consolidation. The term is also used to refer to a number of noninfectious disorders of the lung parenchyma characterized by varying degrees of inflammation and fibrosis (e.g., idiopathic interstitial pneumonias).[8]

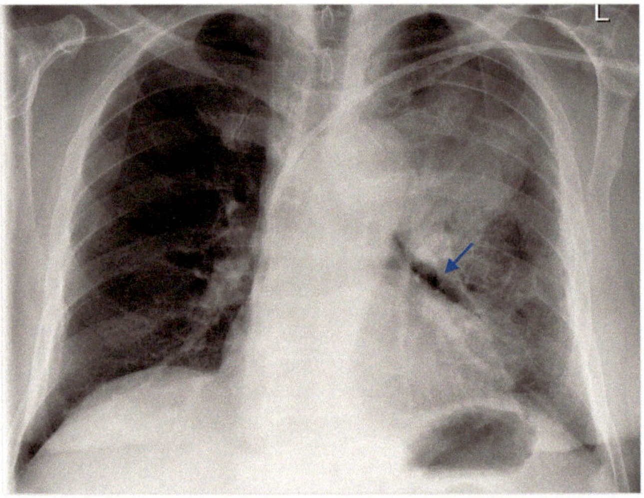

Fig. 25.54 Chest radiograph shows pneumopericardium (*arrow*).

Pneumopericardium

Pathology—Pneumopericardium is the presence of gas in the pericardial space. It usually has an iatrogenic, often surgical, origin in adults.

Radiographs and CT scans—Pneumopericardium is usually distinguishable from pneumomediastinum because the lucency (low attenuation) caused by air does not extend outside the pericardial sac (▶ Fig. 25.54). (See also *pneumomediastinum*.)

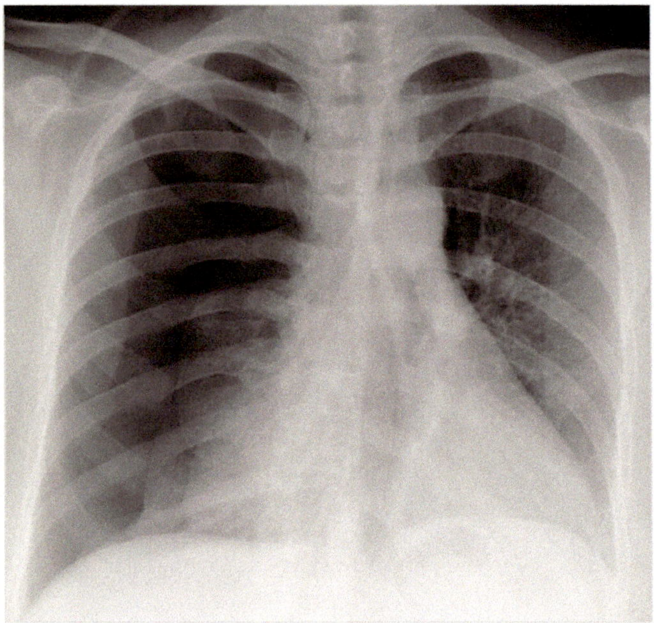

Fig. 25.55 Chest radiograph shows tension pneumothorax.

Pneumothorax and tension pneumothorax

Pathophysiology—Pneumothorax refers to the presence of gas in the pleural space. Qualifiers include spontaneous, traumatic, diagnostic, and tension. Tension pneumothorax is the accumulation of intrapleural gas under pressure. In this situation, the ipsilateral lung will, if normal, collapse completely; however, a less than normally compliant lung may remain partially inflated.

Radiographs and CT scans—On chest radiographs, a visceral pleural edge is visible (▶ Fig. 25.55) unless the pneumothorax is very small or the pleural edge is not tangential to the X-ray beam. Tension pneumothorax may be associated with considerable shift of the mediastinum and/or depression of the hemidiaphragm. Some shift can occur without tension because the pleural pressure in the presence of pneumothorax becomes atmospheric, while the pleural pressure in the contralateral hemithorax remains negative.

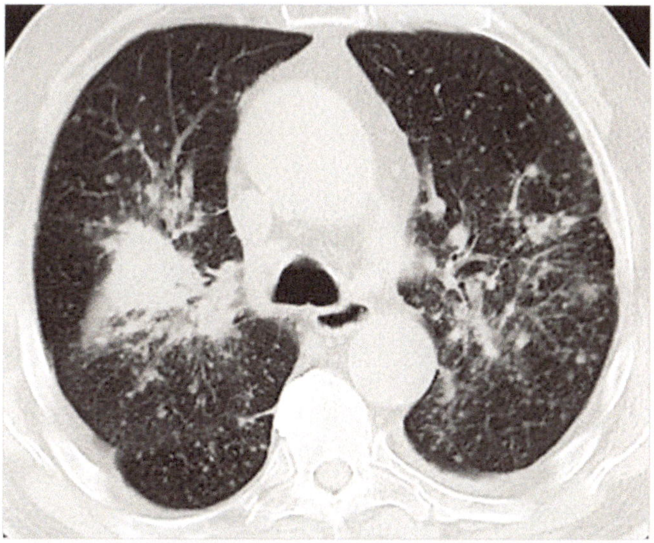

Fig. 25.56 Chest radiograph shows progressive massive fibrosis.

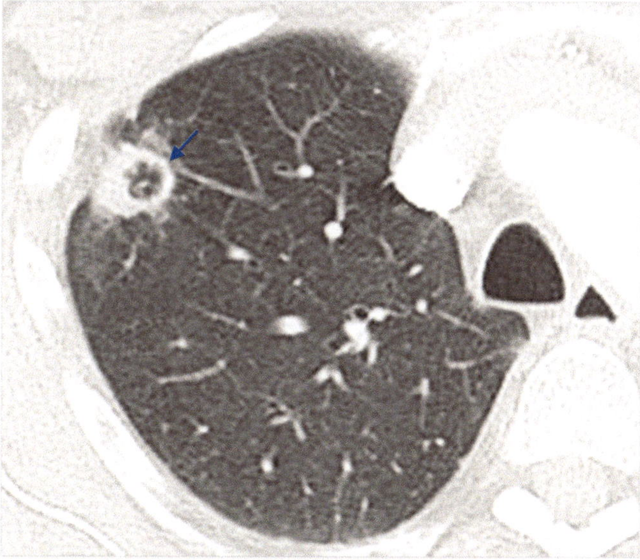

Fig. 25.57 Transverse CT scan shows pseudocavitation in a pulmonary nodule (*arrow*).

Progressive massive fibrosis

Pathology—This condition is caused by slow-growing conglomeration of dust particles and collagen deposition in individuals (mostly coal workers) heavily exposed to inorganic dust.[111]

Radiographs and CT scans—Progressive massive fibrosis manifests as masslike lesions, usually bilateral and in the upper lobes (▶Fig. 25.56). Background nodular opacities reflect accompanying pneumoconiosis, with or without emphysematous destruction adjacent to the massive fibrosis.[112] Lesions similar to progressive massive fibrosis sometimes occur in other conditions, such as sarcoidosis and talcosis.[112,113]

Pseudocavity

CT scans—A pseudocavity appears as an oval or round area of low attenuation in lung nodules, masses, or areas of consolidation that represent spared parenchyma, normal or ectatic bronchi, or focal emphysema rather than cavitation. These pseudocavities usually measure less than 1 cm in diameter. They have been described in patients with adenocarcinoma (▶Fig. 25.57)[d,114] and benign conditions such as infectious pneumonia.

[d]Dag Wormanns' note: The bronchioloalveolar carcinoma mentioned in the original publication[4] is now obsolete and regarded as a subtype of adenocarcinoma; therefore, it has been omitted here.

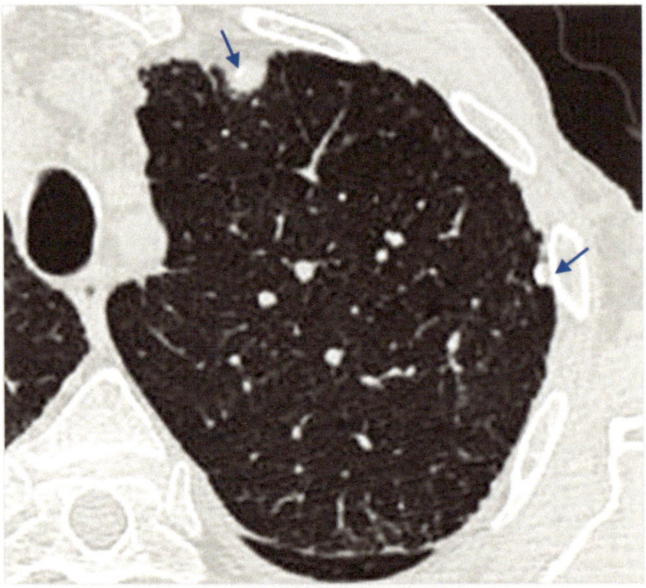

Fig. 25.58 Transverse CT scan shows pseudoplaques (*arrows*) in a patient with silicosis.

Pseudoplaque

CT scans—A pseudoplaque is a pulmonary opacity contiguous with the visceral pleura formed by coalescent small nodules. It simulates the appearance of a pleural plaque. This entity is encountered most commonly in sarcoidosis (▸Fig. 25.58), silicosis, and coal workers' pneumoconiosis.[89]

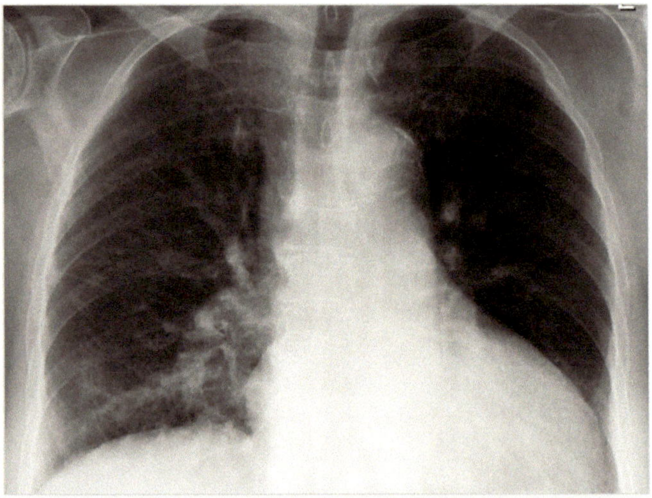

Fig. 25.59 Chest radiograph shows redistribution of blood flow to upper lung zones.

Pulmonary blood flow redistribution

Pathophysiology—Pulmonary blood flow redistribution refers to any departure from the normal distribution of blood flow in the lungs that is caused by an increase in pulmonary vascular resistance elsewhere in the pulmonary vascular bed.

Radiographs and CT scans—Pulmonary blood flow redistribution is indicated by a decrease in the size and/or number of visible pulmonary vessels in one or more lung regions (▸Fig. 25.59), with a corresponding increase in number and/or size of pulmonary vessels in other parts of the lung. Upper lobe blood diversion in patients with mitral valve disease is the archetypal example of redistribution.[115,116]

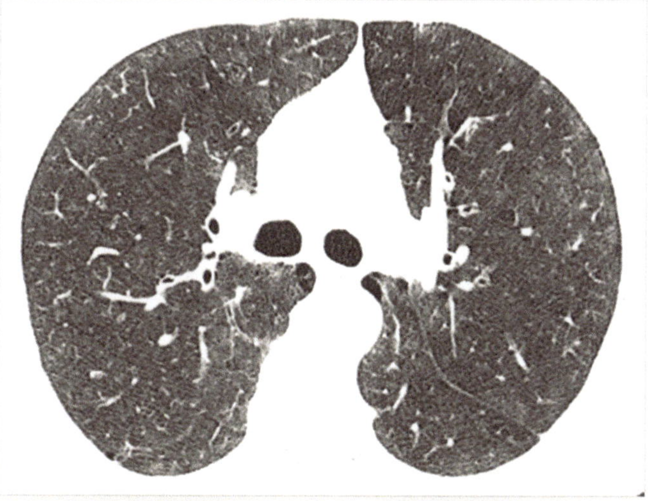

Fig. 25.60 Transverse CT scan shows centrilobular micronodules and patchy ground-glass opacity typical of respiratory bronchiolitis–interstitial lung disease.

Respiratory bronchiolitis–interstitial lung disease, or RB-ILD

Pathology—RB-ILD is a smoking-related disease characterized by inflammation (predominantly by macrophages) of the respiratory bronchioles and peribronchiolar alveoli,[8] sometimes with elements of or overlap with nonspecific and desquamative interstitial pneumonias.[117]

CT scans—RB-ILD typically manifests as extensive centrilobular micronodules and patchy ground-glass opacity corresponding to macrophage-rich alveolitis (▶Fig. 25.60), with or without fine fibrosis.[118,119] It is often accompanied by bronchial wall thickening and minor centrilobular emphysema. Areas of air trapping reflect a bronchiolitic component.

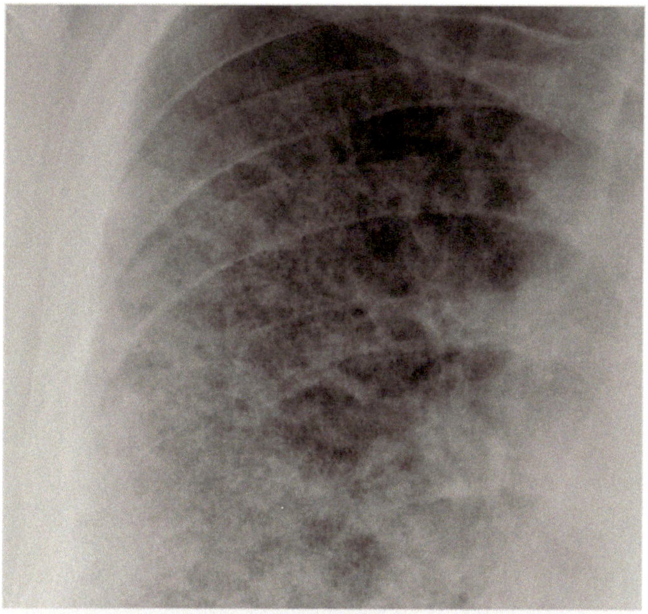

Fig. 25.61 Magnified chest radiograph shows reticular pattern.

Reticular pattern

Radiographs and CT scans—On chest radiographs, a reticular pattern is a collection of innumerable small linear opacities that, by summation, produce an appearance resembling a net (synonym: reticulation) (▶Fig. 25.61). This finding usually represents interstitial lung disease. The constituents of a reticular pattern are more clearly seen at thin-section CT, whether they are interlobular septal thickening, intralobular lines, or the cyst walls of honeycombing. (Reticular pattern and honeycombing should not be considered synonymous. See also *honeycombing*.)

25

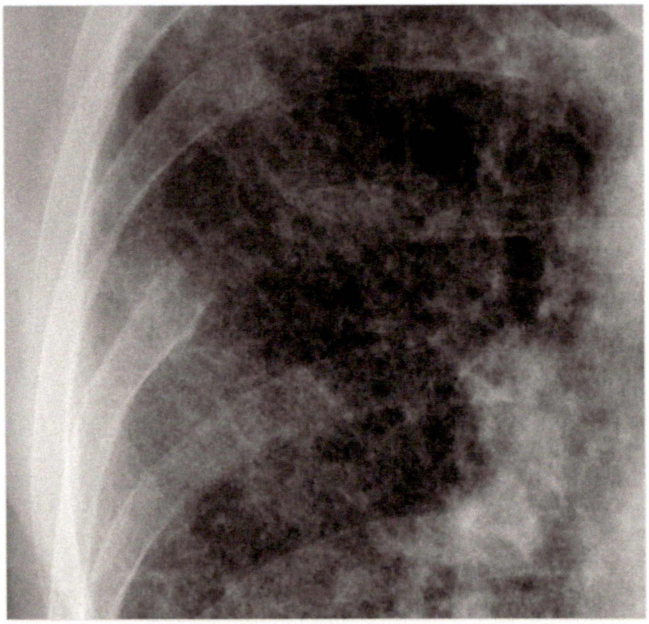

Fig. 25.62 Magnified chest radiograph shows reticulonodular pattern.

Reticulonodular pattern

Radiographs and CT scans—A combined reticular and nodular pattern, the reticulonodular pattern is usually the result of the summation of points of intersection of innumerable lines, creating the effect on chest radiographs of superimposed micronodules (▶Fig. 25.62). The dimension of the nodules depends on the size and number of linear or curvilinear elements. (See also *reticular pattern.*) On CT scans, the pattern appears as a concurrence of reticular and micronodular patterns. The micronodules can be situated in the center of the reticular elements (e.g., centrilobular micronodules) or superimposed on the linear opacities (e.g., septal micronodules).

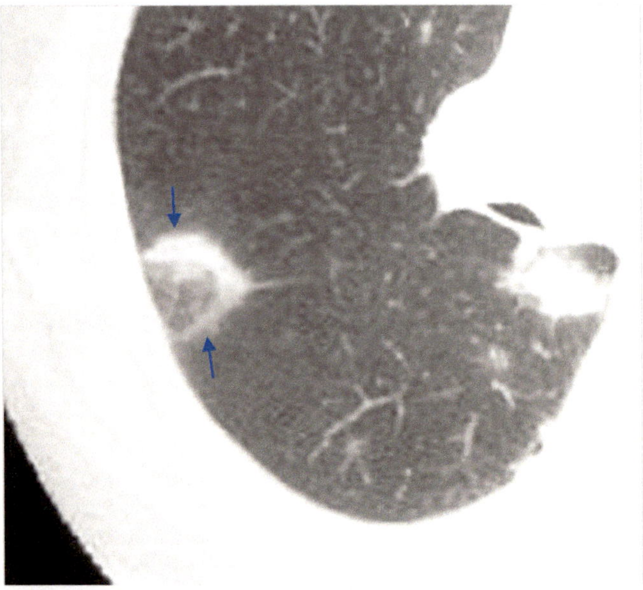

Fig. 25.63 Transverse CT scan shows reversed halo sign (*arrows*).

Reversed halo sign

CT scans—The reversed halo sign is a focal rounded area of ground-glass opacity surrounded by a more or less complete ring of consolidation (▶Fig. 25.63). A rare sign, it was initially reported to be specific for cryptogenic organizing pneumonia[120,121] but was subsequently described in patients with paracoccidioidomycosis.[122] Similar to the halo sign, this sign will probably lose its specificity as it is recognized in other conditions. (See also *halo sign.*)

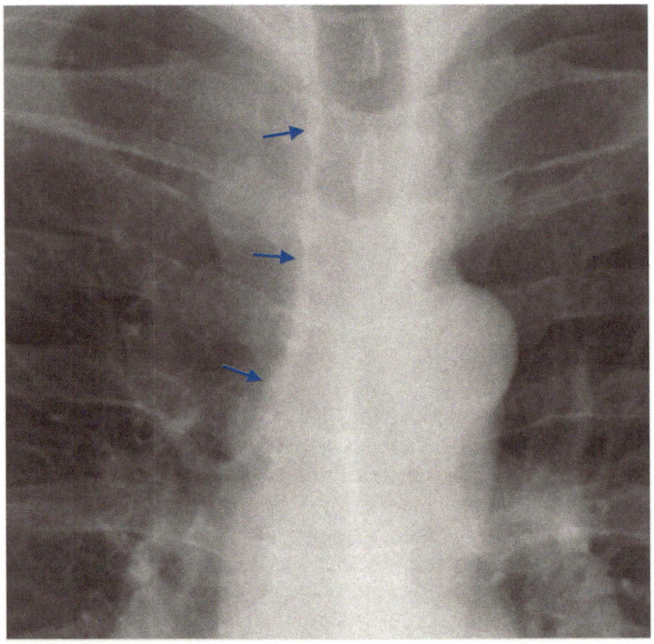

Fig. 25.64 Magnified chest radiograph shows paratracheal stripe (*arrows*).

Right paratracheal stripe

Anatomy and radiographs—The right paratracheal stripe is a vertical, linear, soft-tissue opacity less than 4 mm wide. It corresponds to the right tracheal wall, contiguous mediastinal tissues, and adjacent pleura (▶Fig. 25.64). The stripe is 3 to 4 cm in height and extends from approximately the level of the medial ends of the clavicles to the right tracheobronchial angle on a frontal chest radiograph.[123] It is seen in up to 94% of adults but is widened or absent in individuals with abundant mediastinal fat. The commonest pathologic cause of widening, deformity, or obliteration of this stripe is paratracheal lymph node enlargement.

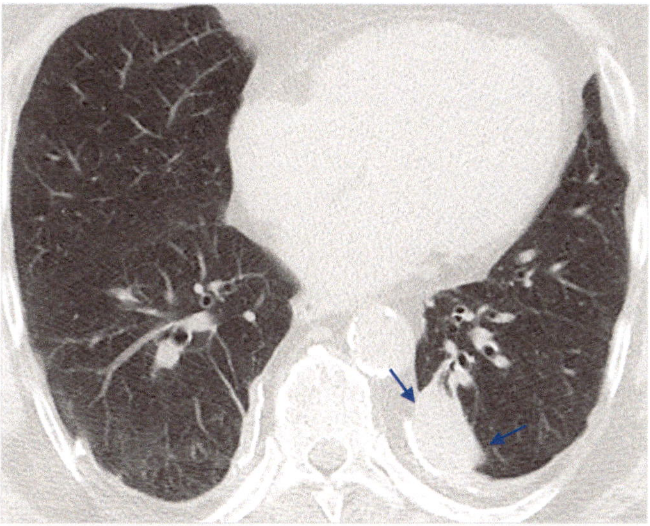

Fig. 25.65 Sagittal CT scan shows rounded atelectasis in left lower lobe.

Rounded atelectasis

Pathology—Rounded atelectasis is rounded collapsed lung associated with invaginated fibrotic pleura and thickened and fibrotic interlobular septa. Most frequently, it is the consequence of an asbestos-induced exudative pleural effusion with resultant pleural scarring,[124] but it may occur with any cause of pleural fibrosis.

Radiographs and CT scans—On chest radiographs, rounded atelectasis appears as a mass abutting a pleural surface, usually in the posterior part of a lower lobe. Distorted vessels have a curvilinear disposition as they converge on the mass (the comet tail sign). The degree of lobar retraction depends on the volume of atelectatic lung. It is almost invariably associated with other signs of pleural fibrosis (e.g., blunting of costophrenic angle). CT is more sensitive for the detection and display of the characteristic features of rounded atelectasis[125,126] (▶ Fig. 25.65). An additional sign is homogeneous uptake of contrast medium in the atelectatic lung. Synonyms include folded lung syndrome, helical atelectasis, Blesovsky syndrome, pleural pseudotumor, and pleuroma.

Secondary pulmonary lobule

See *lobule*.

Segment

Anatomy—A segment is the unit of a lobe ventilated by a segmental bronchus, perfused by a segmental pulmonary artery, and drained by an intersegmental pulmonary vein. There are two to five segments per lobe.

Radiographs and CT scans—Individual segments cannot be precisely delineated on chest radiographs and CT scans, and their identification is made inferentially on the basis of the position of the supplying segmental bronchus and artery. When occasionally present, intersegmental fissures help to identify segments.

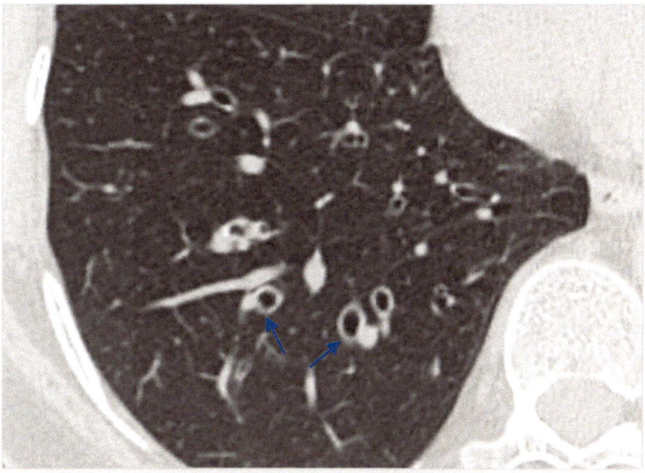

Fig. 25.66 Transverse CT scan shows signet ring sign (*arrows*).

Signet ring sign

CT scans—This finding is composed of a ring-shaped opacity representing a dilated bronchus in cross section and a smaller adjacent opacity representing its pulmonary artery, with the combination resembling a signet (or pearl) ring[127] (▶ Fig. 25.66). It is the basic CT sign of bronchiectasis.[30,128] The signet ring sign can also be seen in diseases characterized by abnormal reduced pulmonary arterial flow (e.g., proximal interruption of pulmonary artery[129] or chronic thromboembolism[130]). Occasionally, the tiny vascular opacity abutting a bronchus is a bronchial, rather than a pulmonary, artery.

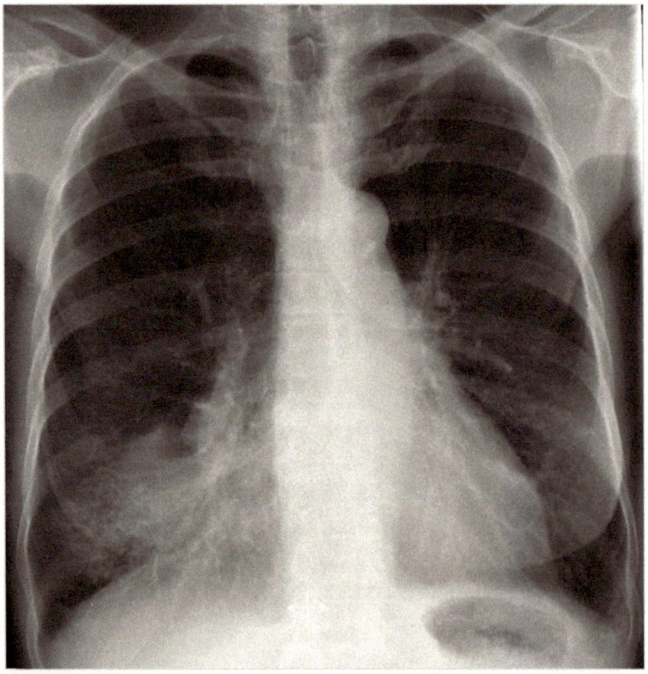

Fig. 25.67 Chest radiograph shows silhouette sign, with obscuration of right border of heart.

Silhouette sign

Radiographs—The silhouette sign is the absence of depiction of an anatomic soft-tissue border. It is caused by consolidation and/or atelectasis of the adjacent lung (▸Fig. 25.67), by a large mass, or by contiguous pleural fluid.[131,132] The silhouette sign results from the juxtaposition of structures of similar radiographic attenuation. The sign actually refers to the absence of a silhouette. It is not always indicative of disease (e.g., unexplained absence of right border of heart is seen in association with pectus excavatum and sometimes in healthy individuals).

Small airways disease

Pathology—This phrase is an arbitrary term used more frequently in thin-section CT descriptions than in the pathophysiology literature, where it was first coined.[133] Small-airways disease now generally refers to any condition affecting the bronchioles, whereas bronchiolitis more specifically describes inflammation of the bronchioles.[134]

CT scans—Small airways are considered to be those with an internal diameter smaller than or equal to 2 mm and a normal wall thickness of less than 0.5 mm.[35] Small-airways disease is manifest on CT scans as one or more of the following patterns: mosaic attenuation, air trapping, centrilobular micronodules, tree-in-bud pattern, or bronchiolectasis.

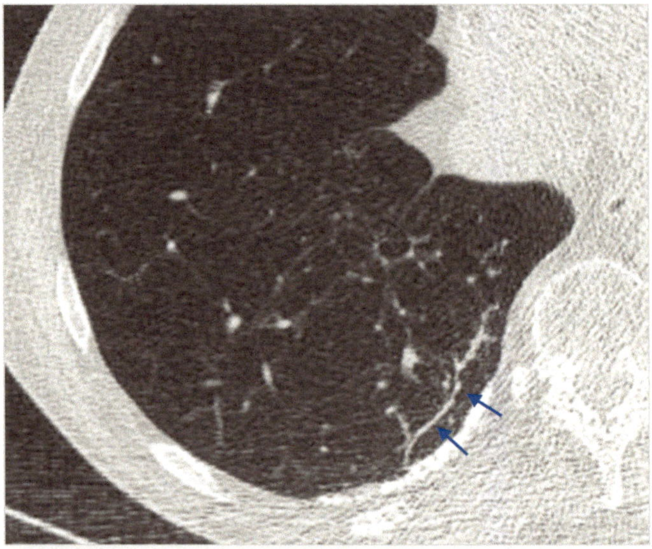

Fig. 25.68 Transverse CT scan shows a subpleural curvilinear line (*arrows*).

Subpleural curvilinear line

CT scans—This finding is a thin curvilinear opacity, 1 to 3 mm in thickness, lying less than 1 cm from and parallel to the pleural surface (▸Fig. 25.68). It corresponds to atelectasis of normal lung if seen in the dependent posteroinferior portion of lung of a patient in the supine position and is subsequently shown to disappear on CT sections acquired with the patient prone. It may also be encountered in patients with pulmonary edema[135] or fibrosis (other signs are usually present). Though described in the context of asbestosis, this finding is not specific for asbestosis.

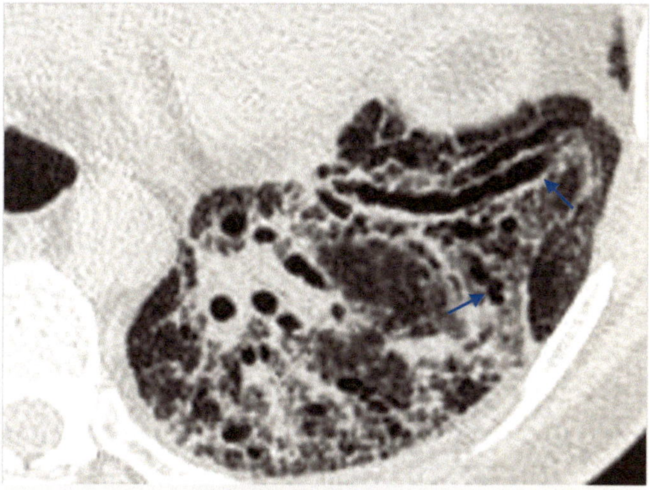

Fig. 25.69 Transverse CT scan shows traction bronchiectasis (*arrows*) caused by retractile pulmonary fibrosis.

Traction bronchiectasis und traction bronchiolectasis

CT scans—Traction bronchiectasis and traction bronchiolectasis, respectively, represent irregular bronchial and bronchiolar dilatation caused by surrounding retractile pulmonary fibrosis.[e,136] Dilated airways are usually identifiable as such (▸Fig. 25.69) but may be seen as cysts (bronchi) or microcysts (bronchioles in the lung periphery). The juxtaposition of numerous cystic airways may make the distinction from “pure” fibrotic honeycombing difficult.

[e]Dag Wormanns' note: In original publication,[4] erroneously referenced as Hogg et al.[133]

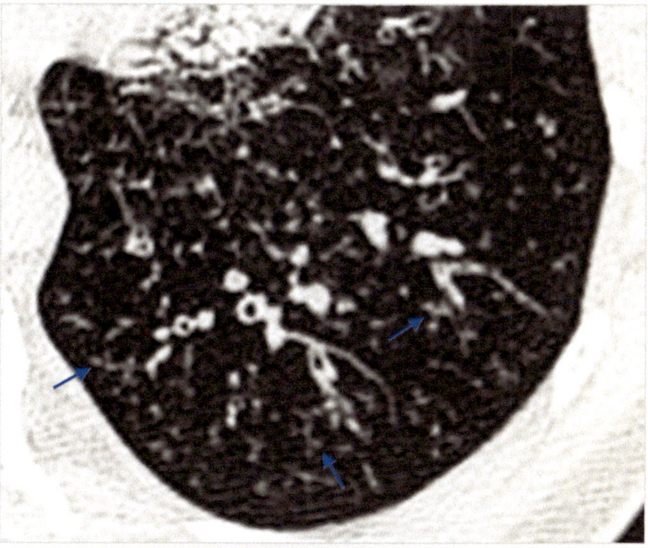

Fig. 25.70 Transverse CT scan shows tree-in-bud pattern (*arrows*).

Tree-in-bud pattern

CT scans—The tree-in-bud pattern represents centrilobular branching structures that resemble a budding tree. The pattern reflects a spectrum of endo- and peribronchiolar disorders, including mucoid impaction, inflammation, and/or fibrosis[137,138] (▸Fig. 25.70). This pattern is most pronounced in the lung periphery and is usually associated with abnormalities of the larger airways. It is particularly common in diffuse panbronchiolitis,[139] endobronchial spread of mycobacterial infection,[140] and cystic fibrosis. A similar pattern is a rare manifestation of arteriolar (microangiopathic) disease.[141]

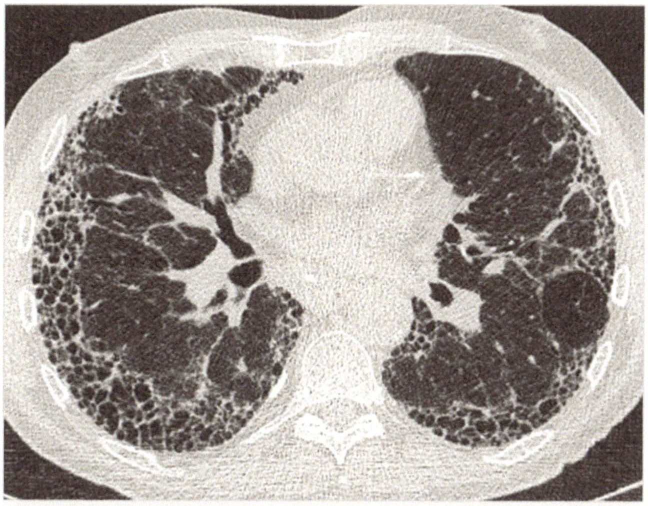

Fig. 25.71 Transverse CT scan shows basal and subpleural honeycombing, indicative of usual interstitial pneumonia.

Usual interstitial pneumonia, or UIP

Pathology—UIP is a histologic pattern of pulmonary fibrosis characterized by temporal and spatial heterogeneity, with established fibrosis and honeycombing interspersed among normal lung. Fibroblastic foci with fibrotic destruction of lung architecture, often with honeycombing, are the key findings.[8] The fibrosis is initially concentrated in the lung periphery. UIP is the pattern seen in idiopathic pulmonary fibrosis, but can be encountered in diseases of known cause (e.g., some cases of chronic hypersensitivity pneumonitis).

Radiographs and CT scans—Honeycombing with a basal and subpleural distribution (▸Fig. 25.71) is regarded as pathognomonic,[66,68] but not all cases of biopsy-proved UIP have this distinctive CT pattern.

25.3 Additional Definitions

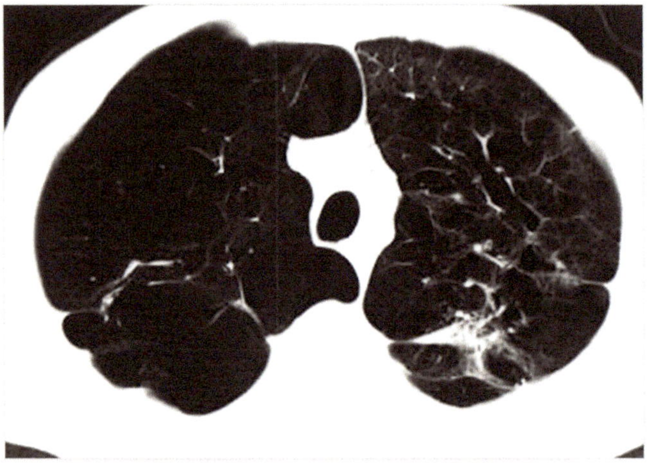

Fig. 25.72 Transverse CT scan shows advanced destructive emphysema.

Advanced destructive emphysema

CT scans—Panlobular lucencies, with hyperexpansion of secondary pulmonary lobules and distortion of pulmonary architecture (▶Fig. 25.72). On CT, it may be indistinguishable from panlobular emphysema.[6]

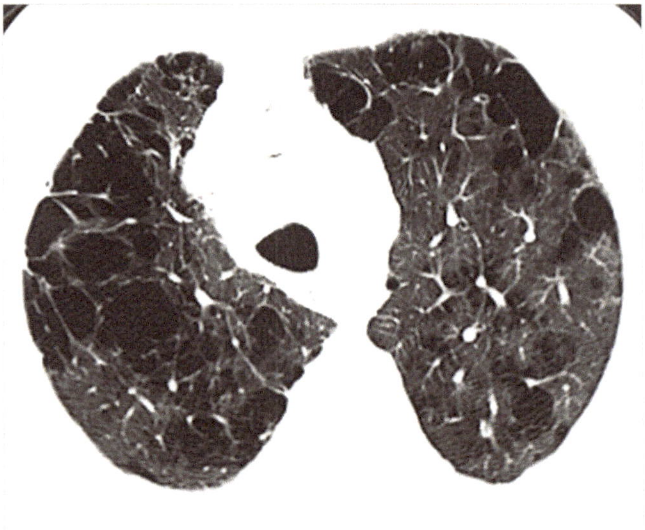

Fig. 25.73 Transverse CT scan shows confluent emphysema.

Confluent emphysema

CT scans—Coalescent centrilobular or lobular lucencies, including multiple regions of lucencies that span several secondary pulmonary lobules, but not involving extensive hyperexpansion of secondary pulmonary lobules or distortion of pulmonary architecture (▶Fig. 25.73).[6]

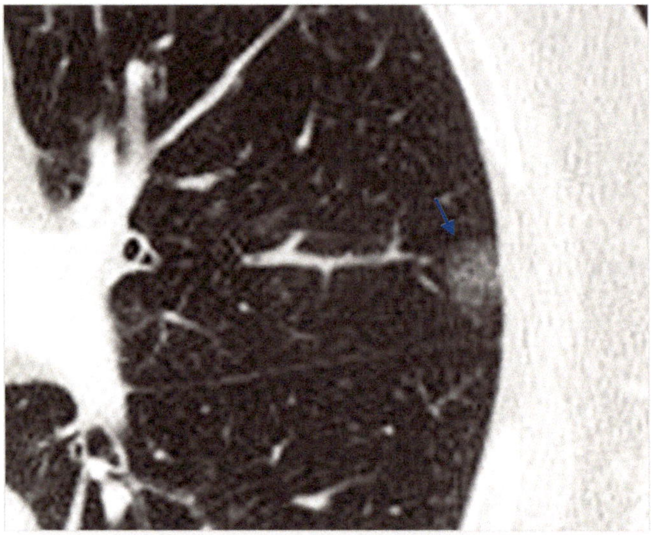

Fig. 25.74 Transverse CT scan shows a ground-glass nodule (*arrow*).

Ground-glass nodule

CT scans—Focal nodular area of lung parenchyma with pure ground-glass attenuation (▶Fig. 25.74).[5]

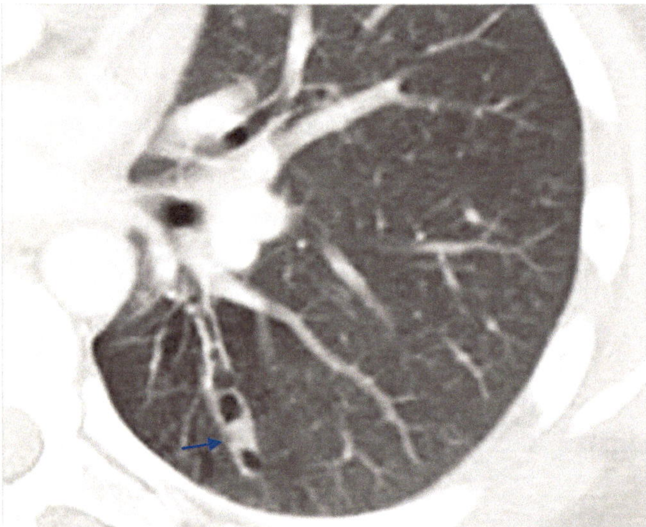

Fig. 25.75 Transverse CT scan shows mucoid impaction (*arrow*) in cylindric bronchiectasis.

Mucoid impaction

Pathology—Bronchus obstruction due to retained mucoid secretions.*CT scans*—Retained endobronchial mucoid can be depicted at CT as complete bronchus obliteration with material of soft-tissue density (▶Fig. 25.75). Can cause atelectasis.

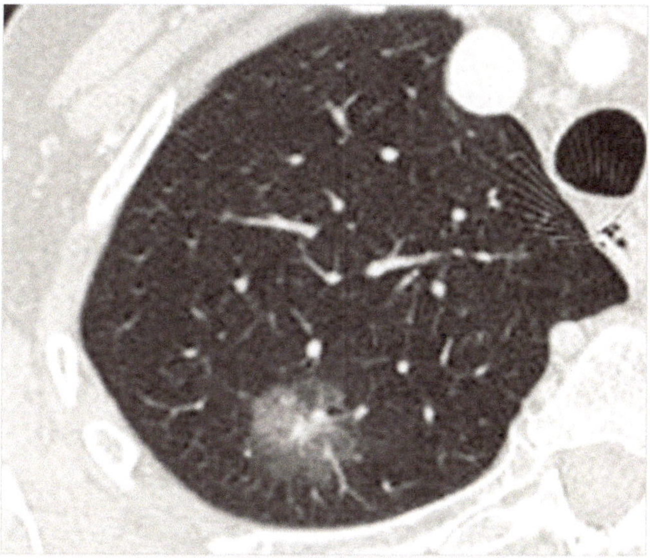

Fig. 25.76 Transverse CT scan shows a part-solid nodule with a central solid and a peripheral ground-glass component.

Part-solid nodule

CT scans—Focal nodular area of increased lung attenuation that include a combination of both ground-glass and solid components, the latter obscuring underlying lung architecture (▶Fig. 25.76).[5]

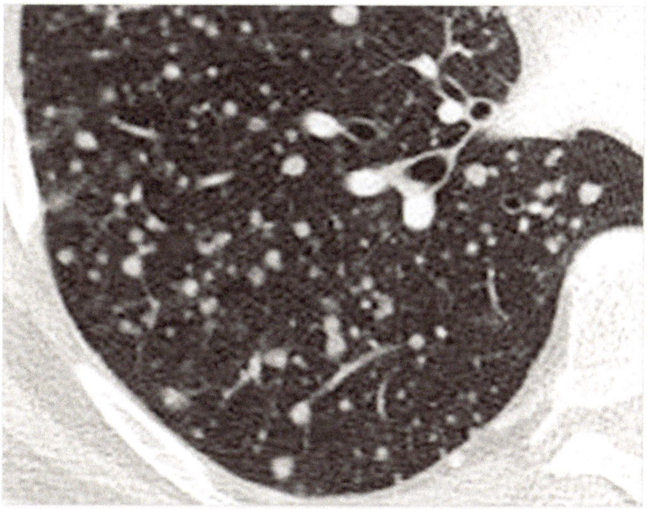

Fig. 25.77 Transverse CT scan shows randomly distributed pulmonary metastases.

Random distribution

CT scans—Distribution pattern of abnormalities with no apparent relation to the anatomic structures of the lobule (▶Fig. 25.77). This pattern is indicative of a hematogenously spread disease (e.g., lung metastases, miliary tuberculosis).

Subsolid nodule

CT scans—A category to describe focal nodular areas of increased lung attenuation with a ground-glass component, containing both pure ground-glass nodules and part-solid nodules.[5]

References

[1] Fraser RG, Mellins RB. The Fleischner Society: a 30th anniversary retrospective. Radiology 2000;214(3):631–632

[2] Tuddenham WJ. Glossary of terms for thoracic radiology: recommendations of the Nomenclature Committee of the Fleischner Society. AJR Am J Roentgenol 1984;143(3):509–517

[3] Austin JH, Müller NL, Friedman PJ, et al. Glossary of terms for CT of the lungs: recommendations of the Nomenclature Committee of the Fleischner Society. Radiology 1996;200(2):327–331

[4] Hansell DM, Bankier AA, MacMahon H, McLoud TC, Müller NL, Remy J. Fleischner Society: glossary of terms for thoracic imaging. Radiology 2008;246(3):697–722

[5] Naidich DP, Bankier AA, MacMahon H, et al. Recommendations for the management of subsolid pulmonary nodules detected at CT: a statement from the Fleischner Society. Radiology 2013;266(1):304–317

[6] Lynch DA, Austin JHM, Hogg JC, et al. CT-definable subtypes of chronic obstructive pulmonary disease: a statement of the Fleischner society. Radiology 2015;277(1):192–205

[7] Webb WR. Thin-section CT of the secondary pulmonary lobule: anatomy and the image--the 2004 Fleischner lecture. Radiology 2006;239(2):322–338

[8] American Thoracic Society. European Respiratory Society. American Thoracic Society/European Respiratory Society International Multidisciplinary Consensus Classification of the Idiopathic Interstitial Pneumonias. This joint statement of the American Thoracic Society (ATS), and the European Respiratory Society (ERS) was adopted by the ATS board of directors, June 2001 and by the ERS Executive Committee, June 2001. Am J Respir Crit Care Med 2002;165(2):277–304

[9] Johkoh T, Müller NL, Taniguchi H, et al. Acute interstitial pneumonia: thin-section CT findings in 36 patients. Radiology 1999;211(3):859–863

[10] Lynch DA, Travis WD, Müller NL, et al. Idiopathic interstitial pneumonias: CT features. Radiology 2005;236(1):10–21

[11] Reed JC, Madewell JE. The air bronchogram in interstitial disease of the lungs. A radiological-pathological correlation. Radiology 1975;116(1):1–9

[12] Abramson S. The air crescent sign. Radiology 2001;218(1):230–232

[13] Buckingham SJ, Hansell DM. Aspergillus in the lung: diverse and coincident forms. Eur Radiol 2003;13(8):1786–1800

[14] Arakawa H, Webb WR. Air trapping on expiratory high-resolution CT scans in the absence of inspiratory scan abnormalities: correlation with pulmonary function tests and differential diagnosis. AJR Am J Roentgenol 1998;170(5):1349–1353

[15] Bankier AA, Van Muylem A, Scillia P, De Maertelaer V, Estenne M, Gevenois PA. Air trapping in heart-lung transplant recipients: variability of anatomic distribution and extent at sequential expiratory thin-section CT. Radiology 2003;229(3):737–742

[16] Arakawa H, Kurihara Y, Sasaka K, Nakajima Y, Webb WR. Air trapping on CT of patients with pulmonary embolism. AJR Am J Roentgenol 2002;178(5):1201–1207

[17] Murata K, Khan A, Herman PG. Pulmonary parenchymal disease: evaluation with high-resolution CT. Radiology 1989;170(3 Pt 1):629–635

[18] Blank N, Castellino RA. Patterns of pleural reflections of the left superior mediastinum. Normal anatomy and distortions produced by adenopathy. Radiology 1972;102(3):585–589

[19] Heitzman ER. The infraaortic area. In: The Mediastinum: Radiologic Correlations with Anatomy and Pathology. 2nd ed. Berlin: Springer; 1988:151–168

[20] Im JG, Webb WR, Han MC, Park JH. Apical opacity associated with pulmonary tuberculosis: high-resolution CT findings. Radiology 1991;178(3):727–731

[21] Yousem SA. Pulmonary apical cap: a distinctive but poorly recognized lesion in pulmonary surgical pathology. Am J Surg Pathol 2001;25(5):679–683

[22] Dail DH. Pulmonary apical cap. Am J Surg Pathol 2001;25(10):1344

[23] Woodring JH, Reed JC. Types and mechanisms of pulmonary atelectasis. J Thorac Imaging 1996;11(2):92–108

[24] Molina PL, Hiken JN, Glazer HS. Imaging evaluation of obstructive atelectasis. J Thorac Imaging 1996;11(3):176–186

[25] Woodring JH, Reed JC. Radiographic manifestations of lobar atelectasis. J Thorac Imaging 1996;11(2):109–144

[26] Heitzman ER. The azygoesophageal recess. In: The Mediastinum: Radiologic Correlations with Anatomy and Pathology. 2nd ed. Berlin: Springer; 1988:276–286

[27] Ren H, Hruban RH, Kuhlman JE, et al. Computed tomography of inflation-fixed lungs: the beaded septum sign of pulmonary metastases. J Comput Assist Tomogr 1989;13(3):411–416

[28] Ryu JH, Swensen SJ. Cystic and cavitary lung diseases: focal and diffuse. Mayo Clin Proc 2003;78(6):744–752

[29] Kang EY, Miller RR, Müller NL. Bronchiectasis: comparison of preoperative thin-section CT and pathologic findings in resected specimens. Radiology 1995;195(3):649–654

[30] Naidich DP, McCauley DI, Khouri NF, Stitik FP, Siegelman SS. Computed tomography of bronchiectasis. J Comput Assist Tomogr 1982;6(3):437–444

[31] Dodd JD, Souza CA, Müller NL. Conventional high-resolution CT versus helical high-resolution MDCT in the detection of bronchiectasis. AJR Am J Roentgenol 2006;187(2):414–420

[32] Grenier P, Maurice F, Musset D, Menu Y, Nahum H. Bronchiectasis: assessment by thin-section CT. Radiology 1986;161(1):95–99

[33] Hansen JE, Ampaya EP, Bryant GH, Navin JJ. Branching pattern of airways and air spaces of a single human terminal bronchiole. J Appl Physiol 1975;38(6):983–989

[34] Buckley CE III, Tucker DH, Thorne NA, Sieker HO. Bronchiolectasis: The clinical syndrome and its relationship to chronic lung disease. Am J Med 1965;38:190–198

[35] Hansell DM. Small airways diseases: detection and insights with computed tomography. Eur Respir J 2001;17(6):1294–1313

[36] Myers JL, Colby TV. Pathologic manifestations of bronchiolitis, constrictive bronchiolitis, cryptogenic organizing pneumonia, and diffuse panbronchiolitis. Clin Chest Med 1993;14(4):611–622

[37] Woodring JH. Unusual radiographic manifestations of lung cancer. Radiol Clin North Am 1990;28(3):599–618

[38] Müller NL, Kullnig P, Miller RR. The CT findings of pulmonary sarcoidosis: analysis of 25 patients. AJR Am J Roentgenol 1989;152(6):1179–1182

[39] Huang L, Schnapp LM, Gruden JF, Hopewell PC, Stansell JD. Presentation of AIDS-related pulmonary Kaposi's sarcoma diagnosed by bronchoscopy. Am J Respir Crit Care Med 1996;153(4 Pt 1): 1385–1390

[40] Oikonomou A, Hansell DM. Organizing pneumonia: the many morphological faces. Eur Radiol 2002;12(6):1486–1496

[41] Seo JB, Song K-S, Lee JS, et al. Broncholithiasis: review of the causes with radiologic-pathologic correlation. Radiographics 2002;22(Spec No, Suppl.):S199–S213

[42] Heitzman ER, Markarian B, Berger I, Dailey E. The secondary pulmonary lobule: a practical concept for interpretation of chest radiographs. I. Roentgen anatomy of the normal secondary pulmonary lobule. Radiology 1969;93(3):507–512

[43] Murata K, Itoh H, Todo G, et al. Centrilobular lesions of the lung: demonstration by high-resolution CT and pathologic correlation. Radiology 1986;161(3):641–645

[44] Webb WR, Stein MG, Finkbeiner WE, Im JG, Lynch D, Gamsu G. Normal and diseased isolated lungs: high-resolution CT. Radiology 1988;166(1 Pt 1):81–87

[45] National Heart LaBI. The definition of emphysema. Report of a National Heart, Lung, and Blood Institute, Division of Lung Diseases workshop. Am Rev Respir Dis 1985;132(1):182–185

[46] Thurlbeck WM, Müller NL. Emphysema: definition, imaging, and quantification. AJR Am J Roentgenol 1994;163(5):1017–1025

[47] Foster WL Jr, Pratt PC, Roggli VL, Godwin JD, Halvorsen RA Jr, Putman CE. Centrilobular emphysema: CT-pathologic correlation. Radiology 1986;159(1):27–32

[48] Leung AN, Miller RR, Müller NL. Parenchymal opacification in chronic infiltrative lung d'seases: CT-pathologic correlation. Radiology 1993;188(1):209–214

[49] Laurent F, Philippe JC, Vergier B, et al. Exogenous lipoid pneumonia: HRCT, MR, and pathologic findings. Eur Radiol 1999;9(6):1190–1196

[50] Kuhlman JE, Scatarige JC, Fishman EK, Zerhouni EA, Siegelman SS. CT demonstration of high attenuation pleural-parenchymal lesions due to amiodarone therapy. J Comput Assist Tomogr 1987;11(1):160–162

[51] Murch CR, Carr DH. Computed tomography appearances of pulmonary alveolar proteinosis. Clin Radiol 1989;40(3):240–243

[52] Rossi SE, Erasmus JJ, Volpacchio M, Franquet T, Castiglioni T, McAdams HP. "Crazy-paving" pattern at thin-section CT of the lungs: radiologic-pathologic overview. Radiographics 2003;23(6):1509–1519

[53] Franquet T, Giménez A, Bordes R, Rodríguez-Arias JM, Castella J. The crazy-paving pattern in exogenous lipoid pneumonia: CT-pathologic correlation. AJR Am J Roentgenol 1998;170(2):315–317

[54] Genereux GP. The end-stage lung: pathogenesis, pathology, and radiology. Radiology 1975;116(02):279–289

[55] Aberle DR, Hansell DM, Brown K, Tashkin DP. Lymphangiomyomatosis: CT, chest radiographic, and functional correlations. Radiology 1990;176(2):381–387

[56] Moore AD, Godwin JD, Müller NL, et al. Pulmonary histiocytosis X: comparison of radiographic and CT findings. Radiology 1989;172(1):249–254

[57] Primack SL, Hartman TE, Hansell DM, Müller NL. End-stage lung disease: CT findings in 61 patients. Radiology 1993;189(3):681–686

[58] Hartman TE, Primack SL, Swensen SJ, Hansell D, McGuinness G, Müller NL. Desquamative interstitial pneumonia: thin-section CT findings in 22 patients. Radiology 1993;187(3):787–790

[59] Cardoso WV, Sekhon HS, Hyde DM, Thurlbeck WM. Collagen and elastin in human pulmonary emphysema. Am Rev Respir Dis 1993;147(4):975–981

[60] Lang MR, Fiaux GW, Gillooly M, Stewart JA, Hulmes DJ, Lamb D. Collagen content of alveolar wall tissue in emphysematous and non-emphysematous lungs. Thorax 1994;49(4):319–326

[61] Foster WL Jr, Gimenez EI, Roubidoux MA, et al. The emphysemas: radiologic-pathologic correlations. Radiographics 1993;13(2):311–328

[62] Remy-Jardin M, Giraud F, Remy J, Copin MC, Gosselin B, Duhamel A. Importance of ground-glass attenuation in chronic diffuse infiltrative lung disease: pathologic-CT correlation. Radiology 1993;189(3):693–698

[63] Remy-Jardin M, Remy J, Giraud F, Wattinne L, Gosselin B. Computed tomography assessment of ground-glass opacity: semiology and significance. J Thorac Imaging 1993;8(4):249–264

[64] Kuhlman JE, Fishman EK, Siegelman SS. Invasive pulmonary aspergillosis in acute leukemia: characteristic findings on CT, the CT halo sign, and the role of CT in early diagnosis. Radiology 1985;157(3):611–614

[65] Primack SL, Hartman TE, Lee KS, Müller NL. Pulmonary nodules and the CT halo sign. Radiology 1994;190(2):513–515

[66] Lynch DA, Godwin JD, Safrin S, et al; Idiopathic Pulmonary Fibrosis Study Group. High-resolution computed tomography in idiopathic pulmonary fibrosis: diagnosis and prognosis. Am J Respir Crit Care Med 2005;172(4):488–493

[67] American Thoracic Society. Idiopathic pulmonary fibrosis: diagnosis and treatment. International consensus statement. American Thoracic Society (ATS), and the European Respiratory Society (ERS). Am J Respir Crit Care Med 2000;161(2 Pt 1):646–664

[68] Hunninghake GW, Lynch DA, Galvin JR, et al. Radiologic findings are strongly associated with a pathologic diagnosis of usual interstitial pneumonia. Chest 2003;124(4):1215–1223

[69] Misumi S, Lynch DA. Idiopathic pulmonary fibrosis/usual interstitial pneumonia: imaging diagnosis, spectrum of abnormalities, and temporal progression. Proc Am Thorac Soc 2006;3(4):307–314

[70] Dalen JE, Haffajee CI, Alpert JS III, Howe JP, Ockene IS, Paraskos JA. Pulmonary embolism, pulmonary hemorrhage and pulmonary infarction. N Engl J Med 1977;296(25):1431–1435

[71] Ren H, Kuhlman JE, Hruban RH, Fishman EK, Wheeler PS, Hutchins GM. CT of inflation-fixed lungs: wedge-shaped density and vascular sign in the diagnosis of infarction. J Comput Assist Tomogr 1990;14(1):82–86

[72] Patterson HS, Sponaugle DN. Is infiltrate a useful term in the interpretation of chest radiographs? Physician survey results. Radiology 2005;235(1):5–8

[73] Kang EY, Grenier P, Laurent F, Müller NL. Interlobular septal thickening: patterns at high-resolution computed tomography. J Thorac Imaging 1996;11(4):260–264

[74] Donnelly LF, Lucaya J, Ozelame V, et al. CT findings and temporal course of persistent pulmonary interstitial emphysema in neonates: a multiinstitutional study. AJR Am J Roentgenol 2003;180(4):1129–1133

[75] Kemper AC, Steinberg KP, Stern EJ. Pulmonary interstitial emphysema: CT findings. AJR Am J Roentgenol 1999;172(6):1642

[76] Weibel ER. Fleischner Lecture. Looking into the lung: what can it tell us? AJR Am J Roentgenol 1979;133(6):1021–1031

[77] Kattan KR, Eyler WR, Felson B. The juxtaphrenic peak in upper lobe collapse. Radiology 1980;134(3):763–765

[78] Cameron DC. The juxtaphrenic peak (Katten's sign) is produced by rotation of an inferior accessory fissure. Australas Radiol 1993;37(4):332–335

[79] Davis SD, Yankelevitz DF, Wand A, Chiarella DA. Juxtaphrenic peak in upper and middle lobe volume loss: assessment with CT. Radiology 1996;198(1):143–149

[80] Westcott JL, Cole S. Plate atelectasis. Radiology 1985;155(1):1–9

[81] Miller WS, ed. The Lung. 2nd ed. Springfield, IL: Charles C Thomas; 1947

[82] Glazer GM, Gross BH, Quint LE, Francis IR, Bookstein FL, Orringer MB. Normal mediastinal lymph nodes: number and size according to American Thoracic Society mapping. AJR Am J Roentgenol 1985;144(2):261–265

[83] Remy-Jardin M, Duyck P, Remy J, et al. Hilar lymph nodes: identification with spiral CT and histologic correlation. Radiology 1995;196(2):387–394

[84] Swigris JJ, Berry GJ, Raffin TA, Kuschner WG. Lymphoid interstitial pneumonia: a narrative review. Chest 2002;122(6):2150–2164

[85] Ichikawa Y, Kinoshita M, Koga T, Oizumi K, Fujimoto K, Hayabuchi N. Lung cyst formation in lymphocytic interstitial pneumonia: CT features. J Comput Assist Tomogr 1994;18(5):745–748

[86] Johkoh T, Müller NL, Pickford HA, et al. Lymphocytic interstitial pneumonia: thin-section CT findings in 22 patients. Radiology 1999;212(2):567–572

[87] Fraser RS, Paré PD. Fraser and Paré's Diagnosis of Diseases of the Chest. 4th ed. Philadelphia, PA: W.B. Saunders; 1999

[88] Heitzman ER. The Mediastinum: Radiologic Correlations with Anatomy and Pathology. 2nd ed. Berlin: Springer; 1988:7–309

[89] Remy-Jardin M, Beuscart R, Sault MC, Marquette CH, Remy J. Subpleural micronodules in diffuse infiltrative lung diseases: evaluation with thin-section CT scans. Radiology 1990;177(1):133–139

[90] Remy-Jardin M, Remy J, Wallaert B, Müller NL. Subacute and chronic bird breeder hypersensitivity pneumonitis: sequential evaluation with CT and correlation with lung function tests and bronchoalveolar lavage. Radiology 1993;189(1):111–118

[91] Brauner MW, Lenoir S, Grenier P, Cluzel P, Battesti JP, Valeyre D. Pulmonary sarcoidosis: CT assessment of lesion reversibility. Radiology 1992;182(2):349–354

[92] Worthy SA, Müller NL, Hartman TE, Swensen SJ, Padley SP, Hansell DM. Mosaic attenuation pattern on thin-section CT scans of the lung: differentiation among infiltrative lung, airway, and vascular diseases as a cause. Radiology 1997;205(2):465–470

[93] Martin KW, Sagel SS, Siegel BA. Mosaic oligemia simulating pulmonary infiltrates on CT. AJR Am J Roentgenol 1986;147(4):670–673

[94] Arakawa H, Webb WR, McCowin M, Katsou G, Lee KN, Seitz RF. Inhomogeneous lung attenuation at thin-section CT: diagnostic value of expiratory scans. Radiology 1998;206(1):89–94

[95] Hansell DM, Wells AU, Rubens MB, Cole PJ. Bronchiectasis: functional significance of areas of decreased attenuation at expiratory CT. Radiology 1994;193(2):369–374

[96] Roberts CM, Citron KM, Strickland B. Intrathoracic aspergilloma: role of CT in diagnosis and treatment. Radiology 1987;165(1):123–128

[97] Erasmus JJ, Connolly JE, McAdams HP, Roggli VL. Solitary pulmonary nodules: Part I. Morphologic evaluation for differentiation of benign and malignant lesions. Radiographics 2000;20(1):43–58

[98] MacDonald SL, Rubens MB, Hansell DM, et al. Nonspecific interstitial pneumonia and usual interstitial pneumonia: comparative appearances at and diagnostic accuracy of thin-section CT. Radiology 2001;221(3):600–605

[99] Lee KS, Kullnig P, Hartman TE, Müller NL. Cryptogenic organizing pneumonia: CT findings in 43 patients. AJR Am J Roentgenol 1994;162(3):543–546

[100] Guest PJ, Hansell DM. High resolution computed tomography (HRCT) in emphysema associated with alpha-1-antitrypsin deficiency. Clin Radiol 1992;45(4):260–266

[101] Spouge D, Mayo JR, Cardoso W, Müller NL. Panacinar emphysema: CT and pathologic findings. J Comput Assist Tomogr 1993;17(5):710–713

[102] Copley SJ, Wells AU, Müller NL, et al. Thin-section CT in obstructive pulmonary disease: discriminatory value. Radiology 2002;223(3):812–819

[103] Akira M, Yamamoto S, Inoue Y, Sakatani M. High-resolution CT of asbestosis and idiopathic pulmonary fibrosis. AJR Am J Roentgenol 2003;181(1):163–169

[104] Akira M, Yamamoto S, Yokoyama K, et al. Asbestosis: high-resolution CT-pathologic correlation. Radiology 1990;176(2):389–394

[105] Johkoh T, Müller NL, Ichikado K, Nakamura H, Itoh H, Nagareda T. Perilobular pulmonary opacities: high-resolution CT findings and pathologic correlation. J Thorac Imaging 1999;14(3):172–177

[106] Ujita M, Renzoni EA, Veeraraghavan S, Wells AU, Hansell DM. Organizing pneumonia: perilobular pattern at thin-section CT. Radiology 2004;232(3):757–761

[107] Colby TV, Swensen SJ. Anatomic distribution and histopathologic patterns in diffuse lung disease: correlation with HRCT. J Thorac Imaging 1996;11(1):1–26

[108] Roberts GH. The pathology of parietal pleural plaques. J Clin Pathol 1971;24(4):348–353

[109] Lynch DA, Gamsu G, Aberle DR. Conventional and high resolution computed tomography in the diagnosis of asbestos-related diseases. Radiographics 1989;9(3):523–551

[110] Quigley MJ, Fraser RS. Pulmonary pneumatocele: pathology and pathogenesis. AJR Am J Roentgenol 1988;150(6):1275–1277

[111] Wagner JC, Wusteman FS, Edwards JH, Hill RJ. The composition of massive lesions in coal miners. Thorax 1975;30(4):382–388

[112] Chong S, Lee KS, Chung MJ, Han J, Kwon OJ, Kim TS. Pneumoconiosis: comparison of imaging and pathologic findings. Radiographics 2006;26(1):59–77

[113] Ward S, Heyneman LE, Reittner P, Kazerooni EA, Godwin JD, Müller NL. Talcosis associated with IV abuse of oral medications: CT findings. AJR Am J Roentgenol 2000;174(3):789–793

[114] Weisbrod GL, Chamberlain D, Herman SJ. Cystic change (pseudocavitation) associated with bronchioloalveolar carcinoma: a report of four patients. J Thorac Imaging 1995;10(2):106–111

[115] Milne EN. Physiological interpretion of the plain radiograph in mitral stenosis, including a review of criteria for the radiological estimation of pulmonary arterial and venous pressures. Br J Radiol 1963;36:902–913

[116] Simon M. The pulmonary veins in mitral stenosis. J Fac Radiol 1958;9(1):25–32

[117] Fraig M, Shreesha U, Savici D, Katzenstein A-LA. Respiratory bronchiolitis: a clinicopathologic study in current smokers, ex-smokers, and never-smokers. Am J Surg Pathol 2002;26(5):647–653

[118] Hansell DM, Nicholson AG. Smoking-related diffuse parenchymal lung disease: HRCT-pathologic correlation. Semin Respir Crit Care Med 2003;24(4):377–392

[119] Heyneman LE, Ward S, Lynch DA, Remy-Jardin M, Johkoh T, Müller NL. Respiratory bronchiolitis, respiratory bronchiolitis-associated interstitial lung disease, and desquamative interstitial pneumonia: different entities or part of the spectrum of the same disease process? AJR Am J Roentgenol 1999;173(6):1617–1622

[120] Kim SJ, Lee KS, Ryu YH, et al. Reversed halo sign on high-resolution CT of cryptogenic organizing pneumonia: diagnostic implications. AJR Am J Roentgenol 2003;180(5):1251–1254

[121] Zompatori M, Poletti V, Battista G, Diegoli M. Bronchiolitis obliterans with organizing pneumonia (BOOP), presenting as a ring-shaped opacity at HRCT (the atoll sign). A case report. Radiol Med (Torino) 1999;97(4):308–310

[122] Gasparetto EL, Escuissato DL, Davaus T, et al. Reversed halo sign in pulmonary paracoccidioidomycosis. AJR Am J Roentgenol 2005;184(6):1932–1934

[123] Savoca CJ, Austin JH, Goldberg HI. The right paratracheal stripe. Radiology 1977;122(2):295–301

[124] Cohen AM, Crass JR, Chung-Park M, Tomashefski JF Jr. Rounded atelectasis and fibrotic pleural disease: the pathologic continuum. J Thorac Imaging 1993;8(4):309–312

[125] Lynch DA, Gamsu G, Ray CS, Aberle DR. Asbestos-related focal lung masses: manifestations on conventional and high-resolution CT scans. Radiology 1988;169(3):603–607

[126] O'Donovan PB, Schenk M, Lim K, Obuchowski N, Stoller JK. Evaluation of the reliability of computed tomographic criteria used in the diagnosis of round atelectasis. J Thorac Imaging 1997;12(1):54–58

[127] Ouellette H. The signet ring sign. Radiology 1999;212(1):67–68

[128] McGuinness G, Naidich DP, Leitman BS, McCauley DI. Bronchiectasis: CT evaluation. AJR Am J Roentgenol 1993;160(2):253–259

[129] Ryu DS, Spirn PW, Trotman-Dickenson B, et al. HRCT findings of proximal interruption of the right pulmonary artery. J Thorac Imaging 2004;19(3):171–175

[130] Remy-Jardin M, Remy J, Louvegny S, Artaud D, Deschildre F, Duhamel A. Airway changes in chronic pulmonary embolism: CT findings in 33 patients. Radiology 1997;203(2):355–360

[131] Felson B, Felson H. Localization of intrathoracic lesions by means of the postero-anterior roentgenogram; the silhouette sign. Radiology 1950;55(3):363–374

[132] Marshall GB, Farnquist BA, MacGregor JH, Burrowes PW. Signs in thoracic imaging. J Thorac Imaging 2006;21(1):76–90

[133] Hogg JC, Macklem PT, Thurlbeck WM. Site and nature of airway obstruction in chronic obstructive lung disease. N Engl J Med 1968;278(25):1355–1360

[134] Müller NL, Miller RR. Diseases of the bronchioles: CT and histopathologic findings. Radiology 1995;196(1):3–12

[135] Arai K, Takashima T, Matsui O, Kadoya M, Kamimura R. Transient subpleural curvilinear shadow caused by pulmonary congestion. J Comput Assist Tomogr 1990;14(1):87–88

[136] Desai SR, Wells AU, Rubens MB, du Bois RM, Hansell DM. Traction bronchiectasis in cryptogenic fibrosing alveolitis: associated computed tomographic features and physiological significance. Eur Radiol 2003;13(8):1801–1808

[137] Aquino SL, Gamsu G, Webb WR, Kee ST. Tree-in-bud pattern: frequency and significance on thin section CT. J Comput Assist Tomogr 1996;20(4):594–599

[138] Eisenhuber E. The tree-in-bud sign. Radiology 2002;222(3):771–772

[139] Akira M, Kitatani F, Lee YS, et al. Diffuse panbronchiolitis: evaluation with high-resolution CT. Radiology 1988;168(2):433–438

[140] Im JG, Itoh H, Shim YS, et al. Pulmonary tuberculosis: CT findings--early active disease and sequential change with antituberculous therapy. Radiology 1993;186(3):653–660

[141] Franquet T, Giménez A, Prats R, Rodríguez-Arias JM, Rodríguez C. Thrombotic microangiopathy of pulmonary tumors: a vascular cause of tree-in-bud pattern on CT. AJR Am J Roentgenol 2002;179(4):897–899

Index

Note: Page numbers set in **bold** or *italic* indicate headings or figures, respectively.

D

E

F

G

H

I

L

M

N

O

P

R

V

W